Wade O. Brinker · Marvin L. Olmstead
Geoffrey Sumner-Smith · W. Dieter Prieur (Eds.)

Manual of Internal Fixation in Small Animals

Springer-Verlag Berlin Heidelberg GmbH

Wade O. Brinker · Marvin L. Olmstead
Geoffrey Sumner-Smith · W. Dieter Prieur (Eds.)

Manual of Internal Fixation in Small Animals

Second revised and enlarged Edition
With 305 Figures, many in Color, and 11 Tables

Springer

Professor Wade O. Brinker
5675 Van Atta Road
Okemos, MI 48864
USA

Professor Marvin L. Olmstead
Professor of Orthopaedic Surgery
Dept. of Vet. Clinical Studies
Ohio State University
601 Vernon L. Tharp Street
Columbus, OH 43210-0950
USA

Professor Geoffrey Sumner-Smith
Everton Cottage
R.R.4 Rockwood
Ontario, NOB 2KO
Canada

Dr. W. Dieter Prieur
Altenwegs Mühle
D-56868 Liesenich
Germany

ISBN 978-3-642-64338-5 ISBN 978-3-642-60288-7 (eBook)
DOI 10.1007/978-3-642-60288-7

Library of Congress Cataloging-in-Publication Data
Manual of internal fixation in small animals / Wade O. Brinker, Marvin L. Omstead, Geoffrey Sumner-Smith (eds.) ; comments by W. Dieter Prieur. - 2nd rev. and enlarged ed. p. cm. Includes bibliographical references and index. ISBN 978-3-642-64338-5 (hardcover : alk. paper) 1. Fractures in animals - Treatment. 2. Internal fixation in fractures. I. Brinker, Wade O. II. Olmstead, Marvin L. III. Sumner-Smith, G. SF914.4.M35 1997 636.089'715 - dc21

Originally published by Springer-Verlag Berlin Heidelberg New York in 1998
Softcover reprint of the hardcover 2nd edition 1998

Production: PRO EDIT GmbH, D-69126 Heidelberg
Cover design: design & production GmbH, D-69121 Heidelberg
Typesetting: Mitterweger Werksatz GmbH, D-68723 Plankstadt

SPIN: 10052164 24/3135-5 4 3 2 1 0 - Printed on acid-free paper

Dedicated to

R. Bruce Hohn
D.V.M.

(1926–1986)

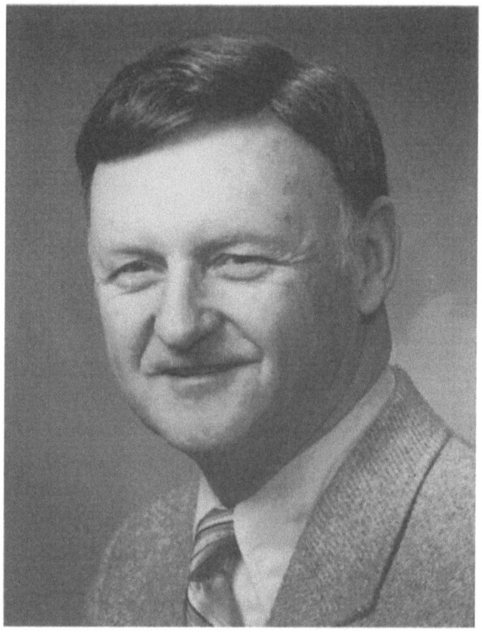

His enthusiasm for educating veterinarians in the fine art and exacting science of orthopedics with a special emphasis on AO principles is the driving spirit of this book. He was one of the primary people responsible for the first edition and it saddens us that he could not work with us on this edition. We take comfort in the fact that he contributed so much to so many and thus his influence will be present for generations of veterinary orthopedic surgeons.

Preface of 2nd Edition

This manual addresses the current techniques used in the implementation of the A.O/ A.S.I.F System in small animal orthopedic surgery.

Fourteen years have passed since the publication, in 1983, of the first edition of the *Manual of Internal Fixation in Small Animals*. During that time philosophical and practical changes have taken place in the treatment of fractures and associated injuries, which are reflected in this new edition.

This edition will serve to inform the experienced surgeon of the current situation and yet, at the same time, be a basic text for the newcomer to veterinary small animals orthopaedies and the A.O./A.S.I.F. system.

The professional artist, Mr Jonathan Clayton-Jones was responsible for the new drawings. He is to be congratulated on his skillful work and his ability to implement the same style and artistic technique used in the First Edition. To Mrs. Bonnie Hamilton we owe a debt of gratitude. She has, without demurring, retyped countless versions of the manuscripts of each chapter and remained cheerful when the light at the end of the tunnel was nowhere near being visible.

Finally, our sincere thanks are due to our editor at Springer-Verlag, Mrs. Gabriele Schroeder, who has guided the manual through its gestation period, and to Mrs. Alison Hepper who had the daunting task of turning the manuscript into a published text.

Fall 1997

Wade O. Brinker
Marvin L. Olmstead
Geoffrey Sumner-Smith
W. Dieter Prieur

Preface of 1st Edition

In 1958 a study group of surgeons in Switzerland formed the *Arbeitsgemeinschaft für Osteosynthesefragen* (AO), known later in North America as the Association for the Study of Internal Fixation (ASIF). The members of this AO/ASIF group studied the then current methods and instrumentation of internal fixation of fractures in human patients, and joined with bioengineers, manufacturers, and basic research specialists to develop new internal fixation devices and techniques of fracture treatment. Through educational courses, now international, they promoted the concept of fracture management through accurate anatomical reconstruction, rigid stabilization, primary bone healing, and prevention of fracture disease through early postoperative weight-bearing.

For best results in treating fractures in animals, the patient should be ambulant shortly after recovering from anesthesia and should have an early return to full function. Until the introduction of the AO/ASIF system to veterinary medicine in the mid-1960s, this goal was unattainable in many cases, particularly in the treatment of complex fractures.

After becoming familiar with the AO/ASIF studies on bone biology, biomechanics, and the metallurgy of internal fixation and their documented results from numerous clinical cases in man, it became obvious that application of the same principles and equipment in veterinary bone and joint surgery would help resolve many of the problems and shortcomings concountered with several existing methods of fracture fixation. We are very grateful to the AO/ASIF group.

Veterinarians have adapted the AO/ASIF principles for internal fixation of fractures, made some modifications better suited to the needs of animals, carried out orthopedic research, developed some new and more versatile equipment, and carefully documented the initial treatment and follow-up results in numerous fracture cases.

The first part of this manual deals with the principles of the AO/ASIF method of stable internal fixation. It covers both the experimental and theoretical aspects, including function and main use of the different implants, use of the different AO/ASIF instruments, operative technique, pre- and postoperative evaluation and care, metallurgy, and postoperative complications.

The second part deals with the AO/ASIF recommendations for the operative treatment of the most common fresh fractures occurring in the various locations in the adult and growing animal.

The third part presents reconstructive bone surgery using stable internal fixation.

This manual is designed to convey to the student and the veterinary surgeon the basic knowledge and techniques of small-animal fracture treatment. The information and procedures presented are those which documentation studies on clinical cases indicate as the most appropriate at this time. Note that we are recommending this as a system of internal fixation of fractures, not as a complete substitute for all fracture treatment. The importance of training, individual study, short courses, documentation, etc. cannot be overemphasized. We wish to express sincere thanks to all who took part in producing this manual, particularly our wonderful artists Georgio Bertoli, Bernhard Struchen, and Andreas Farner.

Fall, 1983

W. O. Brinker
R. B. Hohn
W. D. Prieur

List of Contributors

A. Binnington, D.V.M., M.Sc., Dip. Vet. Surg., D.A.C.V.S.
Associate Professor, Department of Clinical Studies, Ontario Veterinary College, Guelph, Ontario, N1G 2W1, Canada

F. Baumgart, Professor Ing.
AO Research Institute (ARI), Produkteninformation, Clavadelerstrasse, CH-7270 Davos Platz, Switzerland

T. D. Braden, D.V.M., M.S.
Professor, Veterinary Clinical Center, College of Veterinary Medicine, Michigan State University, East Lansing, MI 48824-1314, USA

W. Brinker, D.V.M., M.S., Professor Emiritas
5675 Van Atta Road, Okemos, MI 48864, USA

S. Bruse, Dr. Med. Vet.
Fachtierärztin für Kleintiere, Augenheilkunde, Sonnenweg, D-56203 Hohr-Grenzhausen, Germany

D. G. Clayton Jones, B. Vet. Med., D.V.R., D.S.A.O.
Highlands, Ashford Road, Tenterden, Kent, UK

J. F. Dee, D.V.M., M.S., D.A.C.V.S.
Hollywood Animal Hospital, 2864 Hollywood Blvd, Hollywood, Florida 33020, USA

H. R. Denny, M.A., Vet. M.B., Ph.D., F.R.C.V.S., D.S.A.O.
Cedar House, Wrington, Bristol BS 18 7QD, UK

R. T. Dueland, D.V.M., M.S.
Professor, Dept. of Surgical Science, School of Veterinary Medicine, University of Wisconsin-Madison, 33 N. Randall Ave., Madison, WI 53715-1098, USA

R. Eaton-Wells, B.V.Sc., M.A.C.V.Sc.
West Chermside Veterinary Clinic, 263 Appleby Road, Stafford Heights, Q 4053, Australia

E. Egger, D.V.M., D.A.C.V.S.
The Veterinary School, Department of Clinical Sciences, Colorado State University, Fort Collins, CO 80523, USA

J. E. F. Houlton, M.A., Vet. M.B., D.V.R., D.S.A.O., D.E.C.V.S.
University Surgeon, Dept. of Clinical Veterinary Medicine, Madingley Road, Cambridge University, Cambridge CB3 OES, UK

A. Johnson, D.V.M., D.A.C.V.S.
Professor, Dept. of Veterinary Clinical Medicine, University of Illinois,
108 West Hazelwood, Urbana, IL, USA

Kenneth A. Johnson, M.V.Sc., Ph.D. D.A.+E.C.V.S., M.R.C.V.S.
Professor, Department of Surgery, School of Veterinary Sciences, University of Bristol,
Langford House, Langford, Bristol BS 18 7DU, UK

F. Kasa, Dr. Med. Vet.
D-79539 Lörrach, Bahnhofstraße 11, Germany

G. Kasa, Dr. Med. Vet.
D-79539 Lörrach, Bahnhofstraße 11, Germany

R. Koestlin, Dr. Med. Vet.
Professor, Chir. Univ. Tierklinik, Veterinärstr. 13, D-80539 München, Germany

U. Matis, Dr. Med. Vet.
Professor, Chir. Univ. Tierklinik, Veterinärstr. 13, D-80539 München, Germany

Ron M. McLaughlin, D.V.M., D.V.Sc., D.A.C.V.S.
Associate Professor, Dept. of Clinical Science, College of Veterinary Medicine,
Kansas State University, Manhattan, KS 66506, USA

F. J. Meustege, D.V.M.
Steener Camen 78, N.D. 3721 Bilthoven, The Netherlands

C. Miller, D.V.M., M.V.Sc., D.A.C.V.S.
Associate Professor, Dept. of Clinical Studies, University of Guelph,
Ontario Veterinary College, Guelph, Ontario, N1G 2W1, Canada

M. L. Olmstead, D.V.M., M.S., D.A.C.V.S.
Professor of Orthopedic Surgery, Dept. of Vet. Clinical Studies, Ohio State University,
601 Vernon L. Tharp Street, Columbus, OH 43210-0950, USA

S. M. Perren, M.D., P.D., D.Sc. [h.c.]
Professor, AO Research Institute (ARI), Clavadelerstrasse, CH 7270 Davos Platz,
Switzerland

D. Piermattei, D.V.M., Ph.D., D.A.C.V.S.
Professor (Retd), The Veterinary School, Department of Clinical Sciences,
Colorado State University, Fort Collins, CO 80523, USA

O. E. M. Pohler, M.S. Ph.D.
Metallurgist, Strautec, Ch 4437 Waldenburg, Switzerland

W. D. Prieur, Dr. Med. Vet.
Altenwegs Mühle, D-56858 Liesenich, Germany

G. M. Robins, B. Vet. Med., M.R.C.V.S., F.A.C.V. Sc.
263 Appleby Road, Stafford Heights Q 4053, Australia

J. Schatzker, B.Sc. (Med), M.D., F.R.C.S.(C)
Professor, University of Toronto, Sunnybrook Medical Centre, Department
of Orthopaedic Surgery, 2075 Bayview Avenue, Toronto, Ontario, M4N 3M5, Canada

S. G. Stoll, D.V.M., D.A.C.V.S.
Seattle Veterinary Hospital, 16418 7th Place West, Lynwood, WA 98037, USA

G. Sumner-Smith, B.V.Sc., M.Sc., D.V.Sc.(Liv) F.R.C.V.S.
Professor (Retd), Department of Clinical Studies, Ontario Veterinary College, University of Guelph, Guelph, Ontario. N1G 2W1, Canada

Dr. R. Vanini, Dr. Med. Vet., D.E.C.V.S.
Bessy's Kleintierklinik, Dorfstrasse 51, CH 8105 Watt-Regensdort, Switzerland

L. L. Wallace, D.V.M., M.S.
Professor, University of Minnesota, College of Veterinary Medicine, Dept. of Small Animal Clinical Studies, St. Paul, MN 55108, USA

Contents

Part I
General Considerations

1 Basic Aspects of Internal Fixation

1.1 Aims and Principles

1.1.1 Introduction

Every fracture leads to a complex tissue injury involving bone and surrounding soft parts. Immediately after the fracture and during the repair phase, we see local circulatory disturbances and manifestations of local inflammation, as well as pain and reflex immobilization. These three factors – circulatory disturbance, inflammation, and pain – a result of dysfunction of joints and muscles, lead to the so-called fracture disease (Lucas-Championniere 1907).

Fracture disease is caused by two main pathogenic factors: (1) pain and (2) lack of physiological challenge to the bone-muscle complex by movement and changing mechanical load. In the lower limbs, this means lack of weight-bearing and lack of normal muscle work. Fracture disease is therefore a clinical state manifested by chronic edema, soft tissue atrophy, and patchy osteoporosis. Edema, as such, induces intermuscular fibrosis and muscular atrophy. These fibrotic processes cause muscles to develop unphysiological adhesions to bone and fascia and therefore lead to stiffness of adjacent joints.

1.1.2 Life Is Movement, Movement Is Life

"Life is movement, movement is life": this should be the guiding principle of fracture care. Full, active, pain-free mobilization results in a rapid return of normal blood supply to both the bone and the soft tissues. It also enhances articular cartilage nutrition by the synovial fluid and, when combined with partial weight-bearing, it greatly decreases posttraumatic osteoporosis by restoring an equilibrium between bone resorption and bone formation. A satisfactory internal fixation is achieved when full, active, pain-free mobilization of muscles and joints is possible. This is the AO's main objective and is best achieved by stable internal fixation during the bone-healing process.

Major fractures, particularly of long bones, the pelvis, and the spine, have repercussions on the homeostasis of the accident victim as a whole, but primarily on the cardiorespiratory system.

At the outset in 1958, the AO formulated four treatment principles expected to improve the results of fracture treatment in general and of internal fixation in particular (Müller et al. 1984):

1. Anatomical reduction of the fracture fragments, particularly in joint fractures
2. Stable internal fixation designed to fulfill the local biomechanical requirements
3. Preservation of the blood supply to the bone fragments and the soft tissue by means of atraumatic surgical technique
4. Early active pain-free mobilization of muscles and joints adjacent to the fracture, preventing the development of fracture disease

Some 30 years later, it appears timely to evaluate the extent to which these four principles have stood the test of time.

The first of these principles, *anatomical reduction*, has retained all its importance in reconstituting full function in all joint fractures and is also valuable with regard to length, rotation, and axes of meta- and diaphysis. In diaphyseal fractures, it has received certain corrections with regard to reduction of cortical fragments, where it has become related to the method of operative treatment employed. It is of primary importance in fixation by lag screws with or without protection by neutralization (protection) plates. To achieve optimal mechanical strength, the cortical circumference must be fully reconstructed and placed under both interfragmental and axial compression.

However, there is a precarious balance to be struck between early mechanical perfection and devascularization of the detachment fragments. The idea of "biological fixation" has branched off in two directions. The first involves the application of flexible plates, and the second the application of conventional plates bridging a complex fracture zone with only three or four screws anchored proximally and distally in the intact parts of the fractured bone.

So-called flexible plates were devised in an attempt to avoid the "stress protection" formerly believed to be instrumental in plate-induced cortical osteoporosis. This has clearly been demonstrated to be a misconception. Plate osteoporosis after "flexible plating," rather than being decreased, is increased because of the more marked vascular disturbance caused by the tightly fitting plate. In contrast to conventional plates, the limited-contact dynamic compression plate (LC-DCP) preserves periosteal blood supply (see p. 44), causes less osteoporosis than the dynamic compression plate (DCP) with a flat undersurface, and furthermore allows the cortical bone underlying the plate to develop a thin callus bridge. Clinically, this is probably of limited importance because thanks to rapid remodeling following application of a normal DCP, cortical healing is successful in a large majority of cases. However, the possibility of avoiding cortical osteoporosis underlying the plate is of considerable scientific and even clinical interest.

The second very successful line of thought led to the idea of the bridge plate (Müller and Witzel 1984; Heitemeyer and Hierholzer 1985) and the wave plate (Brunner and Weber 1981). The basic idea is to leave the fracture zone and its fragments undisturbed by fixing the plate to the intact part of the bone distal and proximal to the fragment area. When a multifragmentary fracture area is bridged using a wave plate, two advantageous mechanisms come into play:

1. When the plate spans an extended fracture area, the inner part of the plate, not fixed to the bone, undergoes more distributed deformation, so that sites of excessive deformation prone to fatigue failure are avoided.
2. The plate applied at a distance to the bone permits better vascular access to the repair tissue and benefits more from the mechanical support provided by the repair tissue due to better leverage.

Similar considerations apply to the second principle, *stable fixation.* All methods of operative fixation must provide adequate stability to maintain length, axes, and rotation. Lag screw fixation, with or without neutralization plates, depends on "absolute stability" for optimal healing, which occurs by direct angiogenic (haversian) bridging of the precisely reduced fracture. In these cases, visible "cloudy callus" is indicative of lost stability for which nature has tried to compensate. It shows the need for a reduced challenge to the fracture area by decreased weight-bearing.

The bone-healing pattern is completely different from that of direct angiogenic union when plates are applied in a bridging mode or when medullary pinning or external fixation is used. With these latter methods, a certain amount of interfragmentary movement is inevitable, even desirable, and nature has to supplement stabilization by producing callus to solidify the "welding" of the fragments.

In summary, callus-free healing is not an aim in itself. It is a fascinating biological property of living cortical bone under conditions of absolute stability and good vascularity. It is clinically only relevant in interfragmentary compression by means of lag screws with or without neutralization plates.

Emphasis on the third principle, *atraumatic surgical technique*, has, if anything, increased. It concerns not only the soft tissues, but also the bony fragments and, in particular, their vascularity (Mast et al. 1989).

The fourth principle, *early pain-free mobilization*, has certainly stood the test of time, and proof is at hand that, after most fractures, permanent impairment has significantly decreased with the advent of immediate postoperative mobilization. A new dimension has been added and abundantly documented in the last two decades: the merit of early total care of the severely traumatized patient in the hours following the accident. A good number of pathophysiological events, earlier thought to be caused by trauma, have now been shown to be related to treatment modalities. In particular, if the animal's body lies for an extended period of time in an unphysiological supine position, this can lead to long-lasting cardiorespiratory disturbance, which often ends in multiple organ failure.

In summary, the initial working hypothesis expressed in the four treatment principles has seen certain changes in emphasis but, all in all, has stood the test of time.

1.2 Basic Aspects

A review of bone as a material, its fracture, and its spontaneous healing should help to understand the problems and basic goals of fracture treatment.

1.2.1 Bone as a Material

The *strength* of bone (Fig. 1.1) is about one tenth of that of steel. The apatite structure of bone is forms the basis of its excellent compressive strength. The tensile elements of bone, i.e., the collagen fibers, are generally thought to be weaker. The tensile strength of the tibia, for instance, is about 20 % less than its compressive strength. That of the radius, on the other hand, is 20 % higher (Knets 1980). The strength of cancellous bone is very variable and

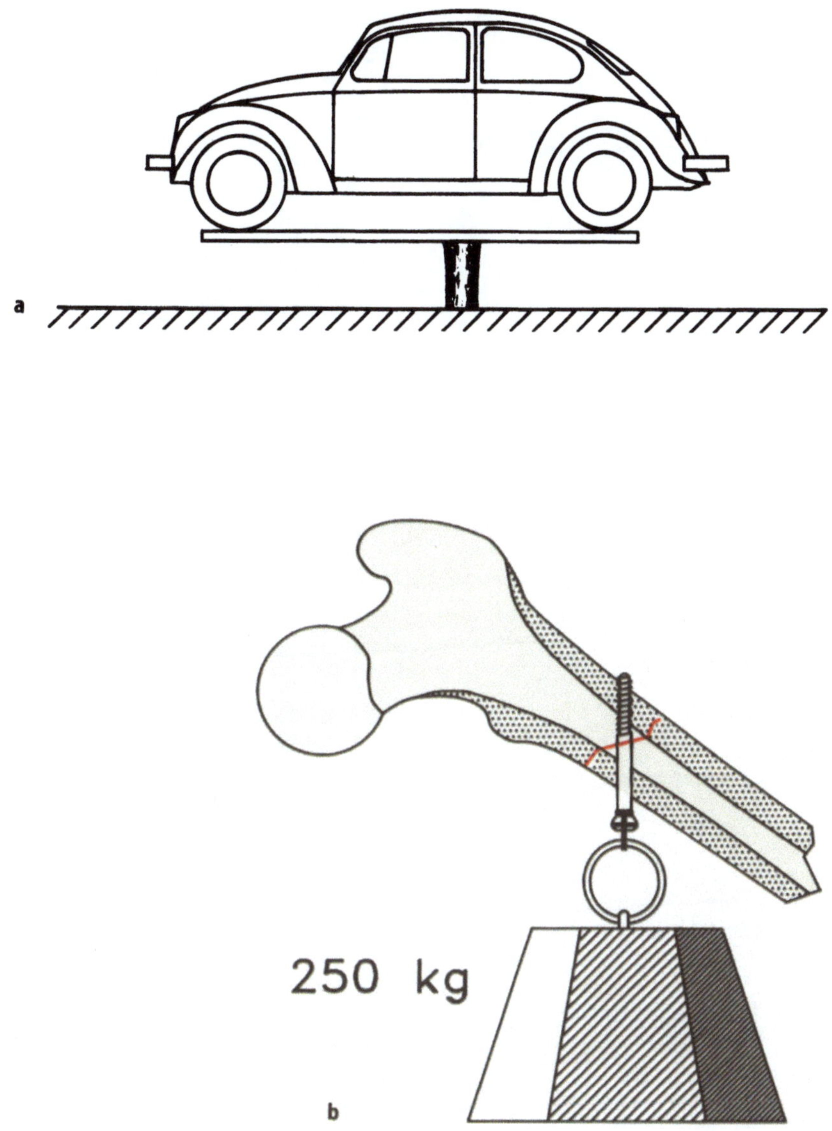

Fig. 1.1a,b. Strength of bone. Bone is a comparatively strong material. Its strength far exceeds the requirements of heavy physical activity. **a** Compressive strength. A short segment of the tibia diaphysis is able to carry the weight of a small car. **b** Holding strength of a screw within cortical bone. A standard 4.5-mm cortex screw, anchored in any one cortex, can withstand 2500 N (the weight of three people)

usually less than one tenth of that of cortical bone (Yamada and Evans 1970).[1] Compression applied to bone using so-called rigid implants is maintained due to the elastic deformability of the bone. A comparably small loss (about 10 %–20 %) is explained by the time-dependent deformation under load ("creep" or, conversely, "stress relaxation"). This phenomenon was earlier attributed to the "viscoelasticity" of bone. A dominant quality of bone is its *brittleness*: bone behaves more like glass than like rubber. When bone is deformed, e.g., elongated, only about 2 % of its length, it breaks.

The anisotropy of bone, i.e., its different mechanical properties along different axes, does not play a major role in internal fixation and will therefore be disregarded here.

Bone serves as a framework for soft organs and allows for locomotion. (It furthermore stores minerals, primarily calcium, a function which will not be discussed here.) To function as a skeleton, the bones must be stiff. As we shall see (see p. 33), this stiffness is the main reason why the stability achieved using internal fixation may be jeopardized

[1] The ultimate tensile or compressive strength of bone is about 1 MPa. A segment of the tibia may therefore be loaded with the weight of a small car without risk of failure (see Fig. 1.1a). For practical purposes, one should bear in mind that a standard 4.5-mm screw anchored, for example, in one femoral cortex is able to resist 400 N per mm cortical thickness. Such a screw could therefore carry the weight of three people.

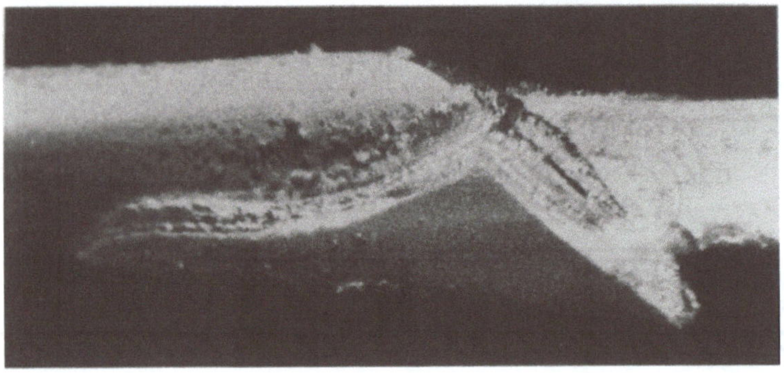

a

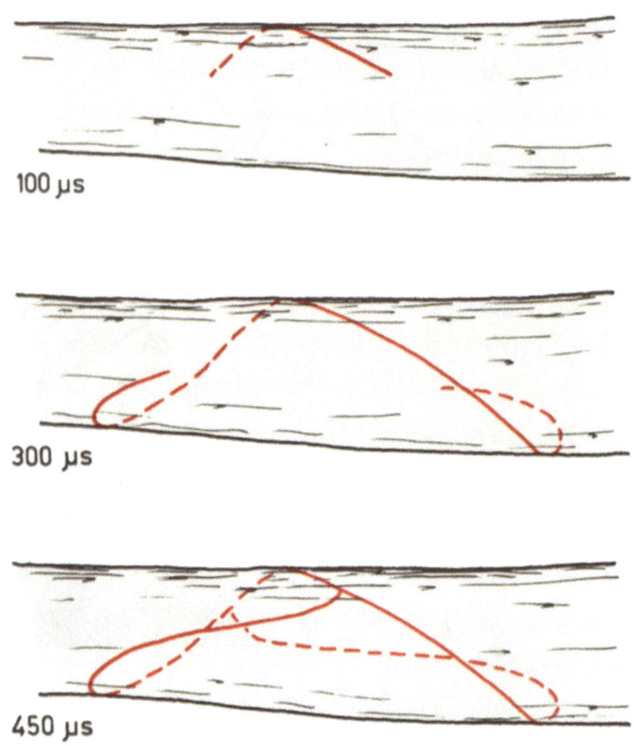

b

Fig. 1.2a,b. The bone fracture. The sequence of events resulting in a spiral fracture with additional (butterfly) fragment analyzed using high-speed cinematography. A human cadaver tibia was fractured using axial torque. The process resulting in a wedge fracture was recorded at 10 000 frames per second (Moor et al. 1989). **a** Tissue trauma. When the applied torque reaches the limit of the strength of the bone, the disruption results in an abrupt opening of a fracture gap. A temporary vacuum is created. An implosion occurs which can be compared in its effect to the process of cavitation in high-velocity gunshot wounds. Marked tissue trauma in the areas of cavitation results. **b** Sequence of events and timing in the process of fracturing. Within 400 µs, the fracture is fully developed. The sequence leading to the dissolution of the butterfly fragment is also shown

by minimal bone fracture surface resorption.[2] During normal activity, and much more so during sports activity, bone has to resist large forces.

[2] Young's modulus of axial stiffness of cortical bone amounts to 20 GPa. As a practical example, a tibia loaded by body weight shortens about 60 µm or six cell layers only. The stiffness of a plated and compressed diaphyseal bone segment is such that only 10 µm shortening results from a load of 1000 N being applied axially. Bone therefore corresponds to a very stiff spring, a fact which is of importance in internal fixation. The stiffness of cancellous bone as a material is one fifth to one tenth that of cortical bone in axial compresion. In bending and torque, the geometry plays a more important role, compensating for the difference in material properties.

1.2.2 Bone Fracture

The skeleton provides a rigid frame for physical activity and for the protection of the soft organs. The basic requirement for optimal locomotor function is adequate anatomic shape and stiffness, i.e., resistance to deformation under load.

Bone fractures as a result of mechanical overload. The fracture interrupts, within fractions of a millisecond, the structural integrity and hence the stiffness of the bone (Fig. 1.2; Moor et al. 1989). The shape of the fracture depends mainly upon the type of load exerted and upon the energy released. Torque results in spiral fractures, avulsion in transverse fractures, bending in short, oblique fractures, and axial compression (especially in metaphyses) in impaction, i.e., fractures without contact between the main fragments after restoration of original length of the bone. The degree of fragmentation depends upon the energy stored prior to the process of fracturing; thus wedge fractures and multifragmentary ones are associated with a high energy release. In this context, the rate of loading plays a certain role.

A special phenomenon is the implosion which occurs immediately after disruption. As Moor and coworkers have shown, such implosion (and with it marked soft tissue damage due to cavitation in a similar way as in gunshot wounds) can be observed using high-speed cinematography.

In addition to the diminished blood supply brought about by soft tissue damage, disruption of the intracortical blood vessels running along the bone axis results in a necrotic deeper layer of the fracture surface. The immediate surface is supported by diffusion.

1.2.3 Spontaneous Bone Repair: Healing Without Treatment

Nature is able to unite untreated fractures (Fig. 1.3). In the absence of treatment, however, significant malalignment frequently results, with consequent impaired function of the skeleton.

1.2.4 Basic Aims of Fracture Treatment

Fracture treatment in general strives for complete and early recovery of limb function. Solid union in the *proper anatomical shape* is therefore the basic goal. With respect to diaphyseal fractures, this means at least correct relative positioning of the bone segments which carry the articulations, i.e., restoration of overall length and reduction of flexural and torsional malalignment. In intra-articular fractures, precise reconstruction of the articular surfaces is a goal in its own right. Reconstruction of the anatomy generally offers the best chance for optimal recovery of function and is preferred to "tolerable malalignment."

1.2.5 Aims of Operative Fracture Treatment

Three indications for internal fixation stand out:

1. Long-lasting immobilization of soft tissues, especially around the joints, may result in fracture disease (see p. 1).
2. In the case of a fracture involving the load-bearing articular surfaces, precise reconstruction of these surfaces is of paramount importance. Any incongruity of the articulating surfaces gives rise to areas of high stress and thus promotes post-traumatic arthrosis.

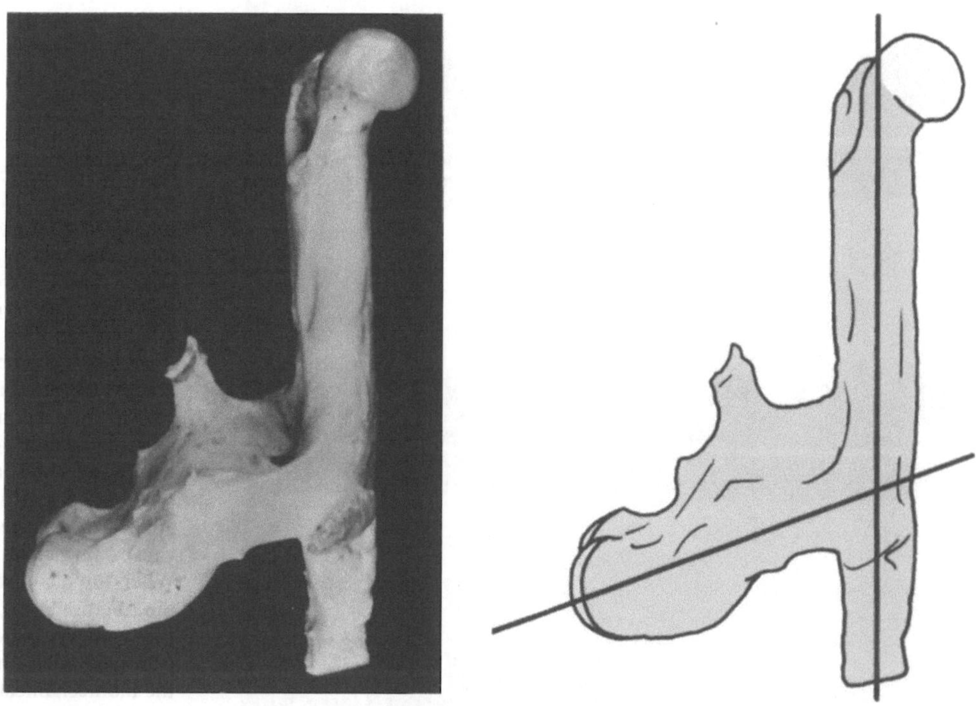

Fig. 1.3. Fracture healing without treatment. The fractured femur of a dog united solidly without treatment; however, marked malalignment resulted. The fracture had been neither reduced nor splinted. (Courtesy of A.G. Binnington)

3. Recovery of function after some fractures of long bones is particularly dependent upon early, exact, and stable reconstruction as well as upon immediate mobilization to prevent permanent impairment.

It should be reemphasized that the goal of fracture treatment is not only solid union, but also (and equally importantly) early and full recovery of limb function, which includes both bone and soft tissue integrity.

The surgical treatment of a reactive (hypertrophic) nonunion aims at restoring the mechanical environment so that, even without direct surgical modification of the interfragmental fibrocartilaginous tissue, uneventful solid healing in an anatomically correct position results (Fig. 1.4). Again, stable fixation allows immediate recovery of pain-free limb function. Solid union following appropriate stable internal fixation is extremely reliable. A rapid rate of union, correction of malalignment, and retaining joint function all lead to optimal results unmatched by nonsurgical treatment. According to the same authors, "most non-unions are more than simply an ununited fracture of a bone: shortening, angulation, joint stiffness, muscle atrophy, neural and vascular disorders, drainage and infection are additional problems needing treatment. It is therefore important to consider a non-union as an injured limb, not simply as an ununited broken bone; e.g. the quality of a certain treatment for non-union cannot be expressed by the rate of ossification only, disregarding angulation, shortening and stiffness."

1.3 Scientific Background to Internal Fixation

Internal fixation requires a sound understanding of the principles and techniques involved for adequate use of the implants and instruments. Understand-

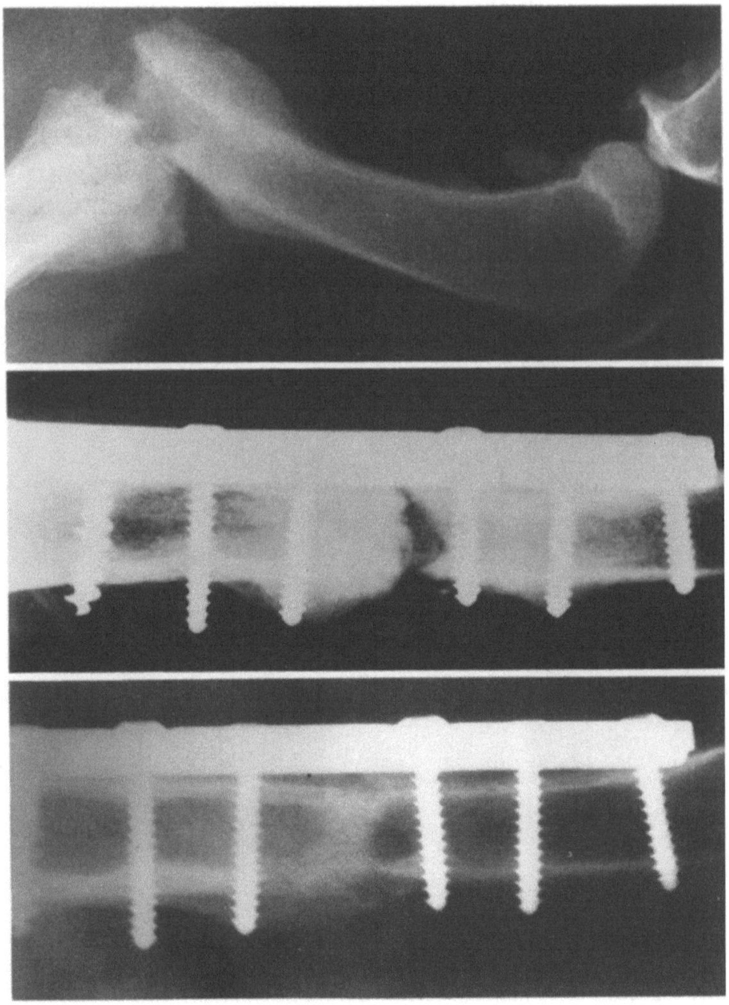

a b c

Fig. 1.4a–c. Surgical treatment of a nonunion after unsuccessful conservative management. In an Appenzeller dog, many attempts to treat the nonunion failed; simple correction of malalignment and stabilization led to prompt healing. **a** Fully developed nonunion. Malalignment has led to an increased bending load which does not allow the repair tissues to stabilize the fracture sufficiently, a prerequisite of solid union. **b** Operative treatment. The surgical treatment consisted in correcting the angulation by the application of a tension band plate to the convex surface of the malalignment. When the plate was put under tension, the fracture straightened out. The interfragmentary tissue was not touched. **c** Prompt, solid union after correction of the biomechanical situation. Once the angulation was corrected and the nonunion stabilized, prompt and solid healing resulted within 3 months ing of the biological reaction to changes in the environment (e.g., forces, blood supply) is essential in order to achieve the desired result and to avoid complications.

The following section on scientific background is intended to convey an understanding of fracture treatment; it is not intended to be a complete overview of the science underlying the present-day art of internal fixation. Thus many distinguished contributions in this field could not be considered.

1.3.1 Technical Background

In fracture healing, a close relationship exists between mechanical input and biological reaction. Internal fixation requires a good knowledge of the mechanical factors that provide the optimal environment for reliable and undisturbed fracture healing and for functional restitution of the injured limb as a whole.

1.3.1.1 Stability

The stability of a fracture (spontaneous or after fixation) determines most of the biological reactions during the process of healing. If the blood supply is adequate, the type of healing and the occurrence of delayed union or nonunion depend mainly upon mechanical conditions related to stability. Stable reconstruction of the fractured bone, e.g., by exact adaptation and compression, minimizes the load to be carried by the implant. Stability of fixation is therefore a critical parameter with respect to implant fatigue and corrosion. The term "stability of fixation" and the factors determining the degree of stability will therefore be discussed.

The use of the term "stability" differs in medical and technical sciences. Stability in internal fixation is used to describe the degree of immobility of the fracture fragments. Stable fixation means a fixation with little displacement under load. A special condition is described by the term "absolute stability." This defines complete absence of relative displacement between (compressed) fracture surfaces. Within the same fracture surface, areas of absolute and relative stability may be present simultaneously (see Fig. 1.7).

Stability, Strain, and Fracture Healing. The degree of instability is best expressed as the magnitude of strain[3] (deformation of the repair tissues). Relative motion between bone fragments is compatible with initial fracture healing, provided that the resulting strain remains below the critical level for the formation of that repair tissue (Perren and Cordey 1977, 1980). It goes without saying that if strain is too low, mechanical induction of tissue differentiation (by irritation) fails. In stably fixed fractures with low strain, internal remodeling of bone seems to be induced by necrotic areas.

The critical parameter determining the effect of instability upon cellular elements is the resulting strain. Strain characterizes the condition of deformation of the tissue elements, taking into account both the degree of displacement and the gap width (relative deformation $\delta L/L$).

Analyzing fracture healing in terms of strain of the repair tissues is more appropriate than judging it merely by the displacement (instability), because strain expresses the deformation of the tissue element (e.g., cell) and allows the veterinary surgeon to determine the amount of critical deformation by considering both relative displacement (fracture instability) and fracture gap width.

Analysis of mechanical conditions using the concept of strain allows us to understand why fractures with a single, narrow gap are very intolerant of even minute amounts of displacement (such displacement may not be detected by vision but must be "detected by intellect"). Instability is better tolerated by multifragmentary (comminuted) fractures because the overall displacement is shared between many fracture gaps. At any single gap, the relative displacement is therefore greatly reduced. If the reduction is not precise, the fracture is also tolerant to further displacement as the strain is reduced due to the larger gap width (see p. 11.

The importance of close adaptation and increased stability achieved by means of compression will be discussed (see p. 19) in the light of the fact that close, but insufficient adapation lacking compression may be dangerous. This is due to problems of tissue differentiation under high-strain conditions and large implant load resulting in more corrosion.

Fractures may be inherently stable or may stabilize spontaneously through the biological process of tissue formation, with subsequent differentiation into tissues with increasing stiffness, from granulation tissue to bone. The simultaneous increase in the diameter of the callus provides the repair tissues with improved leverage for stabilization. Motion-induced fracture surface resorption results in widening of the gap and a consequent further reduction of relative tissue deformation (strain).

If the resulting strain within the repair tissues (in and around the fracture) exceeds a critical limit, further differentiation and thus healing may be prevented. The expression of instability in terms of strain within the repair tissues allows for a logical

[3] For a definition of strain, see p. 11.

understanding of the bone-healing process (for the biology of strain, see p. 37). It explains why some fixation methods without total abolition of interfragmentary mobility may allow healing (e.g., in nonunions fixed using intramedullary nailing), while other methods leaving only very small gaps do not tolerate even macroscopically invisible displacement.

Living bone reacts to high-strain conditions at a bone–bone or bone–implant interface by surface resorption (see Fig. 1.30; Perren et al. 1975). Thus, in healing under conditions of relative instability (see Figs. 1.8, 1.9), the distance between the surfaces is widened, meaning that for a given amount of displacement, the resulting strain of the individual tissue element (cell) is reduced (see Figs. 1.8, 1.9).

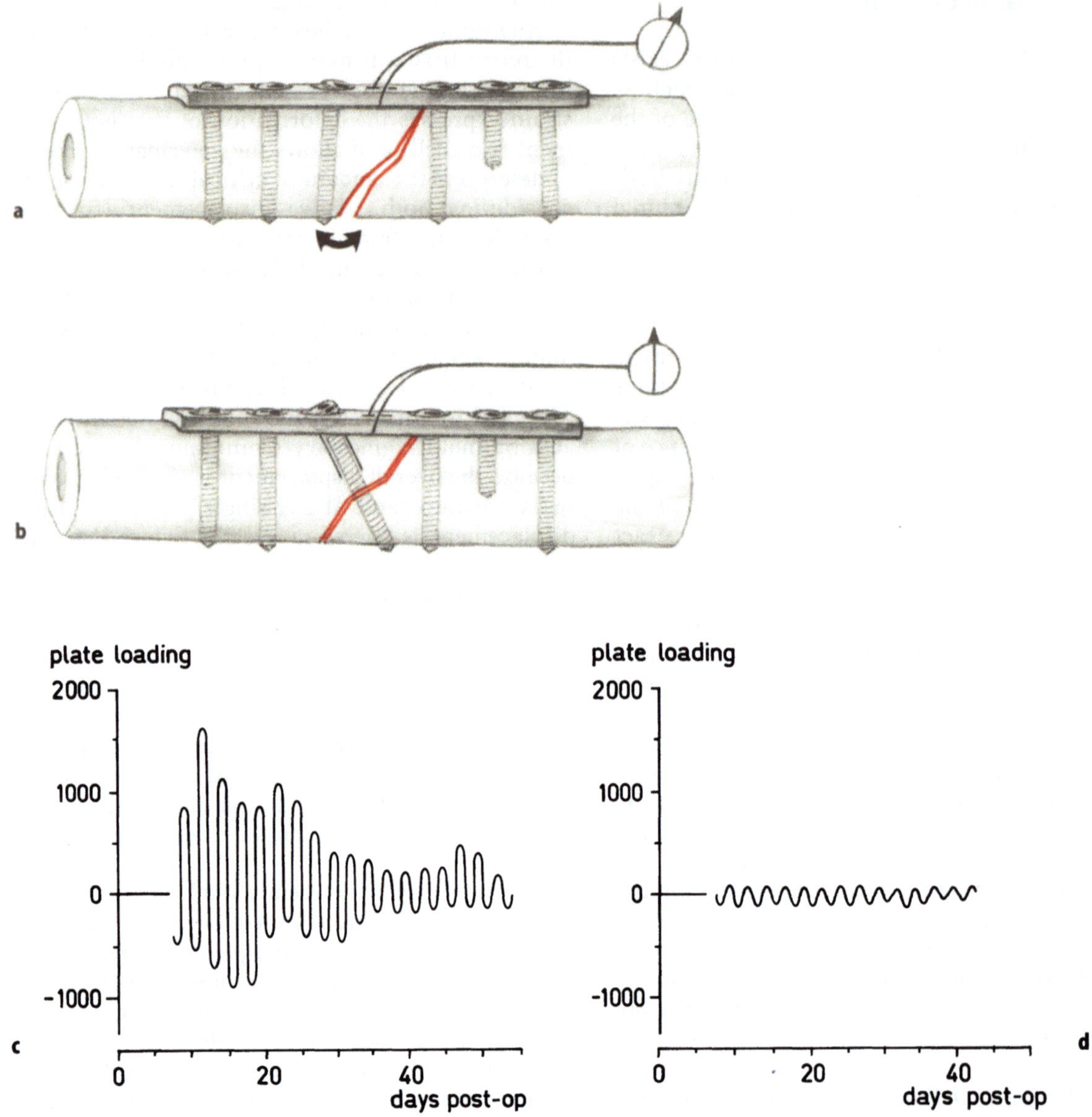

Fig. 1.5a–d. The effect of stability of fixation upon implant loading. Short, oblique osteotomies of sheep tibial diaphyses bridged by plates (Klaue et al. 1985). **a** In one group, only a plate is used to merely bridge the fracture (splinting plate); no lag screw is used to produce interfragmental compression. **b** In another group, a lag screw – here applied through the plate – provides additional stability. **c** The initial *bending load* of the plate (*ordinate*, microstrain) is markedly larger without lag screw. Bone union eventually reduces the load (*abscissa*, days after surgery). **d** The bending load of the plate is continuously smaller when a lag screw is applied. This explains why the technique of application rather than metallurgy determines fatigue failure

Stability and Implant Loading. The degree of stability achieved has a determining effect upon the amount of load borne by the implants used for fixation (Fig. 1.5). The load carried by the implant is critical with respect to possible fatigue failures and/or to (fretting) corrosion.

Fatigue. Stable fixation of adapted fragments restores the "structural continuity" by the recovery of the load-bearing capacity of the fractured bone. It therefore reduces the load placed upon the implants. According to B.G. Weber, (personal communication), "the bone must protect the implant." The relative increase in load resulting from incorrect use of an implant is much larger than the relative increase in strength provided by metallurgical improvements of the implant. A bad surgeon will by far outweigh a good metallurgist – the surgeon changes the loading of the implant by a factor of two to four, while the metallurgist may only improve the strength of the metal by up to 30 %. The latter is often achieved at the expense of give (ductility) or of tissue tolerance of the material.

Measurement of bending load placed upon an internal fixation plate, as carried out by Klaue et al. (1985), shows an important effect of stability in protecting implants from overload.

Corrosion. The most important type of corrosion (practically the only one remaining) for implant materials conforming to today's international standards (International Standards Organization, ISO[5]) is fretting corrosion. Fretting is produced by a changing load applied across and displacing an interface between two metal components of an implant, such as a screw and a nail. The more dynamic the load carried by the implant, the more likely fretting is to cause repeated disruption of the protective "passive layer." Stable fixation helps to reduce corrosion.

In addition to the influence of stability upon the pattern of fracture healing and solid implant-to-bone contact, which avoids biological loosening (see pp. 27, 28, 33), stability of fixation exerts an influence upon the mechanical performance of the implant and upon corrosion. The latter determines the biological tolerance of the implant.

[5] Technical Committees TC 150 on "Surgical Implants", TC 164 on "Biocompatibility Testing."

1.3.1.2 Force, Stress, Strain, and Stiffness

Force (N)[6] acting upon a material results in a state of internal *stress.* The unit of stress (σ), force/area, is N/m^2. Force deforms a material. The deformation ratio, *strain* ($\varepsilon = \delta L/L$) has no units and may be reported as the percentage change of the original dimension (Fig. 1.6). The relationship between the acting force and the resulting deformation is called *stiffness*: the less the stiffness, the larger the deformation. The term "rigidity" is often used synonymously with stiffness in the medical literature.

All three elements – force, stress, and strain – may be split into static (constant) and dynamic (changing over time) components[7](Fig. 1.6c).

1.3.1.3 General Aspects of Load

Load may consist of up to three components of forces and three components of moment; it acts upon a material or a device.

Types of Mechanical Load. Load may or may not change (appreciably) with time. A load which does not change with time is called *static,*[8] while periodically or intermittently changing load is *dynamic* in nature. The compression exerted by an implant applied under tension is static. The forces generated by the function of the limb, e.g., locomotion, are dynamic or functional forces.

None of the components under consideration is evenly distributed over the fracture area; they are affected by the following:

1. The static force generated by the implant
2. The dynamic force resulting from function of the limb (which tends to destabilize the fracture)
3. The amount of contact surface upon which the forces act

At different sites, therefore, different mechanical conditions may exist (Fig. 1.7a,b). According to the different mechanical conditions, locally dissimilar types of fracture healing are observed (Fig. 1.7c) within the same fracture area.

A simple mechanical analysis shows that the tension band wiring (Fig. 1.7a) and the tension band plating as outlined by Müller et al. (1963), if performed without lag screw application, result in conditions which vary with time and location.

[6] Forces are expressed in newtons: 10 N $\approx$ i kp $\approx$ 2.2 lbf. Moments are expressed in newton meters: 1 Nm $\approx$ 10 kp·cm $\approx$ ft·lb/1.37.

[7] In the technical sciences, the terms "static" and "dynamic" are used to define the equilibrium of a situation.

[8] A more appropriate term would be "stationary."

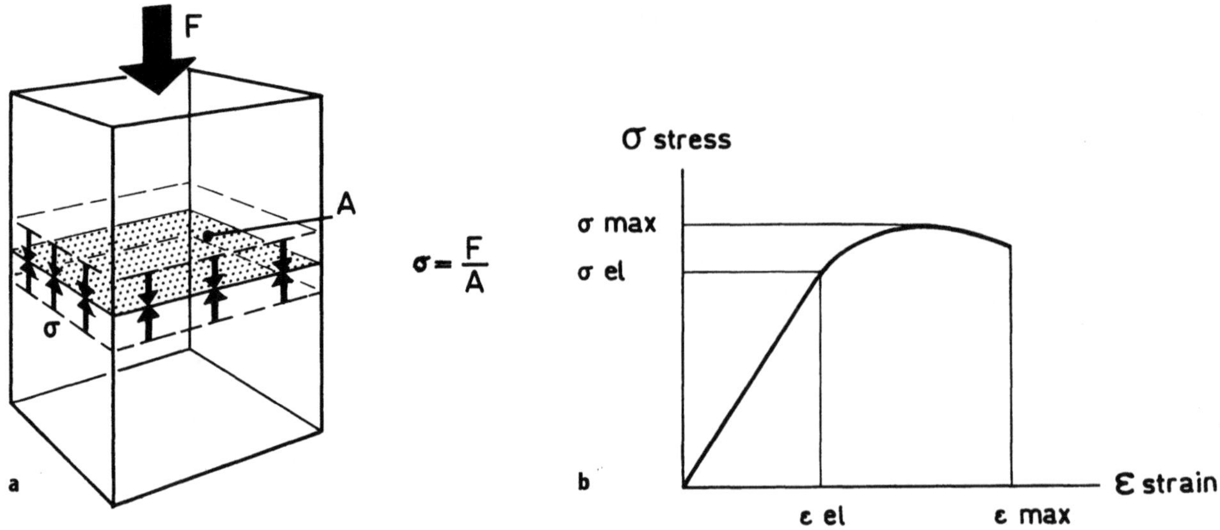

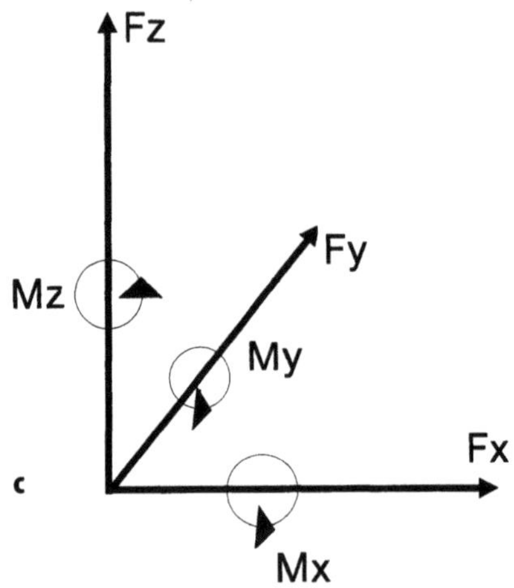

Fig. 1.6a–c. Force, stress, and strain. **a** An externally applied force *F* results in a deformation δL of a body and in an internal state of stress *F*/*A* (σ, force/area). The limit of failure can be described by strength as well as by strain ε (elongation at rupture).[4] **b** The mechanical behavior of a given material can be characterized by a stress–strain diagram. The stress and strain interdependence is plotted. The limit of failure can be described by the strength (limit of stress δ_{max} – strain at rupture ε_{max}). **c** The three components of forces (*Fx, Fy, Fz*) and three components of moments (*Mx, My, Mz*) which describe the loading of a device

The different *mechanical conditions* are the following:

1. A site immediately adjacent to a compression plate may experience a high compressive load (which could eventually exceed the strength of the bone cortex, leading to irreversible deformation such as localized microfractures; Rahn et al. 1971). A minimal dynamic component may be superimposed.
2. A site a little farther from the plate may experience a high static load but within the limits of strength of the bone and with a small component of dynamic load superimposed (stable condition).
3. A site even farther from the plate may exhibit a balance, with lesser stabilizing and greater destabilizing forces resulting in intermittent contact.
4. At the opposite cortex, the fracture gap may remain open continuously, with a changing gap width as the varying (dynamic) tensile forces continuously exceed the compressive stabilizing forces.

The mechanical conditions which prevail within the fracture surface cannot be described with one term only, as at different places (or at different times at the same place) a multitude of changing conditions may exist simultaneously.

The *bone reaction* may vary accordingly within the same fracture (Fig. 1.7c). The different types of healing are:

1. Internal remodeling or "contact healing" of overloaded contact areas. It is especially interesting

[4] The state of stress can be "visualized" by applying an imaginary cut. To reestablish the previous balance of forces, a force must be applied to the cut surface. The amount of force per unit area of the cut surface corresponds to the amount of previous internal stress (σ).

to note that areas which have undergone local overload, but which remain stably fixed by adjacent contact areas, exhibit direct internal remodeling as demonstrated by Rahn (see above).
2. Internal remodeling or "contact healing" of intact contact areas (see p. 41).
3. Fracture surface resorption and indirect healing (see p. 42).
4. Delayed healing. The nonunited gap will eventually fill by indirect bone formation (see p. 42).

The *effect* of load consists of deformation[9] of an intact bone and/or of providing varying degrees of stability of a fracture. Static compression generally stabilizes, while dynamically applied tension or shear tends to result in instability of the interface. The effect of combined forces depends upon their relative values at a given time and place, as outlined above. The surgeon will aim to apply enough static compression to maintain stability in the presence of any opposing dynamic tensile forces which may act upon the fractured bone. Small areas of local overload are not of basic concern, as the bone as a whole is able to resist high loads. Generalized overload exerted prior to onset of bone union, however, results in the mechanical breakdown of the internally fixed fracture. The French term "débricolage" (see p. 53) seems to be appropriate to describe a condition in which the fragments of a fracture which were previously fixed together simply fall apart. This describes a condition in which no biological reaction plays a role. Two possible causes can come into play: the construction may be too weak, or the load excessively large.

Load applied to bone or implant, e.g., axial tension, produces an internal state of stress within the material. Stress increases with load, but it decreases with increasing load-bearing surface.[10] Increasing stress may reach a critical level of strength of the material, and the material may fracture. Here the critical condition of the fracture is described in terms of strength (e.g., ultimate tensile strength).

Load applied to a material produces stress within the material and thus invariably results in deformation (strain) of the material. Strain (Figs. 1.8, 1.9) is expressed as relative (e.g., percentage) increase or decrease in length in relation to original length (see p. 13). Increasing load (stress) may reach the critical level of strength. Deformation may also reach the critical level of *elongation at rupture* (or strain at rupture), and the material may fracture. In the initial stages of fracture healing, when strength and stiffness of the repair tissues do not play a relevant role, it is more appropriate to specify the critical condition of the tissues involved in fracture healing in terms of *tolerated strain* (see Table 1.1) than in terms of stress.

When the load-bearing surface is large, the critical limit of load at fracture is best expressed as stress (stress equal to or smaller than strength). When the load-bearing surface is small, and hence the contribution of the tissue to stabilization minimal, the critical limit is best expressed in terms of strain (limit of strain tolerance). The former condition is defined by load, and the latter by deformation. Although the two characteristics represent two aspects of the same condition, critical mechanical conditions of tissue differentiation in fracture healing and nonunions are more easily understood using a clear concept of strain.

Bone Failure. As a rule, fractures of previously intact diaphyseal bone occur due to a single state of excessive stress. Failures of initial small bone bridges in fracture healing are best understood as the result of an episode of excessive strain, because the force potentially acting by far exceeds the strength of the tissue. The only critical parameter is the deformation allowed by the width of the gap between the fracture surfaces nearby.

Implant Failure. With respect to the implant, two conditions exist which may lead to failure: (1) a single massive overload or (2) multiple smaller overloads (fatigue). The question therefore arises as to why under certain conditions a thicker plate seems to break more readily.

When an implant bridging a long defect is increasingly loaded, e.g., by increasing weight-bearing, the stress generated may eventually reach the limit of strength and the implant fails. This commonly understood behavior is called "load-driven failure."

Another condition exists in a highly loaded fracture area: when surface resorption with gap widening occurs, then eventually the strain of the implant reaches the critical limit – "deformation-driven failure." Given sufficient load, the failure of a plate, for example, depends upon gap width and thickness of the plate. A thicker plates fails at a smaller angle of bending, because its surface experiences a higher strain for the same angle of bending. This analysis is of importance concerning implant failure, because in internal fixation, deformation-driven conditions often prevail.

[9] The other effect of force, acceleration, is not considered here.

[10] Stress is expressed as force per unit area N/m^2 ($\approx 1\ kp/mm^2 = 10 \times 10^6\ N/m^2 = 10\ MPa$).

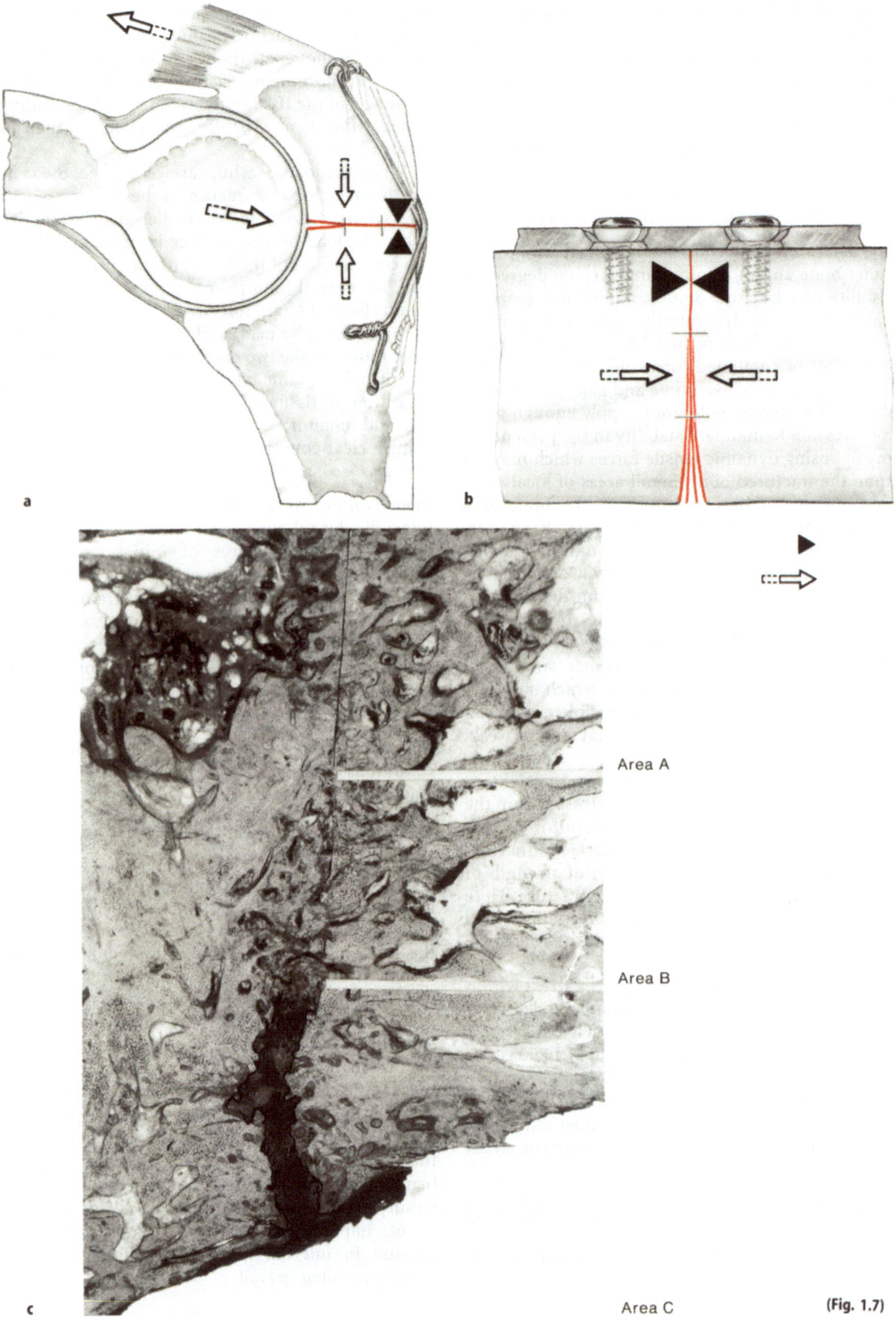

(Fig. 1.7)

◀ **Fig. 1.7a–c.** Different mechanical conditions and types of healing within the same fracture surface. **a** Different conditions within a fracture surface at different times of observation (tension band wiring of the olecranon). The preload exerted by the wire is shown by *black triangles* (static compression); the changing load due to function (pull of the triceps muscle and related articular compression producing additional compression of the fracture surface) is shown by *open arrows*. **b** Different conditions within a fracture surface at different times of observation; tension band plating of shaft fracture without interfragmental compression (either by prebending of the plate or by interfragmentary lag screw) bears an inherent risk of delayed union. The use of plates only, without lag screw or prebending, should therefore be avoided. **c** Different types of healing within the same fracture. This histological section demonstrates within the same fracture area all stages from direct healing to delayed healing. In *area A*, direct bone healing is seen, in *area B*, indirect bone healing, and in *area C*, delayed healing. (Courtesy of J. Craig)

a

b

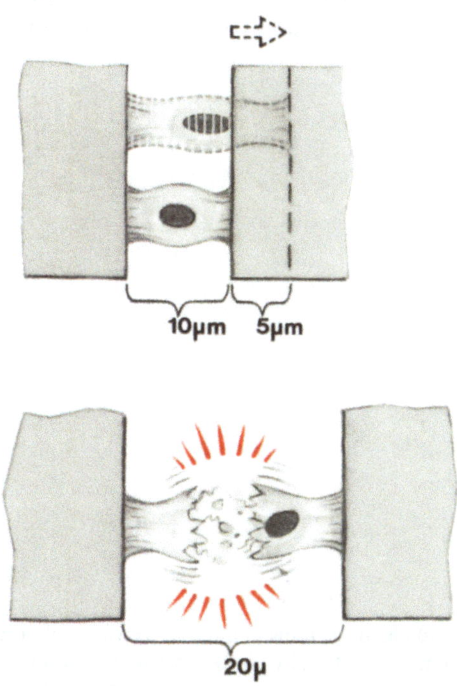

Fig. 1.8a,b. Large strain in small gaps. The deformation of the cells or tissues is critical. It depends not only upon the degree of displacement δL of the fragments (instability), but also (and more importantly) upon the initial width *L* of the fracture gap. For very small gaps, e.g., smaller than 0.1 mm, an imperceptible displacement (0.1 mm) may result in very high strain (>100 %) of any one individual tissue element, e.g., the cell. **a** A small displacement (5 μm) in a small gap between the fragments (here about one cell layer thickness, approximately 10 μm) results in a strain of 50 %. **b** A somewhat large displacement (10 μm) in a small gap reaches the limit of strain tolerance of the cell. The change of the gap width from 10 to 20 μm is not visible to the naked eye, i.e., the surgeon does not see such instability

Table 1.1 Critical strain levels of repair tissues

Tissue	Elongation at rupture (%)
Granulation tissue[a]	100
Dense fibrous tissue	20
Cartilage	20
Cancellous bone	2
Lamellar bone	2

Values taken from Ymada and Evans (1970).
[a] The value of parenchyma has been taken to replace the missing data for granulation tissue.

1.3.1.4 Physiological Load

Physiological activity of a limb consists of movements by muscle forces and weight-bearing. Both result in bone loads with complex patterns of static and dynamic components of torque, bending, and axial load. The effect of physiological load may again be analyzed as consisting of three components of forces and/or three components of moments (see p. 12). Loading of a fracture surface statically by the implant and dynamically by functional load results in a complex pattern in which areas of overload, areas of reversible deformation, areas of intermittently open gaps, and areas of constantly open gaps of changing size can exist simultaneously. An example of such a complex loading situation is the condition produced by a tension band wiring of a fractured olecranon or patella (Fig. 1.7a, see pp. 14). Hertel (1984) has demonstrated that the stress generated within a conventional plate is increased 14 times if a plate hole is placed on top of an open defect (open fracture gap). If, in addition, a screw hole near the fracture is left open, i.e., not fixed to bone, the plate experiences 0.3 times higher stress at this site. Plate holes with and without screws did not show relevant differences in measured loading when the bone was perfectly adapted and was thus able to carry load.

1.3.1.5 Principles of Surgical Stabilization

There are two fundamentally different mechanisms of fracture fixation: *splinting* and *compression*. The two differ in the mechanism of stabilization and in the degree of stability achieved.

Splinting. Fixation by splinting (Fig. 1.10) consists in connecting a (more or less) stiff device to the fractured bone. This device reduces the mobility of the fracture in proportion to its stiffness. Splinting is achieved using a great variety of methods, ranging from external splints, i.e., plaster fixation, to internal fixation by plates and medullary pins and

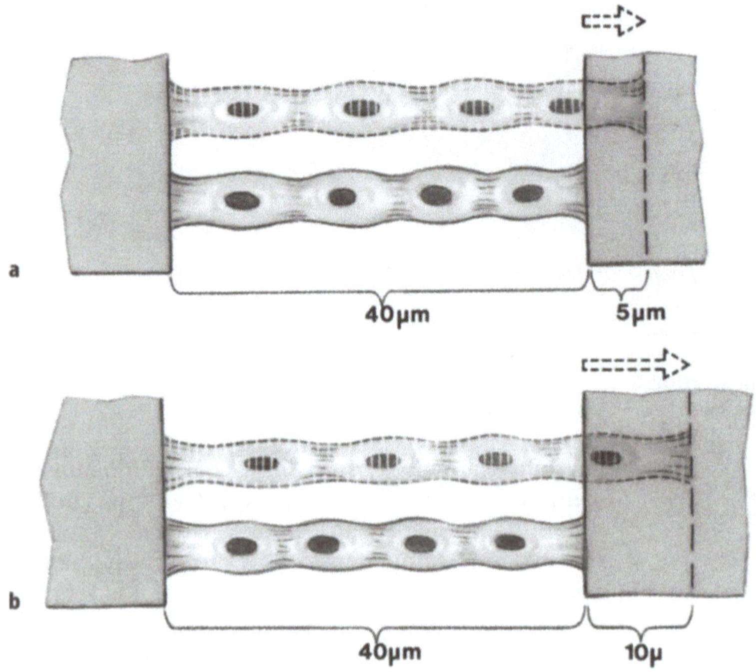

Fig. 1.9a,b. Small strain in large gaps. Strain of the individual tissue element, e.g., ce the repair tissue within the fracture gap (and adjacent to it) may be reduced by widening of the gap (from 10 μm in Fig. 1.8a to 40 μm in Fig. 1.9 by bone surface resorption) and/or by shearing the overall displacement by multiple serial gaps. Both conditions are usually seen in multifragmentary fractures. **a** A small displacement (5 μm, same as in Fig. 1.8a) within an initially wide gap (40 μm) results in strain (approximately 12 %) which is tolerated by dense fibrous tissue. **b** A somewhat larger displacement (10 μm, same as in Fig. 1.8b) within an initially wide gap (40 μm) results in strain (approximately 25 %) which is tolerated by granulation tissue

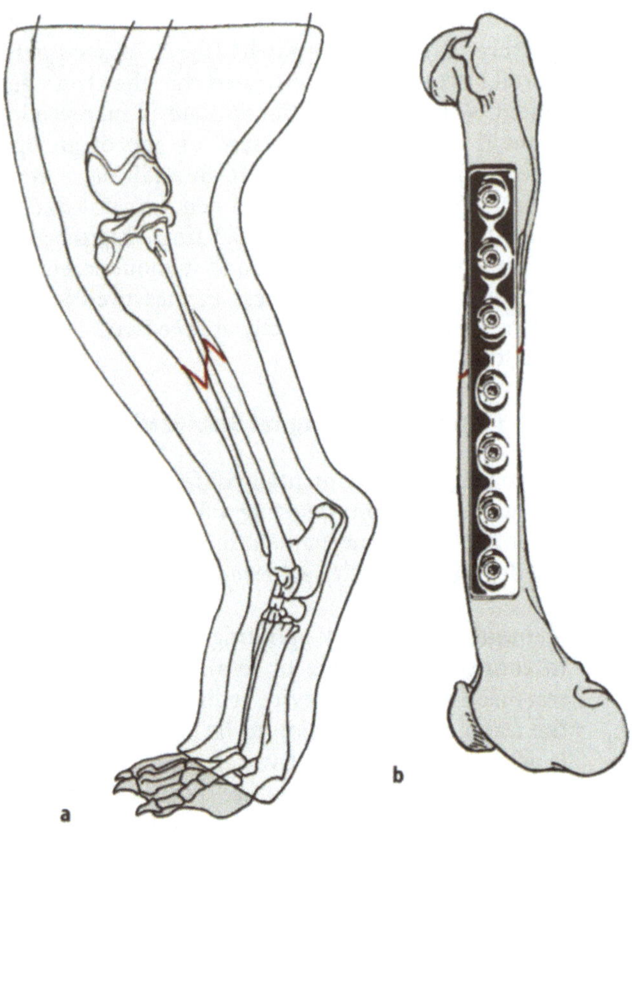

Fig. 1.10a,b. Basic tools in internal fixation: splinting. **a** External splinting by plaster cast relies upon the same basic mechanisms as splinting for emergency care. A splint is indirectly fixed to the bone. Because of its stiffness, it reduces (but does not completely abolish) the mobility of the fracture fragments. A splint by necessity carries part or all of the load, particularly if contact is missing between the fracture fragments. Coupling between plaster cast and bone is comparatively loose due to the interposition of the soft tissues. **b** Plate used as a splint. The plate may theoretically be used to keep the fracture fragments apart. The plate carries full functional load until solid union occurs. Coupling between the plate and bone is very tight; plate fixation of simple fractures (to meet the goal of reliable and undisturbed fracture healing) does not tolerate fracture surface resorption well (locking splint)

also includes the transcutaneous splints: the external fixators. The effect of splinting is to reduce, but not abolish fracture mobility. Thus pain is reduced and the limb is protected from excessive deformation. Some people advocate the use of plates made of a material of stiffness similar to that of bone. As fracture mobility depends proportionally upon the stiffness of the splint, however, there is no point in using such a plate.

A special type of splinting is called *buttressing*, where a stiff splint serves to maintain the shape of a bone after a complex fracture or in the presence of a defect. The implant bridges the segment of the bone which cannot carry the load. The implant is then subjected to full functional load until the bone resumes the load. In this case, special precautions have to be taken to avoid failure of the unprotected implant.

Coupling of Splints. As mentioned above, the splint must be connected (coupled) to the fractured bone. The effectiveness of a splint fixed to bone depends to a great extent upon the stiffness of the softest element within the chain: bone – coupling by soft tissues – splint. Plaster as such is very rigid due to its large dimensions. However, it provides very limited stabilization of the fracture, due to the flexible coupling between plaster and bone by soft tissues. While a plaster cast is very effective in nonoperative treatment (Böhler 1938; Latta et al. 1980; Sarmiento 1980), it will hardly ever unload a stable internal fixation, because it allows significant angulation of the bone fragments and, in addition, increases inertial loading. When a fracture which is fixed by lag screw and plate is deformed by an applied bending load, the screws pull out at a very small overall deformation. A plaster cast does not, therefore, reliably prevent screws from pulling out, nor does it prevent a plate from failing in fatigue, should the surgeon fail to reduce external loading. Stripping of threads occurs at bending angles which are smaller than the angulation allowed for by the plaster.

Coupling in stable external fixators depends mainly upon the stiffness of the pin. Here the thread offers much less stiffness than the shaft of the pin, the flexural and torsional stiffness changing with the fourth power of the critical diameter. The critical diameter is the core diameter of the thread or the outer diameter of the shaft.

Enhancement of Splints. A plate is known to be flexible and, due to its asymmetric positioning, not strong enough to carry the full load of limb function. Müller and Witzel (1984) and Mast et al. (1989) have proposed supplementing a minimal internal fixation with a temporary external fixator (Fig. 1.11). The large lever arm of the external fixator allows for efficient unloading of the internal fixation until bone healing can take over its function of contributing stiffness and strength.

Unloading of Bone by Implanted Splints. Classical splints are the pin and the external fixator. Special consideration is given here to the plate as splint. As we will see, plate splinting is used to reduce the physiological load placed upon, for example, a screw fixation. Unloading of the plated bone segment is a prerequisite of the function of the neutralization plate and the buttress plate. Most other implants act in a similar way and unload, or protect, fractured bone from excessive physiological forces so as to permit undisturbed fracture healing during early functional treatment and to prevent mechanical breakdown of the incompletely healed fracture. On the other hand, a mechanically reconstructed bone, because of its "structural integrity," protects the implant, e.g., from repeated bending and thus from fatigue failure.

Gliding and Nongliding Splints. There are two basic splinting principles: one which allows gliding of the fragments along the implant, and the other which prevents it (Fig. 1.12). An intramedullary pin allows for gliding of the bone along the pin because the friction between pin and bone is generally small. A plate, as a rule, does not allow gliding because the friction resulting from the plate screws is large (each screw produces compression between plate undersurface and bone in the range of up to 3000 N).[11]

A plate applied to a simple fracture, without additional measures (such as interfragmental compression), would not provide sufficient stability to prevent fragment and resorption induced by micromotion between the fragment ends. When such shortening occurs, the high friction between plate underside and bone surface does not allow for coaptation. The plate then bears all the load placed upon the bone and is prone to fatigue failure. Plate fixation therefore requires the use of interfragmental compression by screws and/or axial compression by the plate with or without prebending of the plate (or contact brought about by functional load) to ensure bony contact able to carry load without intermittent displacement. As a rule, the plate should not be used to stabilize a fracture of a

[11] If a frictional coefficient (metal to bone) of 0.4 is assumed and if three screws are applied in each fragment, the surface undergoing a normal force of up to 3000 N per screw is able to resist more than 3600 N of tangentially applied force (on each side of the fracture) without sliding.

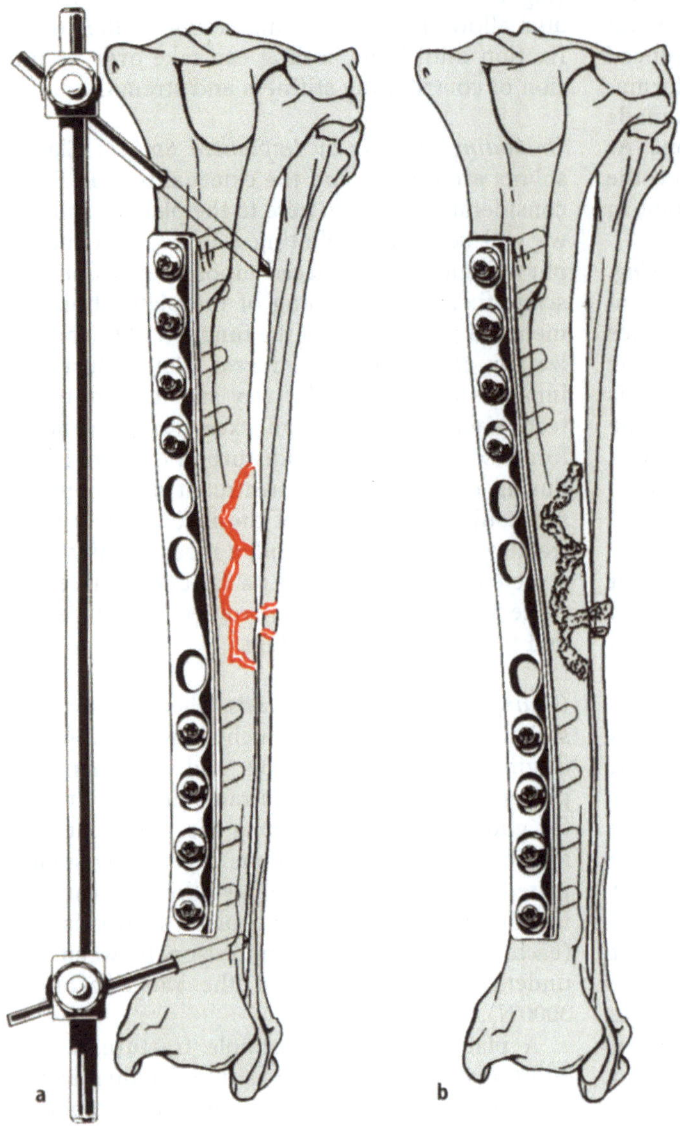

Fig. 1.11a,b. Enhancement of the splint. In practice, for biomechanical reasons, the external fixator is usually placed in the craniomedial plane. For the sake of clarity, it is shown in the lateral plane here. As soon as the callus provides support, the external frame is removed. Thus the time until transcutaneous connection occurs is minimized, and the internal fixation is adapted to the healing process

weight-bearing bone, but to unload (protect) a fracture stabilized by other means (e.g., lag screws); a fracture is splinted to be partially unloaded (protected), provided that bone contact has been restored. When a fracture gap beneath the splint remains open, the bone at the fracture area is completely unloaded by the splint.

It is an important goal of the use of a plate to at least partially unload the fractured bone which has been previously fixed using screws. Stress shielding is, therefore, a prerequisite, and not primarily a disadvantageous side effect of the treatment. This fact has often been misunderstood in recent years.

A further fact to be mentioned here is that, with respect to axial loading, the stiffness of a so-called rigid internal fixation plate made of steel is equal to that of the tibia, for example. However, the plate is many times less stiff than the bone in bending and torque.

Compression. Compression is a very elegant tool to stabilize a fracture because efficient stabilization is achieved with minimal amounts of implanted material. Compression fixation consists in pressing two surfaces (bone-to-bone or implant-to-bone) together.

According to its alteration with time, two different types of compression are distinguished:

1. Static compression, i.e., compression which does not change with time. Once applied, static compression remains virtually unaltered.

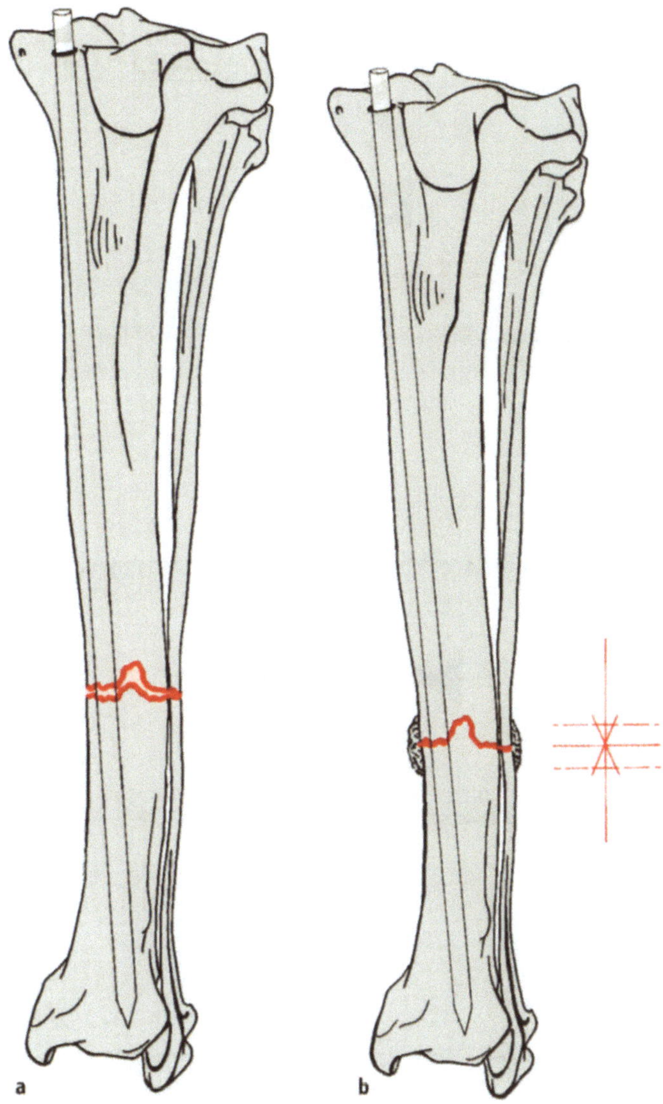

Fig. 1.12. a Intramedullary pin alone allows the fragments to close a fracture gap. Rotational stability is achieved by interlocking of the fragments. **b** Callus formation adds further stability

2. Dynamic compression: limb function, for instance, results in periodic partial loading and unloading of the contacting surfaces due to dynamic forces resulting from function. The wire or plate applied as a tension band transforms the functional tension into compression. A fixation results which allows some load-induced movement.

The effect of compression is twofold:

1. Compression produces preloading, i.e., the surfaces remain in close contact as long as the compression applied remains larger than any opposite-acting force, e.g., tension from physiological load which results in bending (Fig. 1.13a).
2. Compression produces friction, i.e., the compressed surfaces resist sliding displacement as long as the friction produced by compression remains larger than the shearing force applied (Fig. 1.13b,c). Local shear at a transverse fracture results mostly from torque applied around the long axis of the bone, while inclined surfaces such as oblique fractures undergo shear when the bone is loaded along its long axis, e.g., by weight-bearing.

Different methods are used to produce compression. They differ not only in the implant used, but also in the mechanism by which compression is applied and in the efficiency of the compression.

Interfragmentary Compression Applied by Lag Screw. A fracture may be compressed by application

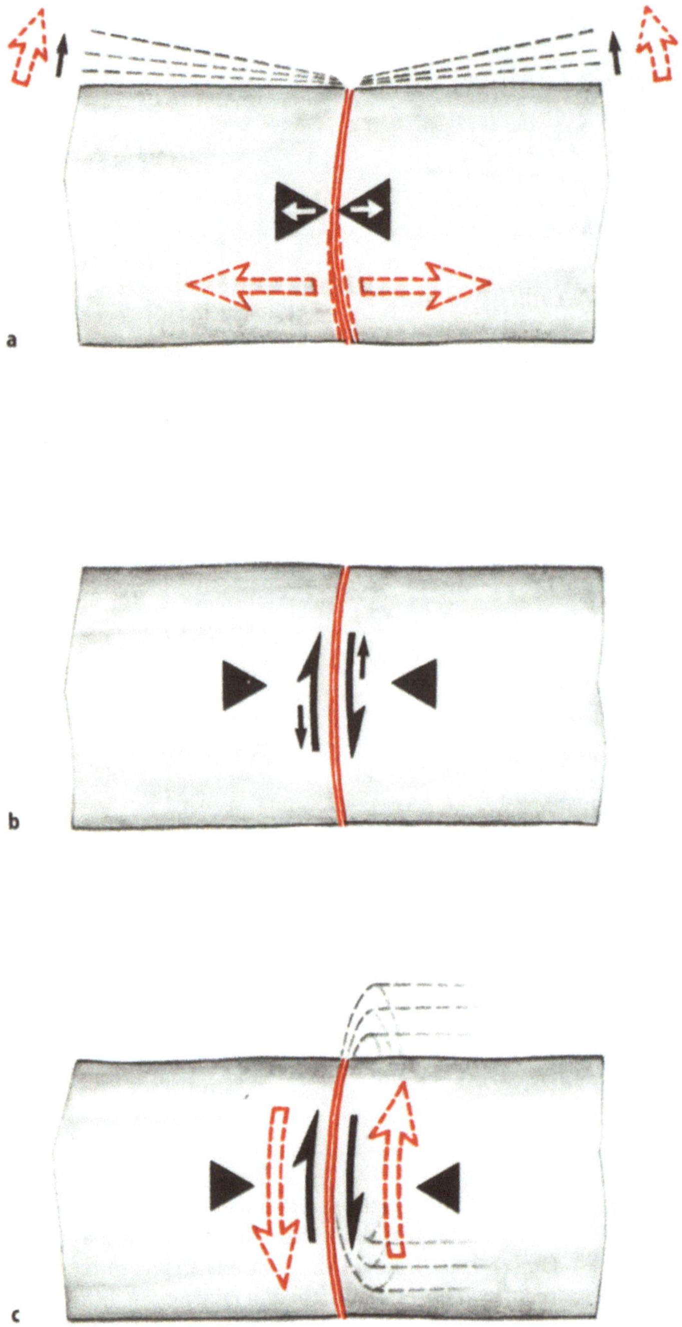

Fig. 1.13a–c. Basic tools in internal fixation. **a** Stabilization by compressive preload. Preload is effective whenever the compression that stabilizes the interface exceeds the tension induced by bending (Perren 1971). **b** Compression stabilization by sufficient friction. Compression of an interface produces friction, which opposes displacement by shear. This mechanism is most important in stabilization of interfaces of a structure placed under torque load. No displacement occurs. **c** Loss of compression stabilization by insufficient friction. If the friction generated is too small and/or the torsional (shear) load placed upon the fracture too large, the surfaces slide along each other, resulting in instability

of a screw across the fracture (Fig. 1.14), whereby the screw thread is anchored within the fragment near the tip of the screw. Thus, when the screw is tightened, this fragment will be pressed against the fragment retained by the head of the screw (Fig. 1.14b). For the lag screw to function, the bone fragment near the head of the screw must not be coupled to the thread of the screw. This may be achieved by using a screw with a partial thread or by removing the thread within the bone fragment near the head of the screw by overdrilling (gliding hole). For a gliding hole to function properly, the screw must be positioned in the axis of the drill hole, i.e., forces acting perpendicular to the long axis of the screw will lead to engagement of the screw thread with the wall of the gliding hole and thus to loss of lag screw effect.

The compression exerted by a lag screw is very efficient because (among other reasons) it is relatively large. Brennwald et al. (1975) and von Arx

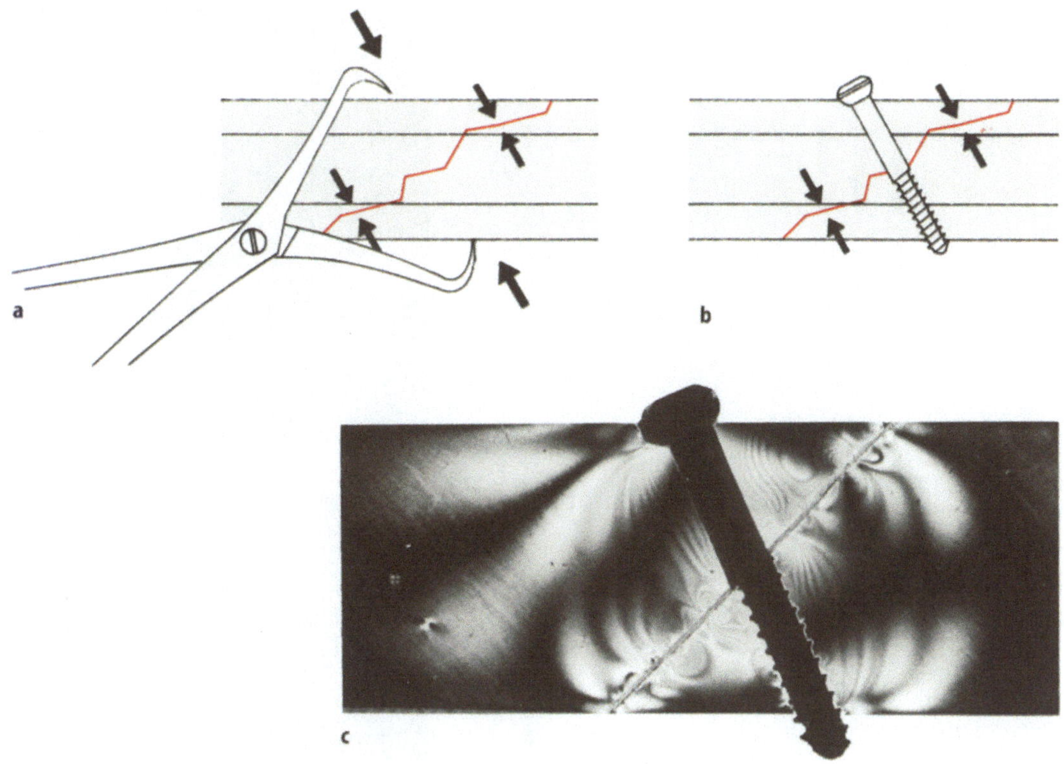

Fig. 1.14a–c. Principles of lag screw technique. **a** In order to find the best location and inclination, forceps compressing the fracture temporarily substitute for the function of the lag screw. They are also adjusted to prevent shear of the fracture. **b** The lag screw replaces the forceps in location and position (inclination) for best stabilization. **c** Photoelastic analysis shows that the range within which compression acts is relatively small. This explains why rotation cannot be countered by a single lag screw

(1975) have determined that the force applied by expert surgeons using a plate screw amounts to 2000–4000 N. It is important to note that the force exerted by the lag screw acts from within the fracture surface (Fig. 1.14c), in contrast to the compression exerted by the plate (see below).

It is noteworthy that the direction along which the compression acts (inclination of lag screw) must coincide fairly well with a perpendicular to the fracture surface. As Johner et al. (1989) have shown, sliding occurs if the compression applied to a smooth osteotomy is inclined only 20° in relation to an axis perpendicular to the fracture surface.

The presumption that an axial load acts along the long axis of the bone shaft is only correct for short stretches within a complex loading pattern. It is therefore safest to select an inclination of a lag screw such that it is perpendicular in respect to the "average" inclination of the fracture surface.

A further important aspect of lag screw fixation consists in the comparatively limited range of action of the lag screw; the stress generated across the fracture tapers off quite quickly with the distance to the screw axis. A single lag screw therefore does not offer good stabilization with respect to torque acting within the fracture plane.

Lag screw fixation provides rigidity, but the strength offered is often considered to be inadequate, i.e., functional loads applied may result in displacement. A single overload applied to lag screw fixation can result in irreversible loss of compression. Therefore, the lag screw fixation is often protected by a plate with neutralizing function. The combination of lag screw and neutralization plate fixation has been studied by Barraud (1982) and Eisner et al. (1985). Diehl (1975) analyzed stability and strength of different types of internal fixation of femur and tibia with respect to early rehabilitation.

Axial Compression Exerted by the Compression Plate. Compression using a plate (Fig. 1.15a,b) is produced by applying a pretensioned plate to the bone. For the application of this compression, the bone fragments need to be in contact and thus to be able to carry load.

Compression by Prebending of the Plate. When a plate which is exactly contoured to the bone exerts

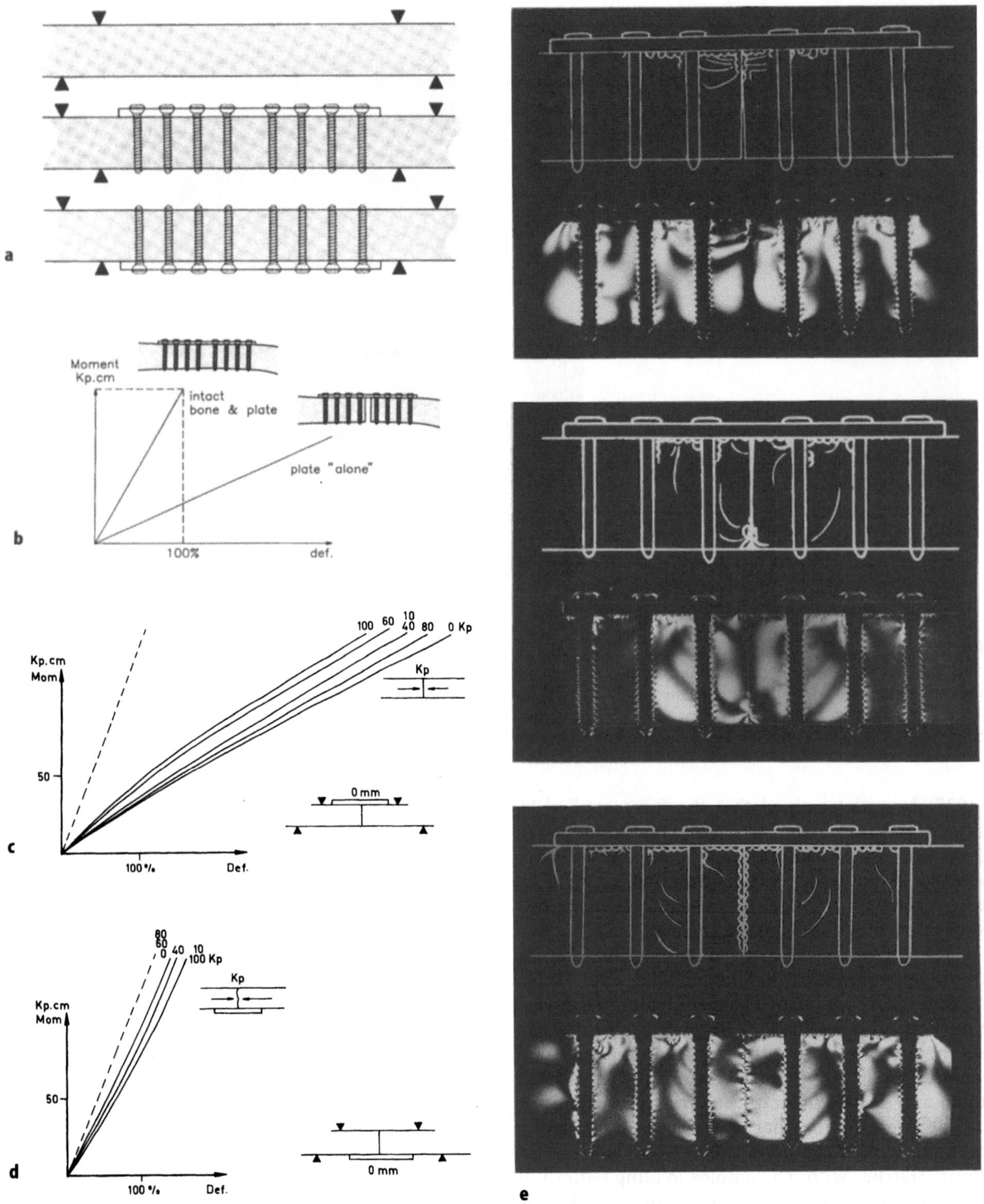
a
b
Moment
Kp.cm
intact
bone & plate
plate "alone"
100%
def.
c
100 60 10 40 80 0 Kp
Kp.cm
Mom
Kp
50
0 mm
100 %
Def.
d
80 60 0 40 10 100 Kp
Kp
Kp.cm
Mom
50
0 mm
100 %
Def.
e

(Fig. 1.15a–e)

◀ **Fig. 1.15a–e.** Compression exerted by the plate. A plate provides stable fixation only under very special conditions. **a** Method of test. First, the stiffness of the plated intact bone is determined. Stiffness is then determined with the plate fixed to the tension side and finally with the plate fixed to the compression (bending) side. **b** Method of evaluation. The deformation produced by the bending moment applied is plotted. The slope of the curve for the plated intact bone is taken as reference for maximal stability, the one for a plate bridging a defect is taken as reference for minimal stability. **c** A plate placed at the tension side provides good stability of fixation. **d** A plate placed at the compression (bending) side provides minimal stability. **e** Axial compression without prebending (*top*) results in compression near the plate only. Prebending without axial compression (*center*) results in adaptation of the far cortex only. The combination of axial compression and prebending (*bottom*) results in compression of the whole cross-section

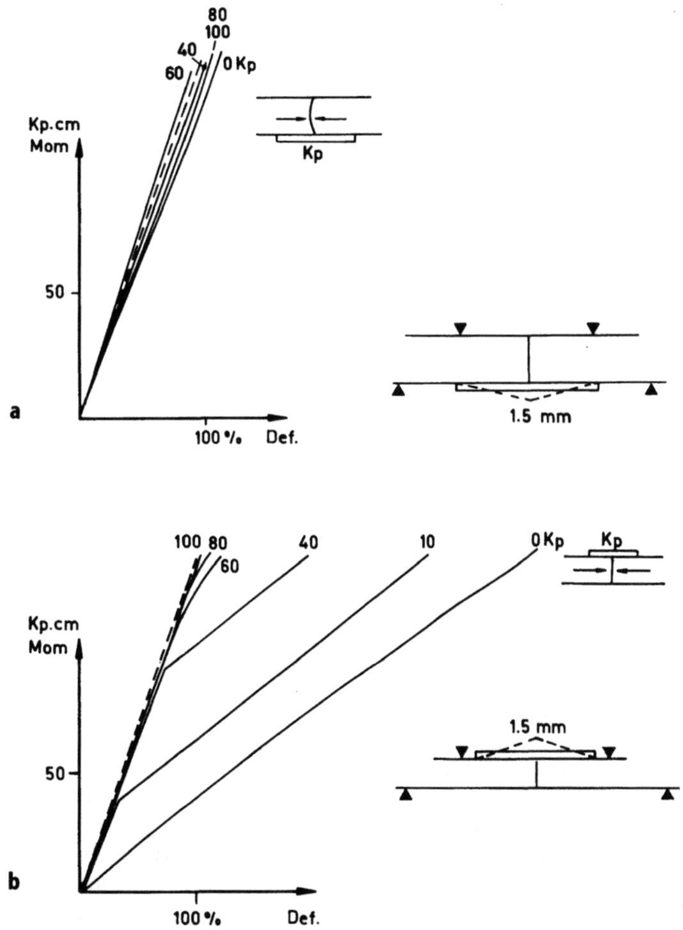

Fig. 1.16a,b. Effect of axial compression superimposed on that of prebending. **a** Plate placed on the tension side; initial stable conditions for all degrees of load and compression. **b** Plate placed on the compression (bending) side; no compression, no stability. Increasing range of stable conditions with increasing compression

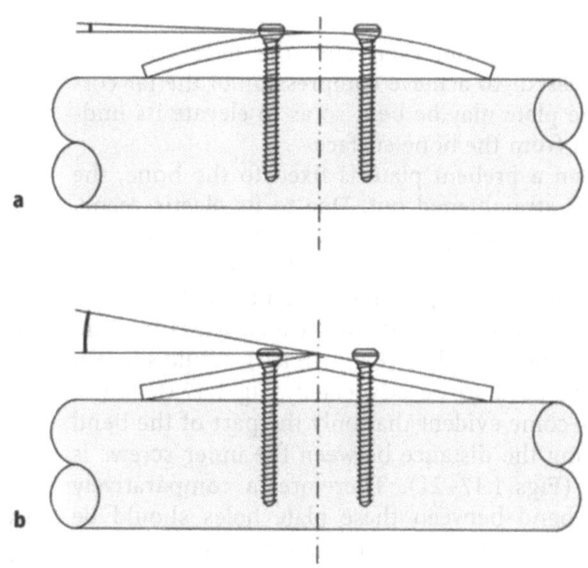

Fig. 1.17a,b. Effect of shallow versus sharp bending. **a** A shallow bend has a minimal effect, as only the bend enclosed within the inner screws is active. **b** A sharp bend is effective

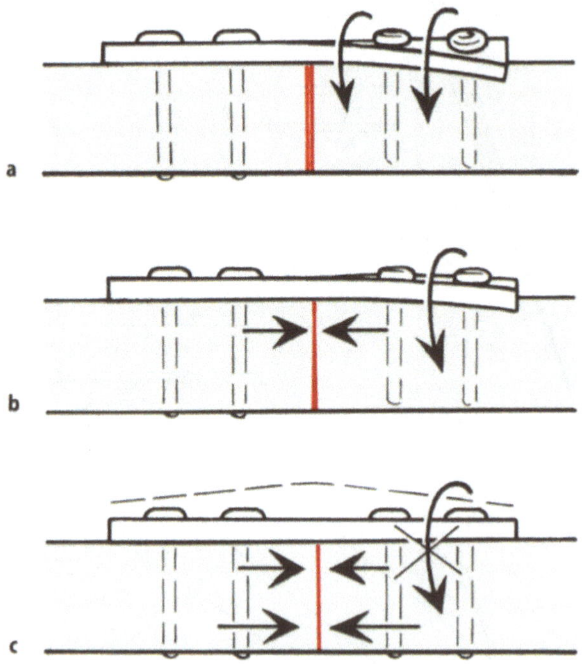

Fig. 1.18a–c. Effect of prebending upon stability under torque load. **a** Torque applied without contact at the fracture surfaces produces shear. The axis of rotation is within the plate. **b** Pure axial compression is ineffective with respect to torque load. The friction produced by axial compression is located near the plate and has a small lever arm. **c** Prebending produces friction far from the plate, i.e., with good leverage

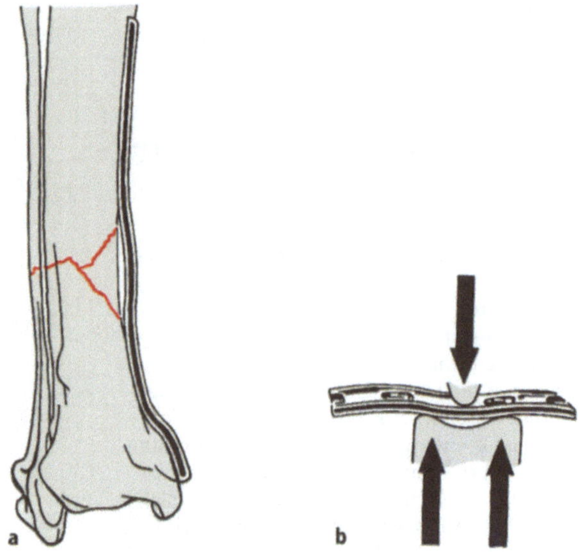

Fig. 1.19a–d. (see p. 25) Practical application of prebending. ▶ **a** A comparatively sharp bend should then be applied. **b** The plate should first be contoured to fit the bone surface snugly. **c** The midsection is therefore elevated (p25). **d, e** When fixed to the bone, the plate compresses the far cortex as well

axial compression, then only the near cortex is compressed. To achieve compression of the far cortex, the plate may be bent so as to elevate its midsection from the bone surface.

When a prebent plate is fixed to the bone, the bend is straightened out. Due to its elastic recoil, the plate has a tendency to recover the bend which was applied by plastic (irreversible) deformation. It therefore exerts a bending moment which tends to close and to compress the far (transcortex) fracture gap opposite the plate (Fig. 1.16 a,b). While smooth bending used to be advocated (Fig. 1.17a), it has now become evident that only the part of the bend spanning the distance between the inner screws is active (Figs. 1.17–21). Therefore, a comparatively sharp bend between these plate holes should be applied. The angle of bend should be such that an eight-hole, 4.5-mm small DCP is elevated about 2 mm from the bone surface. The effect of this method depends upon the balance of the prebend and axial compression applied (Fig. 1.17–21). It should be noted that compression which is equal in both cortices is not an aim in itself. Good stability only requires that the far cortex be compressed enough to maintain contact under physiological loading without being overloaded. The compression of the far cortex is important with respect to stabilizing against torque and shear resulting from it. Displacement of a plated transverse osteotomy under torque load occurs around an axis near or within the plate. In this context, the lever arm of the far cortex is many times larger than the one of the near cortex.

The advantage of prebending over the lag screw is that single overload, which opens the fracture gap, usually does not result in plastic deformation of the plate. Once the load has subsided, the fracture is again stabilized due to the elastic recoil of the plate.

Prebending increases stability and may be combined with the interfragmentary lag screw. It is especially efficient in bones of small diameter and/or in soft bone. The disadvantage of prebending is that the elastic recoil of a prebent plate may disturb the reduction achieved.

The effect of prebending a plate on compression of the fracture surface and stability has been determined by Hayes and Perren (1971), Perren et al. (1974), and Aeberhardt (1973). Gotzen et al. (1981) analyzed extensively the prebending of plates, while Gotzen et al. (1980) and Haas et al. (1985) also

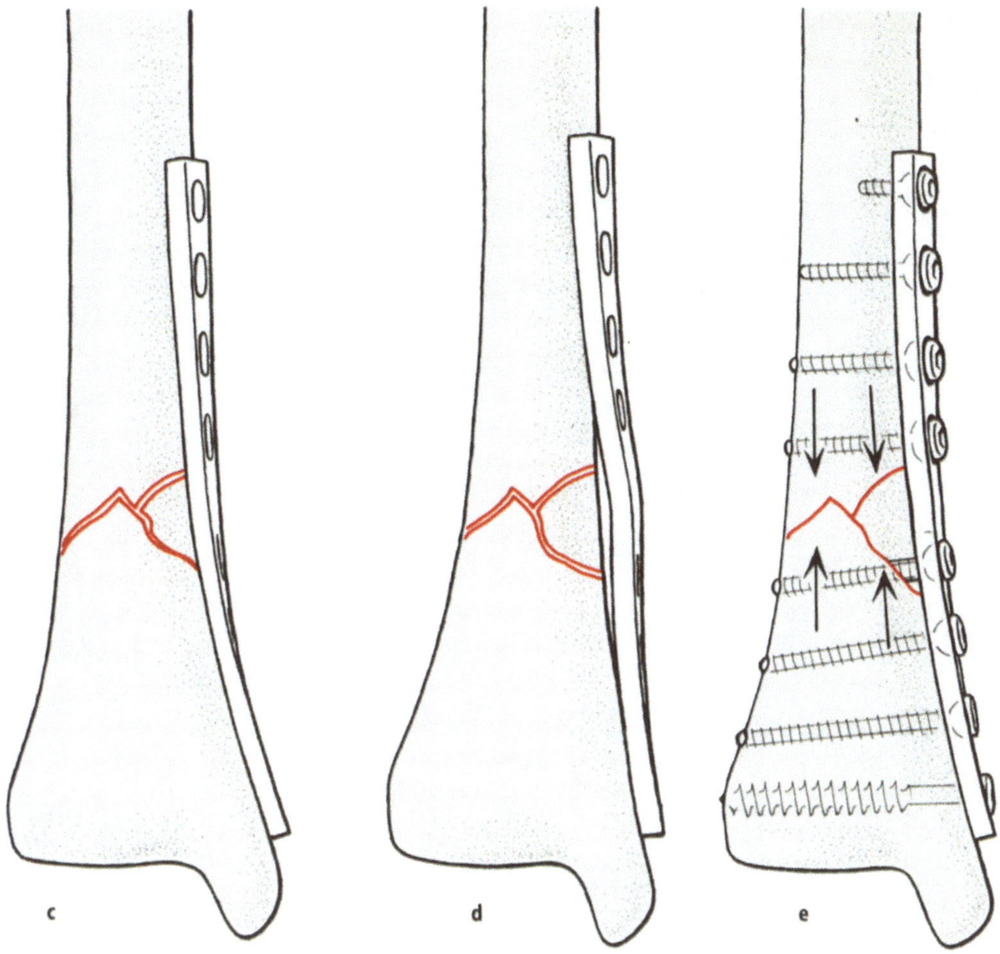

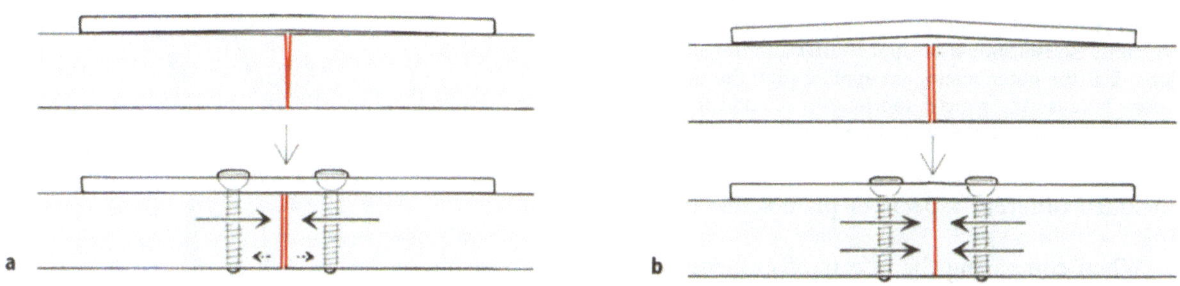

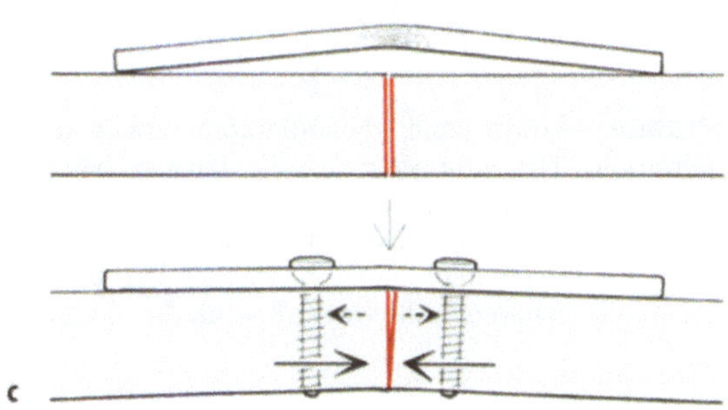

Fig. 1.20a–c. The correlation between prebending and amount of axial compression. The amount of axial compression is kept constant. **a** A small amount of prebending results in minimal compression of the far cortex. **c** If too large an amount of prebending is applied, the near cortex is not compressed efficiently. **b** The goal is to balance the two principles

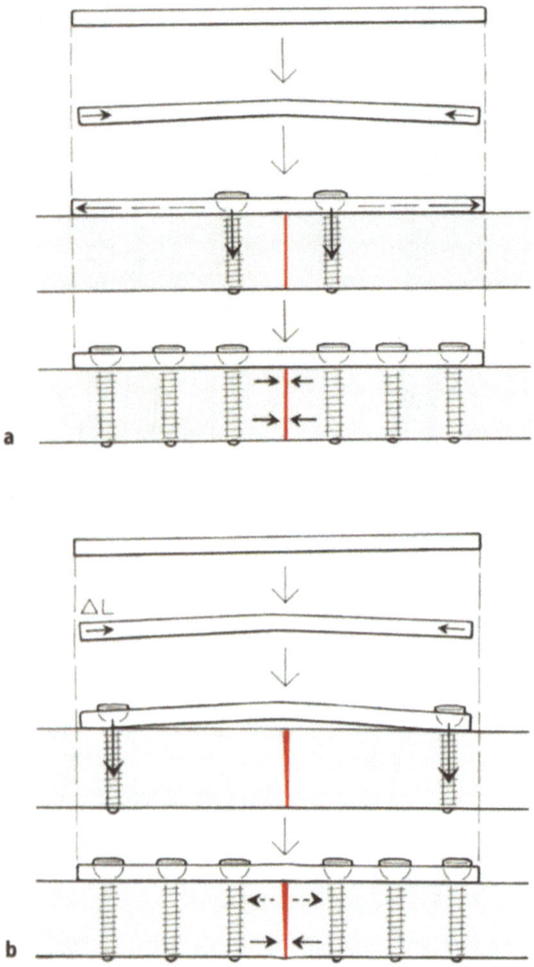

Fig. 1.21a,b. The appropriate sequence of application of the screws in a prebent plate. **a** To fix a prebent plate to the bone, the inner screws should be applied first and the outer thereafter. **b** If the outer screws are applied first, the near cortex opens because the plate is too long in relation to the bone spanned between the outer screw holes

included different aspects of plate screw positioning.

When comparing the effects of prebending and lag screws, Claudi et al. (1979) and Regazzoni (1982) observed that prebending is superior for small bones and for porous bones, while lag screw compression is superior in large and dense bones. A further advantage of prebending is that it tolerates incidences of overload. After overload, the prebent plate returns to normal function, whereas the screw threads are irreversibly stripped.

Tension Band Fixation. Tension band fixation (Fig. 1.22) relies upon compression produced by the dynamic component of the functional load. The classic example of a tension band consists of a wire

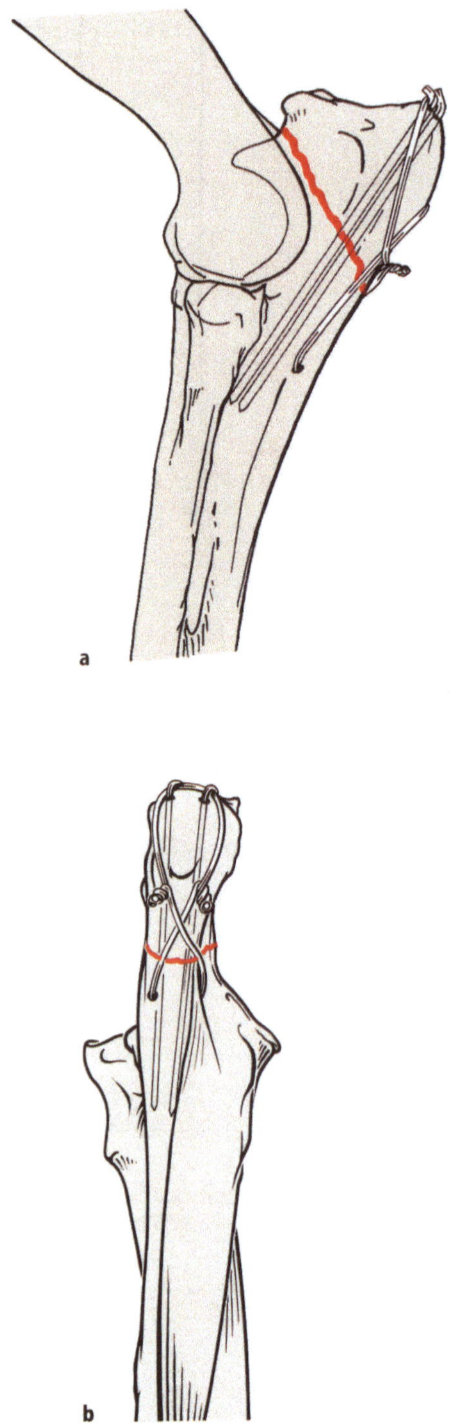

Fig. 1.22a,b. Tension band: dynamic compression used for stabilization. The wire provides the tension band effect directly countering tension loads applied to the bone by muscle pull or weight bearing. **a** Countering tension loads creates compression loads along the fracture line. **b** If tension loads are not countered, the fracture would be distracted

applied to the caudal surface of a fractured olecranon. This wire, together with the supporting condyles, transforms the tension applied by the triceps muscle into dynamic compression acting at the fracture.

The tension band allows for some load-induced movement. Such fixation is often used at the metaphyses, where cancellous bone is less affected by small amounts of instability and reacts faster than is the case for cortical bone of the diaphysis.

Comparison of Compression by Screw and Plate. A cortical bone screw tightened by the average surgeon produces around 3 kN of compressive force. A plate used for axial compression results in about 0.6 kN. The compression produced by the screw is not only large, it also acts from within the fracture surface and results in more or less even compression of the fracture surface. The compression exerted by a straight plate contoured to fit the bone surface in turn acts asymmetrically from outside the fracture surface. The resulting compression is high near the plate (where it may even exceed the strength of bone; Rahn et al. 1971) and low within the fracture surface in the far cortex. The fracture gap may open in the cortex opposite to the plate. The asymmetric effect of the plate may be offset by prebending it (Bagby and James 1957). Prebending, however, is only efficient if the plate is not too soft.

1.3.1.6 Mechanics of Interfaces

In fracture treatment by internal fixation, contact zones are established between bone and bone and between bone and implants. The bone reaction at these interfaces depends upon mechanical conditions, which therefore play a determining role in the outcome of the healing process. The mechanical condition of the interface has two facets: one is the load transmitted, and the other is deformation of the tissue between the bone fragments.

Deformation of repair tissues results in a relatively large displacement of the fracture fragments if the tissues between the fragments are soft. To describe the mechanical condition of relative displacement at the fracture gap, the term "stability" is used. More or less stability is synonymous with less or more relative displacement, which describes different grades of relative stability. When the fracture surfaces are adapted and compressed, the immediate contact surfaces do not displace. This is known as "absolute stability."

Unstable Interface. A bone placed under (repeated) dynamic load deforms cyclically, a behavior which is explained by the spring-like characteristic of the bone (Fig. 1.23). This deformation has been used experimentally in vivo to produce displacement between a plate and bone so that the effect of instability can be studied. A screw (or bolt) inserted at the free plate end is subjected to periodic unloading, while the other end of the plate is rigidly fixed to the bone by two screws under high common preload. This results in intermittent minimal displacements at the contact surface between the unloaded screw (or bolt) and the bone cortex.

Two observations appear to be noteworthy:

1. Investigating the hypothesis that interface instability induces bone resorption, Ganz et al. (1975) produced conditions of minute amounts of instability between a screw and the threaded hole within the bone. Their method consisted of the fixation of an instrumented plate to a functionally loaded bone, whereby only one end of the plate was fixed by inserting screws tightly. The other plate end was left "free" by inserting the experimental screw with only a small amount of torque in order to maintain the correct position rather than to use it for fixation of the plate to the bone. Functional compressive loading shortens the plated bone segment by less than 10 μm. This displacement results in inclination of a screw which is not tightly driven into bone. Figure 1.24 illustrates a simplified version of the same experiment (J. Brennwald, personal communication, 1976), in which a short fixed bolt was used instead of the tilting screw. The displacement and the resulting bone resorption are displayed. Initial minute instability led to secondary massive instability, in both experimental models, due to bone resorption.
2. Stadler et al. (1982) used a hydraulically operated plunger to study bone surface reaction to high interface strain (Fig. 1.24). High interface strain produced by the plunger hitting the bone surface intermittently led to bone surface resorption, while low strain conditions – in which the plunger displaced the same amount, but at a distance to the bone surface – did not.

Thus initially small instability will, by the process of micromotion-induced bone surface resorption, lead to secondary gross instability.[12]

[12] The relationship between applied compression, resulting shortening, and effect of minimal resorption is visualized in Fig. 1.16. It can be seen that a load of 1000 N results in about 10 μm shortening of the compressed segment. Minimal surface resorption completely abolished the compression.

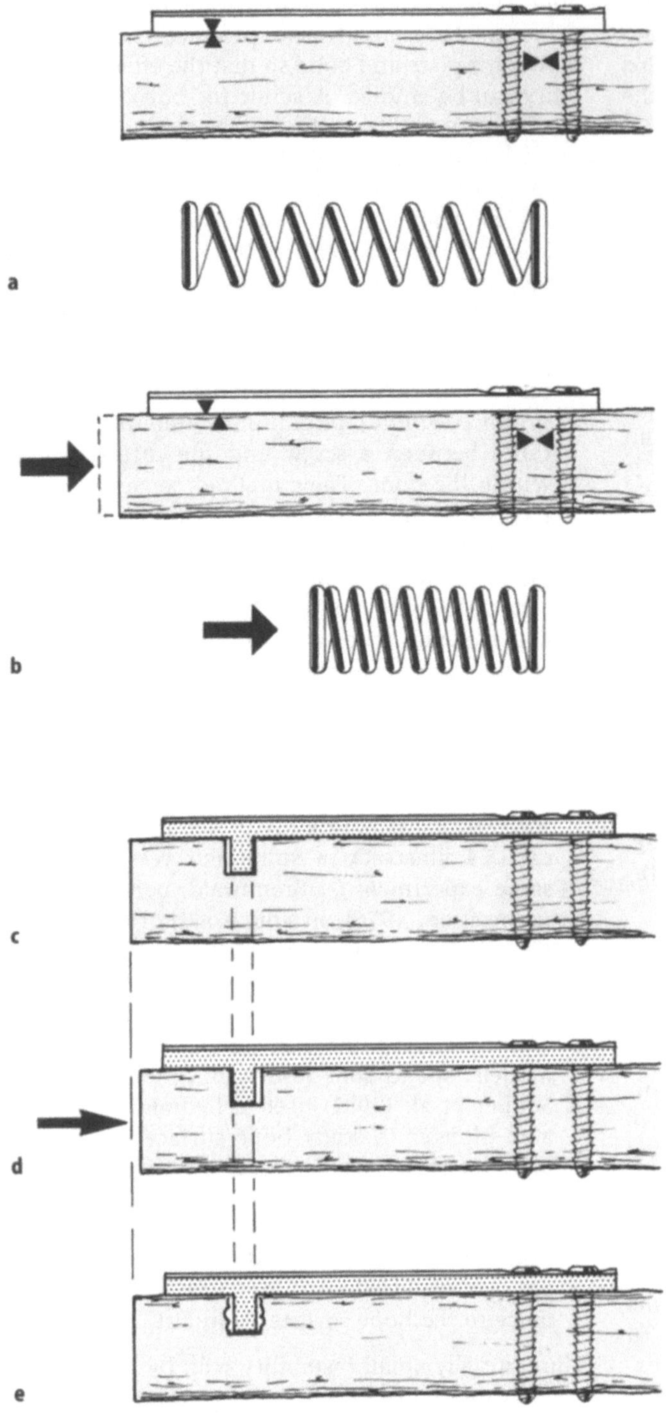

Fig. 1.23a–e. Method of producing instability in an experiment. To study the effect of controlled instability upon implant loosening by bone surface resorption, advantage was taken of the fact that bone shortens cyclically under weight-bearing during walking. Comparing bone with a stiff spring demonstrates how relative displacement can be brought about between the free end of a plate and the underlying bone. The displacement amounts only to a few micrometers. The plate is solidly fixed at the other end by two screws under high common preload. **a** Non-loaded and **b** loaded situations of a plate fixed only at one end to the bone. Bone shortens under axial compression, and a relative displacement between the free end of the plate and the underlying bone results. **c** Initial situation without functional load; the unloaded bone has its original length. A small amount of compression preloads the inner surface of the cylinder to produce bone contact. **d** Situation with functional load; the loaded bone is now shorter. The small initial compression is unloaded, the inner surface opens temporarily, and the outer experiences intermittent contact. **e** Biological reaction to intermittent unloading and instability. In spite of the fact that the above-mentioned displacement amounts to only a few micrometers, bone surface resorption is initiated. Thus a small initial instability results in gross loosening due to the biological reaction

Mechanically Induced Pin Loosening in External Fixation. The pins used with external fixators often loosen at the pin–bone interface. Huiskes et al. (1985) felt that this was due to mechanical failure of bone due to local overload. While this may occur in metaphyseal bone, there is now good evidence that, in cortical bone, surface resorption induced by micromotion is much more common (see p. 37). Two methods to decrease micromotion have been used empirically in the past (F. Behrens 1982, personal communication; Behrens 1989):

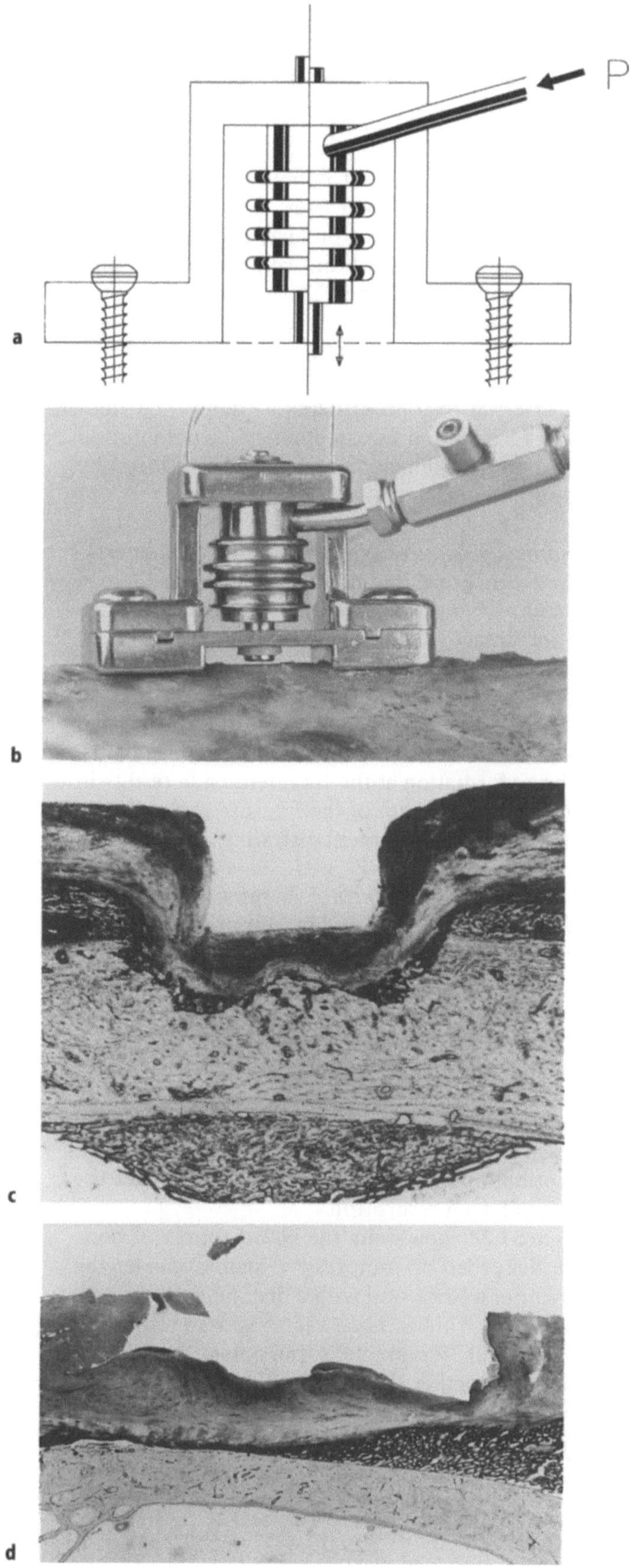

Fig. 1.24a–d. Experimental method used to study bone reaction at unstable interfaces (Stadler et al. 1982). **a** Hydraulically operated bellows with plunger mounted within a U-shaped jig. **b** X-ray showing the apparatus applied to the proximal metaphysis of the tibia. **c** Cross-section of the tibia; the histological section shows marked bone surface resorption in the vicinity of an intermittently contacting plunger surface. **d** Cross-section of the tibia; no resorption in the case of a plunger which cycled at a distance from the bone surface

1. The pins were prebent before they were fastened to the longitudinal rods (bending preload).
2. The size of the pin shaft was selected so that its diameter was larger than the drill hole (radial preload).

Experiments carried out by Hyldahl et al. (1988) (Figs. 1.25, 1.26) have cast doubts on the effectiveness of bending preload, but they have clearly demonstrated that radial preload can significantly reduce surface resorption compared to pins inserted without preload. They showed that the range of possible misfit between the borehole and pin diameter was much smaller than hitherto assumed (see p. 37).

In external fixation utilizing a frame - particularly in fusions and in osteotomies - micromotion of the parallel Steinmann pins can be reduced by bending the pins against each other.

Mechanically Induced Nonunion. Unstable interfaces between bone fragment ends may result in a mechanically induced nonunion even in the presence of intact biological reactions (reactive or hypertrophic nonunion; Weber and Cech 1973). In this case, the tissue differentiation from soft to more stiff tissues and the increase in cross-section are unable to reduce the mobility of the fragments. The bone formation at the fragment ends results in reduction in the width of the fracture gap and thus increases the interfragmental strain.

Stable, Compressed Interface. Screws submitted to bending and thus stabilized by compression (at the interface) were studied in the same experiment in which unstable interfaces were examined. Less bone surface resorption was observed. It is important to note that in this experiment, in spite of very high internal compressive stresses, the bone did not show resorption in the stable areas of contacting interface. Figure 1.27 explains the relationship between compression applied and fracture surface resorption: maintenance of compression proves the absence of such resorption.

Figure 1.28 shows why the blood supply of bone is not disturbed by compressive load. Consider the behavior of a brick wall with a drill hole through its thickness. A rubber hose carrying water through the hole will, for practical purposes, exhibit the same flow whether the brick wall is heavily loaded or not. The flow will change markedly when the brick wall collapses, but not before. The same holds true for blood vessels within the stable framework of hydroxyapatite.

1.3.2 Biological Reactions

Cellular function determines the reliability and quality of fracture healing. In fracture healing with preserved vascularity, this cellular function is primarily controlled by the mechanical environment. The elements of biological reaction to the mechanical environment are outlined in this section.

The mechanical environment is mainly determined by the forces acting on and the resulting deformation leading to displacement of fracture fragments. Two biomechanical events play a role:

1. Cellular function, which results in tissue formation, destruction, and differentiation, is controlled by mechanical input. Tissue deformation (strain) due to instability induces both callus formation and bone resorption at contacting interfaces, i.e., between bone fragments as well as between bone and implant. This resorption in turn results in increased instability of the fracture site. Intense staining of soft repair tissues may necessitate several stages of tissue differentiation, whereby soft tissues which tolerate deformation, e.g., granulation tissues, are replaced by a series of tissues, e.g., connective tissues, which are progressively stiffer and which tolerate less strain. This process is called indirect healing.
   If, on the other hand, small gaps are stabilized by contact surfaces nearby, and if such contact surfaces are maintained in close apposition by interfragmental compression, the gap and the contact surface provide low strain conditions. Under these conditions direct bone formation is possible, and both bone surface resorption and callus formation are absent. This type of healing is called direct healing (contact healing and gap healing). The surface of the contact zones is very small and corresponds to the compression applied multiplied by the strength of bone. The contact zone of a fracture therefore amounts to only a small fraction (a few percent) of the cross-sectional area.
2. Cellular function results in changes in the material properties, in the geometry of the fracture fragments, and in the (soft and hard) tissues connecting the fragments.[13]

[13] The changes in material properties affect the stiffness of the fracture linearly, while the changes in geometry may affect torsional and flexural stiffness in proportion to the cube of the diameter.

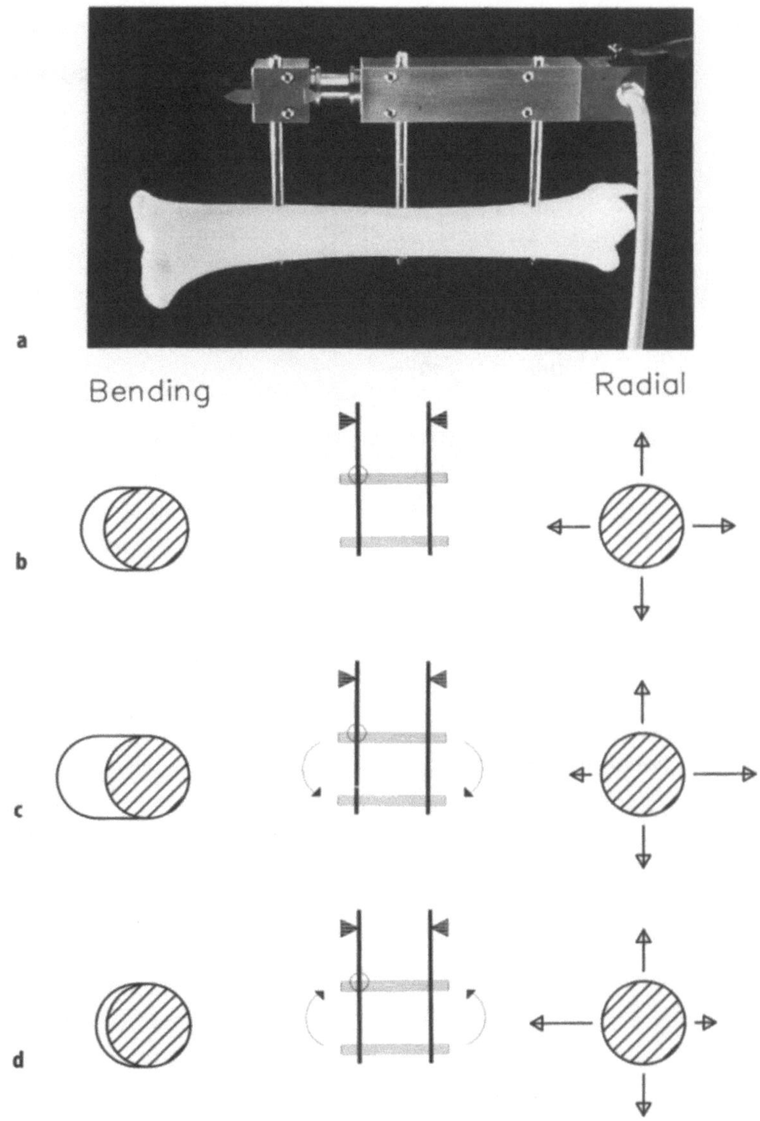

Fig. 1.25a–d. Effect of bending versus radial preload in pins of external fixators. **a** Pneumatically operated external fixator rod, which allows application of a cyclical bending load to the single pin at the right. **b–d** Cross-section of the near cortex. **b** Without additional load, bending produces a tight fit at the right side of the pin, while radial preload results in an equal amount of preload around the pin. **c** With an additional load pushing to the right, the bent pin increases the gap on the left, the radially preloaded one decreases somewhat the preload at the left without displacement. **d** With an additional load pushing to the left, the gap with the bent pin becomes smaller, and the radially preloaded pin does not show displacement

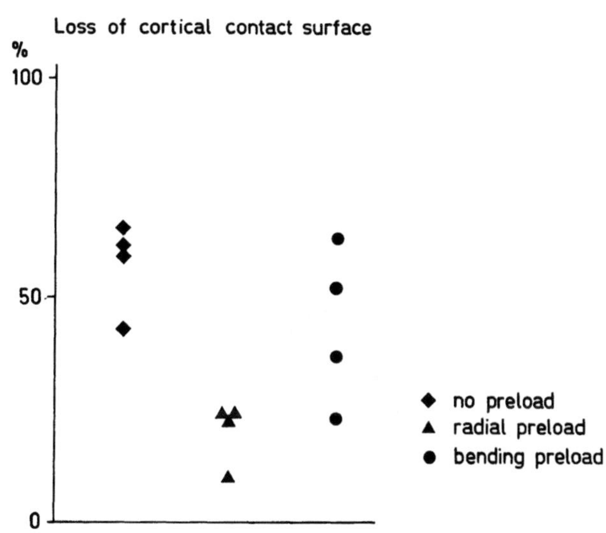

Fig. 1.26. Effect of radial preload of external fixator pins to prevent pin loosening: *Abscissa*, the three groups from left to right: no preload, radial preload, bending preload. *Ordinate*, loss of bone contact surface in percentage. Effect of different conditions of radial preload: *left*, exactly fitting pin with marked resorption of the contact surface; *middle*, slightly oversized pin with minimal resorption; *right*, bending preload was applied. It reduced somewhat, but did not prevent the resorption and loosening

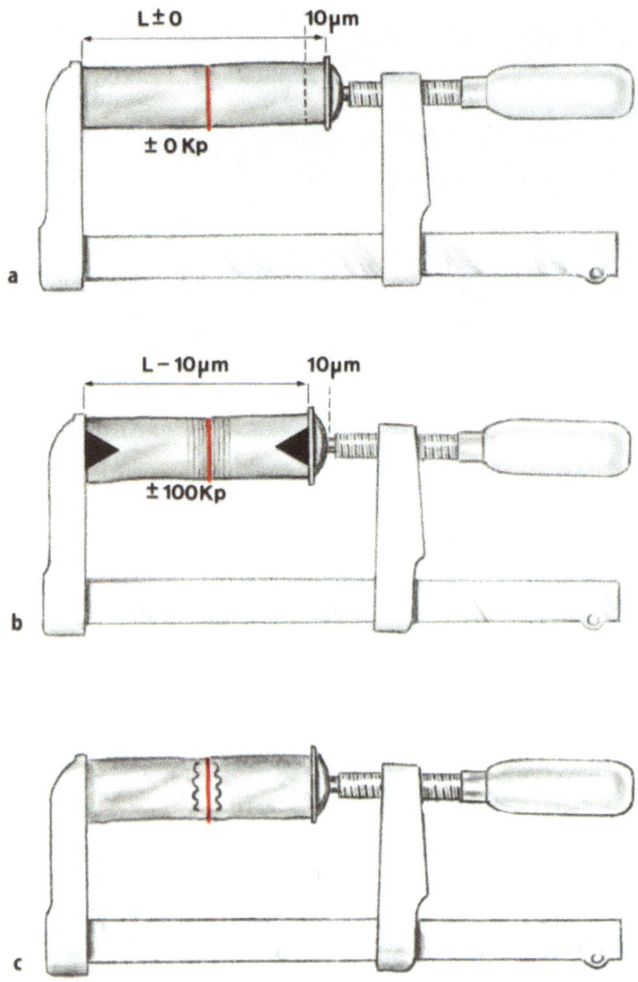

Fig. 1.27a–c. Effect of resorption at the compressed interface upon the amount of compression . **a** A bone segment within a C-clamp of original length *L*, no compression. **b** Deformation (shortening) of 10 µM results in a compression of 1000 N. **c** When the bone segment undergoes shortening of 10 µm due to fragment end resorption at the "fracture site," the compression is abolished

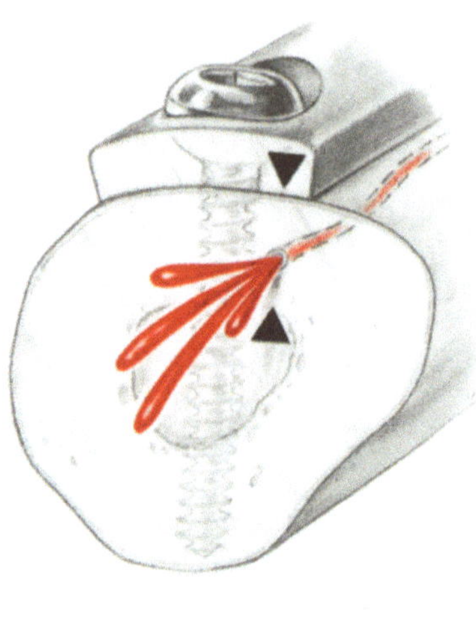

Fig. 1.28. Effect of compression upon blood flow within cortical bone. Large amounts of compression within the bone are well tolerated. However, even minimal compression of the soft tissues at the bone surface results in complete obliteration of periosteal blood supply

1.3.2.1 Stability and Compression

Compression, Behavior, and Effects. For decades, the clinical observation that soft tissues undergo pressure necrosis (pressure sores) when continually compressed led to the belief that bone also underwent pressure necrosis. The observed resorption of the vertebrae near a pulsating aortic aneurysm had been incorrectly explained as resulting from "pressure-induced necrosis." Instead of undergoing pressure necrosis, bone as a tissue is exceptionally well suited to function under mechanical load; its cells and blood vessels are protected by a stiff framework.

Compression by Plate. Using instrumented compression plates, Perren et al. (1969a,b) demonstrated that the static compression applied decreased only gradually over a period of several months (Figs. 1.29, 1.30).

Compression by Screws. The forces exerted by screws, as measured in simulated internal fixation by von Arx (1973), are larger (2–4 kN by screw compared to 0.6–1 kN by plate) and more efficient than the ones produced by "compression" plates. The use of instrumented washers implanted for an extended period of time (Blümlein et al. 1977) demonstrated the maintenance of very high forces applied to a relatively small area of living bone in the sheep (Fig. 1.31).

"Pressure Necrosis". In the experiments using instrumented plates and instrumented screws, the conditions were very sensitive to minute amounts of bone resorption at the compressed interfaces. Thus resorption of a one cell layer thickness of bone (approximately 10 μm) would have resulted in a prompt, noticeable loss of compression (Fig. 1.27). The absence of such reaction demonstrated the absence of induction of bone resorption even by excessive compressive forces. Nevertheless, the incidence of implant loosening, under conditions suggestive of initial instability, led to further studies of "pressure necrosis."

1.3.2.2 Biomechanics of Instability

The effect of instability on bone biology is apparent, especially at the bone surfaces (Fig. 1.32). Instability induces bone resorption, and this in turn increases the instability of fixation, either by plates or screws. Bone resorption induced by even minimal instability at the interfaces may therefore compromise the results of an internal fixation when techniques are applied which require the maintenance of absolute stability of fixation. Such techniques include screws and plates used for the treatment of simple diaphyseal fractures. In a rigid system, applied forces will result in minimal deformation; conversely, a minimal change in geometry (e.g., due to bone surface resorption) results in loss of applied compression.[14]

Induction of Bone Surface Resorption. Using the model of a plate bridging intact and functionally loaded living bone (Fig. 1.23), Perren et al. (1975) demonstrated the effect of relative and intermittent displacement between contacting surfaces of living

[14] The terms "rigidity" and "stability" are often confused. Stability is used here to define a state of absence of relative displacement between contacting surfaces ("bone to bone" or "bone to implant"). Stiffness or rigidity defines the relation between force applied and resulting deformation or displacement. The latter definition correctly implies that some degree of deformation or displacement always results under load in stiff or rigid internal fixation. The term "stable internal fixation" should therefore be used to express the absence of load-dependent displacement at the interface between fragment ends or between bone and implant.

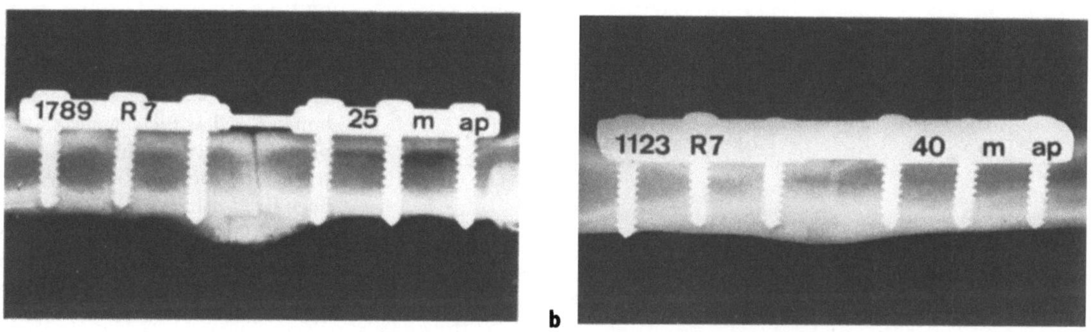

a b

Fig. 1.29a,b. Flexible fixation using plates (Hutzschenreuter et al. 1969). **a** A thin, flexible plate results in callus formation. **b** A thicker, more rigid plate results in smaller, better structured callus and no resorption of the fragment ends

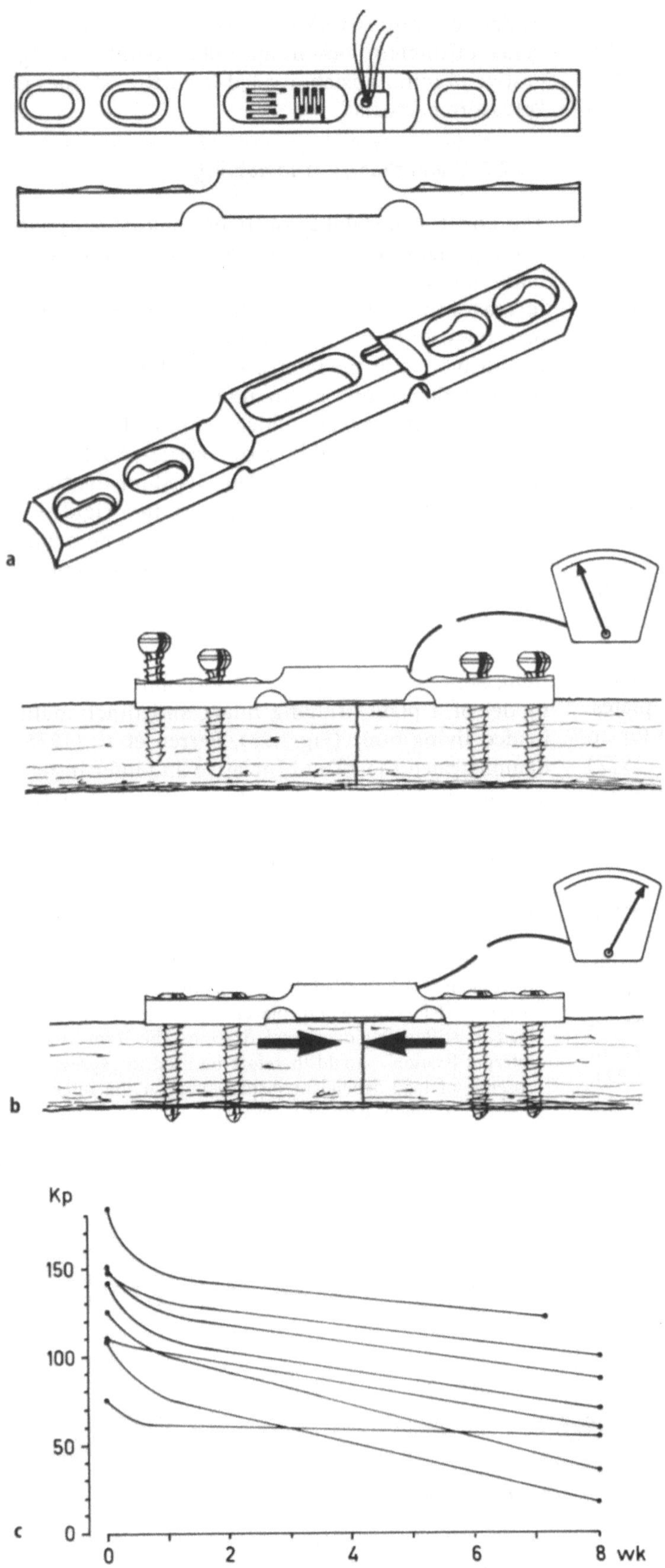

Fig. 1.30a–c. Measurement of plate compression in vivo (Perren et al. 1969a,b). **a** Instrumented plate. An internal fixation plate (dynamic compression plate, DCP) fitted with strain gauges and a wire connection. This plate allowed precise determination of the amount of compression applied to living bone as well as the changes in vivo. **b** Compression measurement in sheep tibia. A transverse osteotomy of a sheep tibia has been fixed using two DCP applied at right angles. (Only one of the two plates is shown here). **c** Compression applied to cortical bone in vivo. The initial value of compression of 1800 N force decreases very slowly. This pattern of change in compression proved that pressure necrosis with surface resorption in the compressed area did not occur

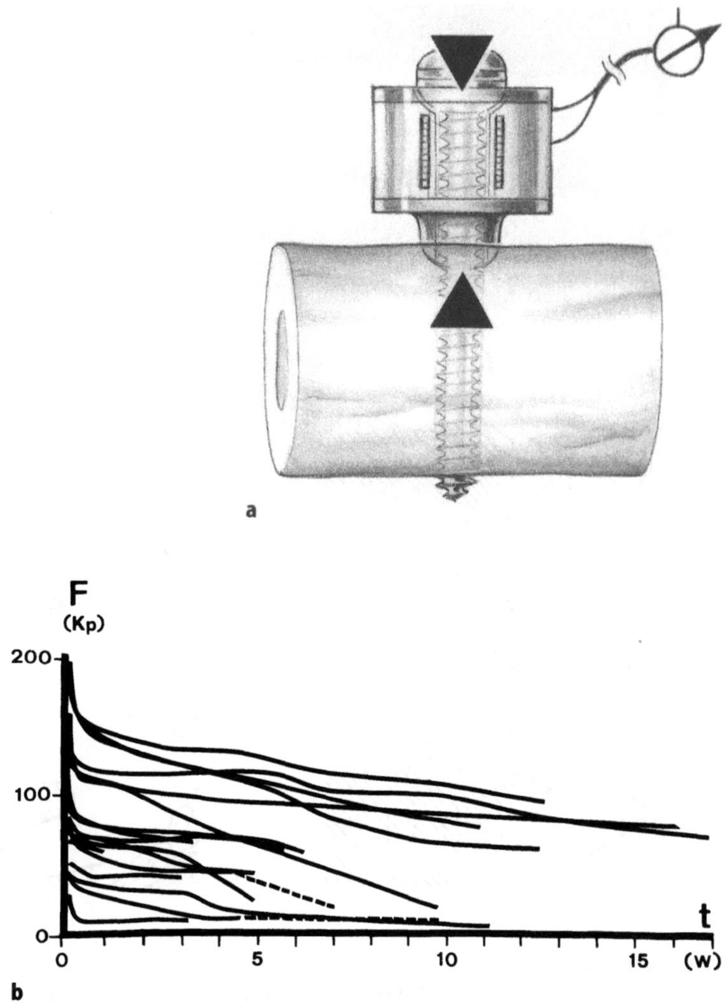

Fig. 1.31a,b. Measurement of screw compression in vivo (Blümlein et al. 1977). **a** Instrumented washer for in vivo measurement of screw compression. A washer is fitted with strain gauges and a transcutaneous wire connection. **b** Recording compression exerted by screws in vivo. Three different groups of initial compression and their changes in vivo are plotted. Over a period of 16 weeks, the compression regressed very slowly

cortical bone (Fig. 1.32). The induction of bone surface resorption was apparent with displacements in the range of less than one cell diameter (1–3 μm). Using hydraulically activated experimental implants in the sheep tibia, Stadler et al. (1982) induced surface resorption with a plunger intermittently contacting the bone surface, even with small forces.

Induction of Callus Formation. It is well known that mechanical irritation of living bone induces "callus" formation (as do other "irritating" factors). In the experiments by Stadler et al. (1982), callus formation was induced when the plunger cycled at a distance from the bone surface. Küntscher (1970) and later Danckwardt-Lilliestrom et al. (1972) demonstrated induction of periosteal callus formation when a corroding metal or plastic was inserted into the bone marrow cavity. Infection is also known to induce the formation of a "cloudy callus" under certain circumstances.

1.3.2.3 Biomechanics of Stability

As we will see when discussing direct or primary healing, compressed bone surfaces do not undergo surface resorption of the fragment ends. Avoidance of such surface resorption is of importance in preventing a "nongliding" implant, such as a plate and screw, from keeping fracture fragments apart and preventing spontaneous stabilization by interdigitation. The latter can occur if the fragments can slide together.

Another situation in which prevention of contact resorption is of importance is the interface between bone and pins of an external fixator. The effects of pin loosening may be:

1. Loss of stability, an effect which, in elastic fixation using external fixators, is not particularly important
2. Pin track infection, a relation that is evident, but not yet clearly proven

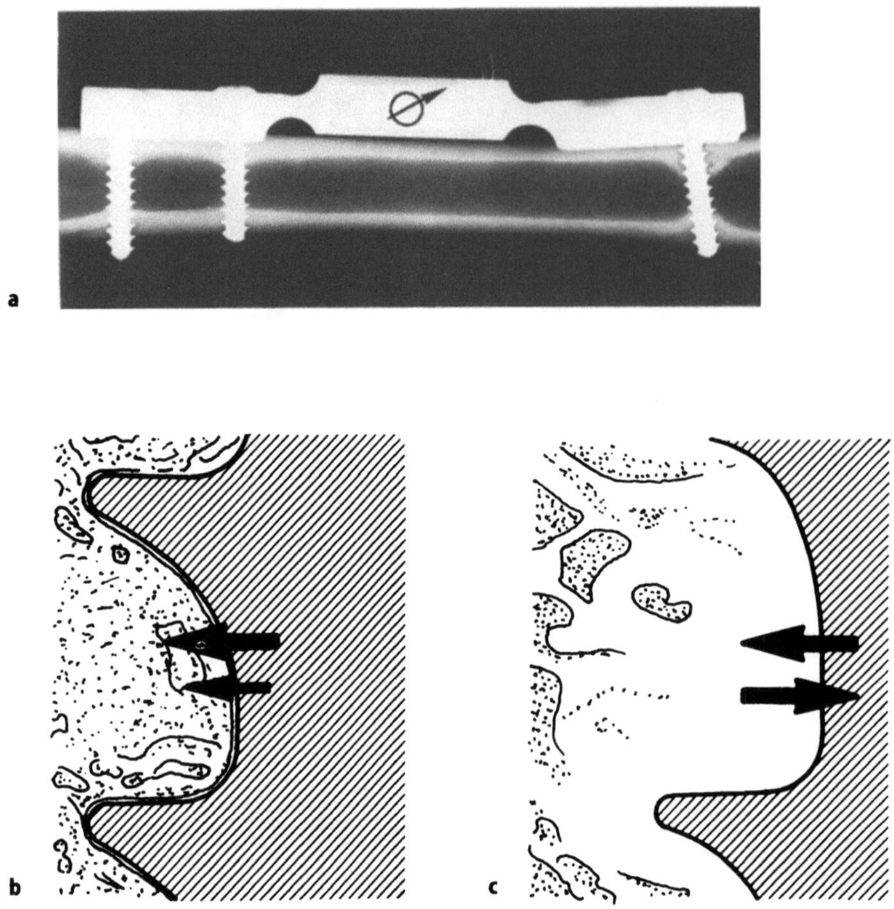

Fig. 1.32a–c. Induction of bone resorption in an experiment. **a** Model according to Fig. 1.23. **b** Stable interface: no resorption. **c** Unstable interface: biological loosening

1.3.2.4 Reaction to Changes in Physiological Loading

The theory that bone structure reacts mainly to changes in functional loading is one of the most widely accepted and unfortunately most often misused theories. Bone adaptation to changes in load according to Wolff's law (Wolff 1893, 1986) applies primarily to cancellous bone; adaptation is slow and less important in cortical bone. In conventional internal fixation using plates, which transmit forces by friction, the unloading of the bone due to the implant is of a temporary nature.

The biological reactions of bone and of hard and soft repair tissues to mechanical influences have recently been studied by Goodship and Kenwright (1985) and Lanyon and Rubin (1985). In fracture healing, the reaction of the cortical bone to mechanical load probably plays a lesser role.

Reaction to Unloading by Implants. Many authors have studied the reaction of cortical bone to unloading by implants, and the mechanical effects of stress shielding are impressive. The cortical bone near a plate, for example, is unloaded. Depending upon the type of load applied, the opposite cortical bone is loaded either less or more than normal (Cochran 1969; Woo et al. 1976; Claes et al. 1982; Cordey et al. 1987; Gautier 1988).

While mechanical unloading has been indisputably demonstrated, and while bone changes are observed after internal fixation, the question remains of which structural changes are due exclusively to the change in mechanical load. To validate the hypothesis that the changes in bone structure seen after internal fixation using straight plates in cortical bone are irrefutably linked to unloading, a close relationship between the mechanical challenge and the structural changes would have to be demonstrated. The apparent paradox is explained by the fact that plates transmitting force mainly by friction based upon compression of the plate to the bone (e.g., the straight plates) lose their close coupling, and therefore their ability to contribute to general unloading, about 6 months after implantation (although they may still protect against peak load).

Reaction to Strain. Strain is defined as relative deformation (strain is the relative deformation by a given stress, or vice versa). The basic assumption of the strain theory is that a tissue cannot differentiate when strained beyond the limit of its tolerance to strain. Thus the relation of *momentary strain* to *tissue-specific strain tolerance* determines the potential for its differentiation. As Pauwels (1965, 1980) has pointed out, the differentiation in failed healing of a fracture does not follow a new direction, it is simply halted at a certain level. There is obviously a lower limit of strain (strain induction level) below which no differentiation is initiated, even though the strain level would be tolerated.

Strain Controlling Fracture Healing. Surgeons are often amazed by the fact that some fractures heal under gross instability, while others do not tolerate even invisible instability. The concept of strain (Perren and Cordey 1977, 1980) considers the deformation sustained by the individual cell. If the deformation present within the repair tissue exceeds the elongation which would lead to tissue (cell) disruption (elongation at rupture) of the next tissue to be developed, then differentiation comes to a halt. A tissue cannot exist under conditions of strain exceeding the elongation at which rupture occurs.

With a grasp of this concept of strain, i.e., deformation expressed independently of geometry (see p. 13), the surgeon can now understand why in some situations (e.g., spontaneous healing of complex fractures) marked instability is compatible with the development of solid union, while under other conditions (closely adapted, but not compressed fractures) even minute amounts of instability may not be compatible with solid union.

Reaction to Interface Conditions Grossly Exceeding the Strain Within the Bone. We have shown that radial preload is a very efficient tool in preventing intermittent displacement at the pin–bone interface. The question therefore arises as to how much misfit can be tolerated mechanically. Again, strain is the critical parameter that allows us to determine the mechanically optimal misfit, i.e., the most favorable relation between the size of the drill hole and the diameter of the pin.

Bilouris et al. (1989) have recently studied this question and have come up with the statement that, when using a 4.5-mm pin, a misfit of 0.1–0.2 mm is optimal; a misfit of more than 0.2 mm results in local mechanical breakdown of the bone at the interface. Instability and surface resorption and/or sequestration of a ring (ring sequestrum) may result. Both processes result in loss of optimal stability at the interface.

1.3.2.5 Disturbance of Blood Supply to Bone

Disturbance Due to Fracture. A fracture induces several different circulatory changes. It disrupts the longitudinal blood vessels, and the open ends of these blood vessels undergo thrombosis. Bone just deep to the fragment ends is no longer nourished and will become necrotic. The ensuing remodeling may lead to demarcation and formation of a sequestrum. Cavitation (see p. 6) at the time of fracture and displacement of the fracture fragments also add to the vascular trauma. In any case, the fracture results in disruption of the longitudinal blood supply within bone. A thin surface layer of bone nourished by diffusion is superimposed on a deeper band of nonperfused and hence necrotic bone.

Disturbance Due to Soft Tissue Trauma. Stripping of the periosteum results in damage to the periosteal blood supply, but particularly in damage to the nutrient artery. The latter is detrimental to the overall blood supply of bone. Stripping of the periosteum may occur due to displacement of the fracture fragments and/or as a result of inappropriate surgical procedures.

Disturbance Due to Implant Contact. Implant-to-bone contact invariably results in damage of the radial perfusion of bone (Fig. 1.33; Rhinelander and Wilson 1982). Gunst et al. (1979) demonstrated a correlation between the implant contact and the damage to blood supply using the method of Lüthi et al. (1982), which was developed to determine the implant (plate)-to-bone contact area.

1.3.2.6 Reaction to Disturbance of the Blood Supply

There are two consecutive effects of damage to the cortical bone blood supply: (1) necrosis and (2) remodeling (Fig. 1.33). Remodeling starts within the adjacent living bone and moves toward the necrotic bone, eventually leading to removal and replacement of the necrotic area.

The blood supply is first disrupted by displacement of the fracture fragments. It is also damaged by the cavitation phenomenon during fracture (see Fig. 1.2). Conservative treatment or open reduction may further compromise the blood supply. External splints may impede the blood supply because the soft tissues are not exercised. Internal splints, e.g., plates or nails, may hinder blood supply by their contact with bone, where they compress the blood vessels which enter or exit from bone (Fig. 1.33). From the experiments by Rhinelander (1978) and Ganz and Brennwald (1987), we know that, if the

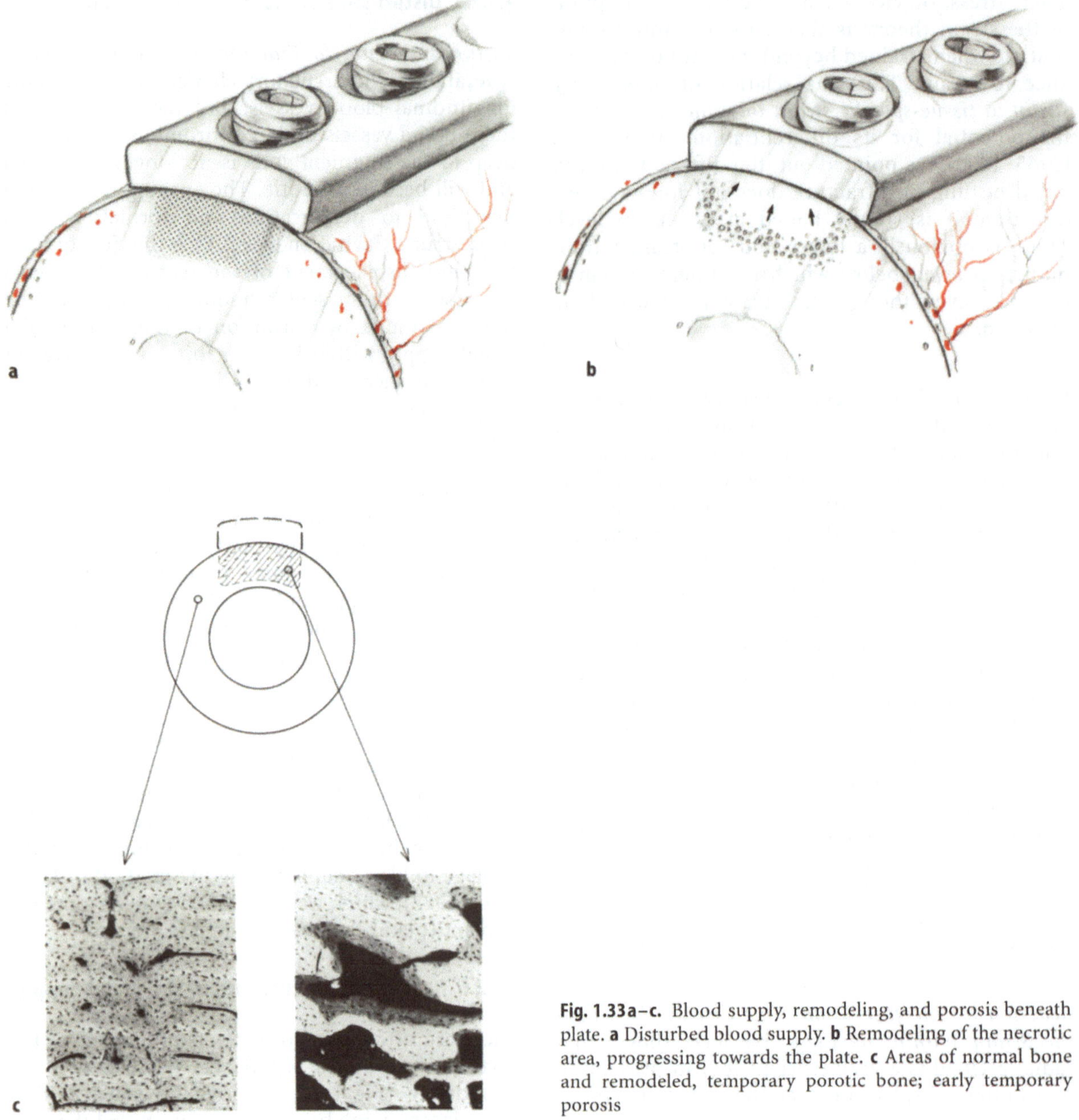

Fig. 1.33a–c. Blood supply, remodeling, and porosis beneath plate. **a** Disturbed blood supply. **b** Remodeling of the necrotic area, progressing towards the plate. **c** Areas of normal bone and remodeled, temporary porotic bone; early temporary porosis

fracture is stabilized, the medullary circulation may recover within 1–2 weeks. With regard to the blood supply, the surgeon must weigh the negative effects (surgical trauma) against the positive effects (faster recovery of blood supply) of different types of treatment.

Early Temporary Bone Loss Near Implants. Uhthoff and Dubuc (1971), Coutts et al. (1976), Moyen et al. (1978), and Matter et al. (1974) reported changes in the structure of long bones in the vicinity of the plate. The bone loss was explained on the basis of Wolff's law (Wolff 1893, 1986), which states that bone adapts its structure to mechanical loading conditions. The work of Woo et al. (1976) and Claes et al. (1980) seems to support the theory of "stress protection" of bone loss in plated bone. Tonino et al. (1976) and Tayton et al. (1982) proposed the use of soft plastic or carbon plates in order to minimize stress shielding.

Possible effects of static compression and tension applied to living cortical bone have been studied by

Matter et al. (1974). They found no statistical difference in the remodeling rate, despite the comparatively large amounts of static forces applied to the bone.

Based on recent experiments, three findings emerge:

1. Early temporary bone loss is seen in the vicinity of all implants, including intramedullary nails (Fig. 1.34) and external fixator pins (Pfister 1983).
2. Early temporary bone loss exhibits a close relationship to the vascular damage brought about by implantation and by the presence of the implant, i.e., implant-to-bone contact. The pattern of early temporary porosis does not show a correlation with any conceivable type of unloading (Gautier et al. 1986).
3. Plastic plates, which were softer than standard metal plates, showed more porosis, contrary to expectations based on the mechanical theory of stress protection (Gautier et al. 1986). Softer plates may adapt more snugly to the bone and result in increased vascular damage.

Early temporary bone loss disappears 3 months following surgery, and at 1 year the cross-section of the bone appears to be nonporous. Some authors have stated that the late changes in bone structure due to unloading by the implant may result in refractures (Kessler et al. 1988; Leu et al. 1989). Using quantitative computed tomography (CT), Cordey et al. (1985) studied the bone structure of the tibia after plate removal in a series of 70 patients. They observed only small changes in bone structure (less than 20 %) when density and geometry were used to calculate expected strength. At the time of plate removal, the plate is no longer rigidly pressed to the bone. Thus force transmission between bone and plate via friction is lost, and the plate induces unloading only at peak load.

Working on the hypothesis that implant-to-bone contact and the subsequent damage to blood supply is the cause of early bone loss, Jörger (1987) and Vattolo (1986) studied the immediate changes in blood supply (Fig. 1.35) and the bone loss under normal and special undercut plates 3 months following surgery (Fig. 1.36). The grooves reduced vascular damage and, as a corollary, also mitigated the bone porosis that accompanies haversian remodeling.

1.3.3 Bone Healing

Healing is defined as restoration of the original integrity. For surgeons, this means regaining the stiffness of the bone structure. For biologists, the microscopic restoration of the original structure may take years of internal remodeling.

A prerequisite for healing is an adequate biological capacity to react. Biomechanical conditions control the activity of the cells, with the mediators being of either a chemical or an electrical nature.

1.3.3.1 Basic Requirements

Fracture healing cannot proceed without adequate biological activity; living pluripotent cells must be available locally. These cells require a blood supply for nutrition and most likely for cellular support. It can safely be assumed that, given biological integrity, the cells surrounding a fracture are pluripotent and able to form bone. The critical parameter, therefore, is whether or not these cells are stimulated to repair the fragment ends with living, solid bone. Adequate blood supply to the repair tissues is crucial.

1.3.3.2 Type of Healing

With the onset of stable internal fixation, a new type of healing was observed. First, "healing by primary intention" (Lane 1913) and "soudure autogène" (Danis 1947, 1979) were observed radiologically, and then "primary bone healing" was observed histologically (Schenk and Willenegger 1963). The term "primary bone healing" is replaced in this paper with the term "direct bone healing" to avoid confusion and to avoid an implicit qualification. Direct healing is based upon the process of angiogenic bone formation (Krompecher and Kerner 1979). Different types of healing are outlined here because they have direct implications upon the rationale for various treatment modes.

1.3.3.3 Spontaneous (Indirect) Bone Healing

Spontaneous (indirect) bone healing consists of three elements (Fig. 1.37):

1. Granulation tissue forms first around the fragments and later between the fragments. This is the callus precursor.
2. The fracture gap then widens due to surface resorption of the fragment ends, i.e., when plates and screws are used for stabilization.
3. Bone formation progresses through a series of different steps from granulation tissue to cortical bone (indirect bone formation).

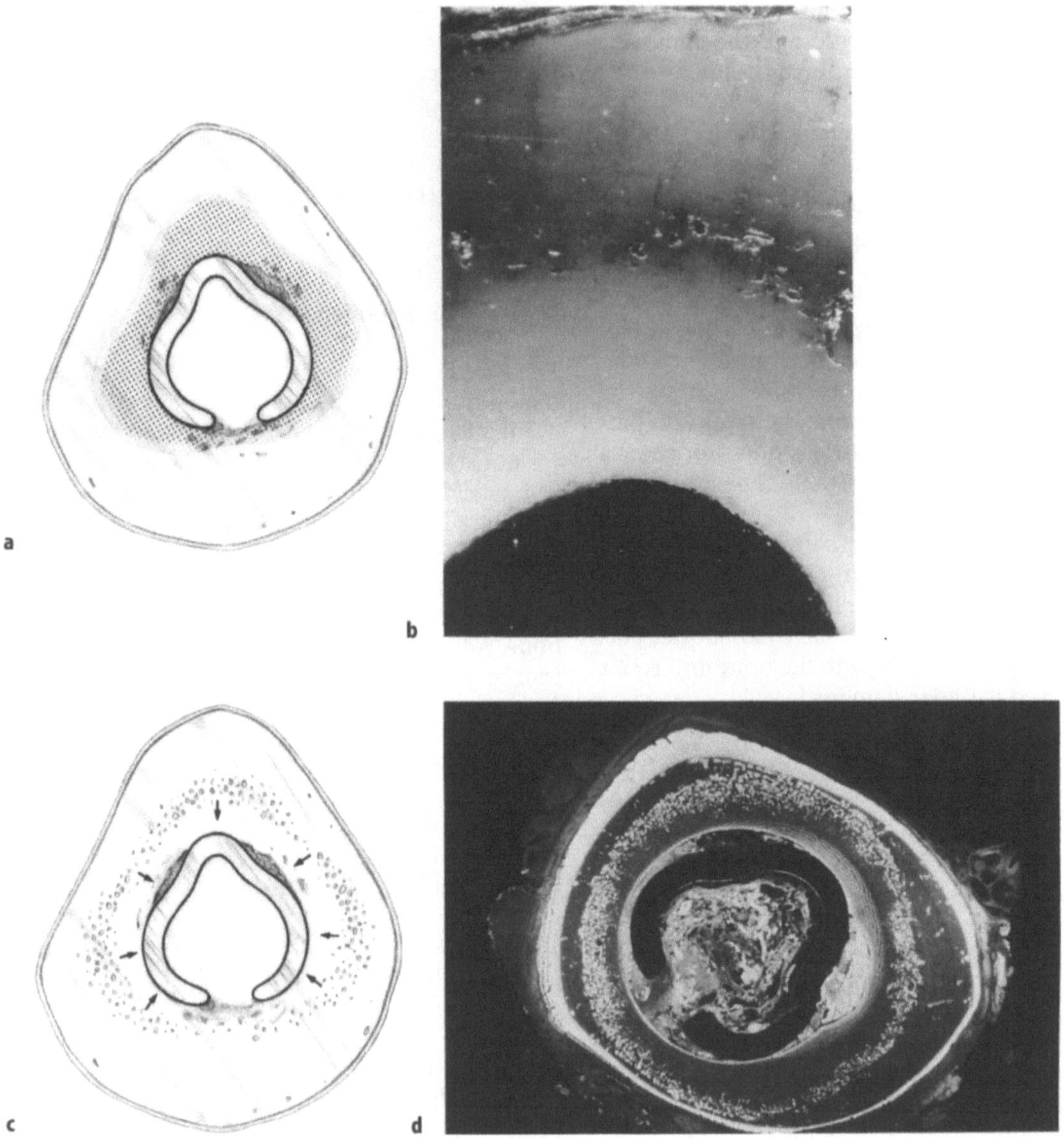

Fig. 1.34a–d. Blood supply, remodeling, and porosis around a nail in the tibia of a sheep. **a** Disturbed blood supply; circular area around nail. **b** Initial remodeling in the demarcation area between necrotic and live bone. Cross-section with disulfine intravital staining of blood supply at higher magnification. Within the demarcation zone, enlarged canals of the osteons are seen. These represent osteons in remodeling with temporary porosis. **c** Remodeling of the necrotic area progressing towards the nail. **d** The rate and direction of the remodeling process were determined using the polychrome sequential labeling method (Rahn et al. 1980).

Radiologically, the process of indirect bone healing is characterized by the appearance of callus, by the widening of the fracture gap, and by the filling of the fracture gap with newly formed bone, which is patchy in appearance at first and gradually acquires a more distinct and dense structure. The latter is achieved by a process of internal remodeling of the haversian system, which may last several years.

1.3.3.4 Direct (or Primary) Bone Healing

Direct bone healing bypasses the different steps outlined for indirect healing and proceeds directly to internal remodeling (Fig. 1.38) in contact zones (contact healing) (Fig. 1.38a) or to filling of stable gaps with lamellar bone and consequent remodeling or plugging (gap healing; Fig. 1.38b). The sur-

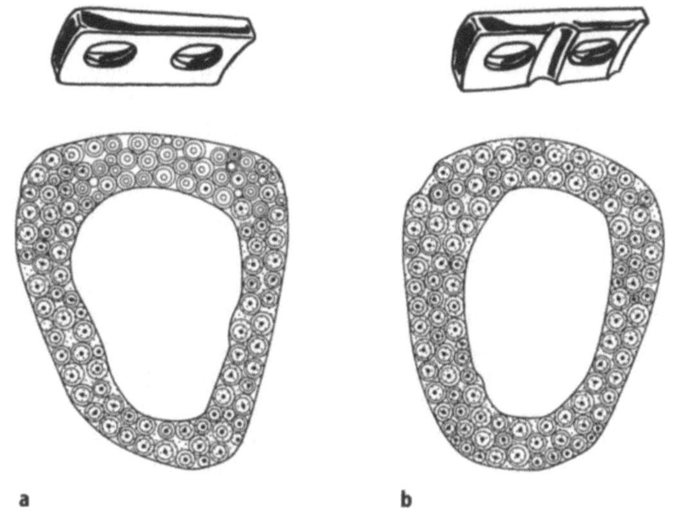

Fig. 1.35a,b. Vascular damage produced by different plates. **a** Plates with smooth undersurface and with grooves, as used by Jörger and Vattolo in their investigation designed to compare the changes in blood flow and in haversian remodeling. The grooves are located between the plate holes, where the conventional plate is excessively strong. **b** Using disulfine blue as a vital marker of blood supply, the cross-sections of the sheep tibias displayed a markedly better blood supply beneath a grooved plate

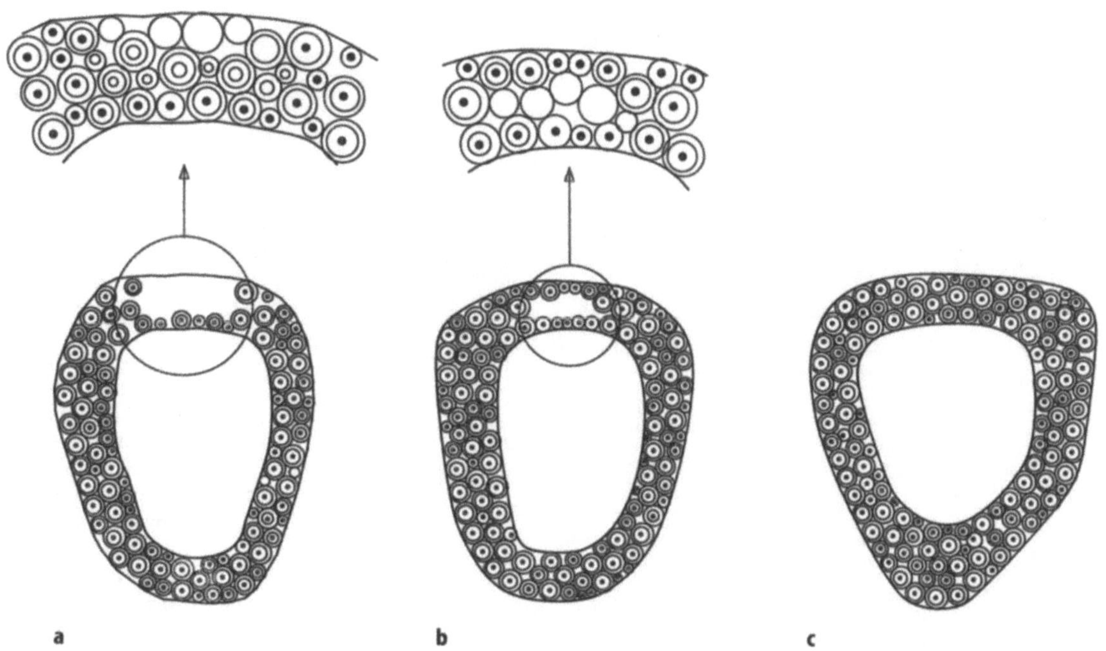

Fig. 1.36a–c. Vascular damage and consequent haversian remodeling. **a** At 12 weeks, a distinct difference in remodeling is seen. The bone is porotic beneath a conventional smooth plate. The porotic area, which in cases of high rates of remodeling may sequestrate, reaches the periosteal surface of the bone, where plate contact retards the revascularization. **b** With grooved plates, the porosis is much less pronounced and does not reach the surface of the bone plated. **c** There is literally no porosis if, under similar circumstances, a plate is applied as an internal fixator, i.e., at a distance from the bone surface

face of immediate contact within a fracture is directly related to the compression applied (Ashhurst 1986). It amounts in reality to only a small fraction (a few percent) of the total cross-section.

In direct healing, no relevant amount of callus, especially of callus which specifically bridges the fracture line, becomes visible radiologically. Fragment end resorption does not occur. The process of internal remodeling of the haversian system, uniting the fragment ends, is the only process resulting in solid union. Direct healing does not lead to faster union. The absence of fragment end resorption may be of utmost importance when nongliding splints are used. The radiological appearance of direct fracture healing is characterized by virtual absence of callus formation. The fracture gap does not truly widen, but may appear to do so due to intense remodeling near the fracture surface. Therefore, the surgeon is guided mainly by the absence of signs of complications, such as callus formation, which would indicate instability and fragment end resorption (shortening). Callus is not considered to be undesirable per se, but its appearance under conditions which require absence of fragment end shortening is a sign of a critical instability.

1.3.3.5 Nonunion

Bone healing may come to a stop (See Fig. 1.4) when one or both of the following elements are disturbed:

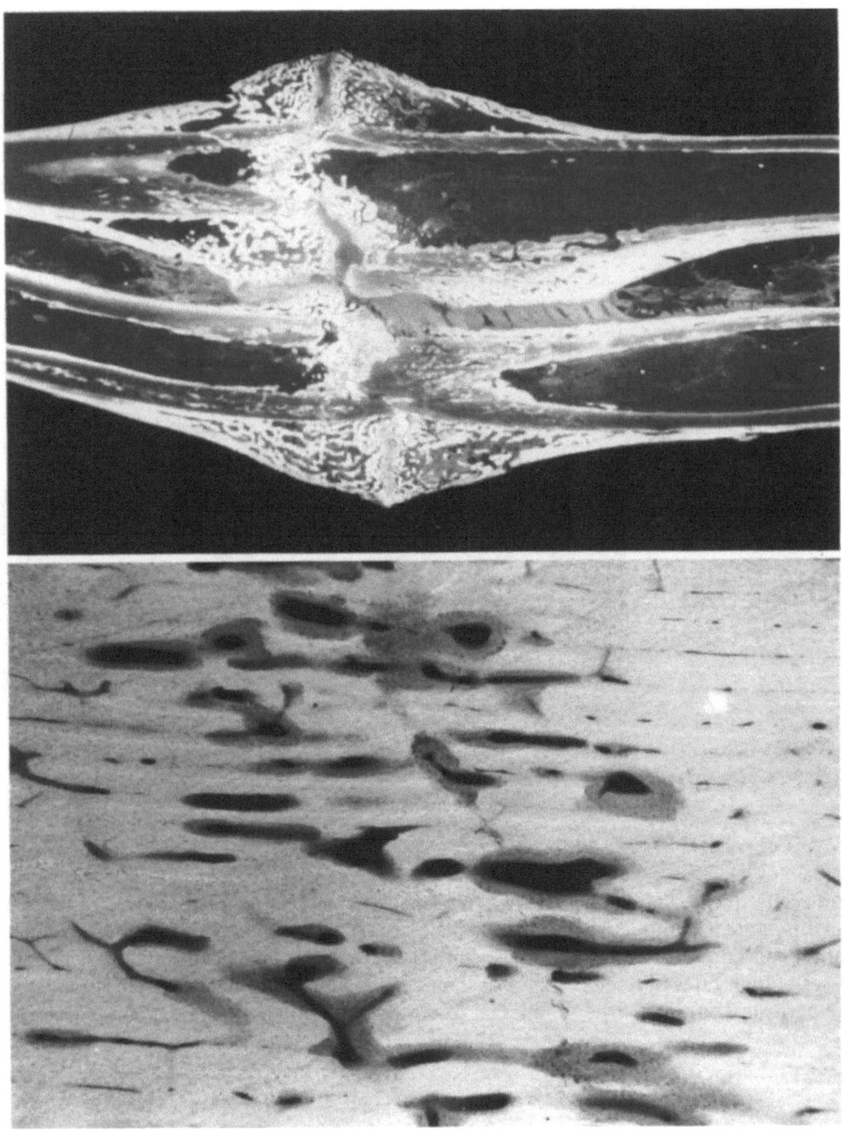

a

b

Fig. 1.37a,b. Healing pattern. **a** Spontaneous (or indirect) healing. Radiography of cortical bone following a transverse fracture without fixation. Abundant callus formation, bridging starts at the lower periosteal side in this figure (Rahn 1987). **b** Direct (or primary) healing. An oblique fracture fixed stably using a lag screw and plate healed by internal remodeling alone. The radiological picture and the histological section of such healing showed neither relevant periosteal nor endosteal callus formation specific to the fracture area. As can be seen in this histological picture, direct healing proceeds without resorption of the fragment end surfaces, i.e., contact healing. This figure shows an extremely precise adaptation achieved under experimental conditions. In reality, contact zones are comparably infrequent and therefore contribute little to the strength of healing

1. Mechanical conditions of strain
2. Capacity for biological reaction

In the first case, a hypertrophic nonunion is seen (Fig. 1.4a). Treatment (Fig. 1.4b) must then aim to correct the mechanical instability by using an internal splint. In the second case, a nonreactive or atrophic nonunion is present. Treatment here consists in inducing bone formation by applying a living bone graft as well as providing mechanical stability.

1.3.3.6 Relevance of Different Types of Healing

The different types of bone healing are of considerable scientific interest. The clinician in charge of fracture treatment may argue that the only goal of treatment is the solid union of a correctly reduced bone with maintained joint function (thus avoiding soft tissue complications). The important difference between direct and indirect healing is that direct healing does not proceed with fragment end shor-

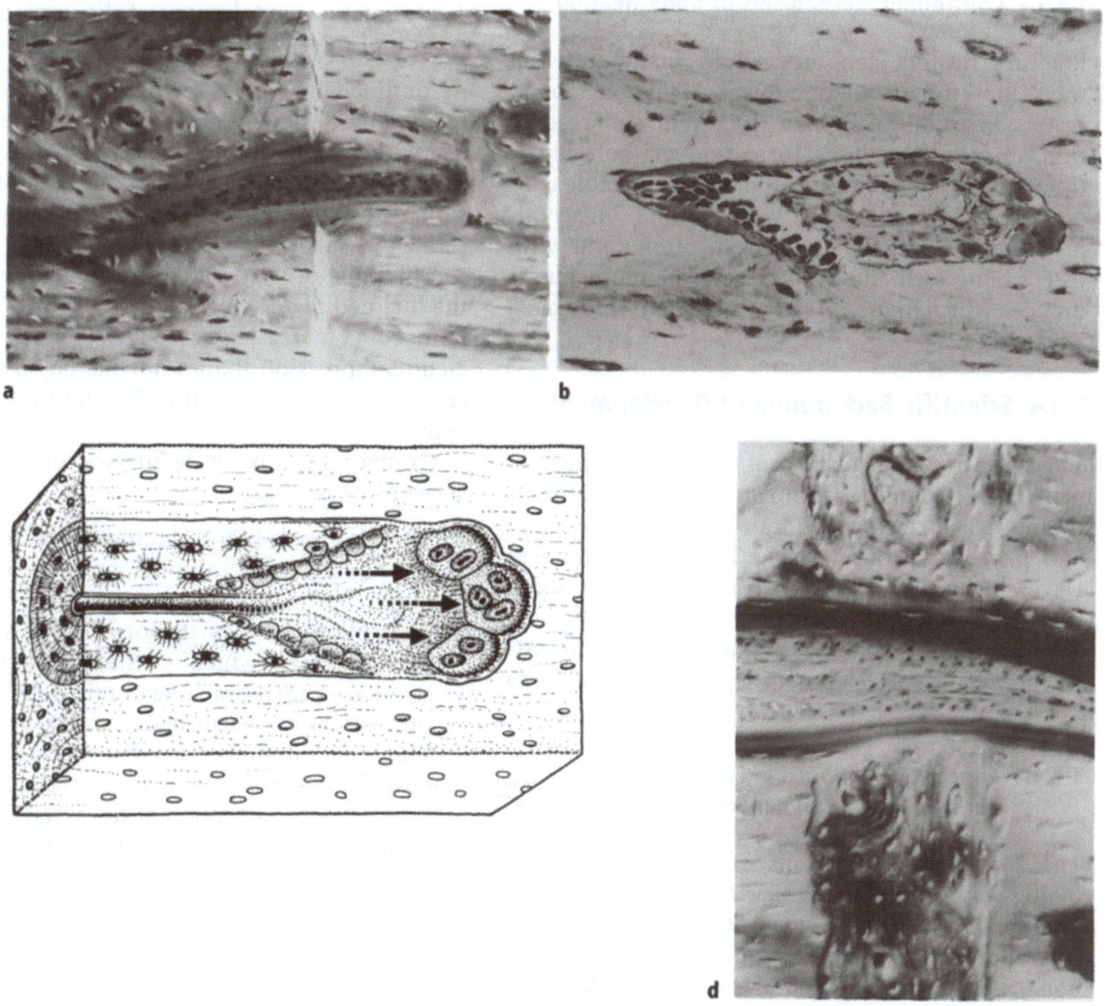

Fig. 1.38a–d. Elements of direct or primary bone healing. **a** Contact healing. The initial direct bone healing and final healing in all cases consist of remodeling of the haversian system. In the case of contact healing, this remodeling is essentially the only element upon which healing relies. The histological section shows the "cutter head" with osteoclasts and osteoblasts at a distance producing a new vascularized osteon (Perren and Cordey 1980). **b** Histological appearance of an osteon tunneling the bone from left to right (Rahn and Perren 1975). **c** The cutter head at the right tip with osteoclasts and the conical surface with osteoblasts towards the left is visualized (Perren and Cordey 1980). **d** Gap healing. Under stable conditions (due to nearby contact), a gap fills directly with mature bone of similar structure, but whose orientation is different to that of the original lamellar bone. This bone is later remodeled to a structure and orientation similar to lamellar bone, i.e., gap healing. The next step in this process consists of internal remodeling through the gap and/or from the gap into the cortex (plugging) (Perren and Cordey 1980)

tening. Such shortening can easily be taken up by a gliding splint, such as the intramedullary nail. Fixation by intramedullary nailing does not require absolute stability. Compression fixation of single fractures by lag screws in combination with a neutralization plate does not tolerate even minimal instability. The type of plate used in the bridge or wave mode ("biological fixation," see p. 4) with preservation of the fragment blood supply neither provides nor requires absolute interfragmental stability and greatly extends the indication for plate fixation.

1.3.3.7 Controlling Mechanisms of Bone Healing

Fracture healing can proceed in many different ways. It is now well documented that instability results in callus formation, fragment end resorption, and indirect bone formation via soft repair tissues. Under conditions of maintained stable contact, bone heals internally with minimal or no callus, without fragment end resorption, and with direct bone formation. The fracture circumstances dictate which type of healing offers the most advantages.

1.3.4 Scientific Background of Development

The specific characteristic of the development of principles, techniques, implants, and instruments by the AO is close collaboration between research and practical surgical work. The AO Institute in Davos (Switzerland), the central research facility of the AO, has recently contributed to the following developments. Similar developments from other AO research and development groups are equally important.

1.3.4.1 Concept of Biological Plating: Limited-Contact Dynamic Compression Plate

The scientific observations of biomechanics and biology of bone led to the new concept of biological plating. The newly designed LC-DCP stands for a new approach to plate fixation: reduced trauma to bone, preservation of blood supply, avoidance of producing stress risers at implant removal, and excellent tissue tolerance were the goals to be realized. The LC-DCP is technically a further development of the DCP (Perren et al. 1969c). It is based mainly on the experimental work of Klaue (1982) and Klaue and Perren (1982), who developed its predecessor, the dynamic compression unit (DCU). In the DCU, the lag screws applied through the plate are about twice as efficient as the conventional inclined lag screws. The symmetrical, self-compressing plate hole and the deletion of the elongated distance between the innermost screw holes make the DCU more versatile for use in any fracture type, disregarding the hitherto "standard" transverse osteotomy in cortical bone rarely treated by plating (Fig. 1.39).

The new concept aims at:

1. Minimal surgical damage to blood supply
2. Improved healing in the critical zone covered by the plate
3. Minimal damage to the bone lining the plate to reduce the risk of refracture following plate removal
4. Optimal tissue tolerance of the implant by selection of pure titanium as an implant material

As outlined in Fig. 1.40, when using a shaft screw (originally designed as an inclined plate screw for use with the DCU or LC-DCP) to replace the fully threaded inclined lag screw, about 50 % of compression – lost due to wedging of the fully threaded screw – is salvaged.

This type of shaft screw, originally designed for the inclined plate screw in the DCU or LC-DCP, can be used as a free lag screw. It provides more efficient compression than a normal lag screw. Again, secondary wedging within the gliding hole is prevented.

Grooves on the undersurface of the LC-DCP serve three purposes:

1. They improve blood circulation by minimizing the damage due to contact between plate and bone.
2. They allow for a small bone bridge beneath the plate at a place which is otherwise weak due to a stress concentration effect of the nonhealed fracture gap at the periosteal surface.
3. They result in more even distribution of the stiffness of the plate than in conventional plates, where the cross-section at the screw holes is softer and weaker, while the full rectangular cross-section between the screw holes is markedly stiffer, i.e., more resistant to bending and torque. The difference in stiffness results in a relatively increased load within the weak spot at the screw holes.

The healing pattern of bone plated with the LC-DCP displays a more abundant bone formation with a circumferential shell of mature callus bone (Fig. 1.41), especially around the fracture site. The fracture gap exhibits a band of remodeling and not fracture surface resorption (which could lead to breakdown of stability). The contact of the plate with the bone is limited, and the plate-induced remodeling is small. The bone porosis induced by the LC-DCP ranges between the extremes shown in

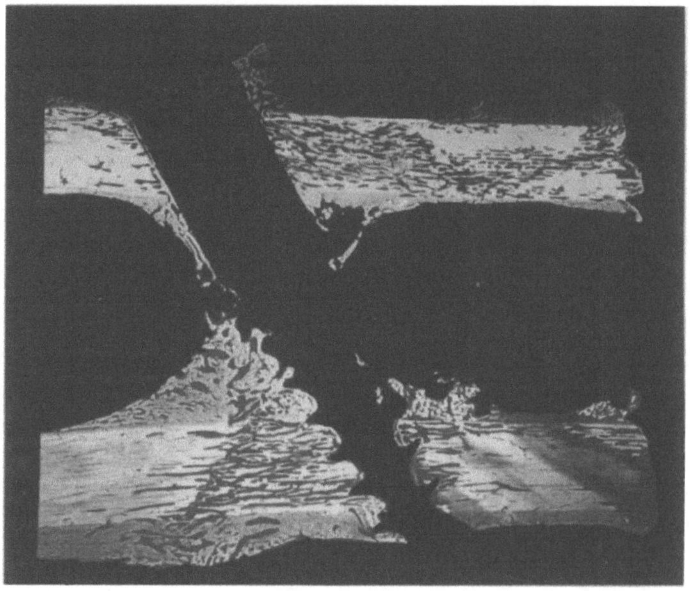

Fig. 1.39. Histological appearance of bone healing with the dynamic compression unit (DCU). Sheep tibia 56 days after surgery (Klaue et al. 1985). Intensive remodeling of the oblique osteotomy is seen mainly as a band lining the osteotomy (*area A*). Little remodeling is seen immediately deep to the plate with smooth undersurface (*area B*). Where the shaft of the screw is in direct contact (*area C*), intensive remodeling is observed. Where the shaft of the screw does not touch the clearance hole (*area D*), minimal remodeling is seen. In the contact area around the thread of the lag screw (*area E*), intensive remodeling is visible. Though the overall pattern of remodeling is "patchy," it best correlates with local conditions of blood supply. It is noteworthy that the band of remodeling providing healing is obviously related to temporary loss and recovery of blood supply rather than to changes of mechanical load or to an unknown signal radiating from the fracture site. Direct or primary healing therefore seems to be a byproduct rather than a direct biological response to the fracture

Fig. 1.36a (conventional plate, smooth undersurface) and Fig. 1.36c (plate does not touch bone at all).

A larger screw hole apparently remains after removal of the shaft screw. However, one should consider that the outer diameter of the hole with a fully threaded screw is the same as that with a shaft screw. The fully threaded screw, however, allows for filling in of the threads. The mechanical difference with respect to the strength of the bone is negligible.

The radiograph of a diaphysis plated with a conventional plate with a smooth undersurface (Fig. 1.42e) illustrates the problem: at the periosteal surface, facing the undersurface of the plate, the fracture gap shows a small defect. Since, whenever possible, the plate is placed at the tension side of the bone for best resistance to fatigue failure and for best stabilization according to the tension band principle, this defect is at the worst possible place, when considering plate removal. The photoelastic model of a beam under bending load with the defect at the tension side is shown in Fig. 1.42 g, the harmful stress concentration is disclosed. The difference in healing resulting from the experimental application of an LC-DCP is shown in Fig. 1.41.

1.3.4.2 Distraction Osteogenesis

Bone defects resulting from infected nonunions, for example, require prolonged treatment with bone grafting in most cases. The most efficient way to produce bone would be autologous grafting with optimal vascular support and soft tissue connection. Bone segment transportation according to Ilizarov (1989) ideally fulfills these requirements. In one or both fragments adjacent to a defect, an osteotomy is performed. The resulting bone segment is then transported (1 mm/day) along the long axis of the bone to close the defect. The newly formed gap behind the segment fills with bone. Once the transported segment has closed the defect, it unites readily with the opposite fragment. This type of autologous local bone grafting has gained wide acceptance for the treatment of very serious cases. Similarly, malformations and malalignment may be treated by bone lengthening and correction.

Ilizarov has achieved, in a clinically reliable and reproducible way, what Kirschner (1916), Bier (1918), Putti (1918), and Anderson (1936) before him demonstrated, but for which they could find no wide application. While Ilizarov's ingenious method is performed with an apparatus that allows

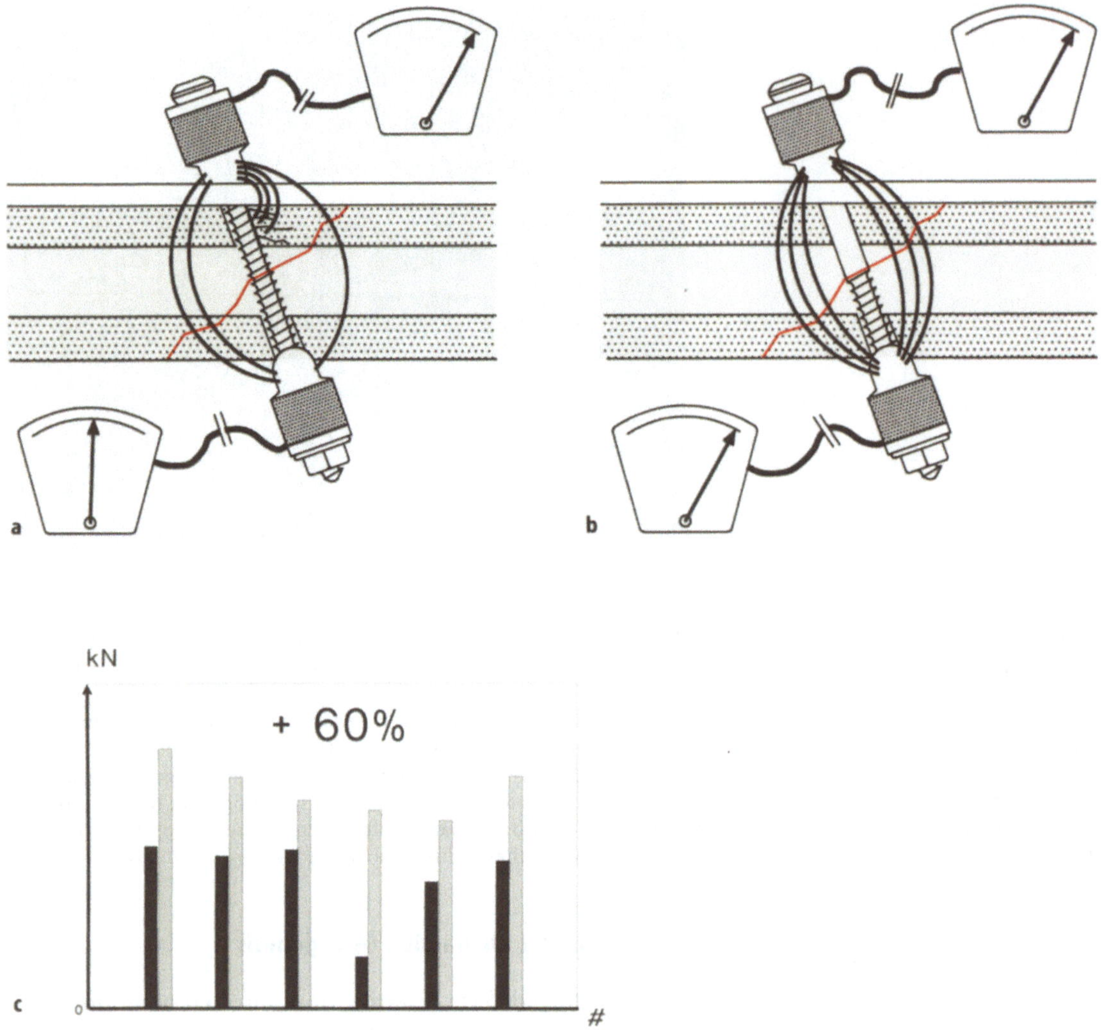

Fig. 1.40a–c. Klaue's experiment demonstrating the loss and recovery of lag screw compression. **a** When a conventional fully threaded lag screw (i.e., a screw within a gliding hole) is applied in an inclined position, wedging of the threads within the gliding hole occurs and a considerable part (more than 50%) of the potential compression is lost. **b** Using a shaft screw with a shaft diameter corresponding to the outer diameter of the screw thread, wedging is avoided and optimal compression achieved. **c** Measured values of interfragmental compression exerted by the two different types of screws. The *black bars* correspond to **a**, the *hatched bars* to **b.** The new shaft screw is 60% more efficient than the fully threaded inclined lag screw

for easy three-dimensional corrections, the requirement of multiple transfixing wires, the comparatively large rings, and the long duration of fixation has led others to study the feasibility of bone transportation with simpler devices that are more able to meet the higher expectations of today's patients. Rüter and Brutscher (1988) have established the clinical usefulness of a device which allows for transportation without transfixing wires. Their procedure completely avoids cutting of the wires through soft tissues. Regazzoni (1989) has recently demonstrated the use of the AO unilateral external fixator supplemented with a simple nut for transportation along the conventional AO spindle.

Rüter and Brutscher (1988) studied the use of wires applied along the bone in animal experiments utilizing full osteotomies and corticotomies. Figure 1.43 shows the result in sheep. Transportation was reliably achieved. Once the transported fragment closed the defect, solid union occurred without further internal fixation. Long-lasting fixation using transcutanously connected external devices was felt to be in need of improvement. Brunner et al. (1990a,b) devised a method of transportation

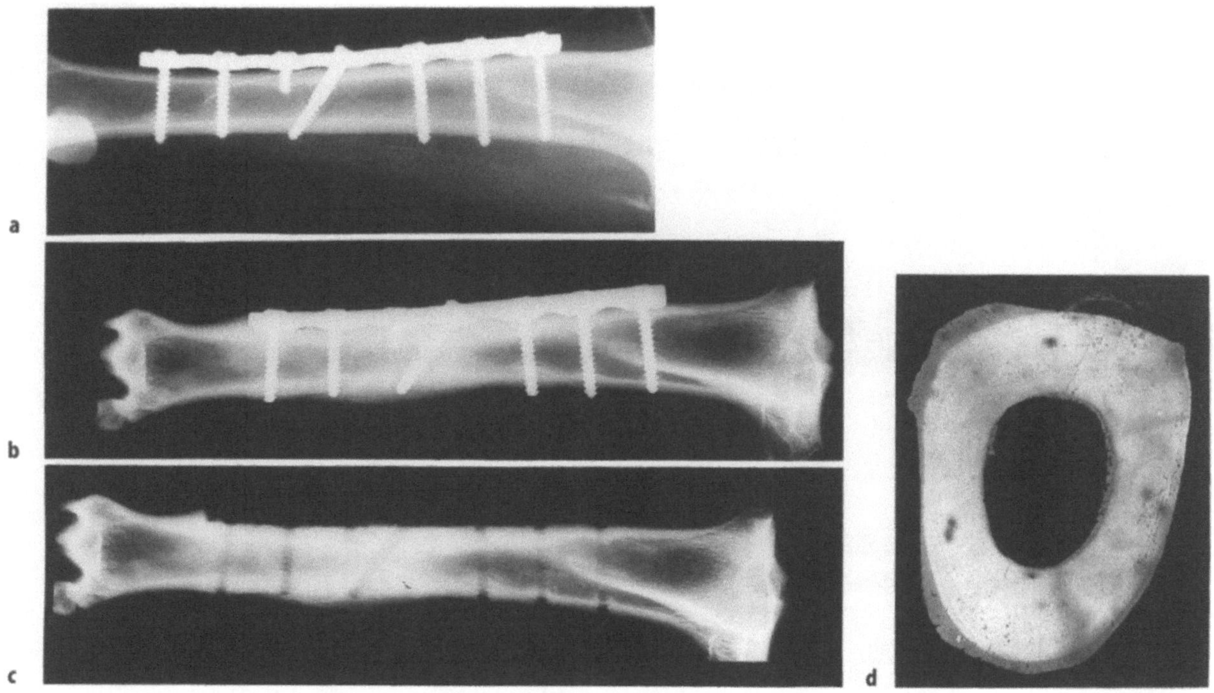

Fig. 1.41a–d. Bone healing and minimal early temporary porosis with the limited-contact dynamic compression plate (LC-DCP). **a** Fracture of sheep tibia plated with LC-DCP. An oblique shaft screw and a nearby single cortex plate screw were used. **b** Three months after the operation: clinical X-ray before the animal was killed. **c** Three months after the operation: X-ray of the dissected bone shows marked bone density in the fracture area. **d** Microradiograph of the undecalcified cross-section shows minimal early temporary porosis beneath the plate and in the next quadrant. A shell of mature callus is seen lining the periosteal surface

using an intramedullary nail, whereby transport is achieved using the method of noncutting wires explained in Fig. 1.43b. The small and simple external frame helps to achieve distraction of the fragments, and the intramedullary rod provides splinting. After transportation has come to an end, the external part is removed and the intramedullary rod left in place. S. Tepic (1989, personal communication) developed a method for continuous transportation of the fragment; it consists of a bar which includes a battery-operated spindle device. K. Korcinek (1989, personal communication) demonstrated the formation of a more homogeneous bone in dogs and in humans with continuous distraction according to Tepic.

1.4 Development

Development involves principles, techniques, instruments, and implants.

1.4.1 Principles and Guidelines

This insight into the fundamental facts that guide development stems from basic and applied research and from practical experience. Knowledge is compiled by careful and open-minded observation of the reaction of the body tissues to different changes brought about by various types of trauma and distinct modes of treatment.

As an example of principles developed, we may quote the principle of *early functional treatment*, which is based on the observation of the reactions of soft tissues to immobilization of the limbs and the analysis of the reactions to early pain-free mobilization. Observations of the effect of suboptimal restoration of joint congruence have resulted in the definition of the principle of *complete restitution of joint anatomy* as a basis for optimal long-term function.

Development within the AO group gives priority to the scientific establishment of basic principles rather than to production of a multitude of implants, one for every bone, location, and fracture conceivable.

A basic guideline for the development of principles within the AO group is that injured bone is understood as being a biological structure that depends on its biological interaction with soft tissues. Bone should not be treated like a piece of broken furniture to be first cleaned and then embel-

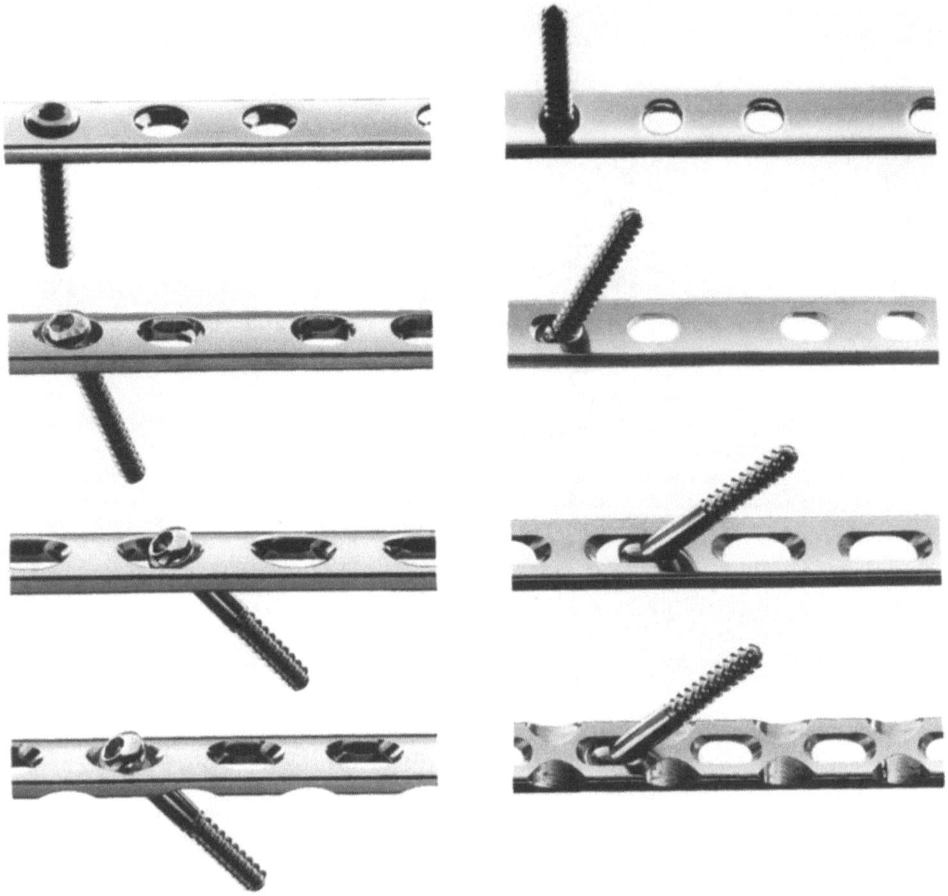

a

b

c

d

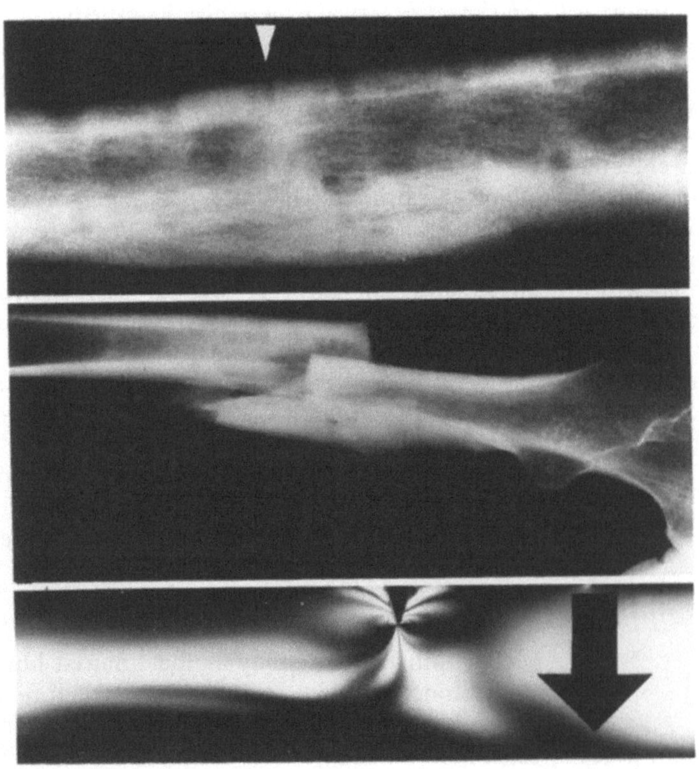

e

f

g

◀ **Fig. 1.42a–g.** Developments in AO internal fixation plates. Upper (*left*) and lower (*right*) surfaces are shown. **a** Round hole plate (Müller et al. 1963). The conically undercut screw head allows for only a perpendicular position of the screw. The distance between the inner screw holes is larger. The plate undersurface is smooth. **b** Dynamic compression plate (DCP) (Perren et al. 1969c). The spherical contact geometry allows for 20° tilting of the screw along the long axis of the bone. **c** Dynamic compression unit (DCU) (Klaue and Perren 1982). The completely symmetric screw holes are distributed at even distances throughout the plate. Symmetric screw holes with oblique undercut for improved range of inclination. **d** Limited-contact (LC)-DCP (Perren et al. 1991) viewed from above: symmetric arrangement of the screw holes without a solid elongation between the innermost screw holes. The screw holes themselves are symmetrical and are provided with two sloped cylinders. Lateral undercuts allow for bone formation at the plate (tension) side of the periosteal surface. Less damage to blood supply results, and the trapezoid cross-section allows for easier and less traumatic removal of the plate. **e** A clinical case in which a plate with a smooth undersurface had been used; defect in fracture healing immediately beneath the plate. This defect acts as a stress riser and increases the mechanical stress locally. (Courtesy of S. Kessler). **f** Following plate removal, a refracture originated at the stress concentration. Removal had been too early for this type of plate. **g** The photoelastic model shows a stress concentration under mechanical loading near a small defect at the surface of a cantilever beam loaded in bending

lished by application of individual, but largely "unnecessary fittings" (B.J. Weber, personal communication).

Decisions regarding principles are taken by physicians and scientists assisted by a competent and creative technical team. This interdisciplinary group forms the general technical commission of the AO.

1.4.2 Techniques

The manner of accomplishing internal fixation according to these principles must satisfy the criteria of simplicity and safety. The different techniques, such as plating, pinning, external fixation, and wiring, rely on an understanding of bone reaction to the prevailing mechanical and biological ("biomechanical") conditions. In conventional plating (with the exception of biological plating, for example), unloading of the plate, degree of corrosion, mechanical fatigue of the implant, type and rate of bone healing, and susceptibility to infection are highly dependent on the degree of stability of fixation achieved.

With respect to the selection of the optimal technique, the type of fracture and the conditions of the soft tissues obviously play an important role. Other factors, such as the skill of the surgeon, the surgical environment (help provided, conditions of asepsis), the instruments and implants available, and patient cooperation are important and variable elements to be taken into consideration.

1.4.3 Instrumentation and Implants

The tools and the implants must be simple and of high quality. The surgeon must have an armamentarium at hand which puts him or her in a position to deal with the widest variety of fractures. The instrumentation must be understood and therefore be taught and learned. The interaction and the function of the set of instruments and implants must satisfy the criteria of simplicity and completeness. Good results depend on the selection of the material, the appropriate grade (e.g., degree of cold work, purity), and high-quality construction. Instruments and implants must be used for the applications for which they have been developed. Only a creative expert may take advantage of other possible uses. The dimensions of the instruments must be carefully adapted to those of the implants. This is why mixing instruments and implants from different producers may lead to unexpected problems, e.g., if the nominal dimensions fit, but the tolerances are different.

We do not recommend repeated use of implants. They are not designed for reuse, and the degree of fatigue the implant has undergone during an earlier period of use cannot be estimated.

1.4.4 Technical Commissions of the AO

Developments under the aegis of the AO are controlled by the technical commissions. The main technical commission sets the long-term goals and guidelines and coordinates the smaller technical commissions. The latter deal with problems in special areas such as small-fragment surgery, maxillofacial surgery, spine surgery, joint surgery, pelvic surgery, and veterinary surgery. An additional group deals with the development of new materials.

At the AO research center in Davos, there is a group responsible for developing prototypes based on the insights provided by the scientists. Each manufacturer of AO products has a group for product development. Coordinating the efforts of all these groups is a further task of the technical commission.

A development is initiated by a single person – either a scientist or a physician – who works with a member of the prototype or product development group. Once such a team has developed something they consider to be worth testing, the technical commission organizes tests in laboratories and hos-

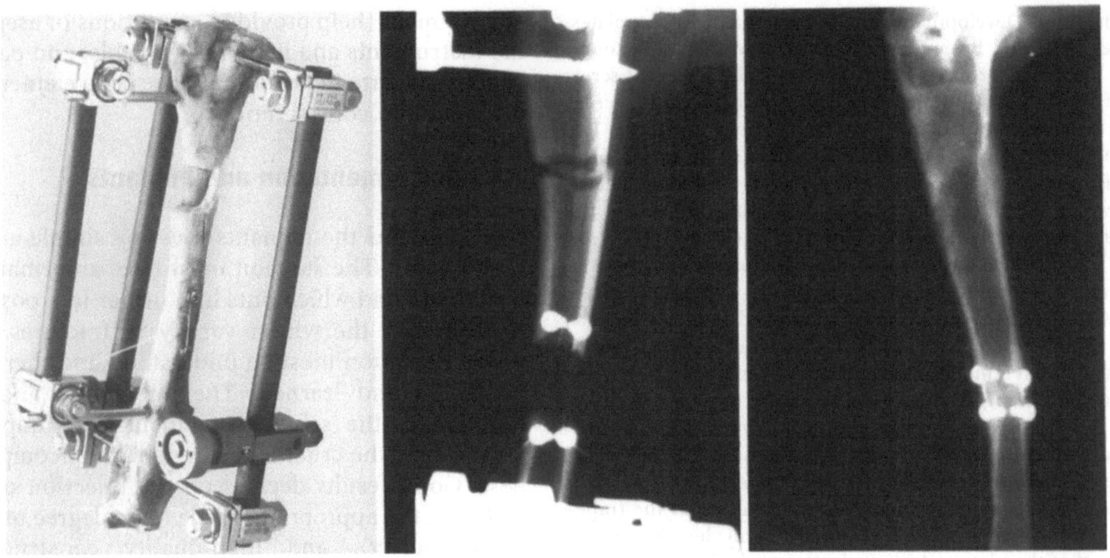

a

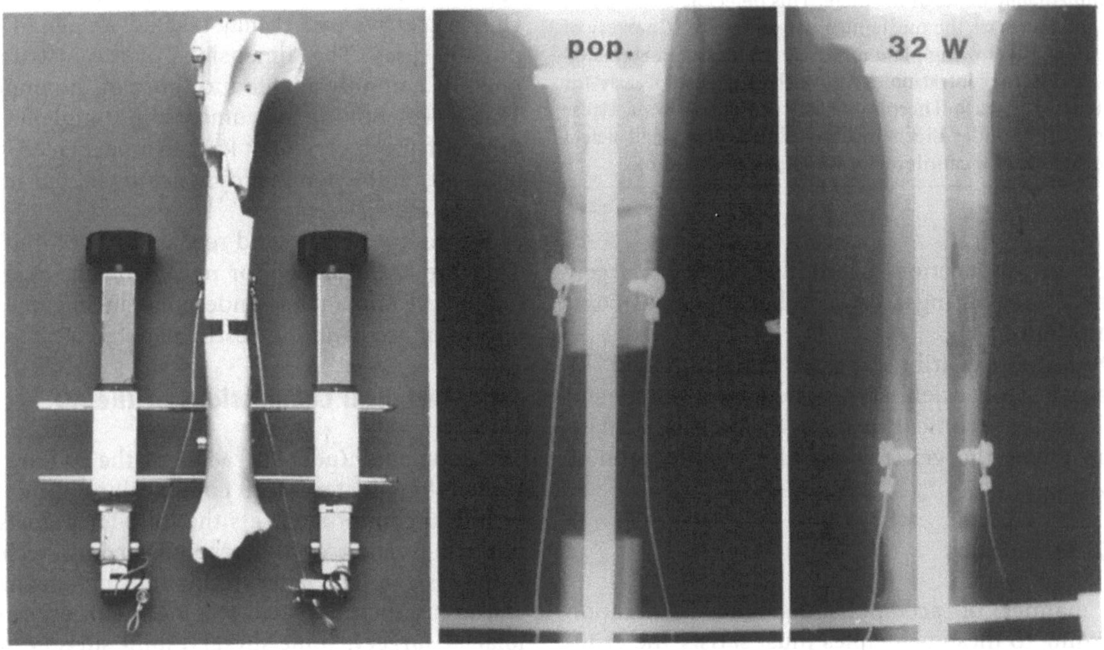

b

Fig. 1.43a–e. Distraction osteogenesis according to Ilizarov. **a** The new method of Rüter and Brutscher (1988) using noncutting wires, with X-ray and computed tomography (CT) immediately after surgery and 3 months later. *Left*, transportation is achieved using elements of the conventional AO external fixator with carbon fiber bars supplemented with two ratchets. *Center*, before transportation. *Right*, after complete transportation. **b** The recent method of Brunner and coworkers combining the above-mentioned method with an intramedullary nail. *Left*, the apparatus consists of a small bilateral AO external fixator frame supplemented with two small Wagner external fixators to allow transport of the segment using a pair of tension wires. *Center*, the situation before transportation of a segment to close a 45-mm-long defect. *Right*, after 32 weeks, the gap has filled with homogeneous, tubular bone. The defect is solidly healed. **c** Rüter and Brutscher radiologically quantified the difference between corticotomy (*filled symbols*) and osteotomy (*open symbols*). A relatively small difference was found. **d** The cross-sections obtained by quantitative CT of the transported segment shown in **b** and **c**. The bone within the gap shows a normal shape with temporarily lesser density (Brunner et al. 1990a,b). **e** Motor-driven rod of Tepic for continuous distraction. The study by K. Korcinek (1989, personal communication) seems to demonstrate the superiority of continuous distraction. At 6 weeks after surgery, the gap is filled with more homogeneous bone

c
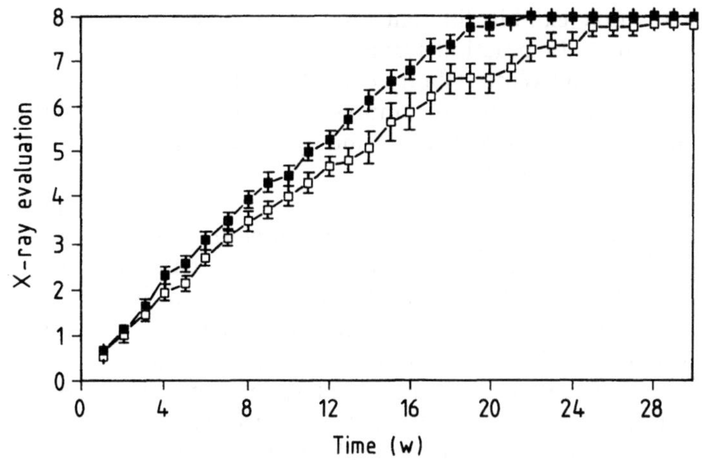

d
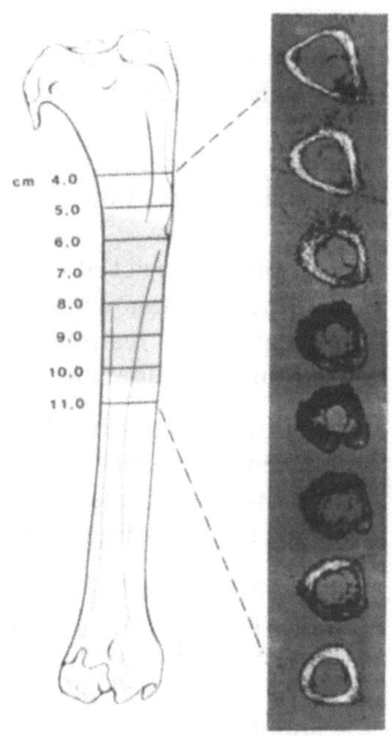

e
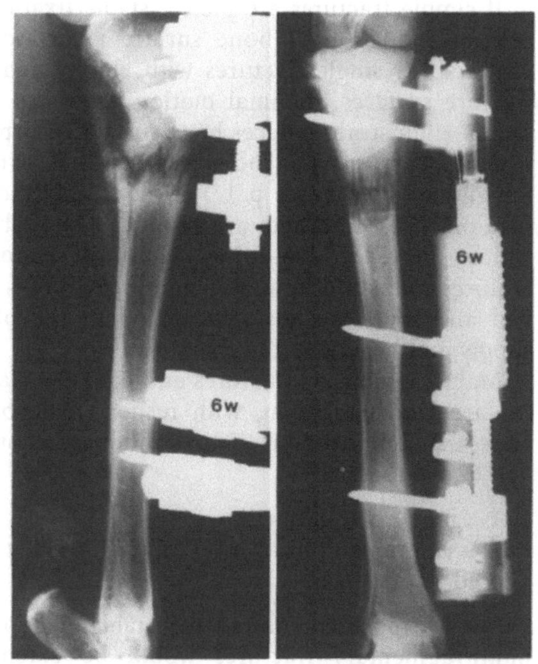

pitals. Care is taken that the clinics selected for performance of the tests provide a complete test of the different intended types of use under realistic conditions. The results are reported to and judged by the technical commission. The AO works as a group; therefore, the inventor's name does not appear on the final product, and there is no private reimbursement (apart from reimbursement of the costs of development) . However, the AO readily supports ongoing research, teaching, and fellowships at the inventor's facility. A safeguard is thus provided against private interests which might impede critical and realistic evaluation of the potential and the possible shortcomings of a technique, instrument, or implant. The AO Prize is awarded for outstanding scientific achievements, and the AO Inventors Prize or the AO Recognition Prize is awarded for inventions.

1.5 Glossary

Absolute stability. The compressed surfaces of the fracture do not displace under applied functional load. The definition of absolute stability applies only to a given time and a given site; some areas of a fracture may displace in relation to each other, other areas of the fracture may not, and different areas may exhibit different displacement at different times. In practical terms, the only method of achieving absolute stability consists in the application of interfragmental compression. The compression stabilizes by preloading and by producing friction (Perren 1972).

Biological internal fixation, biological plating (Mast et al. 1989). In internal fixation, a delicate balance exists between the degree of stabilization and that of surgical trauma. The benefits of each must be weighed against one another. Biological fixation favors preservation of the blood supply and thus optimizes the healing potential of bone and soft tissues. It provides sufficient stability for multifragmentary fractures to heal in correct alignment. For protection of the implants from overload, it relies on early biological reaction (callus formation).

If simple fractures are plated, stable fixation to prevent induction of bone surface resorption is required. In single fractures with closely adapted fracture surfaces, minimal motion generates high strain. High strain induces bone surface resorption in contact areas. When locking splints (see p. 16) or nongliding splints (see p. 17) are used for fracture fixation, reliable results are produced by stability which prevents loosening. Surgical exposure required for stabilization of a simple fracture is limited and therefore less detrimental to the blood supply and healing of the fracture.

Multifragmentary fractures and complex fractures are less demanding with respect to stability. Here, instability produces small amounts of strain due to two factors:

1. Larger fracture gaps
2. Distribution of strain over several serially located fracture gaps

Surgical exposure required for stable fixation of multifragmentary fractures would be extensive, with considerable disturbance of blood supply as a consequence. Therefore, in plating of simple fractures, stability is an important goal to achieve, while in multifragmentary fractures biology takes precedence.

Blood supply to cortical bone (restoration of). Cortical bone which has been completely deprived of blood supply for an extended period of time becomes necrotic. It may be revascularized by regrowth of blood vessels without marked widening of the haversian canals or by newly formed haversian canals. The restoration by neoformation of haversian canals is a process with a marked lag period and relatively low speed (0.1 mm/day; Schenk 1987). Bone may be revascularized by resorption and replacement with newly formed, vascular bone (creeping substitution).

Buttress. When the trauma results in impaction of the bone, e.g., at the distal metaphysis of the tibia, a defect remains after fracture reduction. An implant (plate or external fixator) then temporarily carries functional load while maintaining the shape of the bone.

Callus. A reparative tissue made of connective, cartilaginous, or bony tissue (or any combination thereof). Callus formation may be induced by any irritation – chemical (Küntscher 1970), infection, and/or instability (Hutzschenreuter et al. 1969) or others. In internal fixation, the appearance of callus is therefore little appreciated, being a sign of an unwanted condition. Callus, however, is always welcome as a repair tissue.

Complete articular fracture. The articular surface is completely dissociated from the diaphysis.

Complex fracture. Fracture in which after reduction there is no contact between the main fragments.

Compression. The act of pressing together. It results in deformation (shortening like a spring) and in improvement or creation of stability. Compression is used for the following:

1. To provide stability of fixation where motion-induced resorption must be prevented
2. To protect the implants and to improve their efficiency by unloading them

Unloading is achieved by restoration of the load-bearing capacity of the bone. Any fixation taking advantage of the load-bearing capacity of fragments of a fractured bone can withstand appreciable amounts of load without mechanical failure or temporary micromotion within the fracture. This is the main reason for using careful reduction and application of compression. Compression furthermore helps to restore dynamic loading of the bone fragments, a process for which stable contact of the fracture fragments is essential.

If the implant (screw, plate) bridging the fracture is applied under tension, the fracture focus undergoes an equal amount of compression. The compression is used to help stabilize the fracture. We have not observed any "magic biological effect" of compression.

Contact healing. Healing which occurs between two fragment ends of a fractured bone, at circumscribed places which are maintained in motionless contact. The fracture is then repaired by direct internal remodeling. Contact healing may be observed additionally where the gap is only a few micrometers wide.

Débricolage. A French term signifying the process of mechanical failure of an internal fixation prior to the onset of solid bone bridging.

Direct healing. A type of fracture healing observed with stable internal fixation. It is characterized by:

1. Absence of callus formation specific to the fracture site
2. Absence of bone surface resorption at the fracture site
3. Direct bone formation, i.e., without intermediary repair tissue

Direct fracture healing was formerly called "primary healing" in some countries. The term "primary" is now avoided so as not to grade the quality of fracture healing. Two types of direct healing are distinguished: contact healing (see above) and gap healing (see below).

Extra-articular fractures. The fracture does not involve the articular surface, but it may be intracapsular.

Far (trans-)cortex. The cortex away from the plate. The consequences of a defect within the far cortex are much more serious than those of a defect in the near cortex. The difference is due to the larger lever arm of the far cortex.

Fracture. A sudden rupture of a structure, which occurs whenever the internal stress produced by load exceeds the limits of strength. Depending on the type of load – compressive, flexural, torsional, shear, or any combination thereof – a typical fracture pattern is observed, e.g., impaction, transverse fracture, spiral fracture, avulsion. The complexity of the fracture depends mainly upon the amount of energy stored prior to fracture.

Fracture disease. A condition characterized by pain, swelling, and other signs of dystrophy, such as patchy bone loss and stiffness of joints (Lucas-Championnière 1907). Fracture disease (also called Sudeck's atrophy) can best be avoided by stable fixation to reduce irritation and by early active movement and, when possible, immediate or at least partial weight-bearing on the injured limb (Allgöwer 1978).

Gap healing. The healing process taking place between two fragment ends kept in a stable relative position with a small gap between the fragment ends. Gap healing progresses in two phases:

1. Filling of the gap with lamellar bone of an orientation different from that of the bone of the fragments
2. Subsequent remodeling of the newly filled bone from within the gap into the fragments (plugging) or crossing from one fragment through the newly filled bone into the other fragment (remodeling)

Gliding hole. When a fully threaded screw is used as a lag screw, the cortex under the screw head should not engage. This can be accomplished by overdrilling the near cortex screw hole to at least the size of the outer diameter of the screw thread.

Gliding splint. A splint, e.g., conventional nail, which allows for axial shortening. Such a splint provides the possibility for coaptation under conditions of fragment end shortening due to bone surface resorption.

Goal of fracture treatment. According to Müller et al. (1963), the goal of fracture treatment is to restore optimal function of the limb with respect to mobility and load-bearing capacity. The goal is furthermore to avoid early disturbances, such as Sudeck's atrophy (fracture disease), and late sequels, such as post-traumatic arthrosis.

Healing. Restoration of the original integrity. Theoretically, the healing process after a bone fracture lasts many years, until internal fracture remodeling subsides. For practical purposes, healing is considered completed when the bone has regained its normal stiffness and strength.

Impacted fracture. A fracture in which the cortex or articular surface is driven into the cancellous bone.

Indirect healing. Bone healing as observed in nontreated or nonstably treated fractures. Callus formation is predominant, the fracture fragment ends are resorbed, and bone formation results from a process of transformation of fibrous and/or cartilaginous tissue to bone.

Interfragmental compression (effect of). Static compression applied to a fracture area stabilizes the fragments and thus reduces irritation. Bone surface resorption is then absent. No proof has been found that compression per se has an effect upon internal remodeling of the cortical bone (Matter et al. 1974).

Interlocking nail. A nail provides some degree of stability mainly by its (flexural) stiffness. A conventional nail allows the fragments to slide along the nail; the fracture must therefore be provided with a solid support against shortening. For the treatment of complex fractures, the nail can be interlocked to prevent shortening and rotation.

Lag screw. The lag screw produces interfragmental compression by compressing the bone under the screw head against the fragment in which the screw threads are anchored. Interfragmental compression is reduced by engagement (wedging) of the screw threads with the walls of the gliding hole. Anchorage in the near fragment can be avoided by the use of a shaft screw. This method is required to maintain efficient compression when the lag screw is applied through the plate in an inclined position.

Locking splint. An implant, e.g., plate, acting as splint which, when somewhat loosened by interface resorption, does not allow coaptation. Therefore, when using a locking splint for fixation of a simple and adapted fracture, interfragmental displacement should be avoided to prevent bone surface resorption with consequent biological loosening of the fixation. Such loosening without possible coaptation may result in a mechanically induced nonunion. This is a problem after plating, while after locked nailing the mere removal of the locking pins allows for maintenance of the splinting while gliding along the long axis of the nail is permitted.

Multifragmentary fracture. A term usually reserved for extra-articular and articular fractures which have one or more completely dissociated intermediate fragments.

Near (cis-)cortex. The cortex near the plate. With respect to bending, the near cortex contributes little to stability of fixation. When the distance between the plate and the near cortex is increased, e.g., in wave plate application, the bone and the repair tissues gain better leverage.

Neutralization. An implant (plate, external fixator, or nail) whose action is based upon its stiffness is said to "neutralize" the effect of the functional load. The implant carries a major part of the functional load and thus, for example, protects a screw fixation. It does not actually "neutralize," but does minimize the effect of the forces (see "Protection").

Partial articular fracture. The fracture involves only part of the joint, while the remainder remains attached to the diaphysis.

Pin loosening. The pins of external fixator frames serve to stabilize the fragments of a fracture. Stability depends, among other things, upon the contact between pin and bone. If bone surface resorption at the pin–bone interface occurs, stability is reduced. Pin loosening is less important with respect to loss of stability, but is important with respect to its deleterious effect upon pin tract infection.

Prebending of plate. Exactly contoured plates produce asymmetric compression, i.e., the near cortex is more compressed than the far cortex. The latter may not be compressed at all. With respect to stabilization against torque and bending, compression of the far cortex is more important than that of the near cortex. To provide compression of the far cortex, the plate is applied after exact contouring, but with an additional bend of the plate segment bridging the fracture. The bend is such that the midsection of the plate is elevated from the bone surface prior to fixation to the bone. Prebending is an important means of increasing stability in small and/or porotic bones.

Precise reduction. Exact adaptation of fracture fragments (hairline adjustment). It should result in complete restoration of anatomy and optimal late function. It should be noted that overall stability does not depend on precise reduction, but precise reduction more reliably results in stability and increased strength of fixation.

Preload. The application of interfragmental compression keeps the fragments together until a tensile force exceeding the compression (preload) is applied.

Protection. While the term "neutralization" has often been used in plate and screw fixation, the term "protection" should replace it. In reality, nothing is neutralized. In plate fixation, the plate reduces the load placed upon the screw fixation. It therefore protects the screw fixation from overload.

Pure depression. An articular fracture in which there is only depression of the articular surface without a split.

Pure split. An articular fracture in which there is an articular split without any additional cartilaginous lesion.

Refracture. A fracture occurring after the bone has solidly bridged, at a load level otherwise tolerated by normal bone. The resulting fracture line may coincide with the original fracture line or it may be located remote from the original fracture, but within the area of bone undergoing changes due to fracture and treatment.

Relative stability. An internal fixation construct that allows small amounts of motion in proportion to the load applied. This is the case with a fixation which depends only on the stiffness of the implant (such as a nail bridging a fracture without exerting compression). It will always show deformation or displacement which is inversely proportional to the stiffness of the implant. Such motion is always present, but is harmless in nail fixation. According to the philosophy of the AO/ASIF group, plate fixation is more reliable if motion is prevented. (Callus as a sign of unwanted instability is then absent.)

Rigid fixation. A fixation of a fracture which allows little deformation under load.

Rigid implants. In general, implants are considered to be rigid when they are made of metals. The implant geometry is more important than the stiffness of the material. Most implants made of metal are much more flexible than the corresponding bone.

Rigidity. This term is often used synonymously with stiffness. According to Timoshenko (1941), it should be used when related to shear, e.g., at the plate-bone interface.

Simple (single) fracture. A disruption of bone (diaphyseal, extra-articular, articular) with two main fragments.

Splinting. Reducing the mobility of a fracture by coupling a stiff body to the bone fragments. The splint may be external (plaster, external fixators) or internal (internal fixation plate, intramedullary nail).

Split depression. A combination of split and depression in an articular fracture.

Spontaneous healing. The healing pattern of a fracture without treatment. Solid healing is observed in most cases, but malalignment frequently results.

Stable fixation. A fixation which keeps the fragments of a fracture in motionless adaptation at least for joint movement. While a mobile fracture produces pain with any attempts to move the limb, stable fixation allows early painless mobilization. Thus stable fixation minimizes irritation, which may eventually lead to fracture disease.

Stability of fixation. This is characterized by lack of motion at the fracture site, i.e., little or no displacement between the fragments of the fracture. In technical terms, stability describes the tendency to revert to a condition of low energy.

Stiffness. The resistance of a structure to deformation. The higher the stiffness of an implant, the smaller its deformation, the smaller the displacement of the fracture fragments, and the smaller the straining of the repair tissue. Reduced, but not abolished strain promotes healing.

Stiffness and material properties. The stiffness of a structure depends on its Young's modulus of elasticity. An increasing Young's modulus affects the deformation of the material by its first power.

Stiffness and geometrical properties. The thickness affects the deformability by its third power. Changes in geometry are therefore much more critical than the changes of material properties, a fact which is often overlooked by nonengineers. Thus, if flexible fixation is a goal, it can be achieved better by a small change in the dimensions than by using a "less rigid" material.

Strain. Relative deformation, e.g., of a repair tissue. Motion at the fracture site in itself is not the important feature, but rather the resulting relative deformation, which is called strain ($\delta L/L$). As strain is a relative unit (displacement of fragments divided by width of fracture gap), very high levels of strain may be present within small fracture gaps under conditions in which the displacement may not even be visible. This possibility must always be considered.

Strain induction. Tissue deformation may – among other things – result in induction of callus. This is an example of a mechanically induced biological reaction. For those reactions triggered by strain, such as callus formation and bone surface resorption, a lower limit of strain, the minimum strain, should be considered.

Strain tolerance. This determines the tolerance of the repair tissues to mechanical conditions. No tissue can be formed under conditions of strain which exceed the elongation at rupture of the tissue. Above the critical level, the straining of tissues will destroy the tissue once formed or will prevent its formation.

Strength. The ability to withstand load without structural failure. The strength of a material can be reported as ultimate tensile strength, as bending strength, or as torsional strength. The local criterion for failure of bone or implants is expressed in units of force per unit of area: stress, or (equivalent) deformation per unit length; strain, or elongation at rupture.

Stress protection. This term, initially used to describe bone reaction to reduced functional load (Allgöwer et al. 1969), is now mainly used to express the negative aspects of stress relief of bone. The basic assumption is that bone deprived of necessary functional stimulation by changing mechanical load becomes less dense or strong (Wolff's law; Wolff 1893, 1986). Stress protection is often used synonymously with stress shielding, i.e., in a purely mechanical sense. It is often used to characterize bone loss – implying a negative reaction to stress shielding. With regard to internal fixation of cortical bone, stress protection seems to play a fairly unimportant role compared with vascular considerations.

Early bone loss, which was hitherto attributed to stress protection, can be explained on the basis of a temporary lack of blood supply. The necrotic area is then remodeled by osteons originating from the area with a good blood supply. Remodeling accompanies temporary osteoporosis. Measurements of late bone loss in humans under clinical conditions of internal fixation using quantitative CT show very little bone loss at the time of implant removal (Cordey et al. 1985).

In summary, bone may react to unloading, but this plays a minor role in internal fixation of cortical bone fractures.

Stress shielding. When internal fixation relies upon screws and plates, according to the AO/ASIF group the stability of fixation is achieved by interfragmental compression exerted mainly by the lag screws. Such stabilization by lag screw is very stable, but provides safety under functional load only in certain situations (e.g., long spiral fractures, metaphyseal fractures). A plate providing protection (or neutralization) is therefore often added. The function of such a plate is to reduce the amount of peak load applied to the screw fixation. Protection is provided based upon the stiffness of the plate. The plate shields the fractured and temporarily fixed bone.

Tension band. An implant (wire or plate) functioning according to the tension band principle; when the bone undergoes flexural load and with the implant attached to the convex surface, it carries tensile force; the bone, especially the far cortex, is then dynamically compressed. The plate is able to resist very large amounts of tensile force, while the bone best resists compressive load.

Vascularity. A tissue is vascularized if it contains blood vessels connected to the main circulatory system. Blood vessels may be shut off temporarily from the circulatory system. We consider a tissue to be nonvascular if there are no vessels, as in cartilage, or if the vessels present are not functioning, e.g., obliterated by thrombosis.

Wedge fracture. A fracture with a third fragment in which, after reduction, there is some direct contact between the main fragments.

2.1 Screws

2.1.1 Function

Screws are used either to fasten plates to bone, to maintain bone fragments in their relative position, or – as lag screws – to hold together fragments of bone.

2.1.2 Screw Types

Screws are differentiated by the manner in which they are inserted into bone, their function, their size, and the type of bone they are intended for. Thus we differentiate between self-tapping and non-self-tapping screws, lag screws, and large- and small-fragment cortical and cancellous screws.

One other major differentiation between screws is based on the manner in which they couple with a screwdriver. Thus screws may have a slot, a cruciate recess, a square, and so on. All but the smallest AO screws have a hexagonal recess and require a corresponding screwdriver with a hexagonal tip. The screws couple securely with the screwdriver, which has completely obviated any screw-holding devices on the screwdriver. This feature has proven to be a great advantage at the time of screw removal and insertion. At removal, once the tissue is cleared from the hexagonal recess in the screw head, the screwdriver can be easily inserted into the screw head and the screw turned without the screwdriver jumping out and stripping the recess. At insertion, the torque is transmitted evenly to the screw and there is no danger of tilting and losing control of screw direction or of stripping the recess. There is one further advantage of the secure coupling of the screw head with the screwdriver: at insertion, it is useful, and at times absolutely necessary, to know the exact direction of a screw; by simply inserting the screwdriver into an AO screw, the surgeon has an automatic guide as to its direction.

2.1.2.1 Self-Tapping and Non-self-tapping Screws

Self-tapping screws (Fig. 2.1b) are designed in such a way that once a pilot hole is drilled into bone they can be inserted by simply screwing them in. The pilot hole is somewhat larger than the core of the screw. The resistance to screw insertion may interfere with the accuracy of insertion, particularly if one is trying to insert the screw obliquely into bone to lag two fragments together. It used to be thought that self-tapping screws had a weaker hold in bone. Experimental investigation (Schatzker et al. 1975a–c) has shown that a self-tapping screw can be removed and reinserted without weakening its hold in bone provided that it is carefully inserted. However, if inadvertently angled, it will cut a new path and destroy the thread that has already been

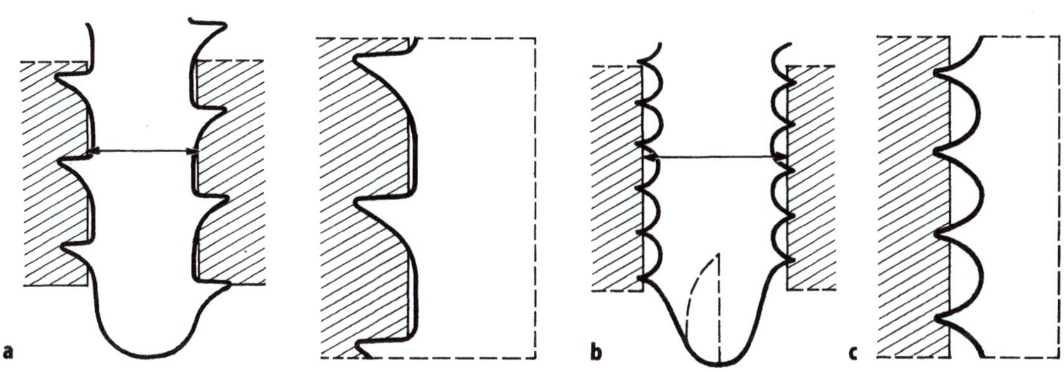

a b c

Fig. 2.1a–c. Non-self-tapping screw (**a**) and self-tapping screw (**b**). The pilot hole for the self-tapping screw has to be larger, and the screw threads do not penetrate as deeply into the bone (**c**)

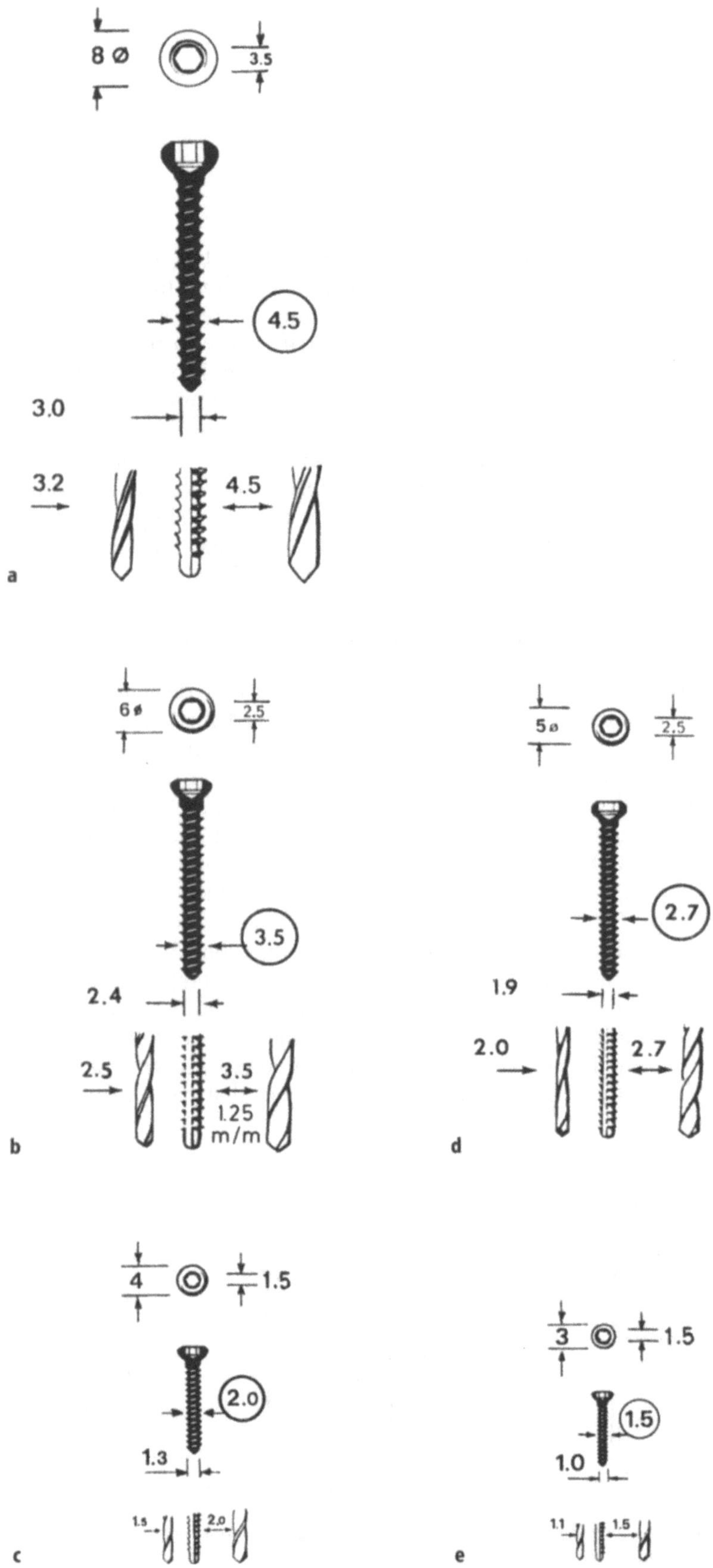

Fig. 2.2a–e. Cortex screws. **a** The 4.5-mm cortex screw. *Top*, fully threaded with a diameter of 4.5 mm and a 1.75-mm pitch. *Center*, screw head 8 mm in diameter with a 3.5-mm hexagonal recess; the core is 3 mm. *Bottom*, the drill bit for the thread hole is 3.2 mm (*left*), the drill bit for the gliding hole is 4.5 mm (*middle*), and the tap has a diameter of 4.5 mm (*right*). **b** The 3.5-mm cortex screw. *Top*, fully threaded with a diameter of 3.5 mm and a 1.25-mm pitch. *Center*, screw head 6 mm in diameter with a 2.5-mm hexagonal recess; the core is 2.4 mm. *Bottom*, the drill bit for the thread hole is 2.5 mm (*left*), the drill bit for the gliding hole is 3.5 mm (*middle*), and the tap has a diameter of 3.5 mm (*right*). **c** The 2.7-mm cortex screw. *Top*, fully threaded with a diameter of 2.7 mm and a 1.0-mm pitch. *Center*, screw head 5 mm in diameter with a 2.5-mm hexagonal recess; the core is 1.9 mm. *Bottom*, the drill bit for the thread hole is 2.0 mm (*left*), the drill bit for the gliding hole is 2.7 mm (*middle*), and the tap has a diameter of 2.7 mm (*right*). **d** The 2.0-mm cortex screw. *Top*, fully threaded with a diameter of 2.0 mm and a 0.8-mm pitch. *Center*, screw head 4.0 mm in diameter with a 1.5-mm hexagonal recess; the core is 1.3 mm. *Bottom*, the drill bit for the thread hole is 1.5 mm (*left*), the drill bit for the gliding hole is 2.0 mm (*middle*), and the tap has a diameter of 2.0 mm (*right*). **e** The 1.5-mm cortex screw. *Top*, fully threaded with a diameter of 1.5 mm and a 0.6-mm pitch. *Center*, screw head 3 mm in diameter with a 1.5-mm hexagonal recess; the core is 1.0 mm. *Bottom*, the drill bit for the thread hole is 1.1 mm (*left*), the drill bit for the gliding hole is 1.5 mm (*middle*), and the tap has a diameter of 1.5 mm (*right*)

cut, which is a disadvantage. Self-tapping screws should therefore not be used as lag screws.

Non-self-tapping screws (Fig. 2.1a) require a predrilled pilot hole and then careful cutting of their thread in cortical bone with a tap which corresponds exactly to the profile of the screw thread. Because the thread is cut with a tap, the pilot hole corresponds in size almost to the core of the screw and the screw thread has a much deeper bite into the adjacent bone. Much less heat is generated when the screw is inserted because there is less resistance. The tap is designed in such a way that it is not only much sharper than the thread of a screw, but it also has a more efficient mechanism of clearing the bone debris, which therefore does not accumulate and clog its threads to obstruct its insertion. This allows one to work with much greater precision, particularly in thick cortical bone. The screws can be removed and reinserted with ease without fear of inadvertently cutting a new channel, as a screw alone is not able to cut a channel in cortical bone. The screws are spun; their core is therefore perfectly straight and their surface is polished. Thus fully threaded screws can be removed easily. Recent investigative work has shown that in extremely thin layers of cortical bone, such as facial bones, self-tapping screws appear to have a better holding power than the non-self-tapping screws of corresponding size (Phillips and Rahn 1989). The non-self-tapping screw is considerably superior except in extremely thin cortical bone, cancellous bone, and in flat bones such as those of the skull, scapula and the pelvis.

2.1.2.2 Cortex Bone Screws

Cortex screws (Fig. 2.2) are fully threaded. In the case of non-self-tapping screws, a tap is required to cut their thread before insertion. Since the holding power of a screw diminishes as the diameter of the screw approaches 40 % of the diameter of the bone, there are a number of different sizes of cortex screws available in the AO armamentarium to enable fixation of bones of different diameters. Each screw size has a corresponding drill bit and tap. Particularly noteworthy is the recently introduced 3.5-mm AO cortex screw. The pitch of this screw is different, as is the ratio of the outer diameter to the screw core. The core is larger (2.4 mm) than that of the corresponding cancellous bone screw (2.0 mm; Fig. 2.3). The increase in the screw core thickness has increased the bending and torsional strength of this screw and has prevented shearing of the screws when used as load screws with the self-compressing dynamic compression plate (DCP).

2.1.2.3 Cancellous Bone Screws

Cancellous bone screws (Fig. 2.4) are characterized by a relatively thin core and a wide and deep thread. This increase in the ratio of the outer diameter to the core gives such a screw considerably increased holding power in fine trabecular bone, which characterizes metaphyseal and epiphyseal areas of bone. Cancellous bone screws are either fully or partially threaded. The fully threaded screws are used for fastening such devices as plates in metaphyseal and epiphyseal areas of bone. The partially threaded screws are used as lag screws. The cancellous bone screws differ not only in the number of threads, but also in size. Thus there are the large 6.5-mm cancellous bone screws (Fig. 2.4a–c) and the fully and the partially threaded 4.0-mm small-fragment cancellous bone screws (Fig. 2.4e). Cancellous bone screws are designed as non-self-tapping screws. Their thread must be tapped only in the near cortex. Tapping of the cancellous bone is unnecessary because the cancellous bone screw can easily cut a thread for itself, and its holding power is increased if its thread is not cut, because it tends to compress the trabeculae together when it is driven in.

If there is a cortex opposite through which the cancellous bone screw can be inserted, the screw should also engage the far cortex, since this significantly increases its hold in bone (approximately six-fold). In the metaphysis, no tapping of the opposite cortex is required. If the far cortex is thick, as might be the case in a young individual, then the far cortex and the intervening cancellous bone may have to be tapped to facilitate the insertion of the screw.

To facilitate the insertion of cancellous bone screws acting as lag screws into fragments of bone, particularly during reconstructions of major epiphyseal or metaphyseal fractures such as the femoral condyles or the proximal tibia or for the fixation of femoral neck fractures of the femur, the AO has recently introduced 3.5- and 6.5-mm cancellous bone screws which are cannulated and can be inserted over Kirschner wires. (In the United States, the large cannulated cancellous bone screw has a thread diameter of 7 mm.)

2.1.3 Screw Fixation

In order to restore the ability of bone to support loads, its structural continuity must be restored. This can be done by the application of a plate to the bone once alignment is restored. As long as there is a gap between the fragments, however small, the load is transmitted via the plate from one fragment of bone to the next. The fracture surfaces by neces-

TAP ∅	PILOT OR THREAD HOLE ∅	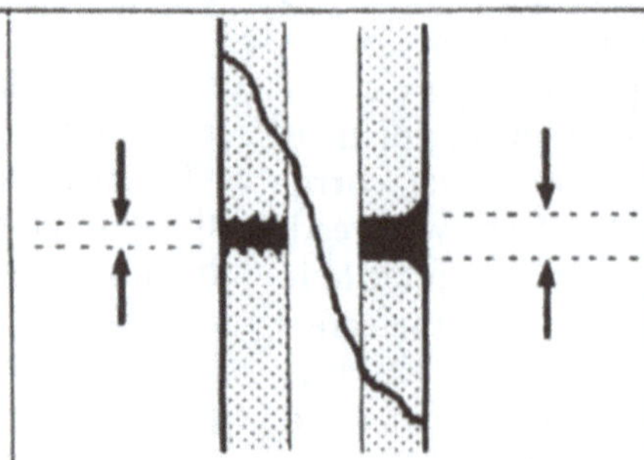	GLIDING HOLE ∅
1.5	1.1	1.5	1.5
2.0	1.5	2.0	2.0
2.7	2.0	2.7	2.7
3.5/1.25mm	2.5	3.5	3.5
3.5/1.75mm	2.5	4.0	—
4.5	3.2	4.5	4.5
6.5	3.2	6.5	(4.5)

Fig. 2.3. Summary of available screws and their corresponding drill bits and taps (see also Appendix)

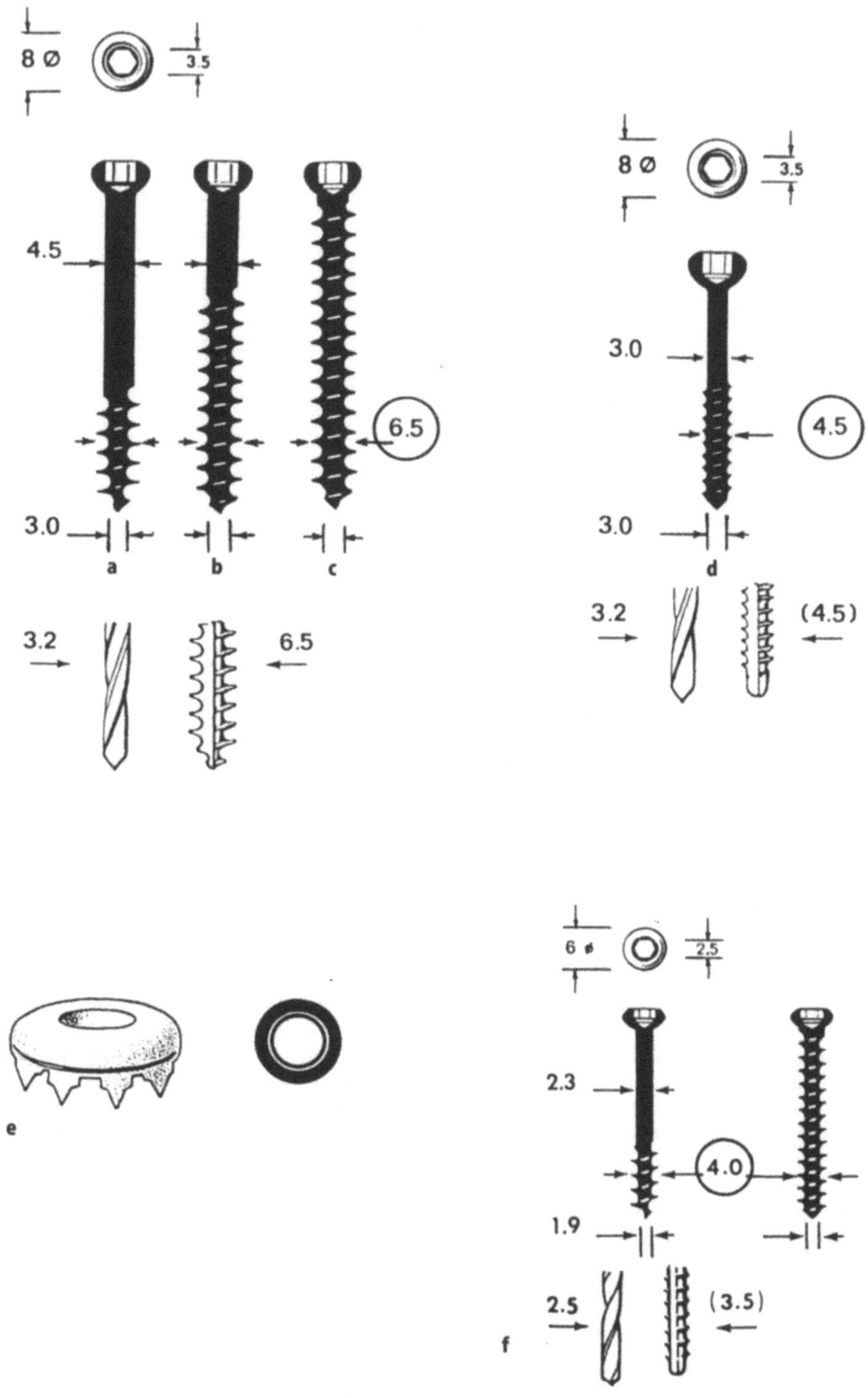

Fig. 2.4a–f. Cancellous bone screws. **a–c** The 6.5-mm cancellous bone screw with an 8-mm spherical head and a 3.5-mm hexagonal recess. **a** Thread length, 16 mm. **b** Thread length, 32 mm. **c** Fully threaded. All have a 6.5-mm diameter, a 4.5-mm shaft, and a 3.0-mm core. All require a 3.2-mm drill bit and a 6.5-mm tap. **d** A 4.5-mm malleolar screw. Its thread has a diameter of 4.5 mm; it is partially threaded, has a trephine self-cutting tip, and a 3.0-mm core. It requires a 3.2-mm drill bit and a 4.5-mm tap. **e** Three sizes of serrated plastic washers are available for ligamentous avulsions and the 13-mm metal washers for 6.5- and 4.5-mm cancellous bone screws. A 7.0-mm washer is available for small cancellous screws. **f** Small-fragment cancellous bone screws: 4.0-mm cancellous bone screws with a 6-mm-wide head and a 2.5-mm hexagonal recess. All have a core of 1.9 mm and a 1.75-mm pitch. All require a 2.5-mm drill bit and a tap for 4.0-mm cancellous bone screws

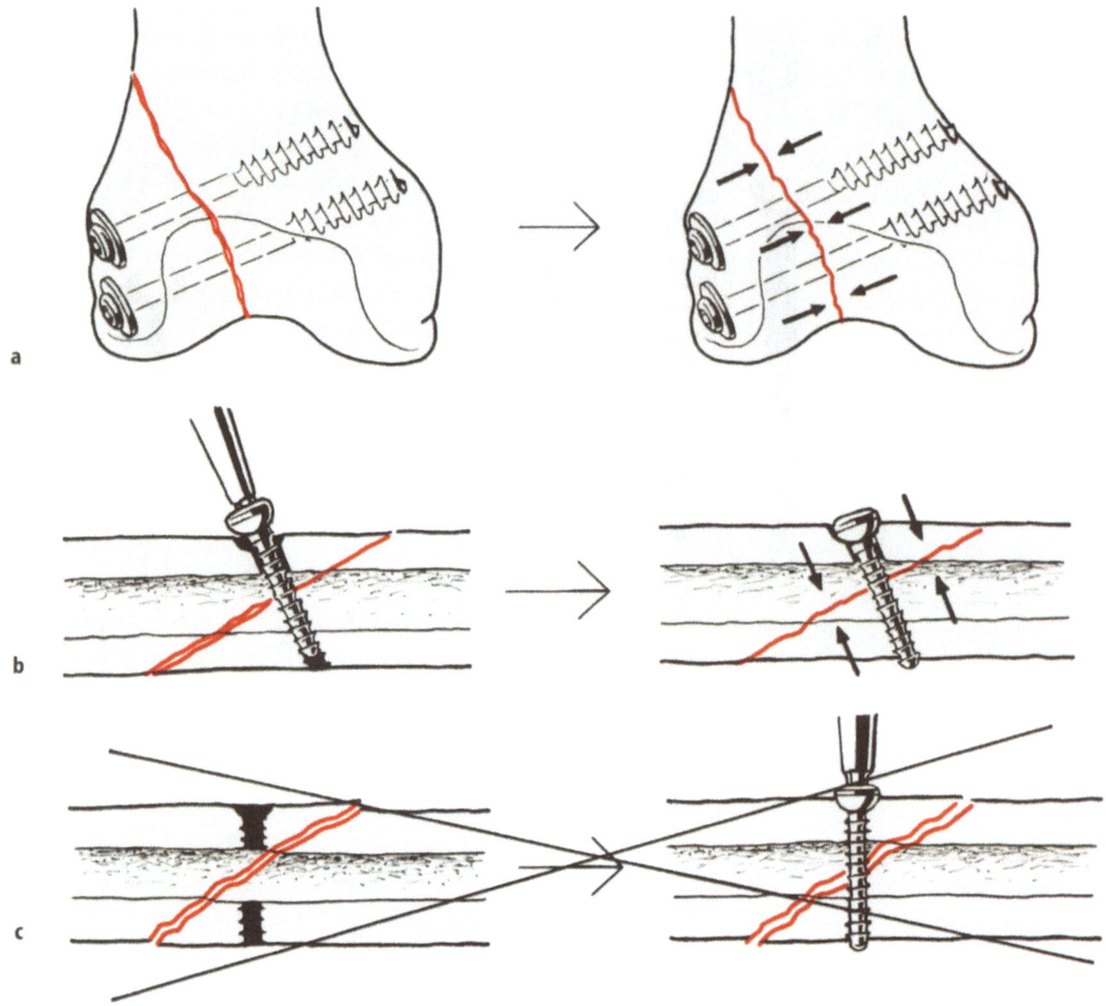

Fig. 2.5. a For a lag screw to compress two fragments, its thread must be engaged only in the far fragment. **b** The cortex in the near fragment must be overdrilled in order to create a "gliding" or a clearance hole. This will ensure that the thread will take purchase only in the "thread hole" in the far cortex. Note also that for maximum compression, the screw should be at 90° to the fracture line. **c** If a screw thread engages both the near and the far cortex, then as it is tightened, no compression is generated because the two cortices cannot come together. In order to achieve maximal compression, the lag screw must be inserted through the center of both fragments and it must be directed at a right angle to the fracture plane

sity will move in relation to each other and the plate will act as a load-bearing device. The stability of the fixation depends on the rigidity of the plate and the holding power of the screws. A fixation device which is subjected to full loads can fail due to mechanical overload or fatigue. Furthermore, the stability thus achieved is never absolute, no matter how rigid the plate is. The most effective way of restoring structural continuity is to bring the fragments of bone not only into contact, but also under compression. This permits direct transfer of load from one fragment of bone to the other, which diminishes the load borne by the fixation device, increases the stability of the fixation, and reduces corrosion. The most effective way to achieve compression between fragments of bone is by means of a lag screw.

2.1.3.1 Lag Screw

A lag screw is a screw whose thread purchases only in the far cortex. This means that the portion of the screw in the near cortex does not purchase, either because the screw shank has no thread or because the hole in the cortex is equal to or actually bigger than the outer diameter of the screw. Thus, when a lag screw is tightened, it causes the two fragments of bone to be compressed (Fig. 2.5). The partially threaded cancellous bone screws may be employed as lag screws. The portion of the screw passing

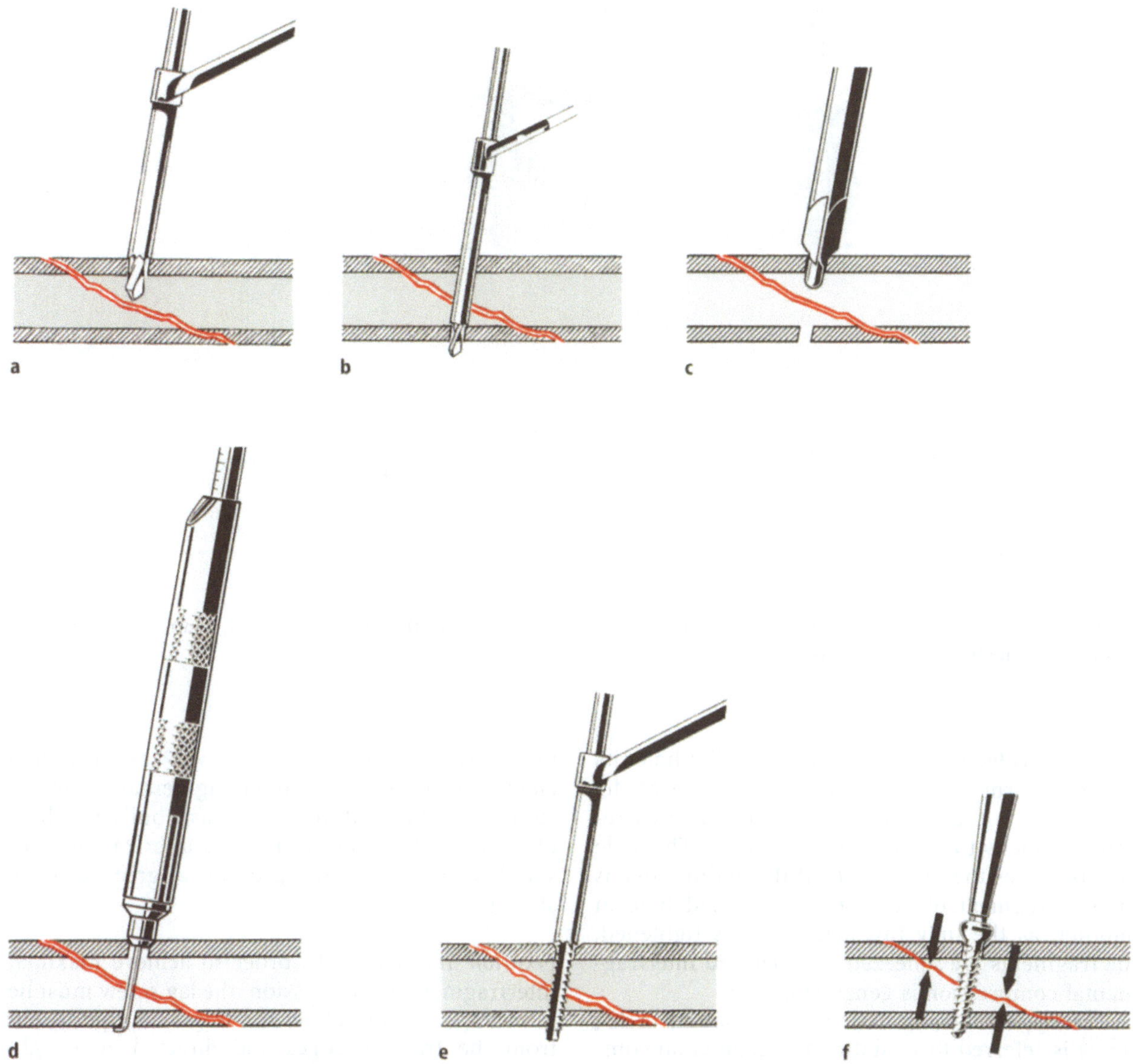

Fig. 2.6a–f. Technique for lag screw fixation after fragment reduction. **a** The gliding hole is drilled the same diameter as the screw thread. **b** The insert drill sleeve with outer diameter of the gliding hole and inner diameter of the thread hole is inserted until the serrated end meets the opposite cortex. This drill sleeve ensures perfect centering of the drill bit even when the holes have an oblique direction. The hole is drilled in the far segment the same diameter as the screw core. **c** To enlarge the contact area betwen the screw head and the bone surface, the hole is countersunk. **d** The screw length is carefully measured with the depth gauge. **e** The thread hole is tapped. **f** The appropriate screw is inserted and tightened. If a screw thread engages both the near and the far cortex, then as it is tightened, no compression is generated because the two cortices cannot come together. In order to achieve maximal compression, the lag screw must be inserted through the center of both fragments and must be directed at a right angle to the fracture plane

through the near cortex does not have a thread and hence will not engage in the near cortex, but the distal portion of the screw is threaded and will, therefore, engage the far cortex. As the screw is tightened, it will approximate the two fragments and interfragmental compression will be generated. This holds true as long as the screw thread does not cross the fracture line to engage in both fragments. If it does, as the screw is tightened it will fail to generate any compression at the fracture (Fig. 2.5c).

If a fully threaded screw is to function as a lag screw (Fig. 2.5b), the near cortex has to be overdrilled so that the hole in it is at least equal in size to the outer diameter of the screw thread. This hole is then called the *gliding hole*. The hole in the far

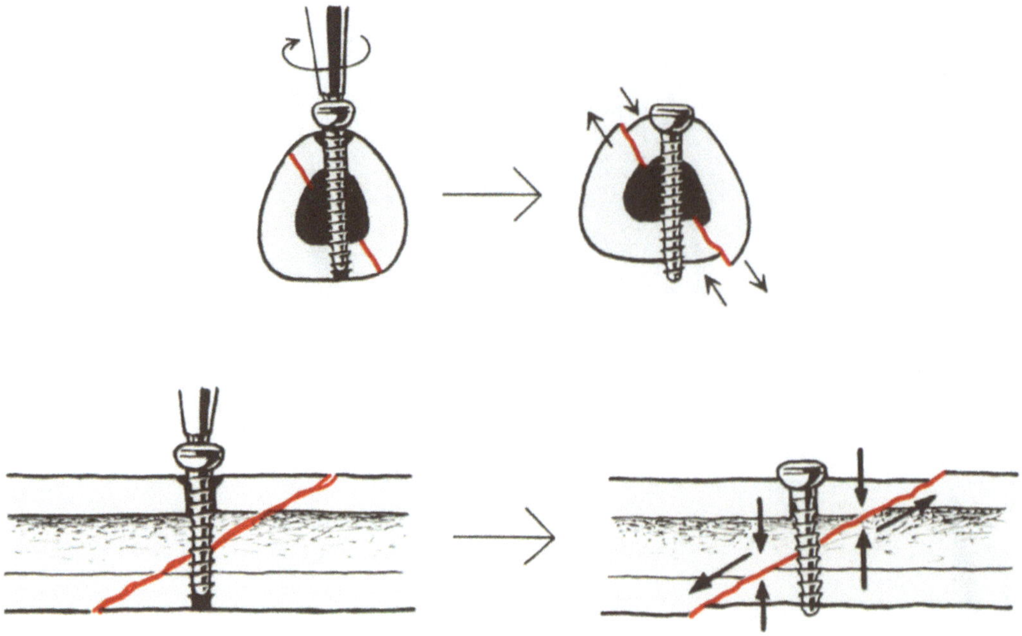

Fig. 2.7. If a lag screw is inserted at an angle other than 90° to the fracture plane, then as it is tightened, it introduces a shearing moment and the fracture may displace

cortex is drilled to the diameter of the pilot hole (its size is determined by the size of the core of the screw) and is then tapped with a tap which corresponds exactly to the thread of the screw. This hole now becomes the *thread hole*. If the gliding hole is in one fragment of bone and the thread hole in another, as the fully threaded screw is tightened, the fragments are squeezed together and interfragmental compression is generated.

The type of compression generated by a lag screw is referred to as static interfragmental compression. It is static because it does not change significantly with load. A lag screw is the most efficient way of achieving interfragmental compression and stability. It forms the basic building block of all stable fixation. It provides interfragmentary stability but does not provide a great deal of strength.

Fixation Techniques. In order to achieve maximal interfragmental compression, the lag screw must be inserted in the middle of the fragment equidistant from the fracture edges and directed at a right angle to the fracture plane (Fig. 2.6a–f). If the screw

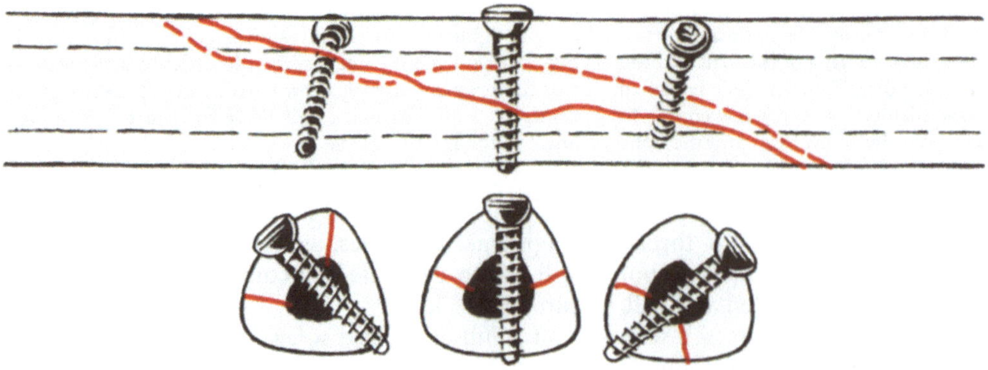

Fig. 2.8. In a spiral fracture which is fixed with more than two screws, the central screw is usually at right angles to the long axis of the bone and is thus able to prevent axial displacement. The other two screws will be at right angles to the spiral fracture plane and will ensure maximal compression

is not inserted perpendicular to the fracture plane, then as it is tightened a shearing force is introduced and the fragments will shift (Fig. 2.7).

Similarly, if a screw is inserted at an acute angle to the fracture plane, then as it is tightened it introduces a shearing moment and tends to displace the fragments (Fig. 2.7). These fundamental errors in screw insertion are often responsible for the loss of reduction. With the loss of reduction, loss of structural continuity and stability are inevitable.

In long oblique, spiral, or multiple fractures, the elements are held in place by lag screws or sometimes by position screws (Fig. 2.8). They are protected from weight-bearing loads by a plate applied in the neutralizing mode.

Indications. As already indicated, whenever there are two fragments of bone whose size and geometry permit lag screw fixation, then this technique should be used. Lag screws are used in the reconstruction of intra-articular epiphyseal and metaphyseal fractures (see Fig. 2.9). The fractures in these areas are usually the result of a shearing or cleaving force, which results in fragments ideally suited for lag screw fixation. In practice, lag screw fixation alone is reserved for short tubular bones and for epiphyseal and metaphyseal fractures.

Countersinking of the Screw Head. The cortex is reamed using the countersink with the object of increasing the contact area between the screw head and the bone, thus preventing microfractures of the cortical surface due to compression. In small-breed dogs and cats, the cortex is very thin. If the countersink area is too deep, the screw head will break through the remaining cortex when tightened. Countersinking is never carried out in areas in which cancellous bone is covered by a thin cortex or soft bone, e.g., in young animals, as the screw head easily breaks through. In order to prevent this, it is advisable to use a washer, which distributes the force over a larger area (Fig. 2.10). Countersinking is carried out prior to measuring the depth of the drill hole.

2.1.3.2 Position Screw

There are times when placing a lag screw will cause a fracture segment to collapse into the medullary cavity. This occurs when the two fracture surfaces can slide past each other and do not abut against each other when the segments are compressed. This is a relatively rare occurrence. If the orthopedic surgeon suspects that this will happen, the effects of compressing the fracture line should be tested prior to the insertion of a screw. By carefullly closing a pointed reduction forceps across the position where the screw is intended to go, the fragments are observed to see whether compression or collapse of the fragments will occur. If collapse of the fragments occurs, then a screw with position function is inserted (Fig. 2.11). In this instance, thread holes are drilled in the cortex of both the far and near fragments. Both holes are tapped to the appropriate size and when the screw is inserted, the position of the two fragments is maintained. There will be an insignificant amount of distraction along the fracture line with the use of a position screw.

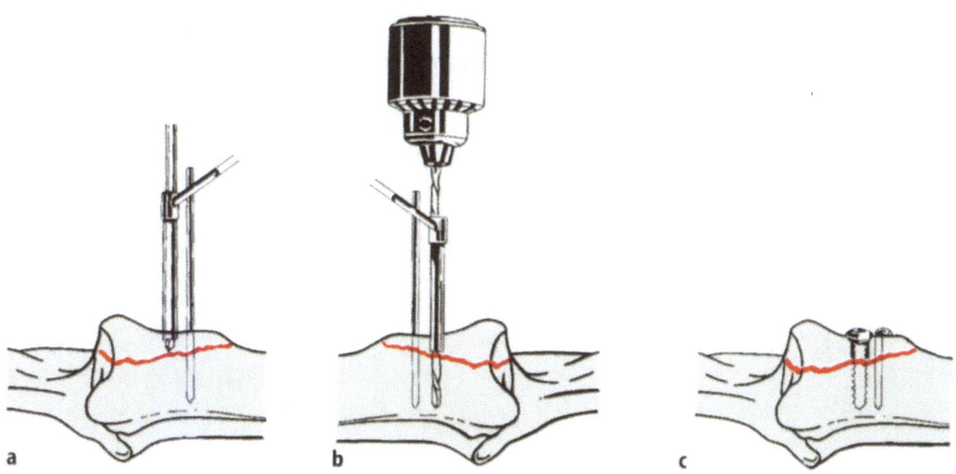

Fig. 2.9a–c. Screw fixation after exact fragment reduction. **a** The fracture is initially reduced and then stabilized with bone forceps and a Kirschner wire to avoid rotation. **b** A glide hole is drilled parallel to the wire. The thread hold is drilled with the aid of the insert sleeve. **c** After the hole has been measured and tapped, a cortex screw is inserted and tightened. The Kirschner wire is bent first and then cut

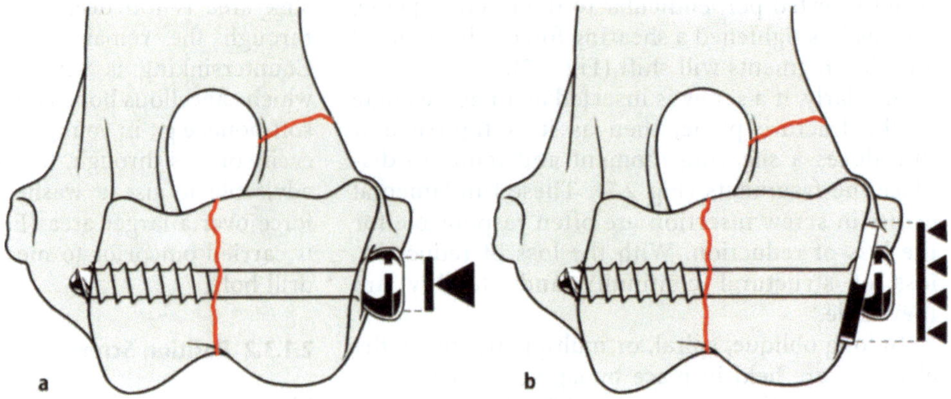

Fig. 2.10. **a** When using a screw in the epiphysis where the cortex over the cancellous bone is very thin, countersinking is to be avoided. **b** In young dogs with soft bony tissue, a washer will distribute the pressure of the screw head to a larger area.

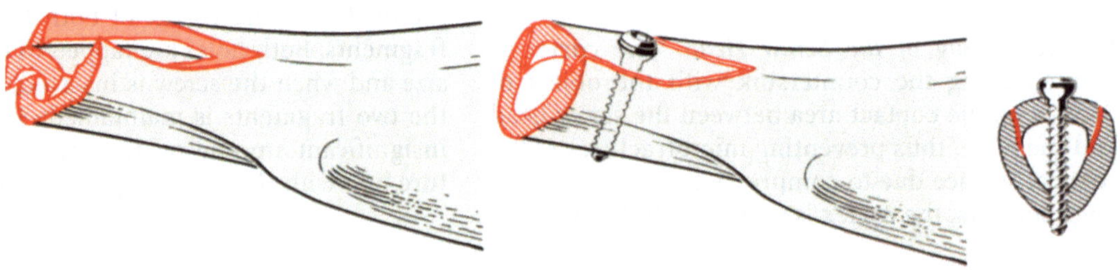

Fig. 2.11. The steps for inserting a position screw. The fragments are reduced and maintained in position. Both fragments are drilled with thread holes, measured, and tapped. The inserted screw will avoid collapsing of the fragment

2.2 Plates

2.2.1 Function

Plates are devices which are fastened to bone for the purpose of providing fixation. They are principally differentiated by their function. Thus there are neutralization plates, buttress plates, static compression plates, and dynamic compression plates. The shape of the plate is an adaptation of the plate to the local anatomy and does not denote any function. A plate may have more than one function in a given fracture repair.

2.2.2 Plate Types

2.2.2.1 Neutralization Plates

Whenever the internal fixation of a diaphyseal fracture consists of a lag screw or screws in combination with a plate whose function is to protect the lag screw fixation, we refer to the plate as a protection or neutralization plate. Lag screw fixation alone is not able to withstand much loading. In order to allow patients early movement of the limbs after internal fixation as well as limited loading, it is necessary to protect most fracture zones fixed by lag screws with a plate. Such a plate protects the interfragmental compression achieved with the lag screw or screws from all torsional, bending, and shearing forces. It is important to emphasize that the lag screw is responsible for interfragmentary stability and not the plate. A plate, even if it exerts axial compression, can never achieve the same degree of interfragmentary stability as a lag screw.

A wedge fracture is first reduced and fixed with lag screws (Fig. 2.12). A carefully contoured plate is then fixed to the two main fragments with a minimum of two to four screws. The type of plate and the number of screws will depend on the bone being fixed and on the quality of the bone. A lag screw can also be inserted through the plate (Fig. 2.13). The combination of lag screws and a plate is the commonest type of internal fixation of diaphyseal fractures when screws and plates are used for their fixation.

It must be appreciated that a plate can perform more than one function at any one time. Thus a neutralization plate can serve as a compression plate if the geometry of the fracture permits (Fig. 2.12). Whenever possible, an implant should

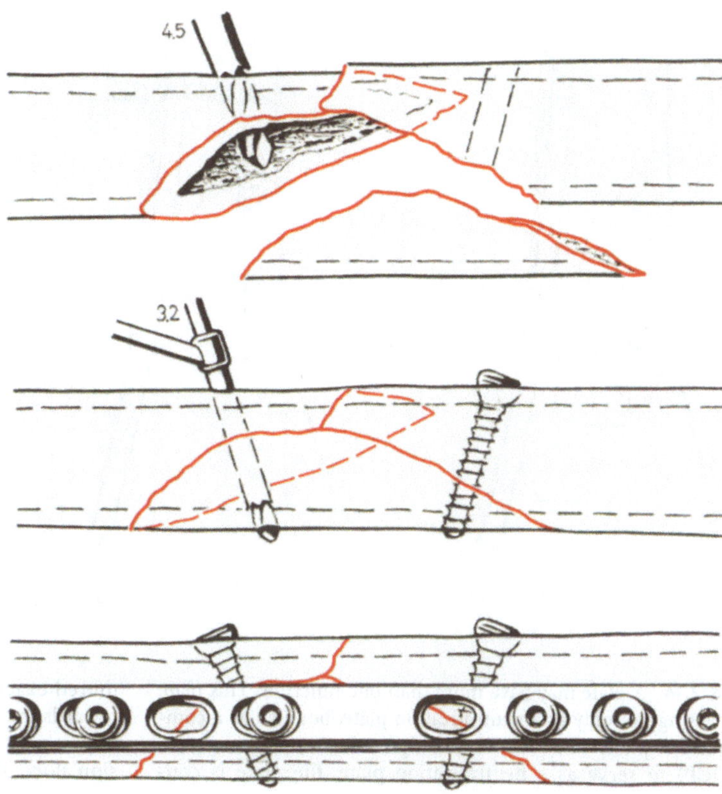

Fig. 2.12. Note that, in this wedge fracture, primary stability is achieved with the lag screws and not the plate. A plate serves only to protect the lag screws

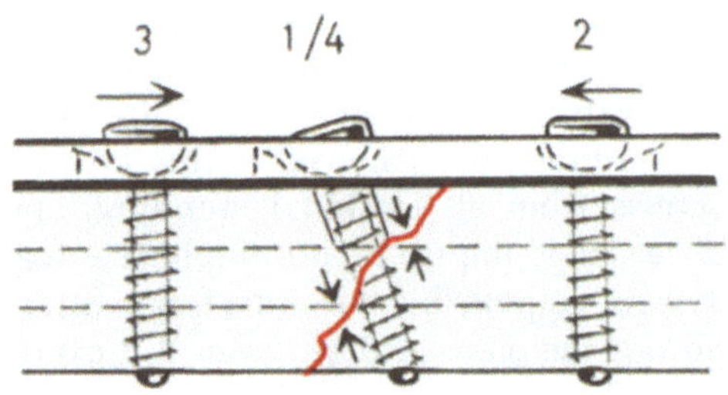

Fig. 2.13. A lag screw can be inserted through the plate once axial compression has been generated. This greatly increases the stability of the fixation

be prestressed. This brings the bone under compression, increases the stability of the fixation, and greatly protects the implant from overload and failure. By virtue of its design, when the fracture is reduced, the DCP automatically exerts some axial compression even with the screws inserted in a neutral position. The plates must not only correspond to the bend in the shaft of the bone, but as the metaphyseal areas are approached, the plates must often follow a twist as well (Fig. 2.14).

2.2.2.2 Buttress Plates

One of the commonest applications of lag screw fixation is in the reconstruction of epiphyseal and metaphyseal fractures. Epiphyseal and metaphyseal areas of bone consist of large areas of cancellous bone surrounded by a thin shell of cortex. As a result of loading, they are also subjected to compressive and shearing forces. If the fracture is in the metaphysis and the cortical shell has been comminuted, the compressive forces tend to lead to an axial deviation or bending. Lag screw fixation cannot overcome these deforming forces of shear and bending. In order to prevent deformity, it is necessary to supplement the fixation with a buttress plate. The function of the buttress plate is simply to prevent axial deformity as a result of shear or bend-

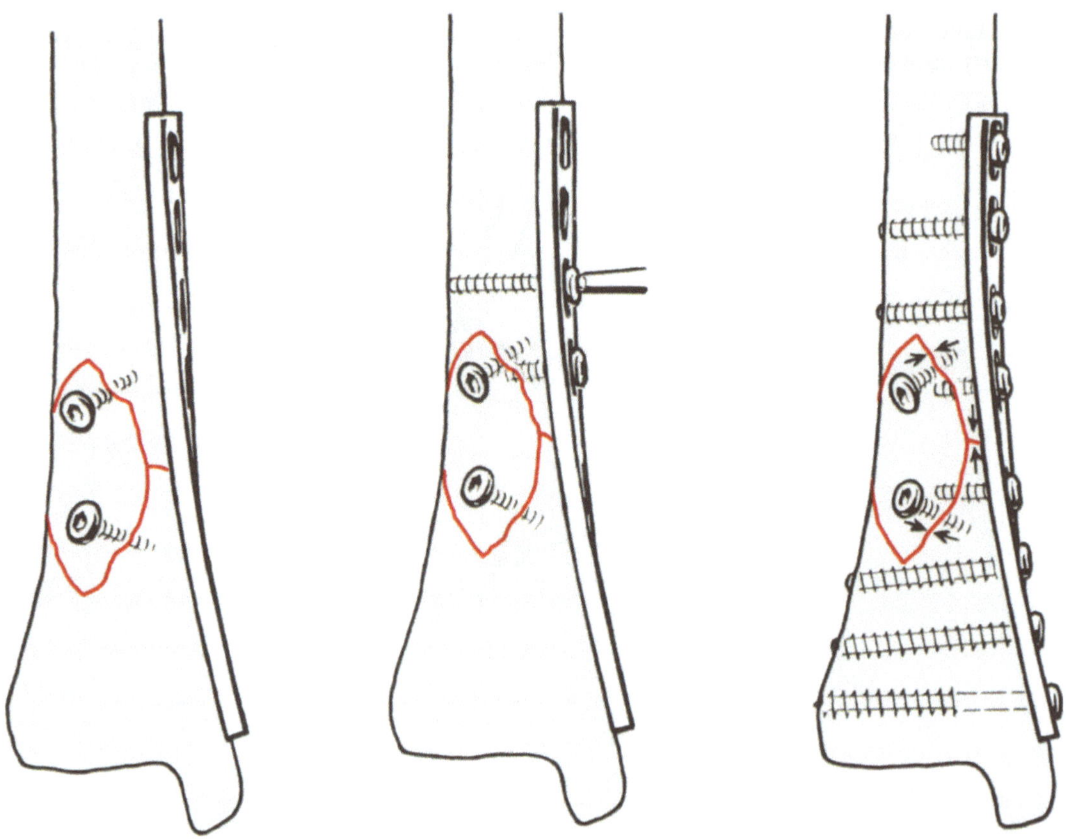

Fig. 2.14. A plate may have more than one function. This plate is acting not only as a neutralization plate, but also as a compression plate. In order for this dynamic compression plate (DCP) to serve as a neutralization plate, the plate is contoured exactly and the screws are inserted from the fracture towards the ends of the plate. As the neutral drill guide places the screws 0.1 mm away from the end of the dynamic compression slope, they cause some axial compression

ing. Thus it must be applied to the area or cortex which has been broken and which is coming under load.

In shaft fractures, the plate with buttress (bridging) function is used when local transmsission surfaces cannot be reconstructed.

The plate maintains alignment of highly comminuted segments of bone. A plate is used in this manner when lag screw fixation of the individual fragments would result in their devitalization or when there is an actual gap and the plate is used to maintain the relative position of the fragments. This type of plate fixation is subjected to full loading. Therefore, every possible effort should be made to maintain all the soft tissue attachments and blood supply of the intervening comminuted fragments, since union will depend on the formation of a bridging callus rather than primary bone union. In these situations, techniques of indirect reduction are particularly useful. Both plate ends have to be solidly fixed to their corresponding part of the bone by two or more screws.

Technical Guidelines for Application. As the function of the buttress plate is to support, it must be firmly anchored to the main fragment, but need not necessarily be fixed with screws to the fragment that it is supporting. It must also correspond very accurately to the shape of the underlying cortex; otherwise, a deformity might ensue. The order and manner in which the screws are inserted through a buttress plate are also important.

The screws must be inserted in such a way that under load there must be no shift in the position of the plate. Thus if the plate which is being used has oval holes, e.g., the DCP, the limited-compression DCP (LC-DCP), or reconstruction plates, then the screws fixing the plate to the shaft must be positioned in the screw holes of the plate close to the fracture (see Fig. 2.19c). In this position, as the load is applied, any tendency for the plate to shift is immediately arrested by the screws.

The recommended method of applying a buttress plate is first to contour it very accurately to the segment of bone and then to begin its fixation to the bone in the middle of the plate and to advance the insertion of screws in an orderly fashion one after another towards both ends of the plate.

It should be noted that any plate that is carefully contoured to the shape of the bone can act as a buttress plate.

Great care must be exercised when buttress plates are used in subcutaneous areas. Problems with wound healing have been encountered in such areas as the medial side of the distal tibia. The surgeon must therefore avoid putting these plates under

Fig. 2.15a–f. Articulated tension device with a pressure gauge and an excursion of 20 mm. The green indicated a compression of 30 kp and the red a compression of 120 kp (colors not shown here). *Note:* This tension device can also be used as a distractor. To be used in this mode, its hook is turned over and the tension device is closed and fixed to bone so that the hook is against the end of the plate. As the tension device is then opened, it pushes against the plate, which is fixed to the other main fragment. This produces distraction of the fracture and can be used to achieve indirect reduction of intermediate fragments by "ligamentotaxis." **b–d** Use of the tension device to compress. **b** The fracture is reduced and the fit of the plate checked. The plate is removed and a 3.2-mm hole is drilled 1 cm from the fracture; its depth is measured through the plate. The hole is tapped and the plate fixed to the bone with a 4.5-mm cortex screw of suitable length. The fracture is reduced and held reduced to the plate with a bone-holding clamp. **c** The hook of the open tension device is engaged in the end hole of the plate and, using the tension device as a guide, a 3.2-mm hole is drilled. After measuring and tapping this hole, the tension device is fixed with a cortex screw to either one or both cortices, depending on the quality of the bone. Osteoporotic bone requires fixation of the tension device to both cortices. With the articulated socket wrench (Kardan key), tightening of the screw of the tension device is begun. This pulls on the plate and causes the fracture to be compressed. **d** Once the tension device is fully tightened, the fracutre is under maximal axial compression. **e, f** Insertion of the remaining screws

Fig. 2.16a–f. Healing of an osteotomy of a dog's radius under compression (drawn from histological material of Schenk). **a** The cortex adjacent to the plate is in contact. There is no ingrowth of mesenchymal cells from either the periosteum or the endosteum. Note that there is a gap in the cortex opposite the plate. **b** The bone ends in contact immediately adjacent to the plate show no changes within the first 3–4 weeks. **c** Opposite the plate, the gap persists. **d** From the fourth week onwards, the bone ends in contact show active haversian remodeling. There is a proliferation of haversian canals, which grow across both living and dead cortex bridging the osteotomy. This is contact healing. **e** The gap in the cortex opposite the plate is invaded by blood vessels, which appear within the first 8 days. These are accompanied by osteoblasts, which deposit osteoid. This gives rise to bone lamellae, which are oriented osteons. This is gap healing. **f** High magnification of a remodeling osteon or "cutting cone" shows resorption and bone formation adjacent to one another. At the head are osteoclasts (*1*) which give rise to a resorption canal, which is then invaded by capillary sprouts (*2*). The circumferentially oriented osteoblasts (*3*) give rise to a new osteon (*4*)

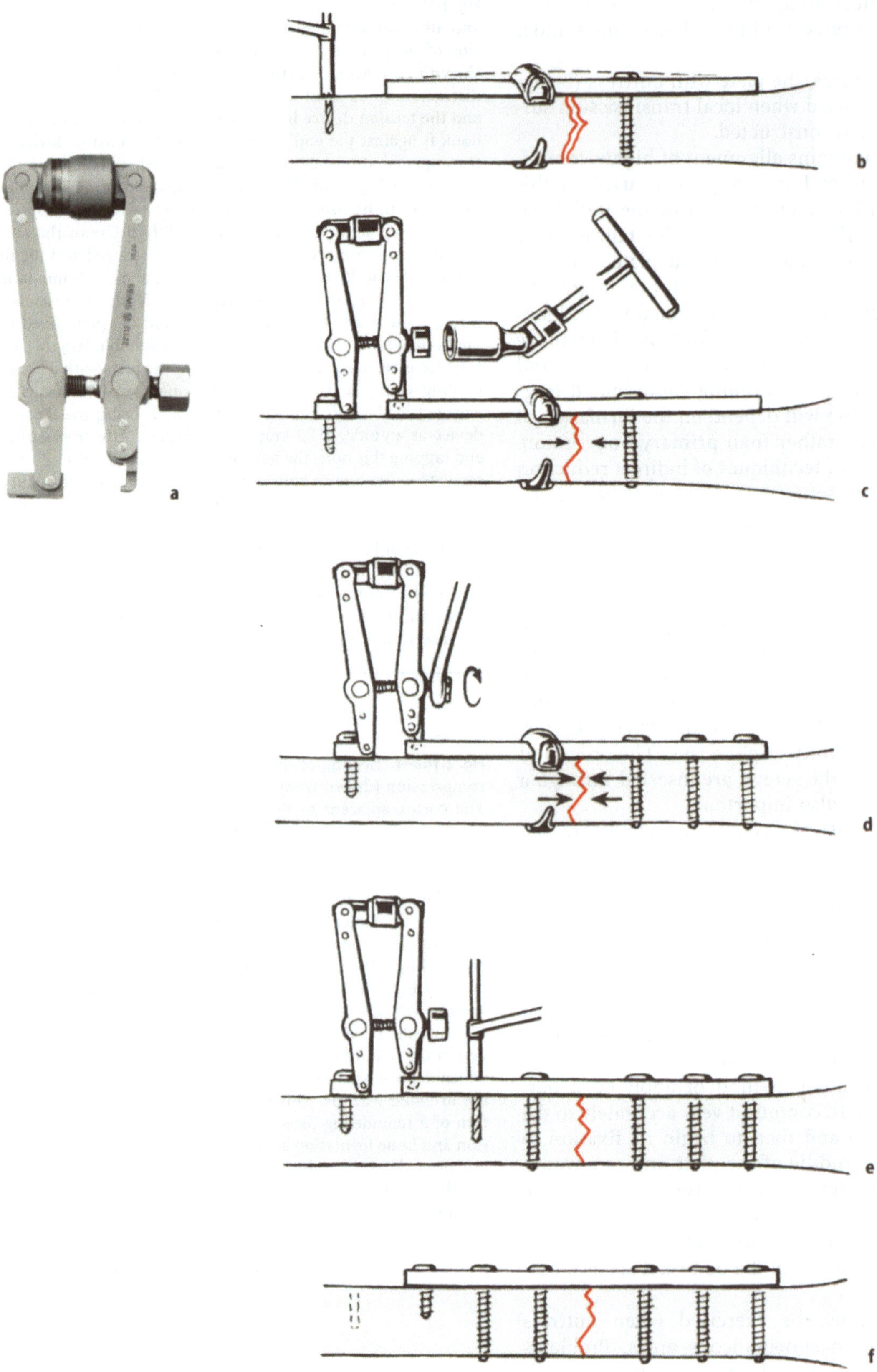

(Fig. 2.15)

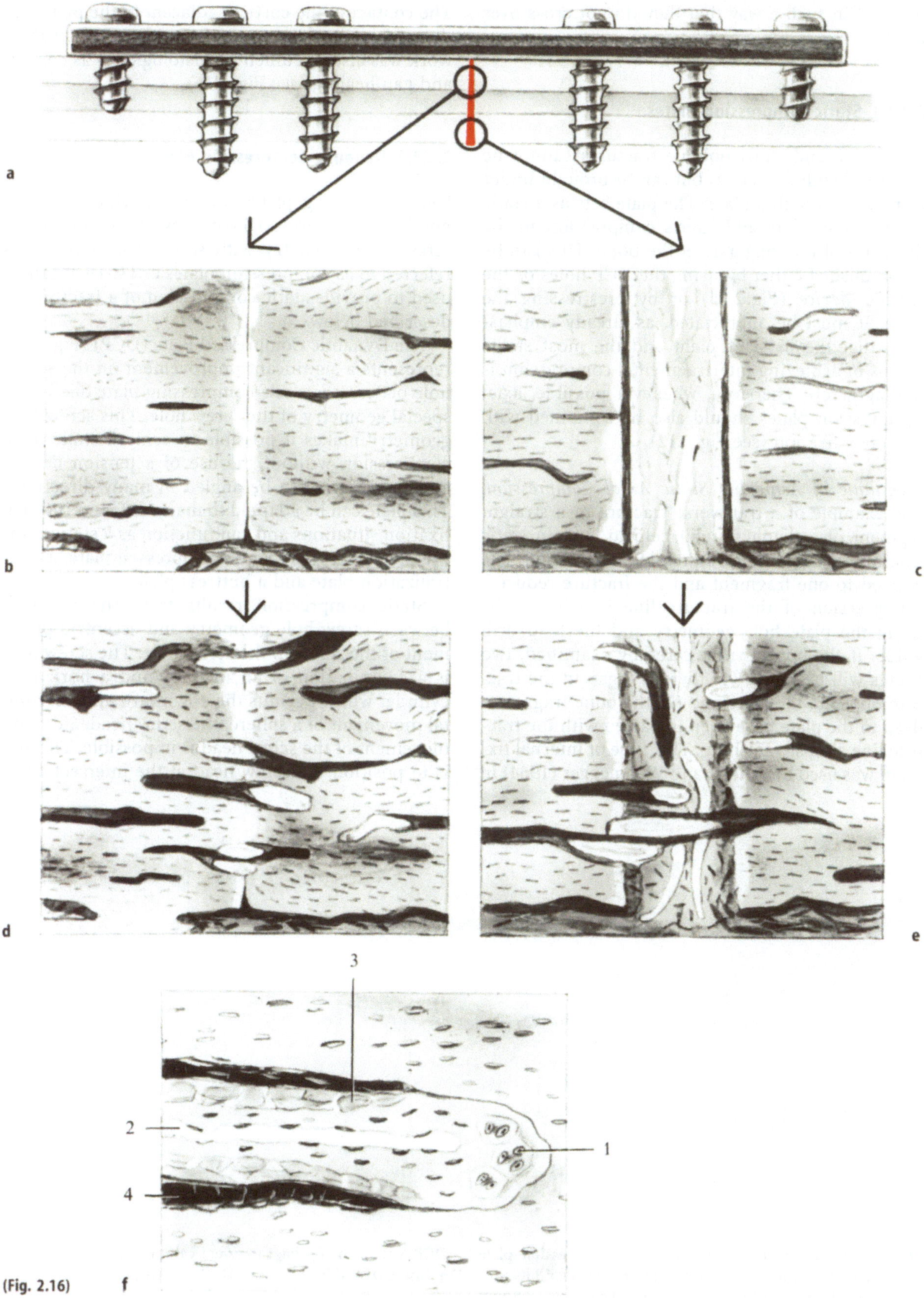

(Fig. 2.16)

badly contused skin flaps, and all incisions must be planned in such a way that they do not cross over plates.

2.2.2.3 Static Compression Plates

Transverse and short oblique fractures cannot be stabilized with lag screws but can be brought under compression with a plate. The plate acts as a static compression plate and exerts compression in the direction of the long axis of the bone. This can be accomplished either by using the DCP holes or the *tension device* (Fig. 2.15) or by prestressing the plate. It must be appreciated, as already emphasized, that the most efficient and the most stable means of achieving interfragmental compression is the lag screw. Therefore, whenever possible, axial compression plates should also be combined with lag screw fixation (see Fig. 2.12).

Technique of Achieving Static Axial Compression. The example of a transverse fracture in a straight segment of a diaphysis will help to explain static axial interfragmental compression. A straight plate is fixed to one fragment and the fracture reduced. Compression of the fracture line is achieved by using the plate hole geometry and the load drill guide. If the bone is now carefully examined, two things will be noted: (1) there is a gap in the fracture opposite the plate and (2) the bone fragments deep to the plate have been impacted with the fracture line almost vanishing. This type of internal fixation was used by Schenk and Willenegger (1964) in their early experiments on primary bone healing. The contact of the cortices adjacent to the plate and the gap in the fracture opposite the plate in their work was also documented histologically as contact and gap healing (see Fig. 2.16).

2.2.2.4 Dynamic Compression Plates

Self-compressing plates are plates which make it possible to achieve axial compression by combining screw hole geometry with screw insertion. Plates referred to as compression plates or LC-DCP can be used to provide static compression of a fracture, as described below.

The Dynamic Compressed Plate (DCP) (Fig. 2.17) represents a significant improvement on the round hole plates. It is a self-compressing plate due to the special geometry of the screw hole. This screw hole geometry makes it possible to achieve static axial compression without the use of a tension device, and the screws can be angled in many directions. This plate can be adapted to many different internal fixation situations and can function as a static compression plate, a dynamic compressed plate, a neutralization plate and a buttress plate.

Static compression results from the interplay between screw hole geometry and eccentric placement of the screw in the screw hole. The screw hole is a combination of an inclined and a horizontal cylinder which permits the downward and horizontal movement of a sphere, the screw head. Sideways movement of the screw head is impossible. The aim is to position the screw head at the intersection of

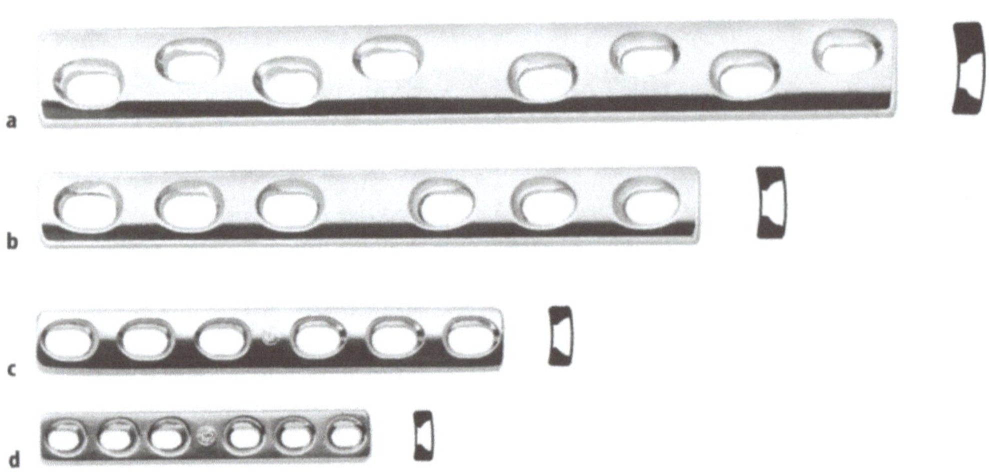

Fig. 2.17. **a** The broad 4.5-mm dynamic compression plate (DCP) and its profile. **b** The narrow 4.5-mm DCP and its profile. **c** The 3.5-mm DCP and its profile. The broad 3.5-mm DCP (not shown) has an identical profile to the narrow 4.5-mm DCP. **d** The 2.7-mm DCP and its profile

the inclined and downward cylinder. At this point, the screw head has a spherical contact in the screw hole, which results in maximum stability without completely blocking the horizontal movement of the screw (Fig. 2.18).

DCP require the use of two drill guides. The neutral drill guide (Fig. 2.19a), which is green, has a central hole for the drill bit. It allows the screw to be inserted in the neutral position, i.e., at the intersection of the two cylinders which make up the screw hole. In this neutral position, the drill guide results in a 0.1-mm loading, so that even when inserted in the neutral position and fully tightened, the screws cause a slight degree of axial compression.

The load guide (Fig. 2.19b), which is yellow, has an eccentric hole for the drill bit, which must be oriented away from the fracture. This results in the load screw being inserted initially 1.0 mm away from the neutral position in the screw hole in the 4.5-mm and 3.5-mm DCP and 0.8 mm in the 2.7-mm DCP. When the screw is tightened, its head slides downwards along the inclined plane of the cylinder as well as horizontally towards the fracture. As the horizontal displacement is resisted by the bone, the horizontal movement results in axial compression of the bone and tension in the plate. Following an anatomic reduction of the fracture with fragment

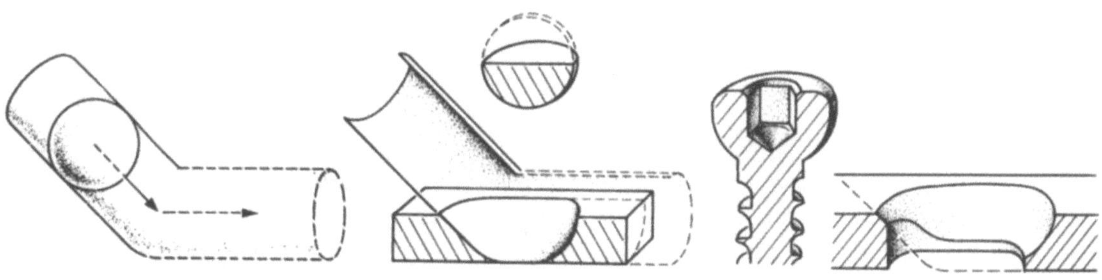

a b c

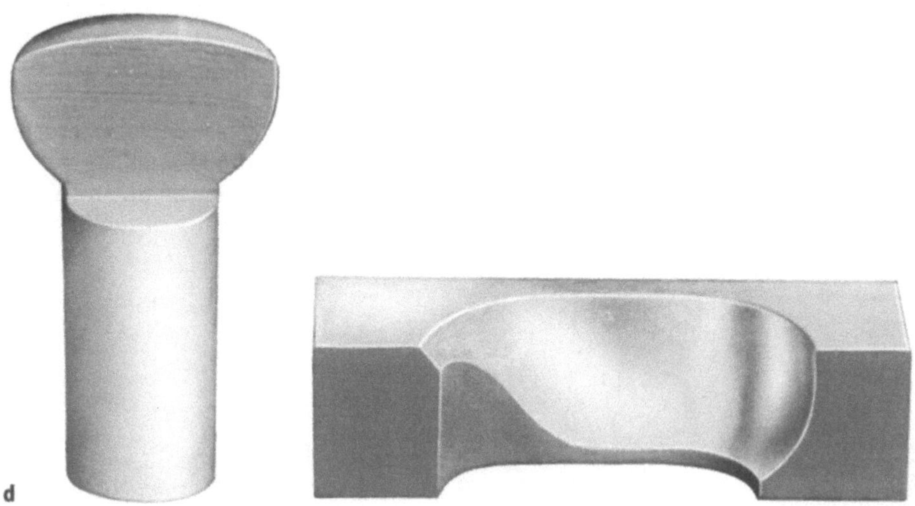

d

Fig. 2.18a–d. The screw hole and the spherical gliding principle. **a** A sphere (the screw head) glides down an inclined cylinder (the screw hole). This combination of downward and horizontal movement of the screw causes a horizontal movement of the underlying bone with respect to the stationary plate. A sideways movement is impossible. The aim is to position the screw head at the intersection of the inclined and horizontal cylinder. At this point, the screw head has a spherical contact in the screw hole, which results in maximum stability without blocking the horizontal movement of the screw towards the fracture. **b** The screw hole is manufactured in such a way that in shape it corresponds to the scheme of the two half-cylinders described in **a.** **c** Here we see the exact representation of the shape of the screw hole. The inclined half-cylinder is for self-compression or self-loading, and the horizontal cylinder is to prevent blocking or obstructing the screw in its horizontal path. This guarantees that only compression will be exerted at the fracture. **d** Sloped gliding hole and its corresponding spherical screw head. In the left portion of the screw hole, we see the inclined load plane, and on the right, the horizontal sliding plane

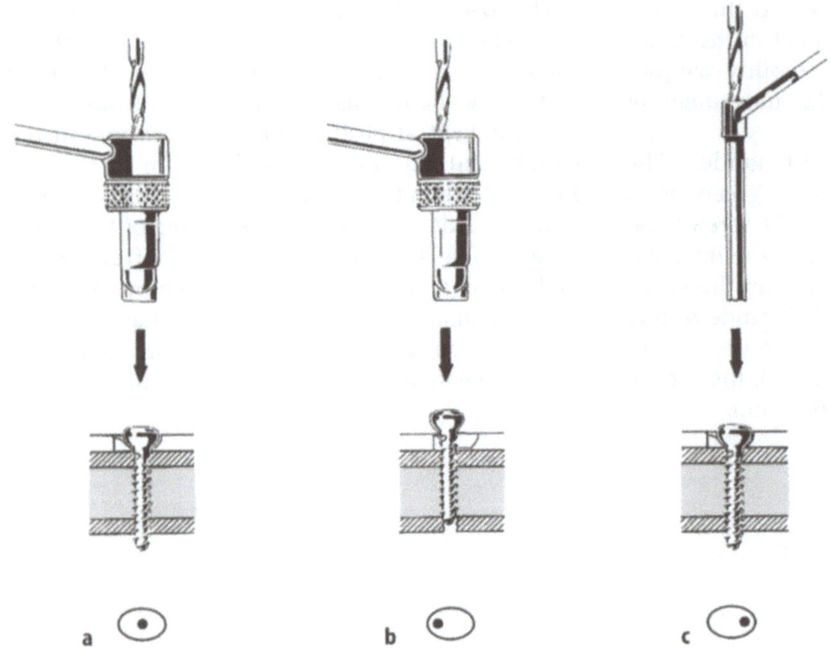

Fig. 2.19a–c. The drill guides for the dynamic compression plate (DCP). **a** Neutral drill guide (green; color not shown here). It places a screw 0.1 mm from the end of the slope, inducing some axial compression. **b** Load drill guide (yellow; color not shown here). It places a screw 1 mm from the end of the slope. **c** The hole for buttress function, drilled using the double drill sleeve

contact, insertion of one screw in the load position results in an axial compression of 50–80 kp. In order to increase the load, i.e., to increase the impaction of the fragments, more than one load screw can be inserted, although this is rarely necessary. When a substantial load is required, as in the case of pseudarthroses, the tension device should be used first.

If the DCP is used as a buttress plate, the appropriate drill sleeve for the cortical screw to be inserted should be used as a drill guide with the sleeve pressed in the end of the screw hole towards the fracture (Fig. 2.19c). The hole is drilled in such a position that when the screw is tightened, its head will be pressed against the plate in the locking position.

As already indicated, the shape of the screw head and of the screw hole in the DCP permits the angulation of screws. This allows a much better adaptation of the screw direction to the particular anatomy of the fracture (Fig. 2.20). It also greatly facilitates the insertion of an oblique lag screw across the plate. It must be stressed again and again that, whenever possible, the stability of the internal

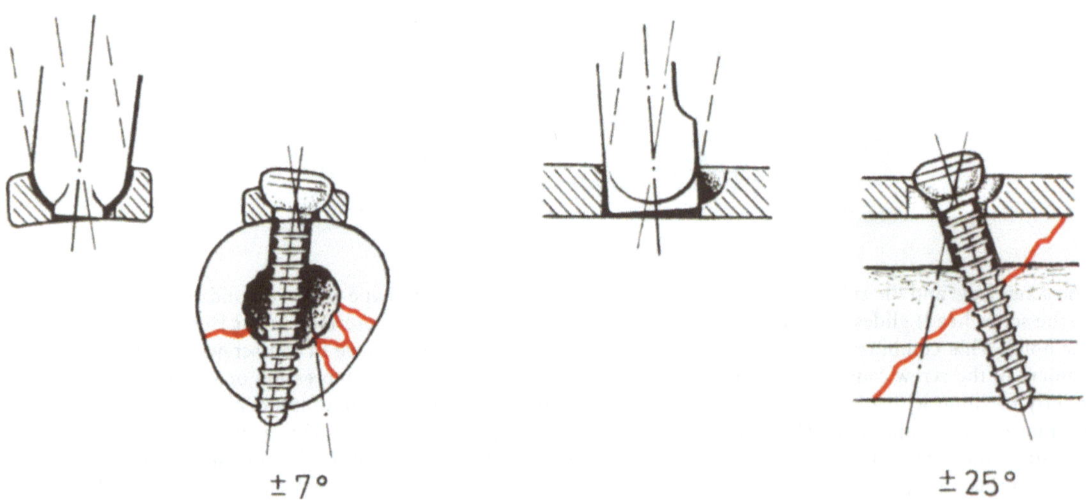

Fig. 2.20. The interplay between the spherical screw head and the geometry of the screw hold permits the angulation of the screws in all directions (maximum 25° longitudinally, 7° sideways)

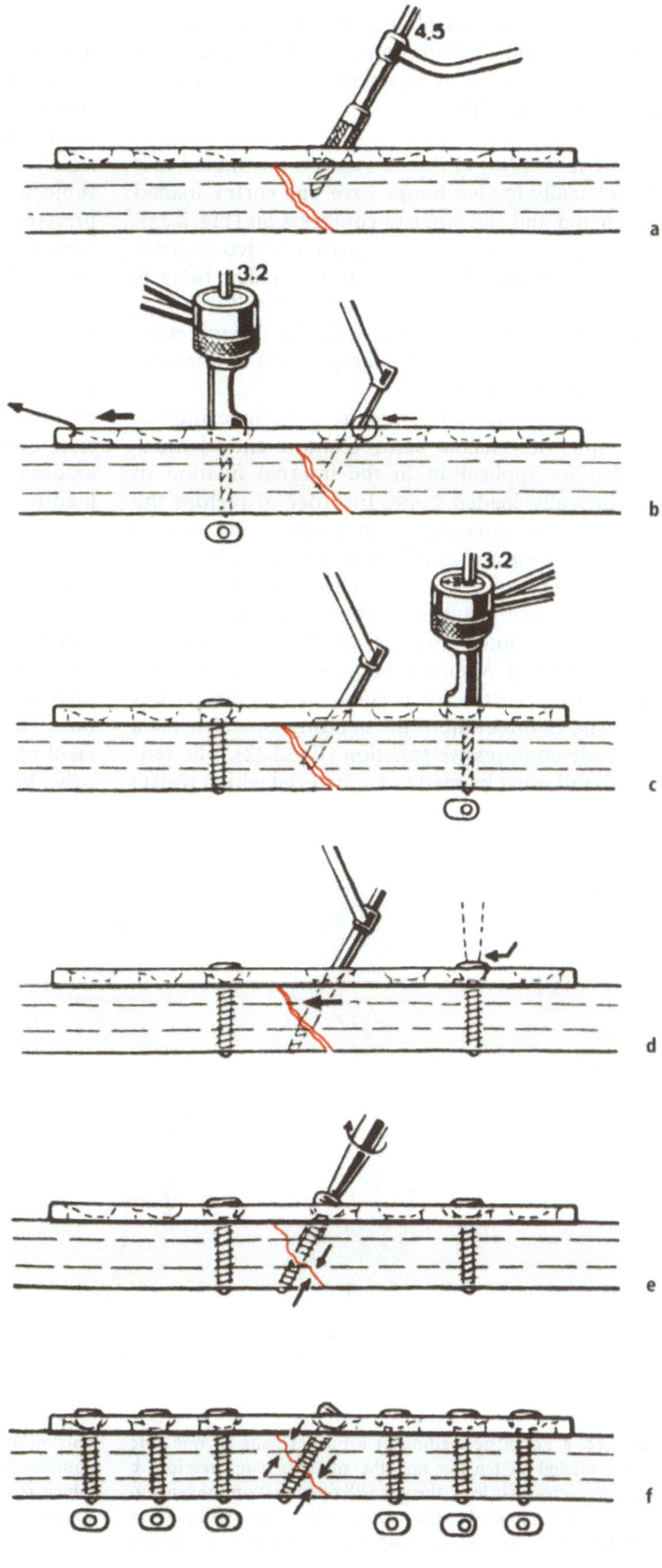

Fig. 2.21a–f. Axial compression fixation of a short oblique fracture with a dynamic compression plate (DCP); maximum angulation, 25° longitudinally, 7° sideways). **a** First the gliding hole is drilled with the 4.5-mm drill bit. **b** The fracture is reduced. The 3.2-mm drill sleeve (3.5/4.5) is inserted through the plate into the predrilled gliding hole and the plate fixed with one screw in a neutral position to the opposite fragment, which subtends an obtuse angle with the fracture plane. Before drilling the 3.5-mm hole, the plate is drawn (*arrow*) towards the fragment so that the 4.5-mm drill guide buttresses against the slope of the plate hole. **c,d** One screw is inserted in the load position into the other fragment. As the screw is tightened, axial compression is generated. **e** The thread hole is drilled for the lag screw. The lag screw is measured, tapped, and inserted. **f** The remaining screws are inserted in the neutral position

fixation should be enhanced by the insertion of a lag screw through the plate across the main fracture line. This applies when the plate is being used as a neutralization plate, but even more so if it is used as a compression plate.

Eccentric Loading of Bones. Pauwels postulated that eccentrically loaded bones have one cortex loaded in tension and the other in compression (Fig. 2.22). This postulate has now been proven in vivo (Schatzker et al. 1980). The eccentrically loaded bone is subjected to bending stresses which result in a typical distribution of stresses, with the tension coming on the convex side and compression on the concave side of the bone.

Pauwels (1935) borrowed from engineering the principle of tension band fixation and demonstrated its application in the internal fixation of eccentrically loaded bone. In order to restore the load-bearing capacity of an eccentrically loaded fractured bone and to minimize the forces borne by the fixation device, it is necessary to absorb the tensile forces, the result of the bending moment, and convert them into compressive forces. This requires a tension band. A tension band is therefore a device which will exert a force equal in magnitude but opposite in direction to the bending force. This is a dynamic compressive function (Fig. 2.22). The tension band must be made of a material which resists tensile forces and which can be prestressed. The bone must be able to withstand compression. This means that the bone must not be comminuted either under or on the opposite side from the tension band. The prestressing of a plate (or wire) in tension will result, as we have already learned, in axial compression of the bone. If such a bone is now subjected to eccentric loading, e.g., the femur, the prestressing of the tension band plate will resist the tensile forces and convert them into compressive forces. This will result in a simultaneous increase and uniform distribution of compressive forces across the fracture. The dynamic component of the compression rises when the bone is loaded and subjected to bending. The prestress in the tension band ensures that the bone remains loaded in compression even when the dynamic component of the loading is removed. Thus the fluctuations in the load magnitude of compression are directly related to cyclical loading (see also Sect. 2.2.4).

As already indicated, the prerequisites for dynamic compression are the following: (a) a plate or wire able to withstand the tensile forces, (b) bone which is able to withstand compression, (c) an intact buttress of the opposite cortex, and (d) a plate (or wire) applied to the tension side of the bone. If the buttress (the opposite cortex) is deficient under load, the plate will be subjected to repetitive bending, will suffer fatigue, and will break.

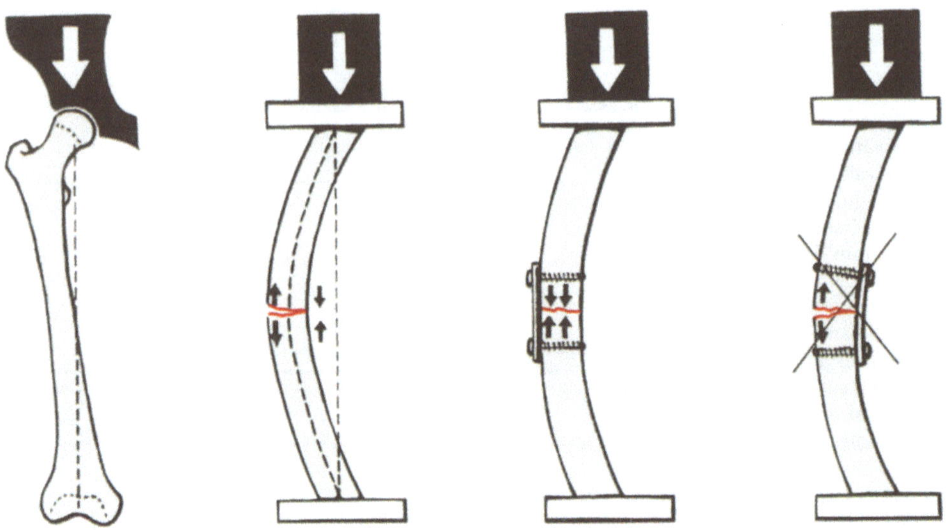

a b c d

Fig. 2.22. **a** Eccentric loading of a bone results in one side being loaded in tension and the other in compression. **b** Under an eccentric load, the gap will open first on the tension side. **c** A plate applied to the tension side of bone will prevent the deformity. As load increases, the plate will be put under tension and the cortex opposite the plate will come under compression. **d** If the plate is applied to the concave side which is under compression, under load the only resistance to deformity is the stiffness of the plate

Shortcomings. The DCP has not only proved to be more versatile than the round hole plate, but has also ensured the elimination of the inconsistencies in achieving successful axial loading which were seen with the round hole plate. Although the DCP has withstood the test of time, over the years certain shortcomings have become apparent.

- *Inclination.* The geometry of the DCP hole is such that, in the long axis, a screw cannot be tilted more than 25° (see Fig. 2.20). This has led to difficulties whenever attempts are made to lag short oblique fractures through the plate and has resulted in less than optimal interfragmental compression.
- *Distribution of plate holes.* The conventional round hole plates had an extended middle segment without holes. When the DCP was designed, this feature was retained without any particular rationale. This middle segment has led to difficulties when a fracture with a zone of fragmentation has to be stabilized. Once the position of the plate has been chosen and the first hole drilled, because the middle segment cannot be displaced, it becomes impossible to shift the plate in the long axis of the bone. The drill hole in bone will not fit the plate holes even if the new position of the plate suits the overall fixation better. Under these circumstances, the only solution for the surgeon is a longer plate.
- *Fragile lining.* Plates with a rectangular cross-section lead to the formation of a comparatively thin bony wall along the length of the plate. These longitudinal ridges add to the strength of the bone when the plates are removed. If the ridges thus formed are thin, they are easily nicked at the time of plate removal. This not only renders the bone less strong, but may also act as a stress raiser and contribute to failure.

Solutions to the Problems. The following solutions to the problems associated with DCP have been proposed:

- *Structured undersurface resulting in improved circulation.* Extensive animal studies have shown that grooves in the undersurface of plates significantly improve the blood supply of plated bony segments (Joerger 1987). To be effective, such grooves must be of adequate depth and width. As a corollary to the improvement in the periosteal blood supply and cortical blood supply, the osteoporosis which was said to have been the result of the so-called stress shielding has disappeared. This plate-related osteoporosis has been shown conclusively to be the result of the initial vascular insult and consequent avascular necrosis which then provoked corresponding florid bone remodeling (Fig. 2.23c).
- *Undercut screw holes.* Each screw hole has been fitted out with oblique undercuts at both ends (Fig. 2.23b,c). This allows a screw to be tilted up to 40° in each direction of the long axis of the bone. This has greatly eased the passing of lag screws through the plate, particularly when lagging short oblique fractures. In addition, it has contributed to a significant reduction in the contact area of the plate with bone.
- *Uniform spacing of screw holes.* The uniform spacing of screw holes and the elimination of the middle segment allows for easy shifting of the plates in the long axis as well as easy changes in the plate length (Fig. 2.23a,b)
- *Trapezoid cross-section.* The trapezoid cross-section of the plate with the smaller surface in contact with the bone has resulted in the formation of lower and broader ridges of bone along the length of the plate than those previously observed with the plates with a rectangular cross-section. Such ridges are less likely to be injured at the time of plate removal (Fig. 2.23d).
- *Additional new compressing principle.* The basic spherical gliding principle of the screw within the screw hole of the DCP has been preserved, but the screw hole has been redesigned so that this feature is present at both ends of the hole. This improves the versatility of the plate when complex fractures are being fixed.
- *Avoidance of bone damage and improvement in compression.* Whenever a lag screw is passed through a DCP screw hole to lag a fracture, it is subjected to a translational force which tends to shift the screw head towards the buttress position as the screw is tightened. This may give rise to one of two complications: (1) either the screw head or thread may abut against the inner wall of the plate hole; because of friction, this may significantly reduce axial compression, and it may also damage the plate or the screw; (2) the thread of the screw may bite on one side into the wall of the gliding hole, which may reduce the lag effect by as much as 37% (Klaue 1982). The use of an elongated and undercut screw hole together with a newly designed partially threaded cortex screw whose shaft diameter equals the outer diameter of the screw thread avoids these complications.

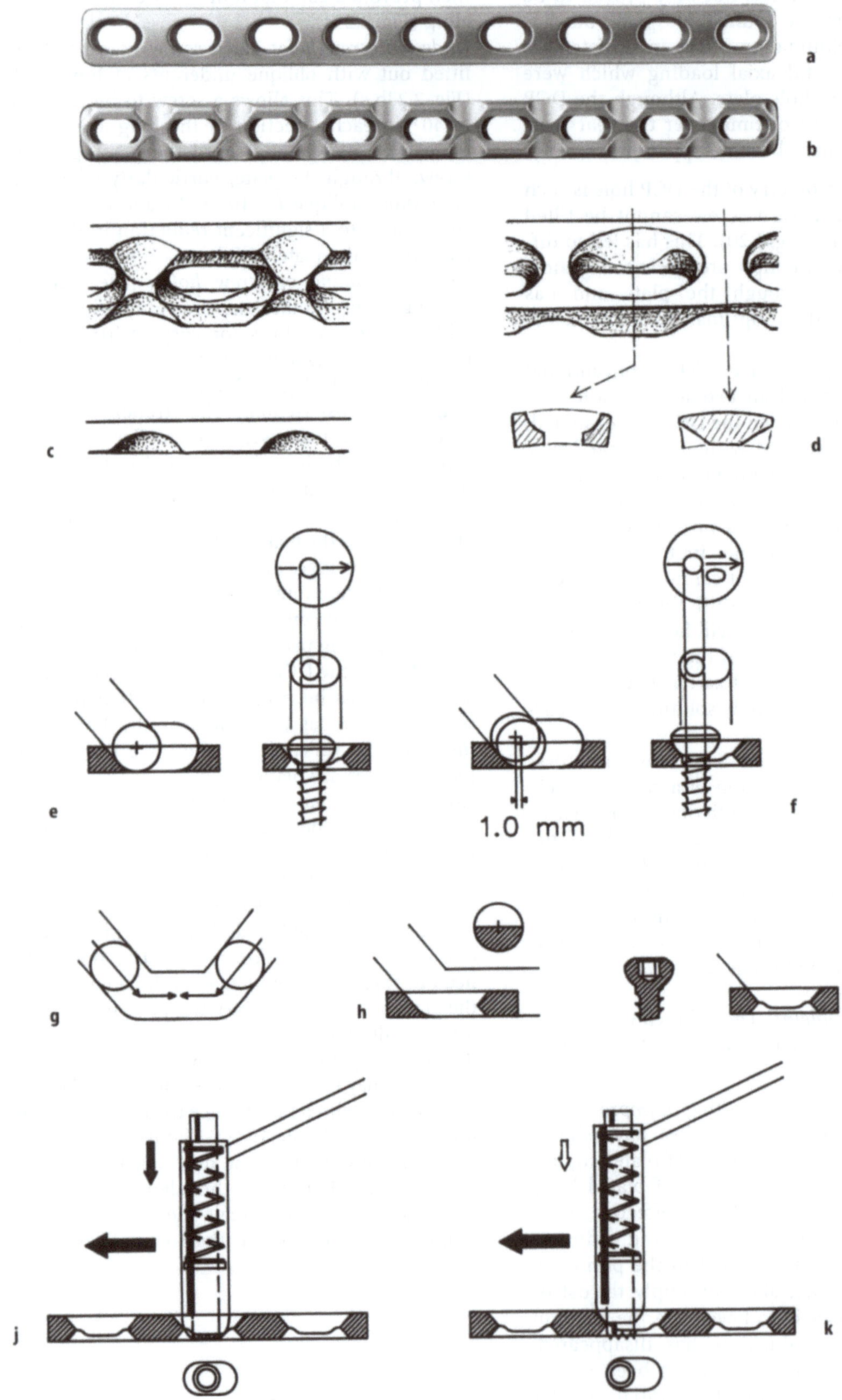
a
b
c
d
e
1.0 mm
f
g
h
i
j
k

◀ **Fig. 2.23a–k.** The limited-contact dynamic compression plate (LC-DCP). **a** Surface of the plate. **b** Undersurface of the plate. **c** Note the oblique undercuts at both ends of each screw hole. This permits a maximum tilting of the screw of 40° in each direction in the long axis of the bone. **d** Note the trapezoid cross-section of the plate and the undercuts between the screw holes. The different undercuts greatly reduce the contact area between the plate and the bone. **e** The LC-DCP screw hole acts in a similar way as that of the DCP: the position of the screw is neutral, i.e., at the intersection of the inclined cylinder with the horizontal cylinder. **f** Using the load guide results in a maximal compressive displacement of 1.0 mm. **g** Detail of the construction of the screw hole composed of three cylinders meeting at obtuse angles. **h** The inclined cylinder of one side and the horizontal one within the plate hole with more marked undercut. **i** The screw with spherical undersurface always provides a congruent fit between screw head and plate hole. The plate hole with two symmetrically opposed inclined compression slides. **j** The universal plate drill guide used for neutral positioning of the screw. When the universal plate drill guide is pressed down, the screw head is positioned onto the horizontal cylinder (neutral buttress position). **k** The universal plate drill guide used for loading positioning of the screw. When the universal plate drill guide is not pressed down, the screw head is positioned onto the inclined cylinder (variable degree of loading; maximum, 1.0 mm)

2.2.2.5 Limited-Contact Dynamic Compression Plates

Conventional Use. The LC-DCP may be used in exactly the same way as the DCP. For the experienced surgeon, there are additional features which provide a definite improvement in plate function.

The plate must be used with the new LC-DCP drill guide (Fig. 2.24–2.27). The old DCP drill guide should not be used. In order to avoid confusion, the handle of the new LC-DCP drill guide is shaped like the plate. A neutral and a load guide are provided within the same instrument. The arrow of both the neutral and the load guide must always point in the direction of the fracture plane to be compressed. The new smooth-shaft screw with its improved efficiency and increased strength should always be used to generate compression either in the load position or as a lag screw (Fig. 2.28c).

Additional Possibilities. The screw hole of the LC-DCP imparts tremendous versatility to the plate. It allows a lag screw to be inclined in an arc of 80° in the long axis of the plate. In addition, it is symmetrical and provides additional compression by taking advantage of the force vector directed towards the fracture line which has been created when the screw head hits the horizontal extension of the screw hole.

Using the neutral LC-DCP drill guide, screws can be inserted in the buttress position. To achieve this, the neutral drill guide is used with the arrow pointing away from the fracture line.

The grooves reduce the stiffness of the plate between the screw holes. This has resulted in a more even distribution of the stiffness of the plate and has made it easier to shape the plate by allowing bending between the screw holes.

Titanium is known to be biologically exceptionally inert and it is therefore well tolerated as an implant material. Commercial pure titanium avoids any potentially toxic components such as vanadium. The mechanical limitations of pure titanium are well known. However, new technical advances in the way titanium is treated have now made it

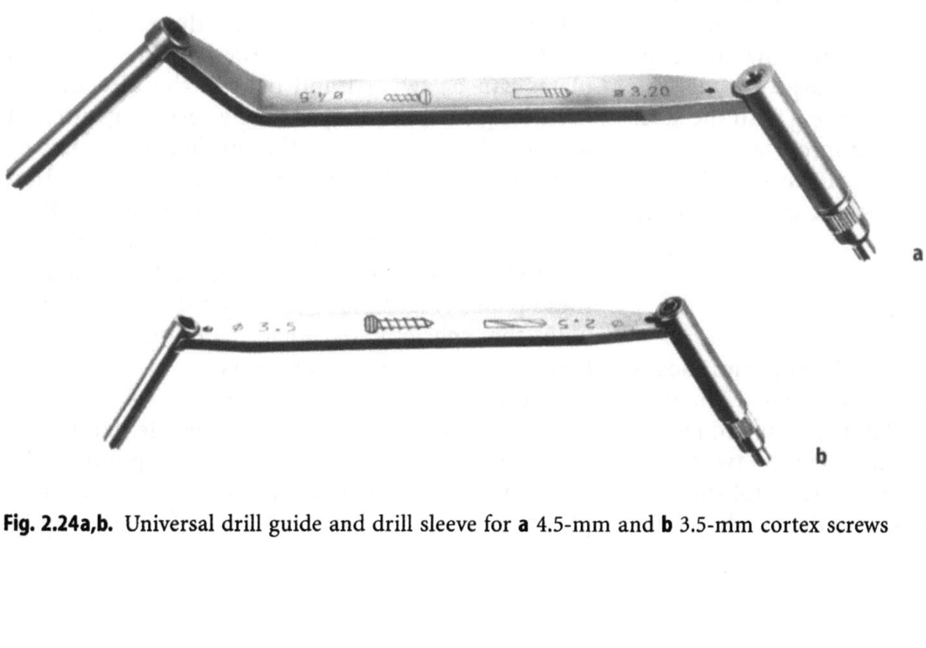

Fig. 2.24a,b. Universal drill guide and drill sleeve for **a** 4.5-mm and **b** 3.5-mm cortex screws

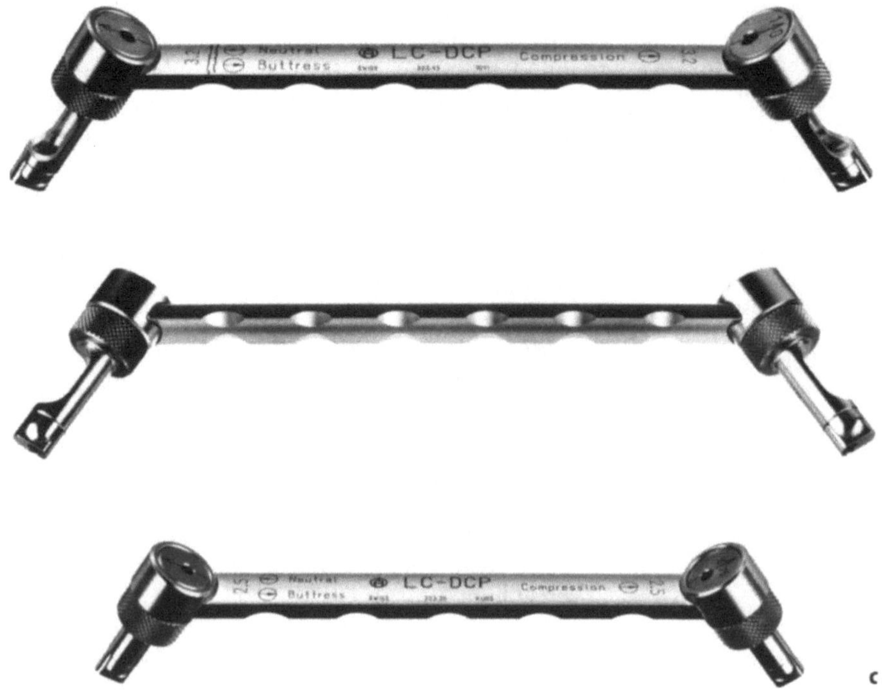

Fig. 2.25a–c. Double drill guide for the 4.5-mm and 3.5-mm cortex screws. Each guide is provided with two inserts, one green one (color not shown here) guiding the drill bit to the neutral position, and one yellow one (color not shown here) guiding it to the load position (1.0 mm). **a** The 4.5-mm drill guide viewed from above. Both drill guides are provided with arrows. These should always point to the fracture or osteotomy. **b** View from below. The undercuts should remind the user that this drill guide should be used with the limited-contact dynamic compression plate (LC-DCP). **c** The 3.5-mm drill guide viewed from above

possible for titanium to reach 90 % of the strength of the stainless steel used for implants. Thus titanium appears to be the best metal from the point of view of tissue tolerance and avoidance of low-grade immunological complications.

The cost of titanium implants and the relatively short life of veterinary patients, in most cases, precludes their use in orthopaedic surgery in small animals. However, as LC-DCP are now made in stainless steel, the veterinary surgeon has the option of choosing to use them, along with the steel shaft screw, where the latter is appropriate.

All these additional features of the LC-DCP are provided without requiring specific changes in the application technique.

2.2.3 Contouring the Plates

Special contouring devices (Fig. 2.29) permit accurate and controlled shaping of the plates. The new shape is the result of plastic deformation and is permanent. With practice, the plates can be twisted at the time they are bent. This is accomplished by inserting the plate at an angle into the bending plier or press. Most of the time, however, the shaping of the plates is carried out using both the bending press or plier and the bending irons. Certain areas of bone, e.g., the pelvis around the acetabulum, the distal humerus, and the mandible, have an extremely complex anatomy, which makes the shaping of normal straight plates such as the DCP extremely difficult. To overcome these difficulties, the AO has developed *reconstruction plates.* Normal plates can be twisted and bent in the direction of their long axis, but they strongly resist any attempt to bend them in the direction of their short axis or width (Fig. 2.30). The design of the reconstruction plate is such that it permits bending about the P–Q axis. Reconstruction plates are available in the 4.5-mm and 3.5-mm configurations. The design of these plates (Fig. 2.31) is such that their contouring with the specially designed bending pliers and bending irons is simple and easy.

The contouring of any plates has been further facilitated by the design of malleable templates. They come in different sizes to correspond to the different plates, such as the 4.5-mm or 3.5-mm plates, and they also come in different lengths

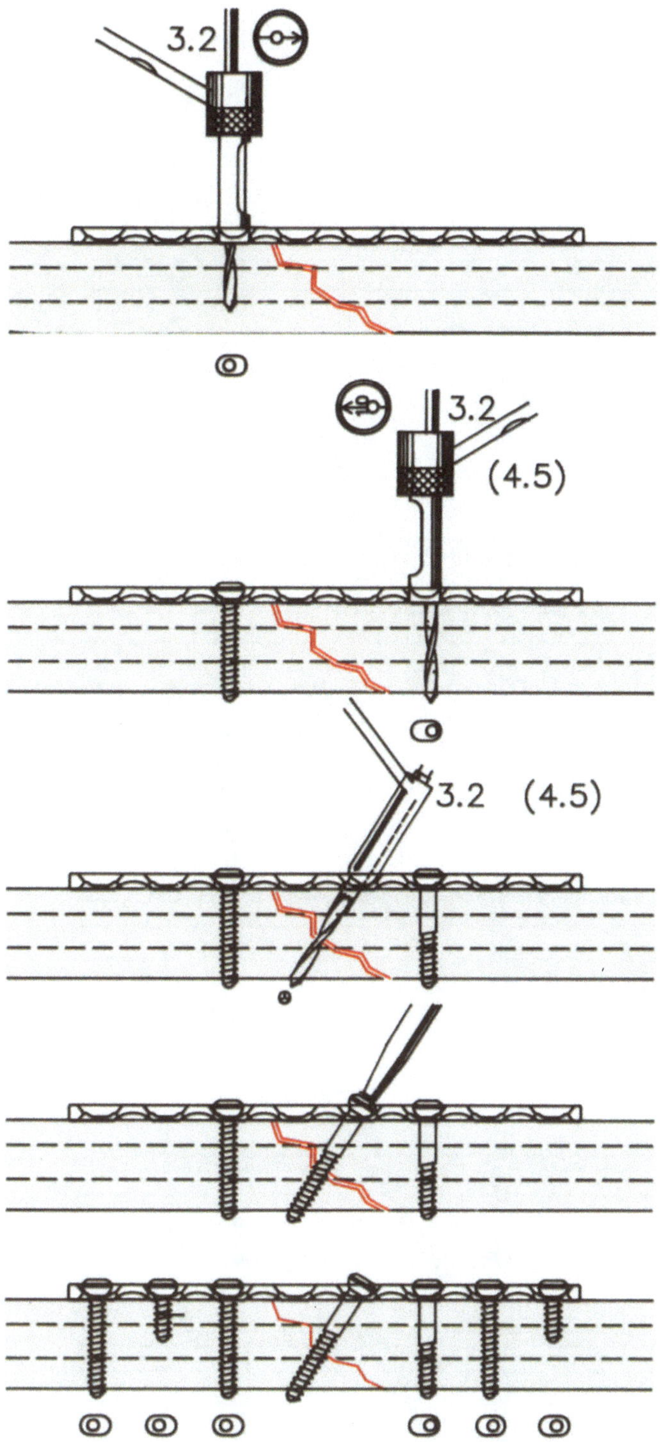

Fig. 2.26a–e. Application of the limited-contact dynamic compression plate (LC-DCP) in steps. Procedure 1. **a** Initially, the fracture is bridged by the plate. Using the neutral drill guide, the first screw is applied to the fragment, which forms an obtuse angle with the fracture near the plate. The resulting space between fracture plane and plate undersurface guides the opposite fragment towards the plate. The *arrow* of the neutral drill guide points towards the fracture. The screw is seated at the neutral position far from the fracture. **b** After adaptation of the fragments, a screw hole for axial compression is drilled in the fragment, which forms an acute angle near the plate. Here the load guide is used. Once again, the *arrow* points towards the fracture line to be compressed. At this position, a shaft screw will be inserted with optimized rigidity and strength (compared with the standard 4.5-mm cortex screw) for axial compression. The same procedure is therefore used as for application of a lag screw. A gliding (4.5-mm) hole and a threaded (3.2-mm) hole are drilled. **c** Using the universal plate drill guide, the threaded (3.2-mm) hole for the lag screw is drilled. It is subsequently overdrilled (4.5 mm) in the near cortex to create a gliding hole. As for any other application in which a drill bit is used in an inclined position, the three-fluted drill bit positions the drill hole more precisely than the conventional two-fluted drill bit. **d** The lag screw and the remaining screws are inserted. **e** Completion of the internal fixation. Some short screws are used if the bone is strong. In porotic and/or small bones, long screws and/or a longer plate may be chosen

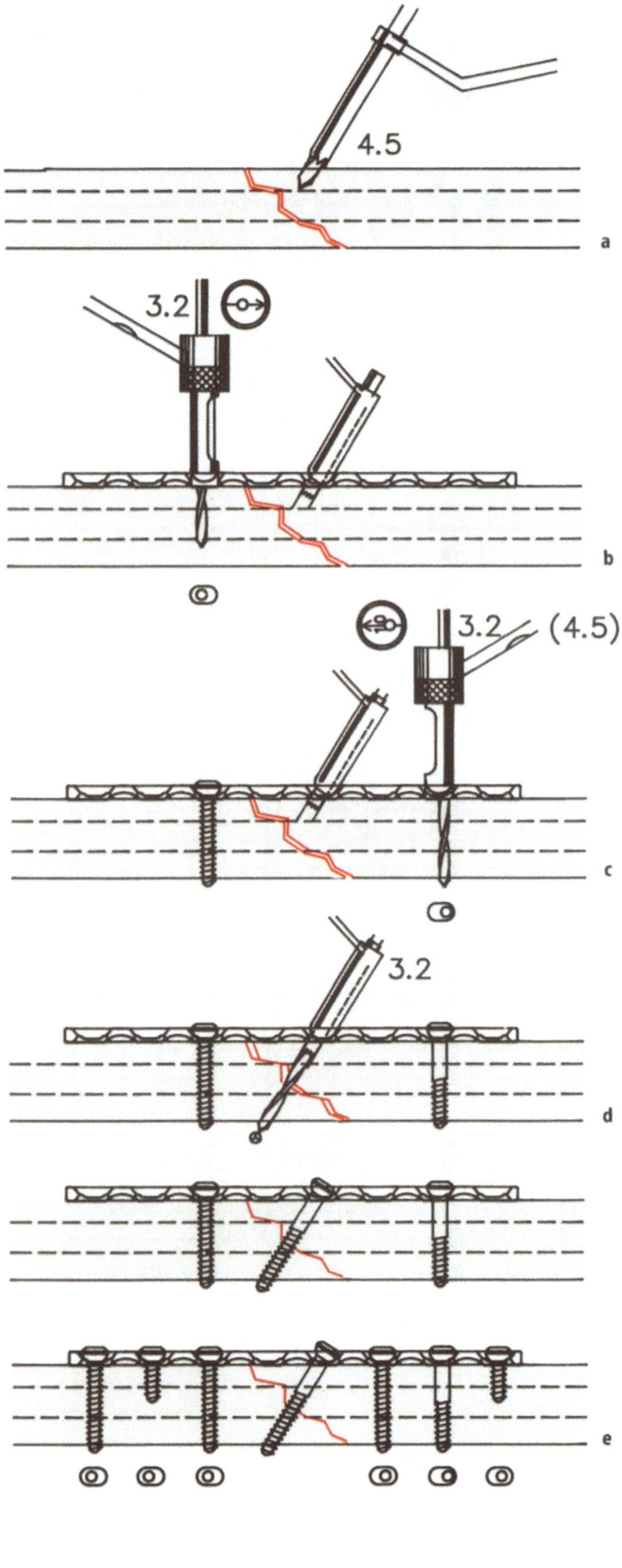

Fig. 2.27a–e. Application of the limited-contact dynamic compression plate (LC-DCP) in steps. Procedure 2. **a** Using the 4.5-mm sleeve connected to the universal plate drill guide, the gliding hole is drilled for the lagged plate screw. **b** The fracture is then bridged by the plate, whereby the tightly inserted universal plate drill guide assures perfect alignment. Using the neutral drill guide, the first screw is inserted into the fragment, which forms an obtuse angle near the plate. The resulting space between fracture plane and plate undersurface guides the opposite fragment towards the plate. **c** With the load drill guide, a screw hole for axial compression is inserted into the fragment, which forms an acute angle near the plate. Here a shaft screw is used. **d** After perfect reduction of the fragments, the lag screw is inserted by drilling the thread hole in the opposite cortex, cutting the thread etc. **e** The subsequent screws are then inserted. Here again, the length and the number of screws chosen varies according to the quality and geometry of the bone and to the pattern of the fracture

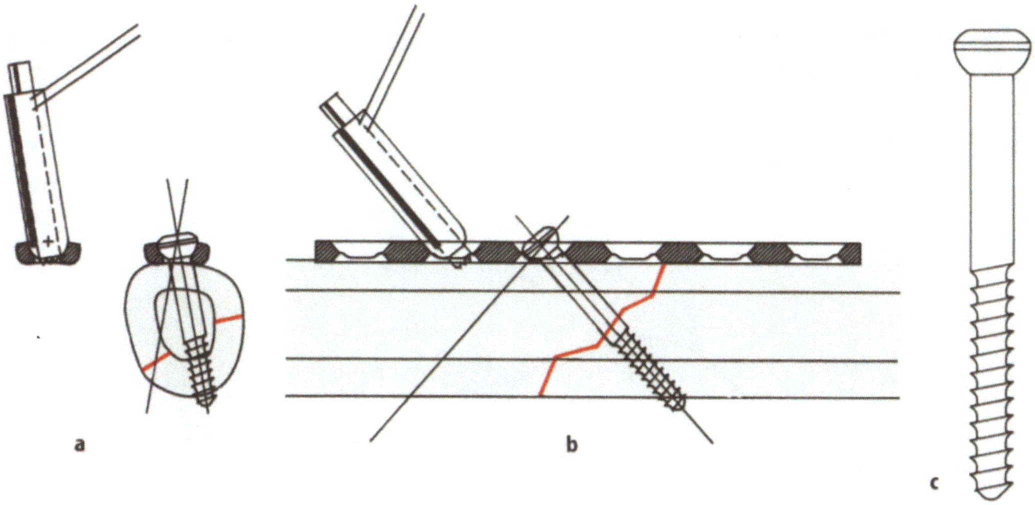

Fig. 2.28a–d. Clinical use of the universal plate drill guide. **a** The universal plate drill guide allows for tilting in a plane perpendicular to the long axis of the plate. It limits the sideways tilting to a maximum of 7 °. **b** It also allows for longitudinal tilting of 40 °. **c** The shaft screw. The thread is 4.5/3 mm wide, and the shaft corresponds to the outer diameter of the thread. This screw offers advantages when used as a lag screw and when used as an axial compression screw (improved stiffness and strength). **d** The equal distance between the screw holes allows easy shifting of the plate at surgery

(Fig. 2.29a). They have been color coded for easy identification. Once reduction has been carried out, the malleable template is laid on the bone and then gently shaped to correspond exactly to the underlying bone (Fig. 2.29). The template is then removed and taken to the contouring device, where the plate is shaped until it corresponds to the template (Fig. 2.29c,f). At the end, the contouring of the plate is checked against the bone and adjusted to make it perfect. In contouring a plate, care should be taken not to bend it back and forth because this weakens the plate.

Radiographs of the opposite normal limb can also be used as an aid to plate contouring. Such radiographs should be taken to show the surface to which the plate is to be contoured.

2.2.4 Overbending

Leaving a gap in the opposite cortex decreases the stability of the fixation. This may result in micromovements with consequent bone resorption. Compression of the opposite cortex can be achieved by overbending the plate, which when pressed against the bone, will act like a spring and close the gap in the opposite cortex (Fig. 2.32). Overbending can be used only when dealing with simple, two-fragment fractures. In complex fractures, overbending will very frequently jeopardize reduction.

When short oblique fractures are fixed with compression plates using the DCP hole and the load guide, the plate must be fixed first to the fragment which subtends an obtuse angle with the fracture plane under the plate (Fig. 2.33). When compression is then applied to the other fragment subtending an acute angle under the plate, this fragment glides under the plate and is pressed against the other fragment, which, by virtue of its fixation to the plate, remains stable.

Biomechanical studies have shown that the bending and rotational stability of "axial compression fixation" of a long oblique fracture can be greatly increased if a lag screw is inserted obliquely through the plate and across the fracture once axial compression has been generated. The increase in stability is due to the greater resistance of the fixation to torsional and bending forces. If there is a transverse or an oblique fracture, fixed with a compression plate, any force which tends to bend the bone and stretch the plate will increase the stability of the fixation. However, if the force is directed in the opposite direction, the only force resisting opening of the fracture is the stiffness of the plate. If there is a lag screw across the fracture, then the tendency of the fracture to open will be resisted by the screw. If the configuration of the fracture is such that the insertion of the screw will interfere with the position of the plate, then the plate should be applied and fixed to the bone as above. The lag screw should then be inserted across the fracture, outside the plate. It still greatly adds to the stability of the fixation, even though it does not go through the plate. One should also remember that axial compression of an oblique fracture by a plate with-

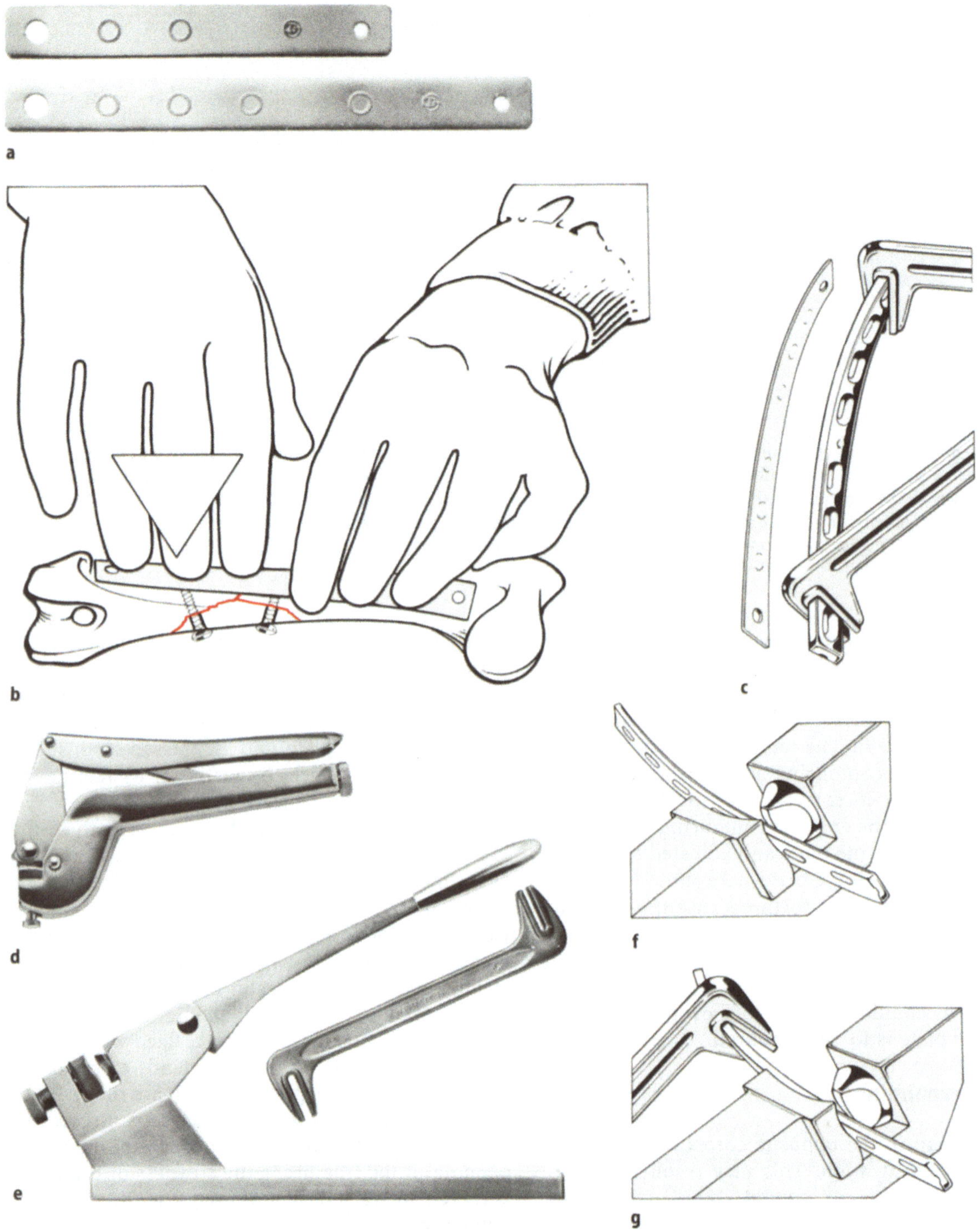

Fig. 2.29a–g. Bending and twisting the plate for a butterfly fracture of the humerus. **a** The colored malleable aluminum templates have the end screw holes punched out. The other screw holes are only marked. **b** After reduction of the fracture and fixation of the butterfly fragment by means of lag screws, the template is placed on the bone and carefully contoured. **c** It will now serve as a template for contouring the plate. **d** Bending pliers. **e** Bending press and twisting irons. **f** The plate is first bent with the bending press. **g** The plate is held in the bending pliers and twisted with the twisting iron. All plates can be bent by means of the bending pliers. If a plate is inserted obliquely into the pliers, both the bend and the twist can be achieved simultaneously

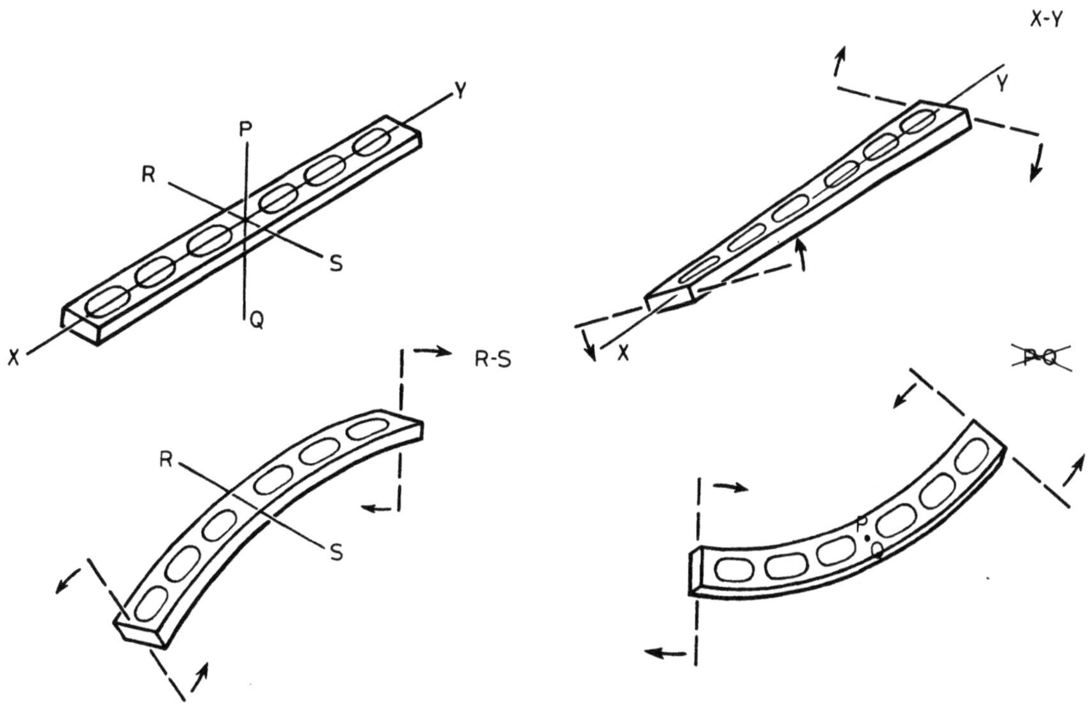

Fig. 2.30. A narrow or a broad dynamic compression plate (DCP) can be twisted about its $X-Y$ axis and bent about its $R-S$ axis. *It resists strongly any attempt to bend it about its $P-Q$ axis*

out an interfragmentary screw may cause the fragments to dislocate. The load must always be applied to the fragment with an acute angle next to the plate. Most of the AO plates can be prestressed. Compression generated using self-compressing plates, e.g., the DCP and LC-DCP, is usually sufficient.

2.2.5 How Many Screws?

Experience has shown that to prevent mechanical failure of plate fixation, a certain number of screws are necessary to secure the plate to the bone. This varies from bone to bone and depends to some degree on the size and weight of the patient and the size and quality of the bone. The number of screws in the plate on either side of the fracture line is very important for the rigidity of fixation of a fracture. A main fracture fragment, under one end of the plate, should never have only one screw in it. This fragment will have only one point of fixation around which it can still rotate. To stop this fragment from rotating, it must have at least two points of fixation and thus at least two screws through two plates holes. Placing two screws beyond the fracture line, in either end of the plate, establishes axial alignment of two main bone fragments. If the mechanical loads acting at the fracture line are potentially high, as occurs with diaphyseal fractures, then two screws per fragment are not adequate. In such a case, a minimum of three screws should be inserted in a fragment. However, if the distance between the end of the bone and the fracture line are insufficient to allow three screws to be placed in the bone fragment, then the minimum number of screws in a fragment becomes two, ensuring axial alignment of the fragment.

One should not feel compelled to fill every hole of the plate with screws. The failure of a plate does not depend on the presence or absence of a screw from a hole, but rather on the presence or absence of a bony defect as well as on its extent. The plate is more likely to fail if the bone defect is short, as this results in considerable stress concentration. This is reflected by the stress concentration around a screw hole in the overlying plate. A plate will fail through a screw hole, since it is the site of the stress concentration as well as the weakest portion of a plate. If the defect in the continuity of the bone is longer, the stresses are distributed over a longer segment and the stress per unit area is correspondingly lower. Thus bridge plating is likely to succeed if the defect is longer, particularly if it is filled with a number of viable bone fragments which will rapidly bridge with callus. If the defect is short, transverse, or oblique, failure is more likely, since there is not

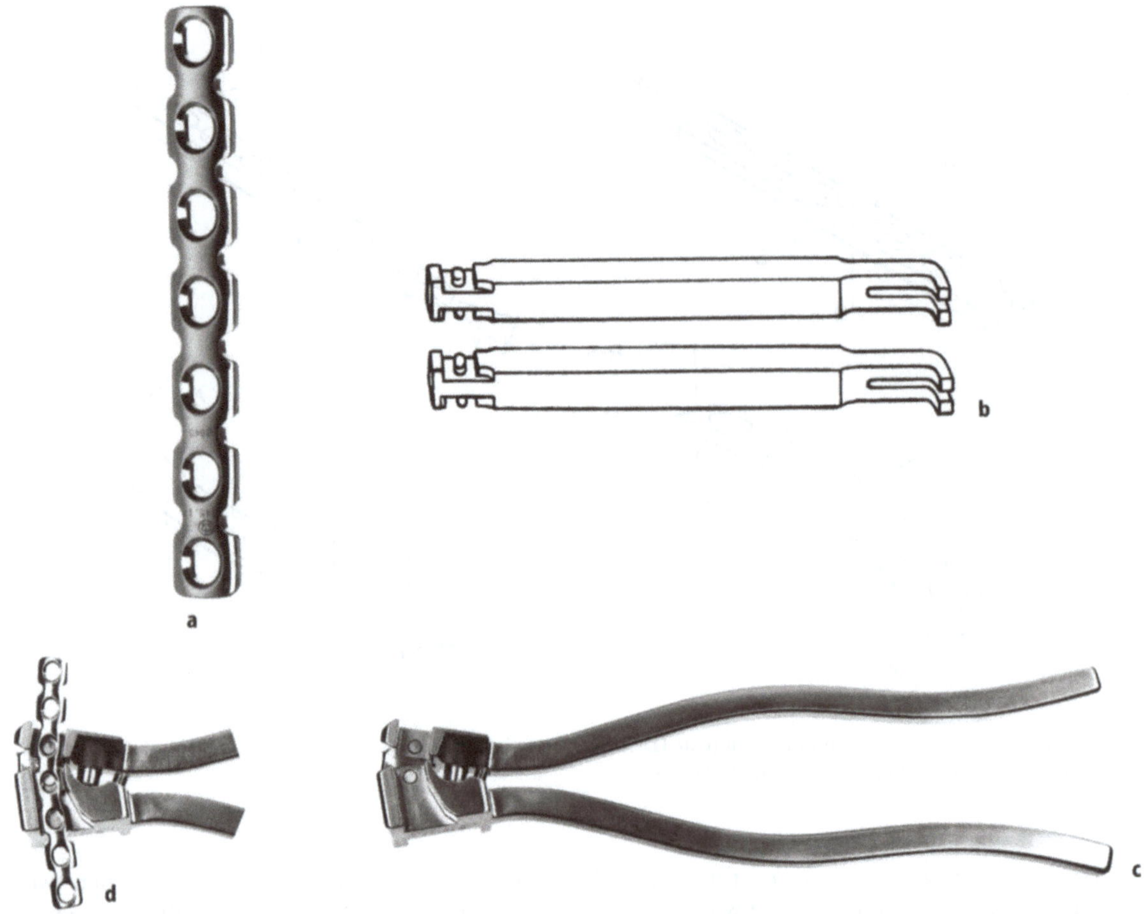

Fig. 2.31. **a** Shape of both the 3.5-mm and the 4.5-mm reconstruction plates. **b** Special twisting irons. These can also be used for bending the plates about their P–Q axis. **c** Special bending pliers. These can be used to bend the plates about their long X–Y and short P–Q axes. **d** Bending of the plates about their short P–Q axis

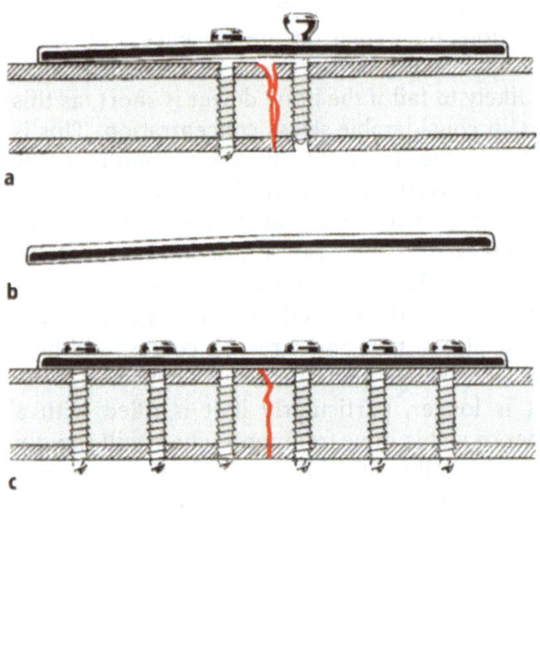

Fig. 2.32. **a** In the contouring process, the plate is prestressed if a slight, but acute bend is made over the fracture site, creating a 1- to 2-mm gap between the plate and the bone on insertion of the first screws at the end of the plate. **b** Insertion of the screws adjacent to the fracture pulls the plate up to the bone, creating static compression between the fracture ends. In order for compression to be achieved, prior anatomical reduction of the fracture is required. **c** Completion of stability is achieved by inserting the remaining screws

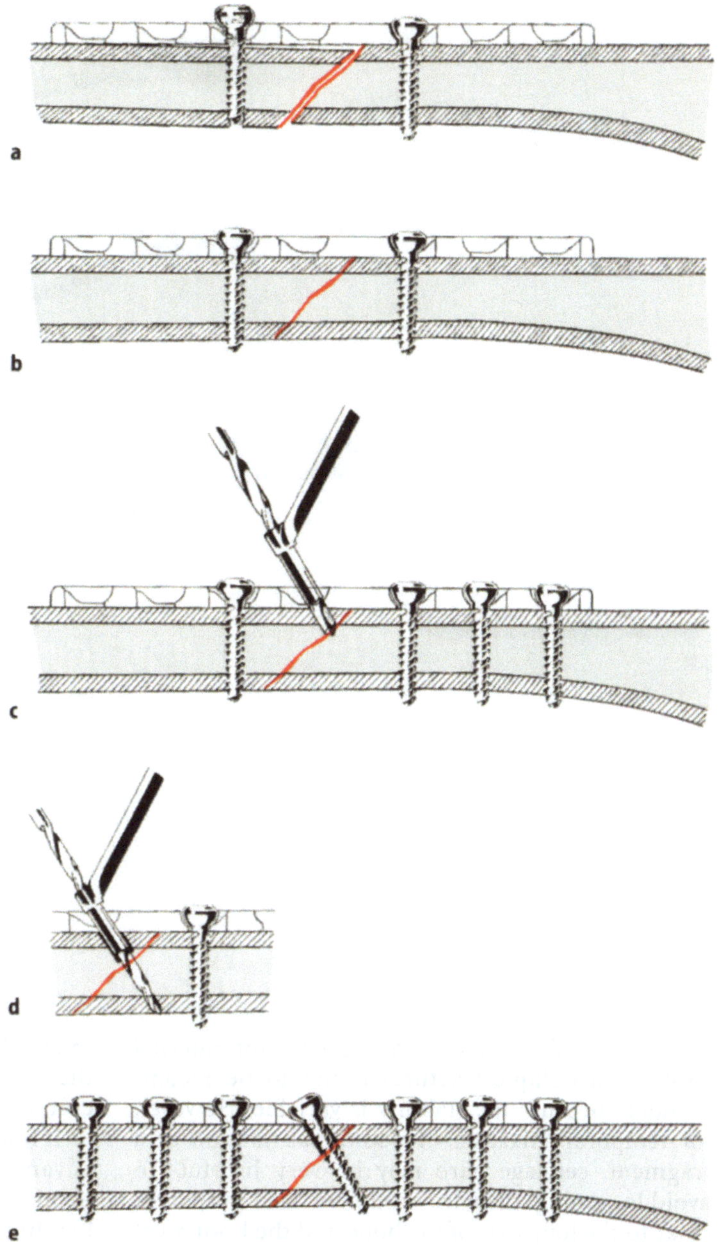

Fig. 2.33. **a** If a plate is fixed to the fragment which forms an acute angle with the fracture, then as axial compression is generated, the fragments displace and reduction is lost. If, however, the plate is fixed to the fragment which forms an obtuse angle with the fracture, then as axial copmression is generated, the spike of the opposite fragment is driven against the plate, and displacement is prevented. **b** Axial compression is achieved by inserting the screw in the "load" position. **c,d** To increase rotation stability and improve resistance to bending, if a force is directed towards the plate, a lag screw should be inserted through the plate whenever possible to lag any short oblique or spiral fracture. **e** The fixation is complete

only a concentration of stresses, but also a considerably longer healing time. If the fragments are small, it is best not to attempt screw fixation since it is likely to result in devitalization of the fragments, a delay in callus formation, and consequently failure.

2.3 Wire

In orthopedic surgery, different types of wire are used. These include the rigid Kirschner wire and the flexible orthopedic wires of different diameters. Various additional instruments for wire fixation are available in the wire instrument set (Fig. 2.34).

2.3.1 Orthopedic Wire

Orthopedic wire is monofilament, soft, and flexible and may be used with the wire-tightener or with the flat-nosed pliers (Fig. 2.35). It is primarily used as cerclage wire or tension band wire.

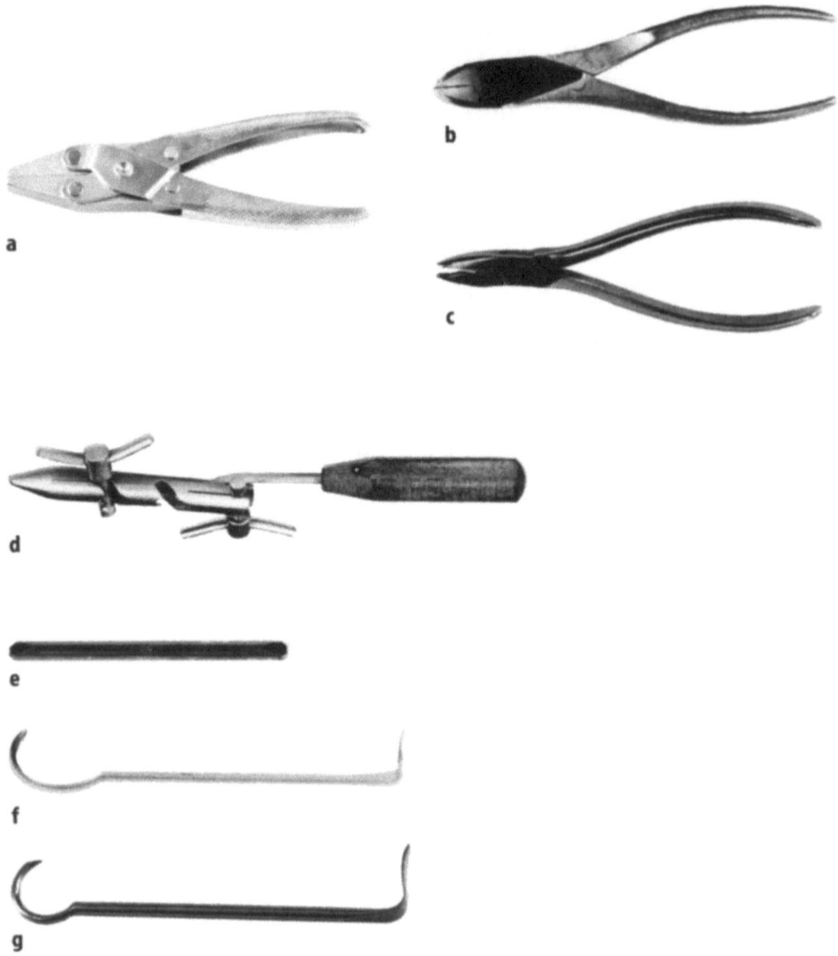

Fig. 2.34a–g. Wire and instruments for wire fixation. Orthopedic wire of different sizes (0.8 mm, 1 mm, and 1.25 mm) is available in rolls and with wire loops. Instruments for wire fixation: **a** Flat-nosed parallel pliers; **b** wire-cutter; **c** wire-bending pliers; **d** wire-tightener with handle; **e** bending iron for Kirschner wires; **f** wire-passer, large; **g** wire-passer, small (25 % of actual size)

The exclusive use of cerclage wire for internal fixation in oblique fractures is not to be recommended, because the stability is variable. However, for temporary fixation or additional fixation of a fragment, cerclage wire may be very helpful. To avoid loosening, the wire should be fixed perpendicular to the long axis of the bone and the knot must be twisted down snugly. Cerclage wire will slip on wedge-shaped bones. Slipping can be avoided by using hemicerclage wire or the figure-of-eight skewer pin technique (Figs. 2.36, 37). Cerclage wires may be applied using the AO/ASIF loops and tightener (Figs. 2.38).

2.3.2 Kirschner Wires

Single-pointed Kirschner wires 0.6–1.6 mm in diameter are used in orthopedic surgery in small animals. They are available up to 3 mm in diameter and also as double-pointed wires. Kirschner wires are used for temporary fixation of fragments and for marking purposes in arthrodeses and osteotomies. They are also used in tension band osteosynthesis, intramedullary fixation in small bones, and certain epiphyseal fractures in young animals.

If full-length Kirschner wires are not needed, it is advantageous to shorten them, as long wires may bend during insertion. If a long wire is needed, bending may be avoided by using the telescoping wire guide.

Kirschner wires should be inserted with a hand chuck or low-speed drill. High speeds increase friction and will heat the wire and surrounding bone, causing necrosis and loosening of the wire. Kirschner wires that are to remain in the bone should be bent at the proximal end, as loose wires may migrate and may be lost in the soft tissue.

2.3.3 Tension Band Wiring

The tension band principle, which involves a combination of orthopedic wire and Kirschner wires, was adopted from the engineering field, where it is used extensively. It was first applied to bone surgery

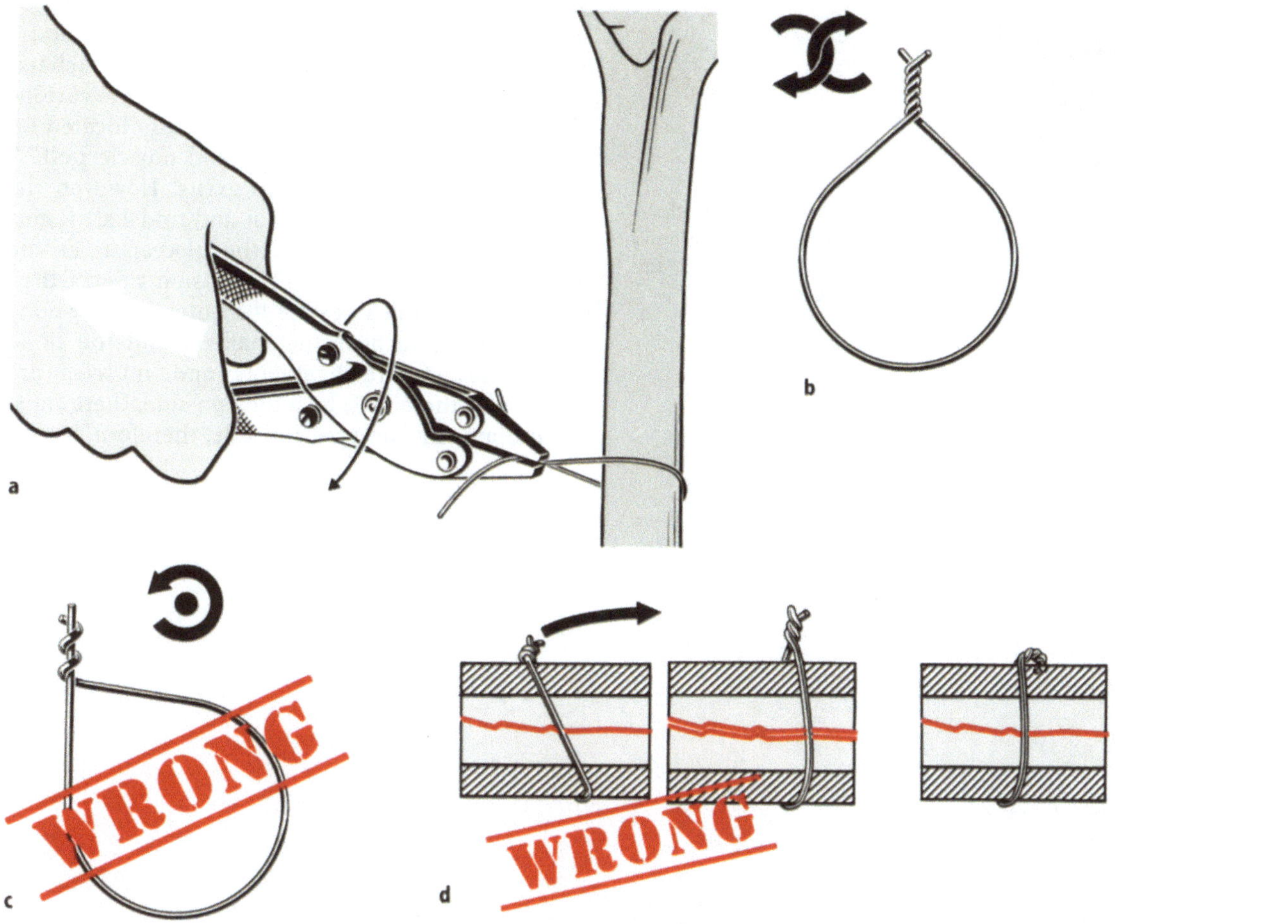

Fig. 2.35. **a** When flat-nosed pliers are used to twist a wire into a cerclage, the wire must be under tension during the process. **b** Correct twist with both wires uniformly wrapped around each other. **c** If the wire is not twisted under tension, one end will swing around the other and the knot will slip. **d** The cerclage must surround the bone perpendicular to the long axis, otherwise it will loosen. The knot should be bent against the bone surface to avoid soft tissue irritation

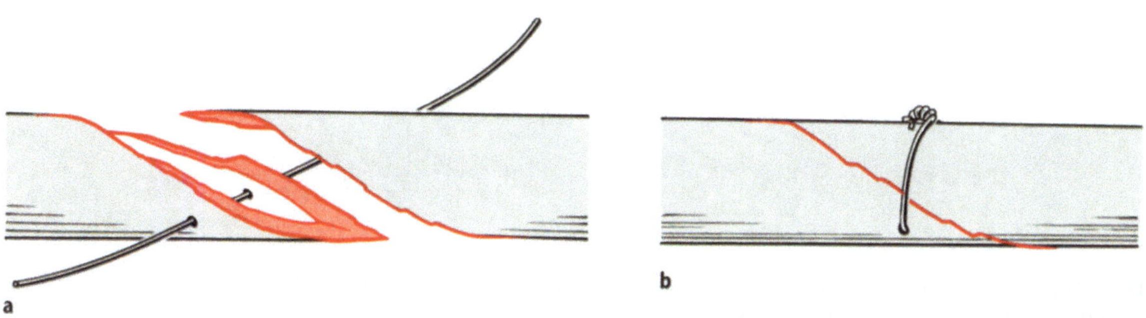

Fig. 2.36a,b. Technique of hemicerclage. **a** Two holes are drilled parallel to the fracture line of one fragment. **b** After reduction, the wire is tightened and the knot pressed against the bone surface

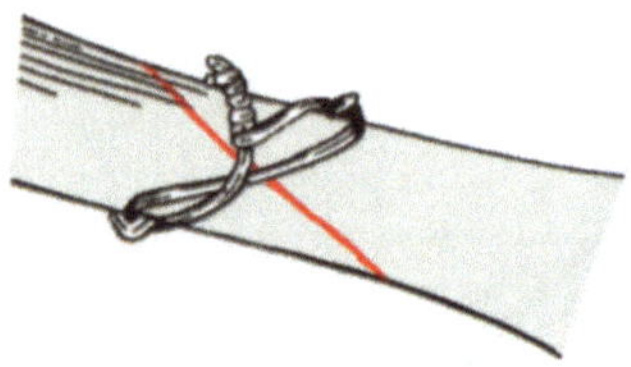

Fig. 2.37. Figure-of-eight skewer pin technique. A Kirschner wire is drilled across the fracture and a wire is passed around the ends, as shown. After reduction, the wire is tightened and the knot pressed against the bone surface

by Pauwels for the treatment of nonunions (Fig. 2.39). Every loaded bone has a tension and a compression side. According to the work of Schatzker et al. (1980), these sides change with the various phases of locomotion and are variously located on the bone according to loading and muscle pull. A constant tension side seldom exists. However, the lateral surface of the proximal and midshaft femur and the caudal surface of the olecranon at the moment of weight-bearing are tension sides. Other, very short tension sides are the outer sides of bony protuberancs, such as the malleoli and the tibial tuberosities, where ligaments and muscles are inserted. If there is to be a tension side, there must be an opposing compression side; therefore, if sup-

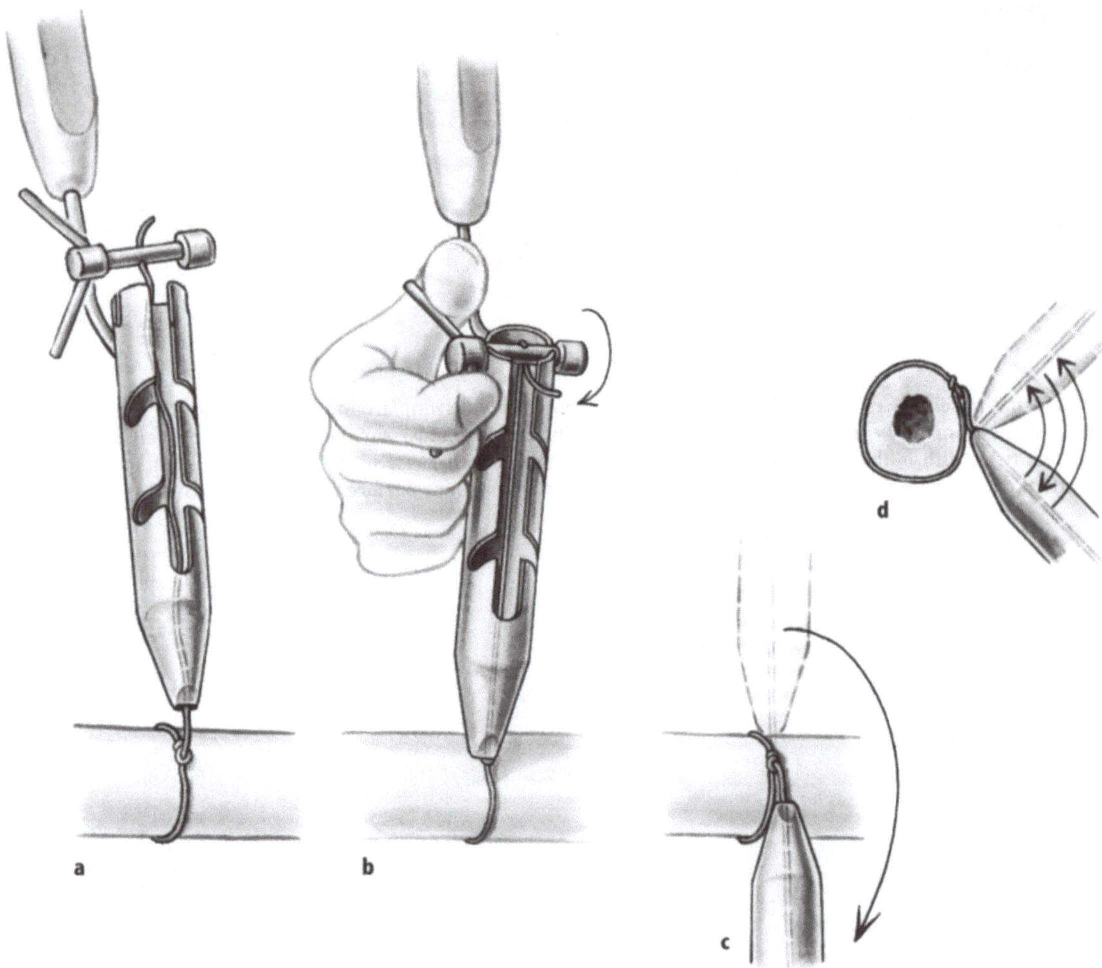

Fig. 2.38a–d. Application of cerclage wires is facilitated by using the AO wire loops in combination with the wire-tightener. **a** The wire is passed around the bone, through the eye of the wire, through the oval hole of the tightener, and finally through the hole in the crank. **b** The wire is slowly tightened by turning the crank in the slit. **c** As soon as the wire is tight, the tightener is tipped through an angle of 90 °, which bends the wire. The tension is released by reversing the turns of the crank. **d** When 1 cm of wire is exposed, the wire is cut with a wire-cutter

port is not present on the compression side, e.g., due to lack of an opposite buttress, the tension band principle is not applicable. With support opposite the implant, tension forces working on the bone are changed to compression forces. Conversely, without support opposite the implant, the latter will be subjected to cyclic loading and fail.

Tension band wiring is a useful technique for stabilizing bone fragments that are under tension in one direction due to the pull of muscles, tendons, or ligaments, such as the olecranon, greater trochanter, and malleoli. The principle is that the Kirschner wires stabilize against rotation and anchor the orthopedic wire, which functions as a tension band (Fig. 2.39).

2.4 Preoperative Planning

A radiograph of the normal side is required in order to have a template on which to plan the procedure. The fracture pattern determines the steps of the internal fixation as well as the choice of plate. The selected plate is drawn in with the help of the templates. The plan should include the order in which the different steps will be carried out, denote the function of the different screws, and indicate whether a gliding hole or a thread hole needs to be predrilled before the reduction is carried out and whether a bone graft is necessary.

The working drawings are made before any surgical procedure is embarked upon. They are of particular importance before corrective osteotomies, because they are the only way the veterinary surgeon can check, preoperatively, the result of the osteotomy and the three-dimensional concept of the procedure.

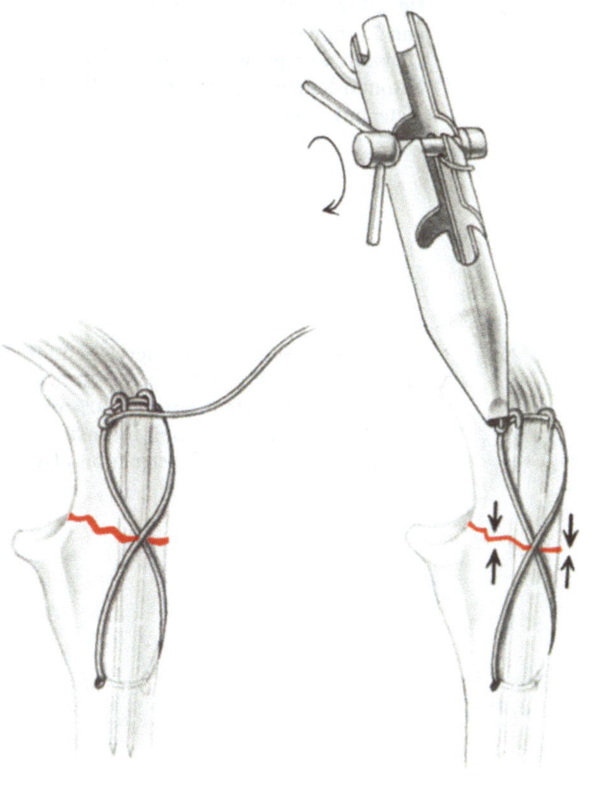

Fig. 2.39. A tension band wire can also be applied using a wire loop and the wire-tightener

2.5 Special Implants

A number of specialized instruments have been developed which greatly facilitate the exact execution of the operation in accordance with the preoperative plan. Neither radiographs nor an image intensifier is a substitute for a three-dimensional concept of the local anatomy, nor will they serve as a guide to the correct insertion of the guide wires. Correct insertion is based on the anatomical landmarks and on the particular device employed for fixation. Radiographs are also useful as a permanent intraoperative record of the position of the guide wires and of all the internal devices as well as of the position of an osteotomy if one is being carried out.

2.5.1 Cannulated Cancellous Bone Screws

For precise placement of cancellous bone screws in metaphyseal and epiphyseal sites, guidance by a guide wire may be advantageous. To this end, large and small cannulated cancellous bone screws are available.

Very often, Kirschner wires, used for temporary fixation, occupy the very position where a cancellous bone screw would have its optimal biomechanical effect. If such Kirschner wires can be used as guide wires for cannulated screws, the problem is solved.

2.5.2 Small-Fragment Plates

Small-fragment plates were originally designed for human hand surgery. These plates are thin and should be used only on bones where there are low bending forces, such as the scapula, pelvis, and sometimes small bones of the distal limb. The plates are designed in a number of shapes in order to suit various fracture types and are used with 2.7-mm screws (Fig. 2.40).

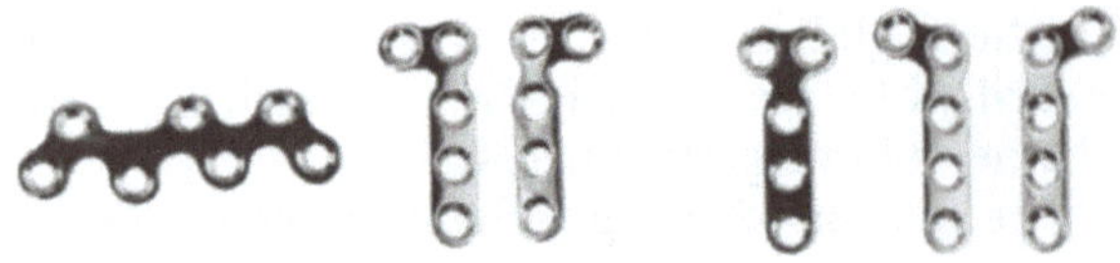

Fig. 2.40. Small-fragment plates are designed for the 2.7-mm cortex screw and have different forms

2.5.3 Miniplates

The mini-fragment plates are designed for use with the 2-mm cortical screw. They may be used successfully in miniature breeds and in small pets such as rabbits. Working with these delicate instruments and implants presupposes some expertise and a steady hand. The miniplates are also available in the DCP type with a special drill guide (Fig. 2.41).

2.5.4 Special-Use Plates

A number of plates have been developed for special purposes in human surgery. Some of these plates are useful in small animal orthopedics, including the 3.5-mm and 2.7-mm reconstruction plates (Fig. 2.42). Some special plates have been developed for veterinary use. These include the 2.7-mm and 2-mm acetabular plates, the double-hooked plate designed for subtrochanteric femoral osteotomy in the dog, and the triple pelvic osteotomy plates (Fig. 2.43).

2.5.5 Veterinary T Plates

Two veterinary T plates are now available: the 2.7/3.5-mm small T plate and the 1.5/2.0-mm mini T plate. They are designed especially for use in metaphyseal fractures in which a small epiphyseal fragment is present. The small T plate may be used in medium-sized and large dogs, and the mini T plate is for use in toy dogs and cats (Fig. 2.44).

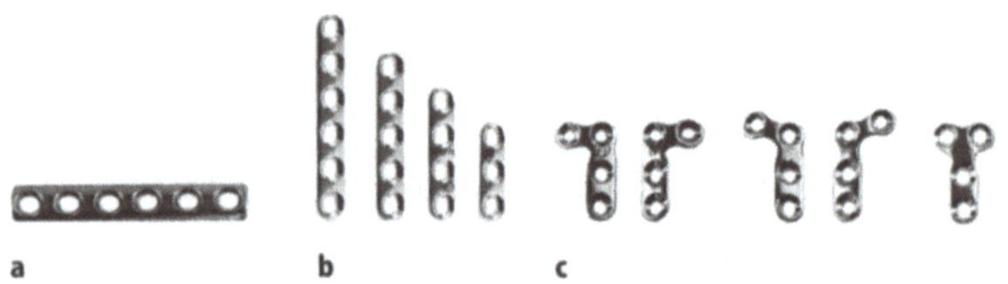

Fig. 2.41 a–c. Miniplates are used with 1.5- and 2.0-mm cortex screws. **a** Mini Dynamic Compression Plate (DCP). **b** Round-hole miniplates. **c** Angled miniplate and T miniplate

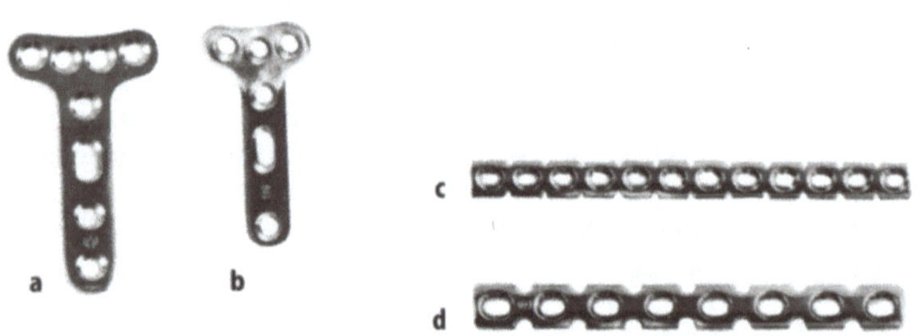

Fig. 2.42 a–d. Special plates developed for human use which may be used in animals. **a** 3.5-mm T plate (four holes). **b** 3.5-mm T plate (three holes). **c** 2.7-mm reconstruction plate. **d** 3.5-mm reconstruction plate

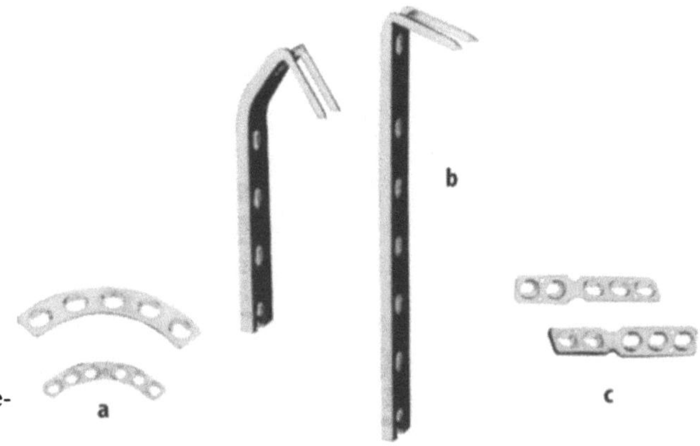

Fig. 2.43. **a** Acetabular plates, 2.7 mm and 2.0 mm. **b** Double-hook plates. **c** Right and left triple pelvic osteotomy plates

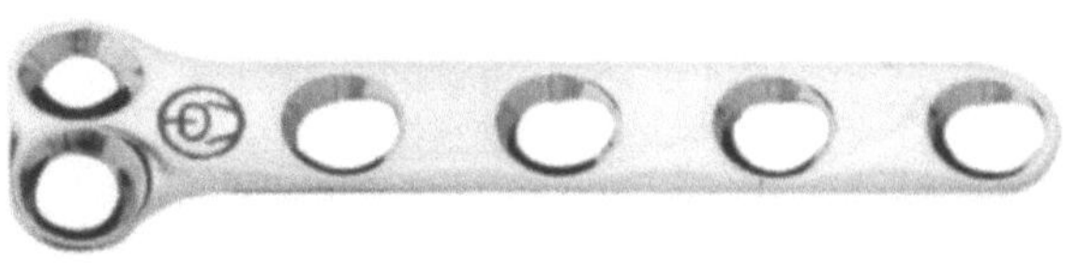

Fig. 2.44. The veterinary T plate comes in 2.7/3.5-mm (*shown here*) and 1.5/2.0-mm sizes

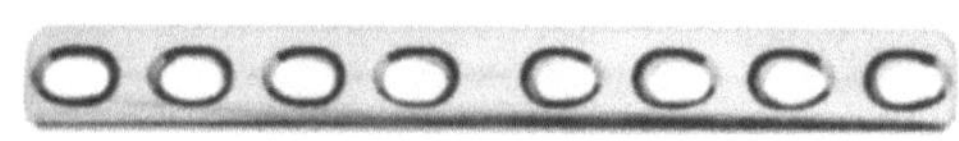

Fig. 2.45. The 3.5-mm broad dynamic compression plate (DCP) expands the 3.5-mm plating technique to include some of the larger canine breeds. The profile matches that of the 4.5-mm narrow DCP; the design and distance between the plate holes conform to those of the 3.5-mm DCP

2.5.6 Broad Veterinary Dynamic Compression Plate

The broad veterinary DCP was especially designed for use in stabilizing fractures in large dogs. It has the same dimensions as the 4.5-mm plate, but takes the 3.5-mm screw. It is thus more rigid and, over a unit length, it has more holes than the 4.5-mm plate. It is recommended for use in long-bone fractures, nonunions, osteotomies, and arthrodeses in medium- to large-sized dogs, weighing 20–45 kg. The plate is especially suited as a buttress (bridging) plate for comminuted fractures in dogs up to 35 kg (Fig. 2.45).

2.5.7 Cuttable Plates

Cuttable plates are versatile plates are designed for use in small animals. They may be custom cut to any length to accommodate a variety of fracture situations. Two sizes are available, and each is manufactured 300 mm long with 50 round holes. The plates may be stacked one on the other using plates with the same hole size; alternatively, the ones with the smaller holes (1.5/2.0 mm) may be placed on top of the one with the larger holes (2.0/2.7 mm). In the latter case, in order to distribute stress risers, the more superficial plate is cut shorter than the one underneath it (Fig. 2.46).

2.5.8 Self-Tapping Screws

Self-tapping screws are made in five sizes: 4.5, 3.5, 2.7, 2.0, and 1.5 mm, in both titanium and stainless steel (Fig. 2.47).

2.6 External Fixators

External skeletal fixation of long bones consists of inserting two or more pins in the proximal and distal bone fragments. The pins are connected by clamps and an external bar. Many modifications have been devised to cover some of the more complex fractures. Rigid aseptic practice is required, whether the splint be applied in connection with

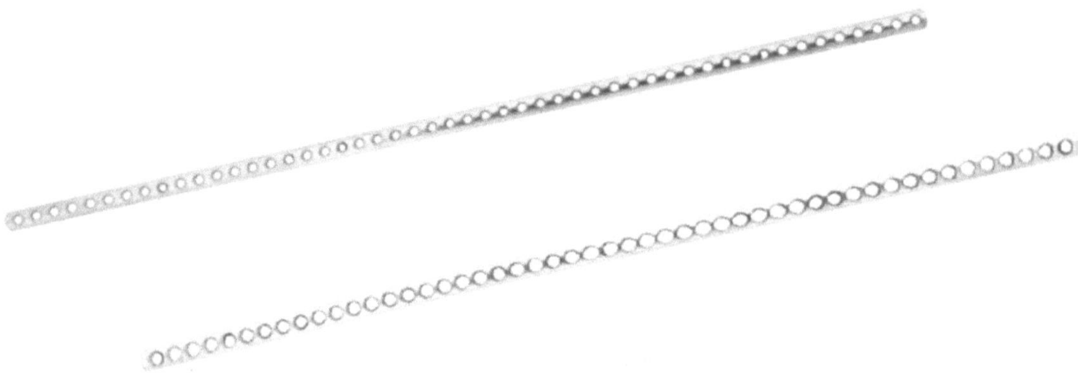

Fig. 2.46. Cuttable plates are made in two sizes: the 1.5 and 2.0-mm plates possess 50 round holes and have dimensions of 1.0×7×300 mm. The plates may be stacked on top of one another, either with a plate of the same size or with a smaller plate (1.5/2.0 mm) on top of a larger plate (2.0/2.7 mm). In such cases, it is recommended that the more superficial plate be cut shorter than the plate which is in apposition to the bone

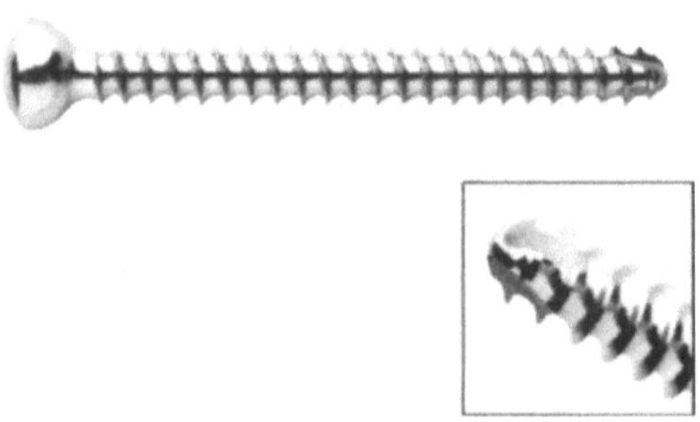

Fig. 2.47. The self-tapping cortex screw is a thread-cutting screw designed to meet orthopedic requirements

closed or open reduction. A sound knowledge of regional anatomy and good tactile sense are helpful in locating bony landmarks for insertion of the pins.

2.6.1 Indications

External fixators are amenable to a wide variety of fractures, both simple and complex. They are especially adaptable to the following: (a) infected fractures, (b) fractures with many small fragments, (c) cases where a supplement to other internal fixation, e.g., intramedullary pins, is required, (d) certain osteotomies (radius curvus), and (e) delayed unions and nonunions.

2.6.2 Methods of Application

With a few exceptions, the fracture should be reduced and maintained in reduction during insertion of the pins into the bone fragments. This brings about proper restoration of the soft tissues to their normal anatomical position. Some of the more stable and easily palpable fractures may lend themselves to closed reduction and application, but most fractures require an open approach for ease and accuracy of reduction. The pins are usually inserted through the skin, underlying soft tissue, and bone by use of a pin chuck, pressure being exerted while quarter-turns are made back and forth (Figs. 2.48, 2.49).

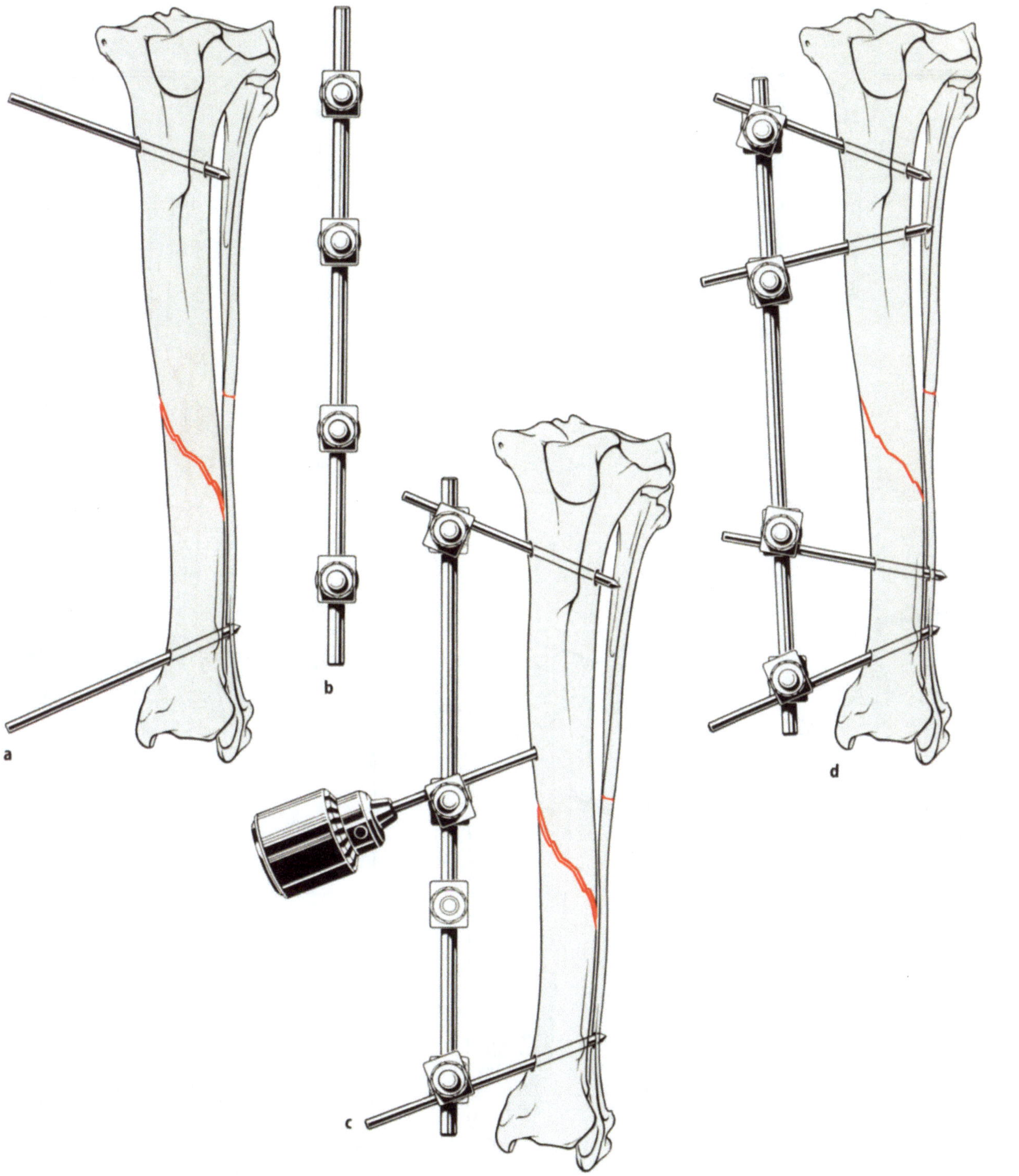

Fig. 2.48a–d. Procedure using one connecting bar. **a** The proximal and distal pins are inserted first. They pass through both cortices, but do not penetrate the skin on the opposite side. They are inserted in the same plane and at an angle of about 35°–40° to each other. **b** The connecting bar and single clamps are assembled. **c** The two outside clamps are attached. **d** The third and fourth pins are then inserted through the clamp holes in approximately the same plane and at an angle of about 35°–40° to the pin in the same fracture fragment. All clamps are then tightened. This procedure lends itself to fixation of fractures of the femur, tibia, humerus, and radius and ulna

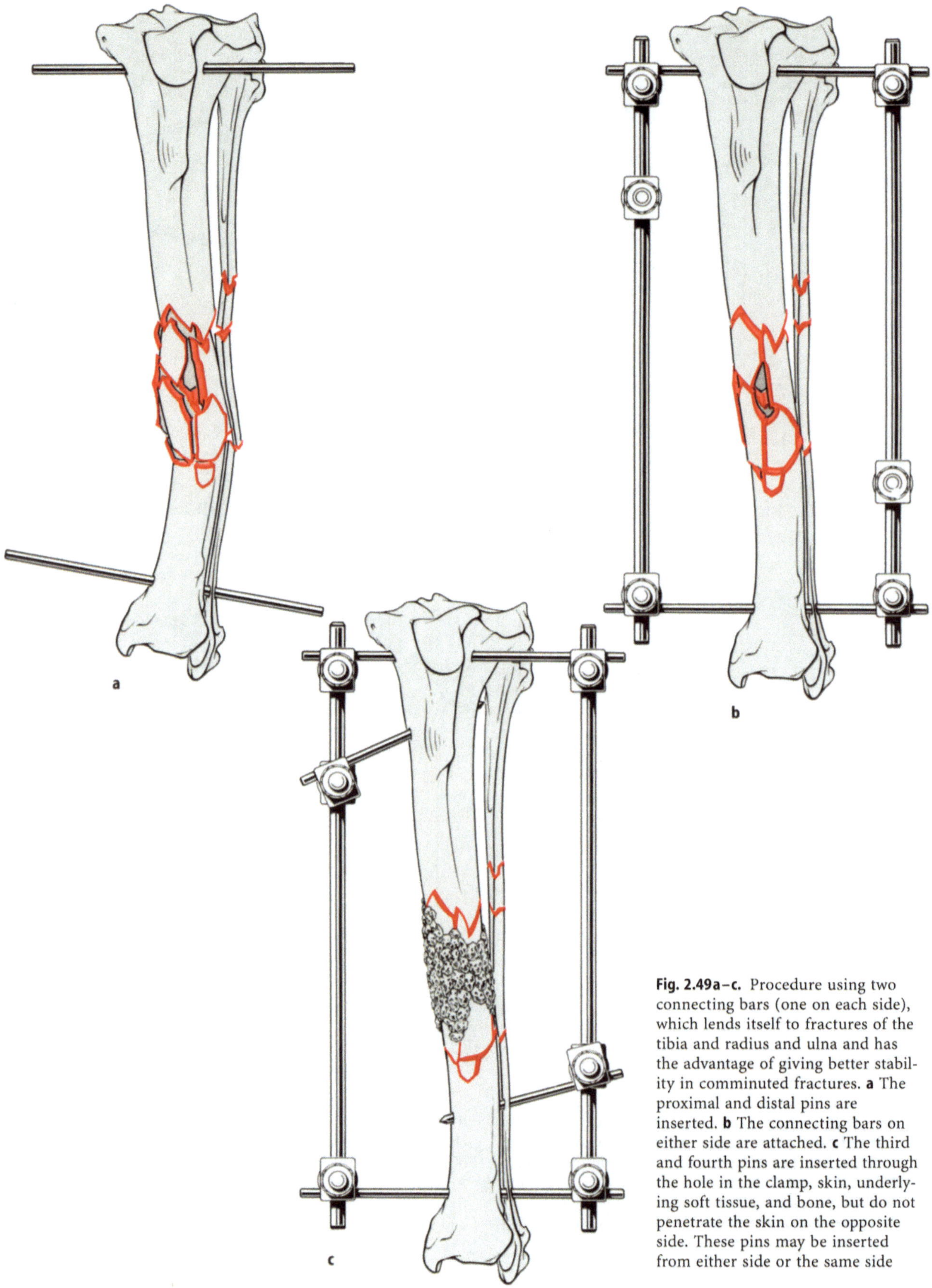

Fig. 2.49a–c. Procedure using two connecting bars (one on each side), which lends itself to fractures of the tibia and radius and ulna and has the advantage of giving better stability in comminuted fractures. **a** The proximal and distal pins are inserted. **b** The connecting bars on either side are attached. **c** The third and fourth pins are inserted through the hole in the clamp, skin, underlying soft tissue, and bone, but do not penetrate the skin on the opposite side. These pins may be inserted from either side or the same side

3 Preoperative, Operative, and Postoperative Guidelines

3.1 Definitions

A *fracture* is a complete or incomplete break in the continuity of bone or cartilage or both. It is accompanied by soft tissue injury and impairment of blood supply and function. *Fracture disease* may be defined as any pathological change in the soft tissues, joint, or bones associated with treatment of a fracture and resulting in impaired limb function. The term *clinical union* indicates a state in which healing bone is sufficiently strong for all fixation devices to be removed. The term *osteosynthesis* is used for internal fixation of a fracture by means of a mechanical device, e.g., pin, screw, plate.

3.2 Cause of Fracture

Causes of fracture include the following:

- *Direct overloading of the bone.* Documentary data indicate that approximately 80 % of all fractures are caused by impact with motorized vehicles.
- *Indirect overloading.* The load is transmitted through bone or muscle to a distant point where the fracture occurs, e.g., avulsion of tibial tubercle, fracture of the condyles of humerus or femur, fracture of the femoral neck.
- *Diseases of bone.* Many diseases of bone may cause destruction and weakening of bone to such a degree that minimal trauma may produce a fracture, e.g., bone neoplasms, certain nutritional diseases.
- *Repeated stress.* Stress fractures are most frequently encountered in bones of the rear or front feet, e.g., metacarpal and metatarsal bones in a racing greyhound.

3.3 Classification

Fractures may be classified according to the presence or absence of a communicating external wound:

- *Closed fracture.* The fracture does not communicate to the outside.
- *Open fracture.* The fracture site communicates to the outside through an external wound.

They may also be classified according to the direction and location of the fracture surface:

- *Transverse fracture.* The fracture is at right angles to the axis of the bone.
- *Oblique fracture.* The line of fracture is a diagonal, extending in an oblique direction to the axis of the bone.
- *Spiral fracture.* The line of fracture is a curve; the bone has been twisted apart.
- *Multiple (comminuted) fracture.* The bone is splintered, fragmented, or crushed, and three or more interconnecting fragments are present.
- *Segmental fracture.* This is a three-piece fracture in which the cylinder of the bone shaft remains complete in the middle segment.
- *Impacted fracture.* One segment is driven into the other.
- *Avulsion fracture.* This involves a fragment of a bone at the origin or insertion of a muscle, tendon, or ligament that is detached due to a traction or tension load.
- *Physeal fracture.* This is a fracture involving the growth plate and occurs only in young, growing animals.
- *Condylar or unicondylar fracture.* The fracture line passes through a condyle or between condyles, e.g., medial or lateral portion of the humeral condyle or the medial or lateral femoral condyle.
- *Fissure fracture.* This involves incomplete longitudinal or spiral fracture lines in the cortex.
- *Wedge or notch fracture.* The fracture is comminuted with two fragments on each side of a main center fragment whose shape resembles a wedge.
- *Greenstick fracture.* The fracture is incomplete and lies in a transverse or oblique plane across the cortex.
- *Bicondylar or intercondylar fracture.* The fracture is situated between the two condyles and diaphysis, e.g., T or Y fracture of the femur.

In addition, fractures may be classified according to stability after anatomical reduction:

- *Stable fracture.* Fragments interlock and resist physiological loads.
- *Unstable fracture.* The fragments do not interlock and move when loaded.

Fracture treatment is classified as follows in this manual:

1. Conservative (limb splint)
   a) Schroeder-Thomas splint
   b) Coaptation splints
   c) Casts
2. Surgical treatment
   a) Without interfragmentary compression (bone splint), i.e., intramedullary pinning or nailing, buttress plates, external skeletal fixation (external fixator)
   b) With interfragmentary compression, i.e., compression plates, lag screws, tension band wires
   c) Combination, i.e., neutralization plate and lag screw, external skeletal fixation and lag screw, intramedullary pin and external skeletal fixator
   d) Other, i.e., adaptation osteosynthesis, Kirschner wires

3.4 General Fracture Treatment

In few surgical specialties is the need for preplanning and preparation greater than in orthopedic surgery. Orthopedics requires teamwork in order to accomplish a surgical procedure successfully and to avoid undue patient trauma and excessive anesthetic time. Many demands are made on the surgical team, both in the preoperative evaluation of the patient and in postoperative care. Bone and joint surgery should only be carried out in operating rooms in which high standards of asepsis can be maintained. Asepsis is vital to preventing the devastating effects of postoperative bone infection. Failure to strive for perfection is soliciting failure.

In addition to the relevant precautions taken in all surgical procedures, there are some rules to be observed in the operating theater in order to reduce the risk of contamination:

- Eliminate unnecessary movement of staff within the operating room after the incision has been made.
- Use surgical hoods rather than routine surgical caps in order to reduce the risk of contamination from the hair of the surgeon or of his or her assistant.
- Use sterile cotton gloves over the sterile surgical gloves or double gloving in order to further reduce the possibility of contamination due to puncture of the surgical glove by bone spicules or sharp instruments. It is advisable to limit contact between the fingers and the bone or tissues and rely on proper instrumentation to accomplish the necessary manipulations.

3.4.1 Preoperative Evaluation

In all surgical procedures, consideration of the patient's well-being is paramount; everything else is secondary. There is often a tendency to concentrate on the obvious pain and make thorough examination of the patient a minimal priority, something which can lead to a calamity. Following a thorough physical examination, it is wise to obtain a hemogram and a blood chemistry profile as a baseline. High-quality radiographs of the affected bone and of the chest are essential in trauma patients for evaluation of the fracture or injury and for making decisions as to treatment.

In multiple fractures, it is advisable to draw the fracture on transparent paper on the radiograph and to delineate all of the fracture lines in order to lay down the method of reduction and fixation with accuracy and with the correct dimensions. This step, in itself, frequently reduces operating time. However, it is essential in every procedure to have an alternative plan in case the primary course of action should prove to be unworkable. Adequate instruments and implants for both options should be available.

The decision to repair a fracture immediately or at a later time is governed by many variables, such as the condition of the patient, the time elapsed since the injury, and whether or not the fracture is open or closed. As a general rule, the sooner the fracture is stabilized, the less trauma there will be to the soft tissues and the vascular supply to the bone. On the other hand, it is not advisable to rush into internal fixation if there has not been proper preparation and if the patient's general condition is not stable. There is some degree of soft tissue injury in all fractures, and frequently it is of such magnitude that it dictates when and how the fracture should be handled. In general, a fracture is best repaired within 48 h of injury. Surgery performed at this time can be done prior to the development of marked edema, swelling, and marked contraction of soft tissues, and reduction can be accomplished in a shorter time and with less trauma to the soft tissue.

Infrequently, contusion of the skin in closed fractures is so great that final surgical repair must be delayed for up to a week while the skin recovers sufficiently to allow surgical intervention, hence precluding the possibility of postsurgical dehiscence. This is particularly true in trauma to the lower portion of the limbs, where blood supply to the skin is not as good as to other parts of the body. External skeletal fixation may be considered as an alternative in these cases or may be used for temporary stabilization until the patient is ready for internal fixation of the fracture. These are general guidelines; however, clinical judgement should always take precedence over generalizations. Disregarding the condition of the soft tissues, particularly in fractures of the lower limb, will jeopardize the chances of successful internal fixation. Edema may often be prevented or reduced by application of a Robert Jones' bandage in lower limb fractures.

Open fractures should be regarded as emergencies and treated soon after presentation. If the patient's condition permits, primary internal fixation can be attempted following proper débridement of the soft tissues (see Sect. 3.8.7).

3.4.2 Operative Procedures

Proper aseptic technique during the operative procedure, coupled with careful manipulation of the soft tissues and bone fragments, reduces the risk of iatrogenic infection and also reduces the healing time. The question as to the use of antibiotics in noninfected fractures has not yet been resolved by experimental data or by clinical findings. The use of antibiotics postsurgically is not necessary if there is neither evidence nor knowledge of a break in asepsis or contamination of the wound during the operation.

3.4.3 Postoperative Considerations

In the 12–24 h following a surgical orthopedic procedure, a rise in body temperature of 1–1½°C (2–3 °F) is frequently observed. This, in itself, is not necessarily evidence of infection, but rather a reaction to tissue damage. Clinical experience has shown that, in the dog, provided that the temperature does not rise above 40 °C (103.6 °F), this is not an absolute indication for the use of antibiotics; the febrile response generally lasts 24–48 h. However, if this temperature persists or rises above 40 °C (103.6 °F), antibiotic therapy should be initiated immediately.

The concept of stable internal fixation of fractures is partially predicated on the early return to function and the elimination of fracture disease. To accomplish this, early ambulation with active movement of the joints above and below the fracture is essential. Unfortunately, when dealing with animals, the degree of movement and weight-bearing cannot be dictated verbally and thus must be controlled by other means, such as restraining devices and/or confinement within a small space. The degree of activity allowed is dependent upon the stability of the fixation. Repair of a fracture using a fixation device is a race between fracture healing and fixation failure. All loaded implants are subject to variable degrees of cyclical stress; therefore, if the fixation is less than optimal, activity must be reduced. This calls for judgement on the part of the surgeon as to the amount of ambulation allowed.

3.5 Biomechanics of Implants and Implant Failure

3.5.1 General Considerations

The implants used for fracture fixation or corrections must reliably support the locomotor system in its function of carrying the load applied by the patient or by nonaccidental external events. The biomechanical investigation of implants is not restricted to the observation of the implant itself, but must take into account the biomechanical conditions of the internal fixation as a whole. Reliable function is based on some important requirements:

- The implant material must be biocompatible.
- The design (with respect to the selected material) must be appropriate to cope with the applied load.
- The application and handling must be appropriate to avoid failure of the biomechanical structure (Fig. 3.1).

In the following, the important parameters influencing the reliable function of an internal fixation implant will be analyzed. The biomechanics of implants cannot be restricted to mechanical aspects alone. Biochemical aspects regarding the materials used must also be considered.

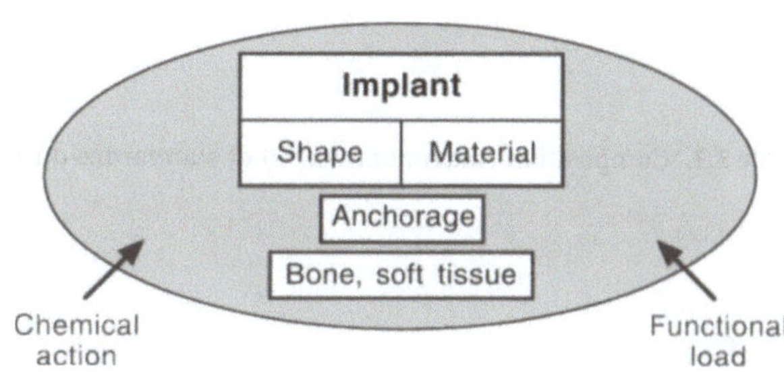

Fig. 3.1. Interaction between implant and environment (biomechanical structure)

3.5.2 Materials

3.5.2.1 Composition

The conventional material used for surgical implants for internal fixation in human beings and in animals is a stainless steel of high purity, strength, and ductility (Table 3.1). The amount of other elements (carbon, phosphorus, sulfur, silicon, copper, and light elements) is restricted to very low levels, i.e., below 1 wt/%.

Unalloyed titanium, containing 99 % titanium, is being increasingly used for implants. The five different grades, according to the ISO standard 5832-2, can be chemically distinguished by the different amounts of light elements they contain, such as oxygen, nitrogen, and hydrogen (Table 3.2). The amount of light elements influences the mechanical properties.

The manufacturers of the AO/ASIF implants specify the properties and the purity of the metallic raw material to narrow limits, which guarantees their high quality.

Although the application of titanium implants in veterinary surgery is still limited, the use of titanium in human beings is increasing. There is no doubt that titanium is superior as a biomaterial.

3.5.2.2 Magnetic Properties

Implant materials containing iron must, in compliance with the standards, be in a so-called *austenitic condition*. These materials are not sensitive to any external magnetic fields to which they might be exposed, e.g., by magnetic resonance imaging (MRI) investigations of the patient.

Table 3.1. Composition of standardized stainless steel

Element	Composition (wt. %)
Chromium	17–19
Nickel	13–16
Molybdenum	2.5–4
Manganese	2 (maximum)
Iron	Balance (i.e., to make up 100 %)

Materials in a *ferritic state* react dramatically to external magnetic fields (such as MRI), which may lead to displacement of the implant. The manufacturers control the magnetic properties (susceptibility) of their raw material to avoid such problems. However, there is no way to control the magnetic properties of an implant in a patient. If the geometry of an implant allows unique identification of its metal properties, this could influence the decision on whether to carry out an MRI investigation. Chemically pure titanium does not show any magnetic susceptibilty.

Instruments, especially cutting instruments such as drill bits, reamers, and chisels, require different material properties. Since these instruments only come into brief contact with the living tissue, corrosion resistance is a secondary consideration compared to strength and wear resistance. In general, these materials have a higher carbon content. which reduces the corrosion resistance but increases hardness and wear resistance. The material is often in a ferritic state.

3.5.2.3 Corrosion

Corrosion resistance, i.e., resistance to chemical destruction of the metal due to chemical processes, is a necessary condition for an implant material. Corrosion in the initial state results in formation and emission, or exchange, of active ions which interact with the body fluid and the tissue.

Ageing, i.e., a change of mechanical properties as a reaction to the environmental conditions in the body, is an undesirable property of a biomaterial. The majority of metallic biomaterials do not show any ageing behavior. Polymeric materials frequently undergo ageing, resulting in increased brittleness caused by cross-linking of the polymer chains.

Degradation of metallic biomaterials is normally prevented by good corrosion resistance. The combined action of high mechanical and chemical forces may lead to local destruction of the material (e.g., fretting corrosion, wear), causing a so-called *metallosis*. Such situations should be avoided by appropriate design. Adequate laboratory tests simu-

Table 3.2. Composition (maximum wt. %) of standardized unalloyed titanium, containing 99 % titanium

Element	Grade 1	Grade 2	Grade 3	Grades 4A and 4B
Carbon	0.1	0.1	0.1	0.1
Iron	0.15	0.2	0.25	0.3
Nitrogen	0.03	0.03	0.05	0.05
Hydrogen	0.0125	0.0125	0.0125	0.0125
Oxygen	0.18	0.25	0.35	0.45

lating these extreme conditions are recommended for newly developed designs.

When an implant undergoes relative motion to another implant or to the surrounding tissue, *wear resistance* is an advantage.

3.5.2.4 Surface Treatment

Electrochemical surface treatment aims to achieve perfect and smooth implant surfaces. Electropolishing is a procedure mainly used for stainless steel implants to create a complex passivation layer on the surface, making the implant more resistant to corrosion.

Anodizing (or anodic oxidation) is another electrochemical process forming a thin oxide layer on titanium implants. The titanium oxide layer is very stable and biocompatible. This layer is extremely thin and produces an optical effect; titanium implants therefore have a specific color.

3.5.2.5 Biocompatibility

The tests for biocompatibility of implant materials are laid down in the ISO 10 993-x standards, which describe guidance for the selection and performing of tests for different investigations, e.g., for toxicity, cytotoxicity, cancerogenicity, and degradation effects. The biocompatibility of metallic materials (alloys) correlates with the content of nontoxic elements and with the corrosion resistance (see Sect. 3.5.2.3). The toxicity of relevant metallic elements has been investigated in a rat femur model.

Allergic reactions to chemically pure titanium are unknown. Allergies to other metals, especially nickel and chromium, are on the increase. Stainless steel is an alloy containing these substances, but the emission rate of ions containing nickel or chromium is very low because of the high corrosion resistance of stainless steel. Therefore, use over many years has proved that the behavior of this material in the body is acceptable. However, in the case of known patient allergy to metals, pure titanium implants should be preferred in order to reduce the potential risk.

3.5.2.6 Standards[1]

The most commonly used metallic biomaterials with accepted biocompatibility are standardized by the International Organization for Standardization (ISO). AO/ASIF experts have contributed for many years to a substantial number of standards related to materials and implants.

The most important material standards for implants for internal fixation are the following:

- ISO 5832-1 Wrought stainless steel
- ISO 5832-2 Unalloyed titanium
- ISO 5832-11 Wrought titanium - 6 aluminum - 7 niobium alloy

There are other ISO standards for biomaterials, such as other titanium alloys, cobalt-based alloys, ceramics, tantalum, and polyethylene, which are relevant to the field of joint replacement and for special applications. In clinical trials, all these materials have been accepted as having sufficient biocompatibility.

3.6 Mechanical Terminology and General Mechanical Properties of Materials

3.6.1 Static Strength

Strength is a material property. It is defined as the stress at which a material fails. (*Stress* is defined as the force divided by the area of the sample on which the force is acting. Normally, the undeformed size of the area is used. We call it *true stress* if the actual size of the area in the deformed stage is used. Units of stress units are N/mm^2 or MPa.) High strength is usually required for biomaterials in order to minimize the necessary volume of an implant. Depending on the kind of applied stress, different strengths are referred to:

- *Tensile strength*, or ultimate tensile strength, is the strength measured in a uniaxial tensile testing machine. The sample is subjected to a uniaxial stress.
- *Shear strength* is the strength measured under uniform shear stress. This pure shear stress state can be approximately realized in a thin-walled torque-loaded tube.
- *Yield strength* is the stress level at which the stress–strain curve exhibits a specified limited deviation from the initial straight part of the curve, i.e., the deformation increases disproportionally more than the force. Both yield strength and force are related to a static or quasi-static loading, i.e., a slow increase of test load until fracture. In the case of dynamic load, an additional characterization of strength properties exists (see below).

[1] Standards are issued by various national standards organizations, e.g., ASTM (USA), BSI (UK), DIN (Germany), AFNOR (France), and UNI (Italy).

3.6.2 Fatigue Strength

If the material is subjected to a time-dependent stress state which does not exceed the static strength limit, failure may occur at a lower stress level. The higher the stress level, the lower the number of loading cycles that the material can resist.

Fatigue strength is the stress level which the material is able to resist for an unlimited number of loading cycles (see Sect. 3.6.6).

3.6.3 Deformation and Strain

Deformation of an implant is a specified geometrical deviation of the implant from its initial shape. This may be measured as a displacement, as an angle, or as strain. Strain is defined as the elongation of a material divided by its resting length. It is a dimensionless measure, often given as a percentage.

Elongation after fracture means the remaining (permanent or plastic) strain after fracture of a test piece in a tensile test. The plastic strain is located in the vicinity of the fracture site (of the metal) and is characterized by a (permanent or plastic) reduction of the cross-sectional area of the test piece.

3.6.4 Elasticity

Perfectly elastic biomaterials do not show any residual deformation after unloading. Elasticity is characterized by the elastic constants of the material (modulus of elasticity, shear modulus). The modulus multiplied by the elastic strain gives the stress; in linearly elastic materials, stress and strain are proportional.

If the stress exceeds the proportional limit, permanent or plastic strain occurs, which can be measured after unloading as the residual strain.

3.6.5 Viscoelasticity

Viscoelastic behavior refers to the time dependency of deformation under constant load or vice versa. Creep and relaxation (decrease of stress if deformation remains constant) are typical effects in polymer or metallic materials loaded under conditions of high temperature.

Under normal environmental conditions (body temperature, environmental temperature), metallic biomaterials do not show any remarkable viscoelastic effects.

3.6.6 Fatigue

Fatigue is the tendency of metallic materials to fail under cyclical loading after a number of cycles at a stress less than the static strength. Fatigue strength is the stress level which the material is able to resist for an unlimited number of loading cycles.

Fatigue tests and their results vary with the load time and process applied. Oscillating (alternating) and increasing – decreasing (monotone) loading processes are in use. A typical test is the rotating – bending test, in which a heterogeneous oscillating stress state is applied to the test piece. The neutral axis is not affected, and the maximum stresses appear at the surface of the cylindrical sample.

3.6.7 Notch Sensitivity

Notches and scratches on the surface of a material cause local stress concentrations. Cracks often start at such high-loaded areas and then run through the healthy material until fracture of the part occurs. Sensitivity to notches is an undesirable property in a material. Brittle materials (materials with low elongation after fracture) are more sensitive to notches. It should be noted that brittleness is not a constant property of a material, but depends upon the applied stress state (three-dimensional states show less deformation after fracture than uniaxial stresses) and is therefore a behavior (not a constant property) of the material under stress.

The notch toughness is a measure of the sensitivity to notches, high strain rate, and three-dimensional stress states.

3.6.8 Specific Mechanical Properties of Stainless Steel and Unalloyed Titanium

An example of the varying properties of stainless steel and unalloyed titanium is given in Table 3.3. The density of the two materials differs: 4.51 g/cm^3 (chemically pure titanium) and 7.95 g/cm^3 (stainless steel).

3.7 Functional Load

3.7.1 Anatomy

An implant should be able to withstand all functional "loads" to which the natural tissue in this area is exposed. The anatomy, i.e., the *mass of the patient* and the *size of the body* including the limbs, considerably influences the functional load acting on the locomotor system, and consequently on the implant.

Figure 3.2, for example, shows the dependency of the knee joint force in jumping for different sized animals, human beings included. There is no doubt that all functional internal loads can be determined

Table 3.3. Mechanical properties of stainless steel and unalloyed titanium

Property	Stainless steel	Unalloyed titanium
ISO standard no.	5832-1	5832-2
Density (g/cm^3)	7.95	4.51
Quality	Sheet, D and E, cold worked	Grade B
Ultimate tensile strength (MPa)[a]	860/1100	680
0.2% yield strength (MPa)[a]	690	520
Elongation after fracture (%)[a]	12	10
Modulus of elasticity (GPa)	NN (approx. 186)	NN (approx. 104)
Fatigue strength (MPa)	NN (approx. 380)	NN (approx. 350)

[a] Minimum.

by similar relationships. This means that large, heavy subjects apply more functional load to the locomotor system than small, light ones.

3.7.2 Fracture Type

The fracture type defines the complexity of the injury. A more complex fracture normally forces an implant to transmit more functional load than a simple fracture. Locked intramedullary nails used for more complicated fractures transmit more load than unlocked nails used in simple fractures.

When selecting implants to be used, this must be taken into consideration by the surgeon; sometimes, a change in the type of internal fixation is necessary.

3.7.3 Activity

The activity of a patient has a twofold influence on functional load: (1) fast-moving (accelerating) subjects apply more force to the implant than slow-moving ones, and (2) an active patient generally applies a greater number of loading cycles to the skeleton than an inactive one. This may influence the life of the implant.

3.7.4 Intended Survival Time of the Device

Each implanted medical device has a certain intended survival time in the body. Thus reliable and safe function during this time interval is required.

Devices for fracture treatment, such as bone plates and screws, are usually temporary devices. They are usually explanted after 2 years or less. However, the possibility of leaving the implant in the body – if the patient does not have any problems with it and/or if he or she refuses implant removal – is an advantage. Therefore, there is now a trend towards using biomaterials which are suitable for long-term use.

K wires and guide wires often used in fracture treatment are very often implanted for a short time and are sometimes removed during the operation.

Instruments such as drill bits, forceps, templates, and scalpels may not be categorized as short-term "implants." The implantation time is very short.

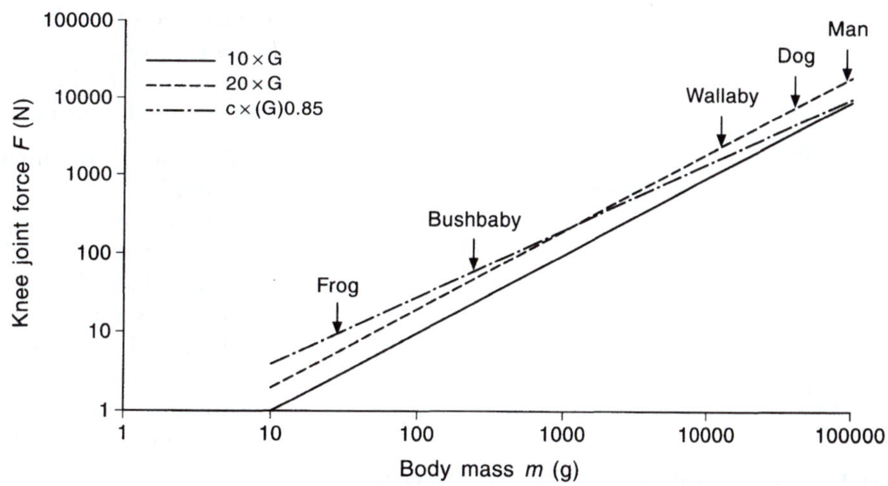

Fig. 3.2. General relationship between internal functional forces and the body weight of vertebrates. Maximum knee joint forces of vertebrates (jumping). Body weight $G = mg$; $g = 9.81\ m/s^2$. (After Alexander 1968–1981)

The standards for these materials do not need to be as strict as for implants.

3.7.5 Anchorage Problems in Natural Tissues

3.7.5.1 General Comments

Sufficient anchorage in the viable tissue is important. Ideally, the tissue adjacent to the implant should not transmit more contact stresses than healthy tissue. High local stresses should be avoided.

The distribution of internal forces depends not only on the elasticity and the shape of an implant, but also upon the external load configuration (e.g., bending, torsion, axial force, and combinations thereof).

3.7.5.2 Anatomical Shape

The anatomical shape of an implant is always a problem. For example, the shaft of an artificial hip joint fills an anatomically empty canal, i.e., there is not any hard tissue at this site. Therefore, a prosthesis can only exist as a foreign body, even if the anatomical shape is perfect. When handling an anatomically shaped implant, it is often desirable to have low contact stresses. This may be obtained even with appropriate nonanatomical designs.

An internal fixation plate is normally adapted to the bone surface by contouring. This procedure aims to achieve exact anatomical reduction of the fragments, good contact, and low stress to the bone, but it induces plastic strain in the implant (Fig. 3.3). Therefore, contouring should be minimized and, in particular, repeated bending or twisting in opposite directions should be avoided.

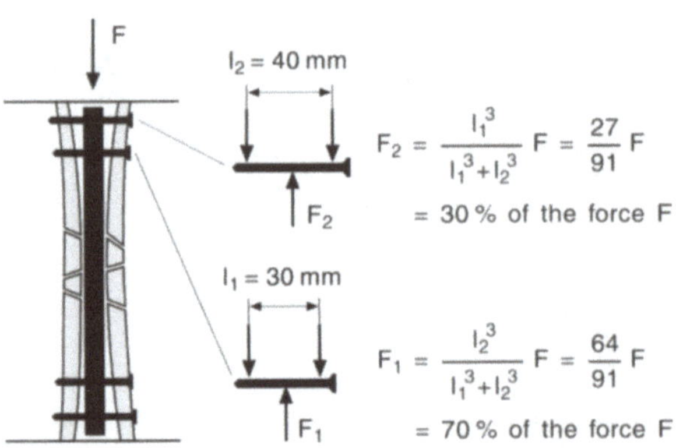

Fig. 3.3. Load distribution for locking bolts: an example

3.7.5.3 Time Dependency of Load

Since all animals permanently change their load configurations relative to the body in time, there is not a fixed configuration of external load. Thus there is also no fixed distribution of internal (functional) forces. Fortunately, the functional loads vary only between certain limits. This allows for an optimization of the implant design in order to deal with the varying loading conditions. However, the search for an optimal implant is a very complex problem and cannot be solved by the choice of the appropriate "ideal" biomaterial alone.

3.7.5.4 Biological Environment/Time Dependency of Tissue Properties

The biological environment of an implant is the body of a human being or an animal. The anchorage of implants in bone depends upon the properties of the bone, and these may change with time. This can affect the stability of the fixation. Anchorage in soft tissues or in organs presents far more difficult biophysical and biochemical problems (e.g., ligaments, tendons, heart valves, vessel implants).

3.8 Open Fractures

An open fracture by definition occurs where there is, or was, communication between bone and the external environment. Open fractures must be considered an emergency situation. Even with proper treatment, this type of fracture has an increased risk of osteomyelitis and/or nonunion. A common cause of failure of internal fixation is the bacterial infection associated with open fractures. In addition, the force involved in the mechanism of injury may result in increased tissue damage. Devitalized soft tissue or bone with the addition of foreign debris decreases the healing potential and diminishes the body's ability to fight infection. The basic principles for the treatment of open fractures include the following:

- Prevention of further contamination of the wound
- Prompt and thorough wound inspection, cleaning, and surgical debridement
- Proper handling of soft tissue and bone to preserve vascularity
- Informed decisions regarding timing of surgery and wound closure
- Adequate stabilization of the fracture with optimal devices depending upon the type of fracture and wound

3.8.1 Classification

The severity of soft tissue and bony injury is classified in order to aid in treatment decisions, prognosis, and for informed client consent:

- *Type I:* Puncture-type wound with skin laceration of less than 1.0 cm. The laceration may be associated with penetration of the skin by a bone fragment. The wound is clean and has minimal tissue damage.
- *Type II:* Skin wound larger than 1.0 cm, with more soft tissue damage caused by the external trauma.
- *Type III:* Skin wound larger than 1.0 cm or multiple wounds with more extensive soft tissue damage, including skin flaps, foreign material wound contamination, degloving, nerve or vessel damage, severe muscle laceration or contusion, or loss of skin, fascia, or muscle. Fractures include increased comminution, periosteal stripping, segmental fracture, and bone loss (Fig. 3.4a). Fractures caused by gunshot (high-velocity or close-proximity shotgun wounds) are included in the type III classification. The extent of soft tissue damage is important for prognosis and treatment planning.

3.8.2 Treatment Guidelines

3.8.2.1 Emergency Treatment

An uncovered open fracture should be immediately covered with a sterile dressing to prevent further contamination. Shock, hemorrhage, or any life-threatening internal injuries are treated immediately. A physical examination is done, including ascertaining the neurological status. After patient stabilization, appropriate radiographs are taken to aid in the treatment plan. All open fractures need adequate wound débridement. Sedation or anesthesia should be administered; if the patient's condition is critical, local or regional anesthetic techniques should be used. The limb is prepared sterilely. Sterile petroleum jelly is used in the wound to protect it from further contamination by clipped hair. In the operating room, enlargement of the skin wound may be necessary to permit adequate wound inspection and treatment. Specimens are taken for culture, sensitivity, and gram stain, and antibiotics are started. Positive evidence of bacteria by quantitative gram staining means that bacteria at a concentration of 10^6 are present and confirms severe wound contamination. Repeating gram stains after débridement can help in judging whether the débridement was adequate.

Systemic antibiotic options are: (a) cefazolin at 20 mg/kg every 6 h for clean types I and II (covers gram-positive bacteria), (b) for types II and III, use either cefotetan 30 mg/kg t.i.d. (covers gram-positive and gram-negative bacteria and 70 % of anaerobes) or gentamicin 6 mg/kg s.i.d. + ampicillin 10 mg/kg q.i.d. + metronidazole 15 mg/kg b.i.d. (covers gram-positive and gram-negative bacteria and anaerobes). Antibiotic therapy should be continued until culture and sensitivity reports are known and then modified or discontinued, as indicated by the reports. If outpatient antibiotics are indicated, either enrofloxacin 5 mg/kg or ciprofloxacin 5 mg/kg + metronidazole 15 mg/kg b.i.d. should be used. The total length of antibiotic treatment varies with the fracture type and cultures; 7–10 days is usual for types I and II, with a longer duration for type III.

Pressure lavage, using either a commercial system (Pulsavac; Zimmer Corp., Ohio) or a 35-cc syringe with an 18-gauge needle, enables bacteria, contaminants, and tissue debris to be efficiently flushed from the wound. An adequate amount of fluid (3–5 l lactated Ringer's solution) is required for flushing. Surgical débridement is carried out with sharp dissection of severely damaged or avascular muscle, fascia, and smaller bone fragments. Large bone fragments should be saved for later rigid fixation. After carrying out wound inspection, pressure lavage, débridement, and evaluation, several major decisions must be made (see 3.8.2.3).

3.8.2.2 Definitive Treatment

If definitive fracture treatment is to be carried out, the following may be considered:

1. *External splints and casts.* These are indicated in selected type I and II fractures below the elbow or the stifle which are minimally displaced or reducible, clean, and biomechanically stable. Frequent reexaminations are necessary during the convalescent period.
2. *Internal fixation.* Intramedullary pins, interlocking nails, or plates may be used for certain type I and II fractures. All are contraindicated if gross contamination/infection (type III) is present in order to prevent spread of infection. Skeletal fixation (external fixator, transcortical pins with acrylic) can be used on all fracture types, especially type III (Fig. 3.4a). The pins are placed some distance from the wound (Fig. 3.4b). Bone plating may be used for all types of open fractures after proper débridement. Delayed plating is indicated for severely infected wounds, after the infection has been controlled. Plating may be

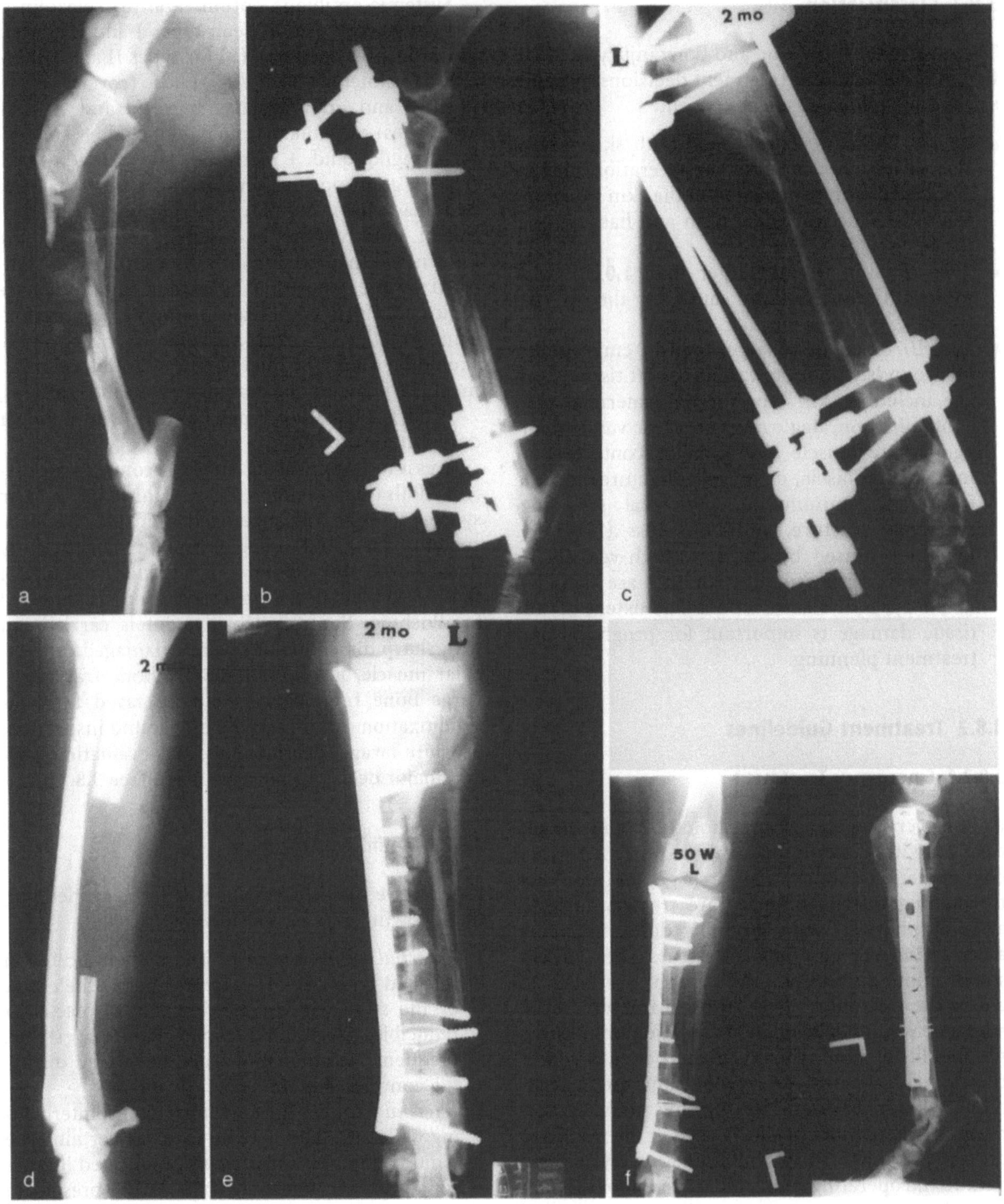

Fig. 3.4a–f. Grade III open fracture. **a** Radiograph of an 8-year-old Springer Spaniel with a highly comminuted tibia/fibula fracture with bone loss caused by a corn-picker accident. **b** Temporary stabilization with an external fixator after thorough débridement. **c** Radiograph after serial débridement and antibiotic therapy, 2 months after the injury. **d** Radiograph shows ulnar donor site where a 6.0-cm autograft was harvested. **e** After removal of the external fixator, the tibial fracture plus ulna and rib autografts were stabilized with a 3.5 broad plate and two cerclage wires. **f** Radiographs show healed fractures and incorporation of autografts at 50 weeks. The plate was removed 18 months after the injury with full return of limb function

used after a temporary external fixator has been removed as long as pin tract infection is not present (Fig. 3.4c,f).

3.8.2.3 Decisions

The following major decisions have to be taken:

1. *Fracture fixation.* Definitive fracture stabilization may be postponed because of the severity of tissue damage (type III), inadequate technical help, or for referral reasons. If further surgery is not to be performed immediately, a sterile supportive bandage should be applied to prevent nosocomial contamination of the open wound and to provide temporary immobilization of the fracture and soft tissue. Definitive stabilization of the fracture immediately after débridement may be performed using appropriate internal or external fixation devices. An external fixator may be applied for temporary fracture stability and to facilitate wound access for serial débridement (Fig. 3.4b).
2. *Is a bone graft needed to aid fracture healing?* If so, should it be immediate or delayed? Types I and II fractures may be grafted at the initial operation using autogenous cancellous or morcellized cortico-cancellous bone. If a fracture has been categorized as a type III fracture because of contamination/infection, then grafting should be delayed until the infection is contolled. This can usually be accomplished in 1–8 weeks. Repeat cultures are necessary. Antibiotic-impregnated methylmethacrylate beads are sometimes installed locally for 2–3 weeks in cases of resistant infection.
3. *Should the wound be closed?* Fracture types I and II are usually amenable to primary closure if the initial wound is clean. Wounds should be left open if the degree of contamination is felt to be significant. Type III should not be closed initially. The timing of the delayed closure depends upon the culture results and the progression of soft tissue healing. In severe cases, the wound or wounds are often allowed to close in by third-intention healing. Open wounds should be dressed with a sterile bandage.

3.9 Design

3.9.1 Shape: Stiffness, Strength

The shape of the implant determines its stiffness and its load-carrying capacity. Stiffness is defined as load divided by deformation, and for elastic materials it represents the proportional factor between these two physical variables. There are indefinite numbers of "stiffnesses" depending upon the defined load configuration and on the deformation considered. For instance, the modulus of elasticity is the stiffness constant of the elastic material itself, representing the relationship between stress ("load") and strain ("deformation"). Bending stiffness defines the relationship between a bending moment and the curvature of the bent strip or plate.

The *stiffness* of implants, for internal fixation, becomes an important aspect if the implant acts as a composite together with living tissue (such as bone) transmitting functional load. In such cases of good or partially good tissue contact (reduction), the distribution of the functional load to the two partners is determined by their stiffness parameters. In general, high stiffness attracts the load, i.e., the stiffer of the two will carry the most load. In human patients, intramedullary locking nails have been used. The shorter (stiffer) locking bolt carries the greater axial load (Fig. 3.5).

Examples include the following:

- The *bending stiffness* of a plate is proportional to the third power of the length of a plate measured in the plane in which the bending occurs. It is also proportional to the width of the cross-section, measured perpendicular to the plane of bending, and is proportional to the modulus of elasticity.
- The *axial stiffness* of a plate is proportional to the cross-sectional area measured in the plane perpendicular to the axial force. It is also proportional to the modulus of elasticity.
- The *torsional stiffness* of a plate is proportional to the third power of the small width of a plate

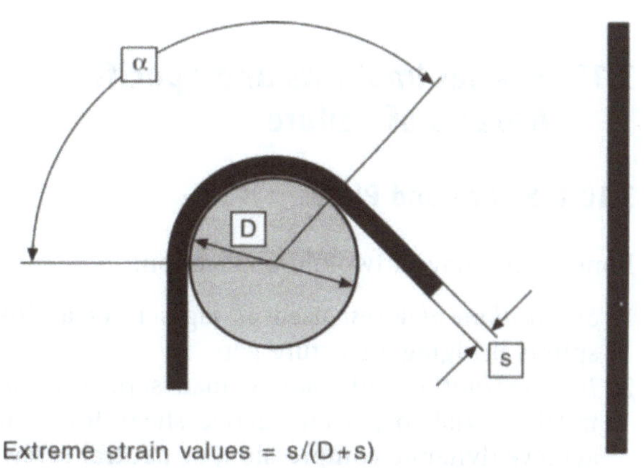

Fig. 3.5. Strain values on the surface of a plate in the case of contouring (bending to a curvature of diameter *D*). Extreme strain values = s/(D + s)

measured in the plane in which the bending occurs. It is also proportional to the greater height of the cross-section, measured perpendicular to the plane of bending, and is proportional to the shear modulus or to the modulus of elasticity.

The *strength* of an implant, in a more general sense, is often identified by its load-carrying capacity, i.e., the maximum force or torque at which the device will fail. The maximum load an implant is able to transmit does not depend upon the modulus of elasticity. It depends upon the strength (or its yield strength) of the material itself and on its shape and dimensions.

Examples include the following:

- The maximum *bending moment of a plate* (bent around the long axis of its cross-sectional area) is proportional to the width and to the second power of the length of the plate and also to the yield strength.
- The maximum *axial force* transmittable by a round bar not showing plastic deformation is proportional to the second power of the diameter and to the yield strength of the material.
- The maximum *axial force* transmittable by a round bar until complete failure is proportional to the second power of the diameter and to the ultimate tensile strength of the material.
- The maximum *torque* of a solid round rod is proportional to the third power of the diameter and also to the yield strength (*note:* tubes and especially slotted tubes obey different rules).

3.9.2 Manufacturing

Manufacturing of implants requires special experience and extensive quality control in order to provide adequate performance of the implant.

3.10 Special Implants and Specific Aspects of Failure

3.10.1 Screws and Plates

Bone screws have a twofold application:

1. *Stand-alone devices:* used as lag screws and/or splints bridging a fracture gap
2. *In combination with plates:* load screws transmitting axial forces and active shear forces to achieve dynamic compression, or neutral screws transmitting axial forces and passive shear forces to achieve firm adaptation of the plate to the bone

Combined application may be possible, i.e., lag screw through a plate hole. The maximum axial force a screw can transmit to the bone is proportional to the outer diameter of the screw and to the strength of the bone (limited by stripping the thread in the bone). The maximum axial force at which the screw fails is determined by the core diameter of the screw and by the strength of the screw material (limited by fracture of the screw). Bone plates are used for internal fixation of fractures bridging the fracture site and replacing the missing bone in this area. Load-transmitting plates may have an additional compressional effect (dynamic compression plate, DCP) or may act as neutralization plates to support fixation by one or more lag screws.

Plates transmit longitudinal forces, bending moments, and torque. Contouring of plates may change their mechanical strength. Additional local stress concentrations can lead to plate fatigue failure, and careful handling of the implants to avoid sharp bends, scratches, and notches is necessary. Single contouring using the appropriate instruments and techniques has proven to be acceptable (Table 3.4).

3.10.2 Wires

Two main functional groups of wires exist:

1. Cerclage wires made from a soft raw material for tension band techniques, fixed mainly by twists
2. Kirschner wires of a certain stiffness used for splinting, guiding, and temporary fixation, available with and without threaded tip.

If at all, very low axial forces are applied. The wires are usually used in a shear-loaded condition. In the

Table 3.4. Mechanical properties corresponding to the solid cross-section of the various plates (maximum tensile strength as maximum load before rupture)

Plate with screws 0.2%	Diameter (mm)	Maximum tensile strength (kgf)	Maximum yield strength (kgf)
Broad DCP	4.5	7500	6900
Narrow DCP	4.5	5000	3225
Small-fragment DCP	3.5	3000	2250
Small-fragment DCP	2.7	2000	1500
Small-fragment plate	2.7	120	90
Miniplate	2.0	50	32

DCP, dynamic compression plate.

case of external fixators, they may also tolerate bending loads. It is evident that sharp edges and knots in wires or repeated bending may cause failure. Scratches and notches should be avoided.

3.11 General Aspects of Implant Failure

Safety and reliability are primary requirements for implantable medical devices. They are not determined solely by the mechanical properties of the biomaterials used. Failure of an implant, which may mean lack of safety under certain circumstances, can occur for a variety of reasons.

The safety of an implant depends on three factors (Fig. 3.6):

1. *The patient* plays a passive and an active role: the anatomy and the type of disease or injury (fracture type) are given properties of the patient and cannot be changed; the activity of the patient should be regulated and controlled in order to achieve the best possible healing and recovery.
2. *The surgeon (and the hospital)* is able to influence the choice of the implant and type of treatment, the quality of application, and the activity of the patient by load-limiting devices and by supervision.
3. *The manufacturer* is responsible for the design, the raw materials, and the reliable manufacturing of the device.

Failure of implants seldom occurs, but in most cases it is caused by dynamic load resulting in fatigue of the material.

Pure static overload by high accident forces or by complex fractures with insufficient bone support seldom occurs. When it does occur, the above-mentioned parameters may play a part, and – as is often the case in accidents – simultaneous exposure to several effects may lead to the load-carrying capacity of the device being exceeding, causing it to fail.

The type of treatment depends upon the anatomy and upon the fracture type. The biomechanical construction must form a stable compound consisting of implant and bone, replacing the missing bone strength in the fracture gap by the tensile strength of the implant and providing additional compression of the fracture gap, if appropriate. Insufficient bone support at important points can lead to load concentrations at the implant site, causing implant failure.

Mishandling of the implants using the wrong instruments for application, producing notches in the surface, or performing repeated contouring (cold forming process) may decrease the safety factor to an insufficient value and lead to fatigue fractures of the implant.

3.11.1 Complications of Internal Fixation

Complications of fracture treatment in small animals are more frequently caused by partial or total

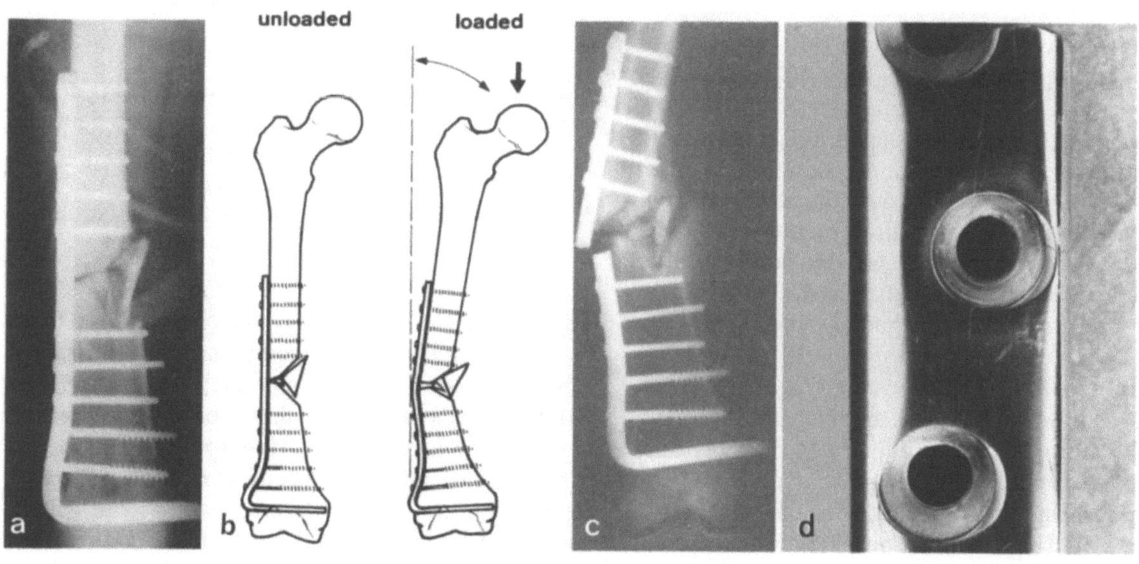

Fig. 3.6a–d. Unstable internal fixation in human femur leading to fatigue fracture of the plate. **a** Postoperative radiograph showing lack of support opposite the plate because of a large, unstablized fragment. **b** Under weight-bearing, bending forces (which cause fatigue failure) are exerted on the plate. **c** Later radiograph showing resorption of the fragment and development of nonunion, which led to increasing instability and implant failure. **d** Fractured plate with fatigue cracks in neighboring holes (compare Figs. 3.7 and 3.8)

collapse of the fixation than by fracture of the implants. This contrary to experience in human orthopedic surgery and indicates that in small animals the bone is usually the weaker component of the bone-implant unit. In comminuted fractures, the fragments are often so tiny that they cannot be stabilized individually, or the screw fixation of a fragment fails because the bone splits. In fractures near joints, the plates often cannot be attached with the necessary number of screws. The breakdown of internal fixation through screw loosening can be caused by a number of different factors:

- Improper fracture repair plan
- Inadequate choice of screws (too small, too large)
- Improper screw direction
- Defective screw seating (e.g., stripped bone threads)
- Poor reduction with subsequent overloading of the screws
- Unstable fixation with subsequent overloading of the screws
- Overloading by secondary trauma or inadequate postoperative treatment
- Necrosis and bone resorption
- Infection

If only one or two individual screws are loose, they can often be replaced by a screw with a larger diameter. However, when the whole fixation breaks down with loss of reduction, reconstruction of the internal fixation is necessary. Occasionally, screws fail due to fatigue fracture.

3.11.2 Implant Fractures

Investigations have shown that implant failures in small animals are caused by the same mechanism as that observed in human orthopedic surgery. Detailed analysis of a series of human clinical cases revealed that implants can fail by fatigue under unstable conditions when the alternating stresses of the loading-unloading weight-bearing cycles are too high or when the number of cycles at relatively low load exceeds a critical value. As an example, Fig. 3.6a shows an unstable internal fixation of a broken femur. Figure 3.6b illustrates how bending forces are exerted on the plate under weight-bearing, leading to fatigue failure of the plate in the fracture zone (Fig. 3.6c,d). Comparison of the fracture morphologies of implants broken in the body with those of fractures generated by different laboratory tests indicates that overload fractures, stress-corrosion-cracking, and corrosion fatigue can be excluded as probable fracture mechanisms.

Fatigue cracking is a critical failure mode for implants, since it is a slowly proceeding, accumulative process. It can even occur when the material is loaded in the elastic range, under stresses which cause only reversible elastic deformation. In such relatively low load ranges, fatigue failures are only possible because metals can be damaged irreversibly in a progressive manner on the free surface. Figure 3.7 demonstrates the development of a fatigue crack on implant material under laboratory conditions. Investigations have confirmed that fatigue cracking takes place in exactly the same manner in the body (compare Fig. 3.7d with Fig. 3.9). The crack propagation into the material is shown in a longitudinal section in Fig. 3.8.

Figure 3.9 shows the fatigue damage structure adjacent to the crack on the surface of a plate broken in vivo, which is similar to that of Fig. 3.7d (from a fatigue experiment). Figure 3.10 gives an overview of the fracture surface of a plate. Higher magnifications show typical parallel fatigue striations created by individual load cycles in the crack propagation zone (Fig. 3.11).

In general, fatigue cracking occurs in a sequence of different steps:

1. Crack initiation:
   a) Deformation structures develop at the free surface. Slip steps of the glide systems of the metal grains protrude through the surface (Fig. 3.7a).
   b) Micronotches form out of certain slip systems during further fatigue damage (Fig. 3.7b).
   c) Nucleation of microcracks which extend over several grains (Fig. 3.7c)
2. Crack propagation:
   a) A main crack forms on the surface (Fig. 3.7d).
   b) The main crack propagates into the depth of the material (longituduinal section, Fig. 3.8; high magnification, Fig. 3.11).
3. Final overload fracture: after the main crack has reduced the cross-section to a critical size, sudden rupture takes place (Fig. 3.10, stage III).

The higher the load under which fatiguing takes place, the quicker the stages described follow each other, with fewer numbers of cycles to failure. The fatigue curves (Fig. 3.12) show the fatigue lifetime to failure as a function of the applied stresses for the different implant material conditions. Curve 1 represents the highly cold-worked material (pins), curve 2 the medium cold-worked material (screw, plates), and curve 3 the soft material. Comparison of curves 1–3 shows that the fatigue resistance of the stainless steel increases with cold work and strength. This behavior is significant for bone plates, which undergo cold-work deformation when

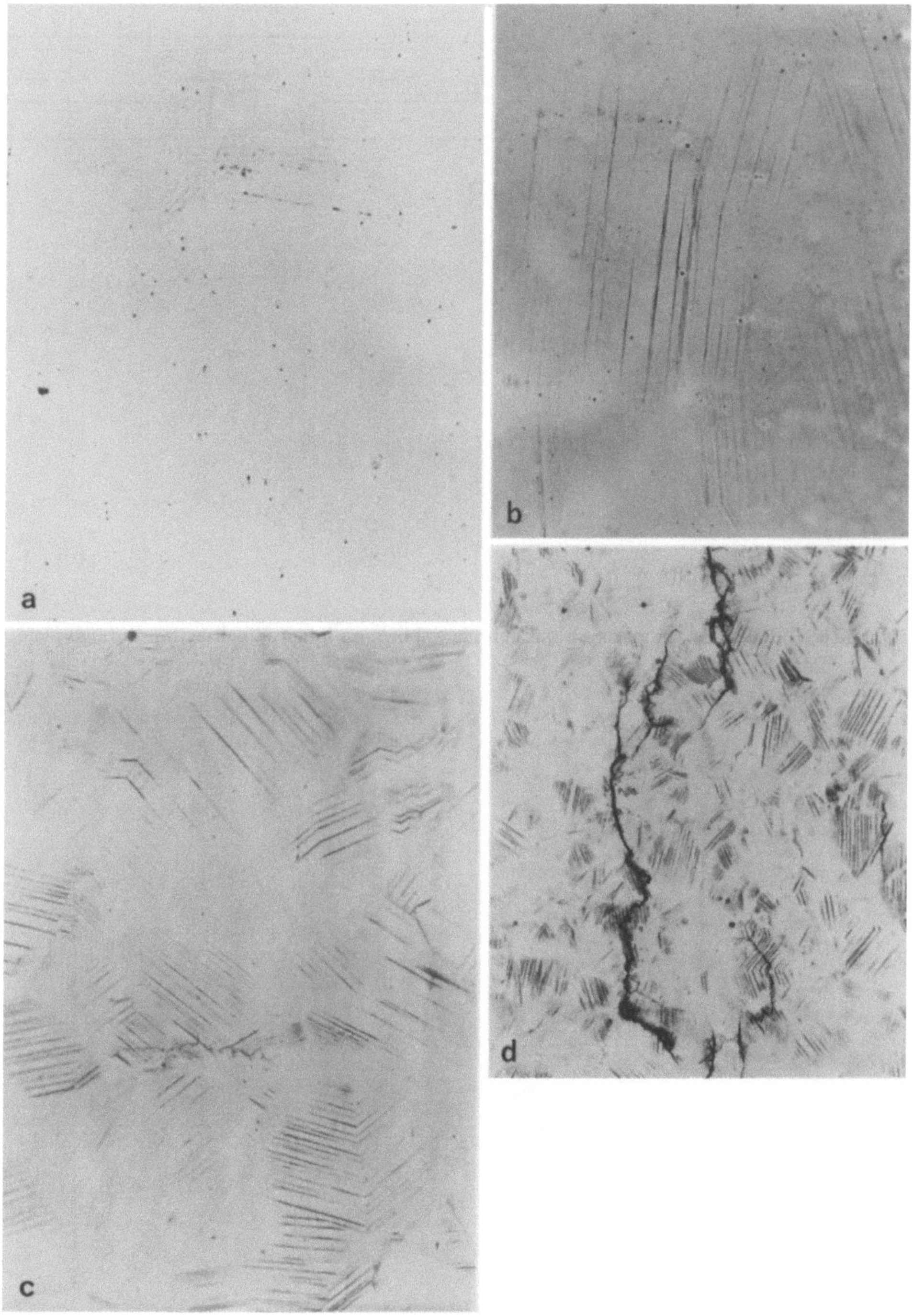

Fig. 3.7a–d. Development of fatigue cracks on stainless steel implant material during in vitro testing in Ringer's solution. (The micrographs show the implant surface after a certain number of load cycles.) **a** After 500 cycles: single slip systems appear. ×275. **b** After 1100 cycles: first extrusions/intrusions (micronotches). ×275. **c** After 29 500 cycles: first visible crack. ×275. **d** After 60 000 cycles: a major crack has developed. ×70

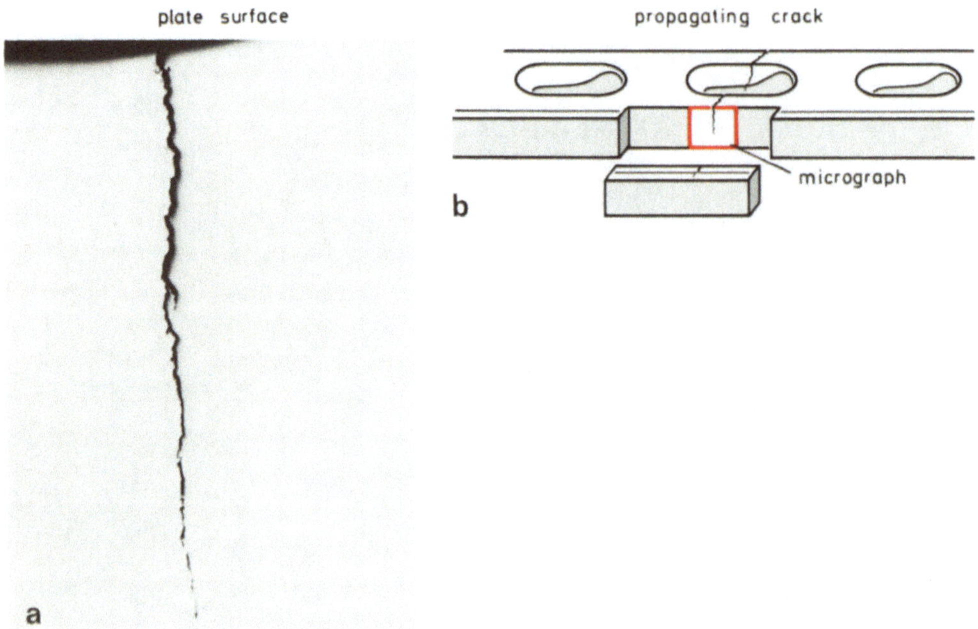

Fig. 3.8a,b. Fatigue crack propagation through plate shown on longitudinal section through plate. ×110

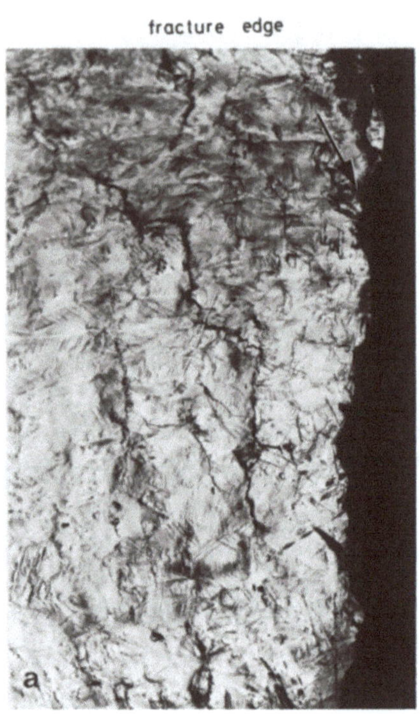

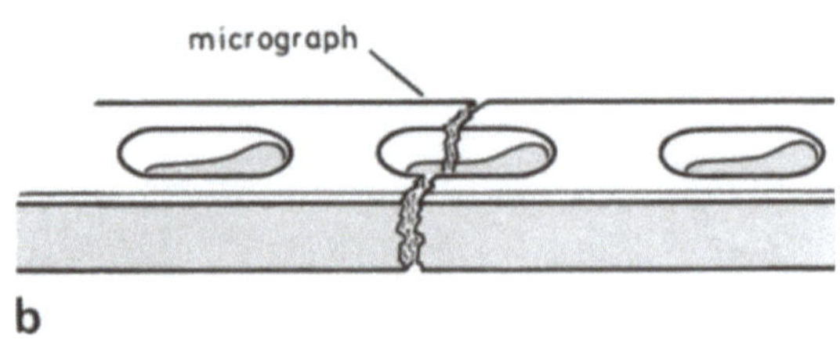

Fig. 3.9a,b. Plate broken in the body by fatigue of plate surface adjacent to fracture with addition minor fatigue crack. ×100

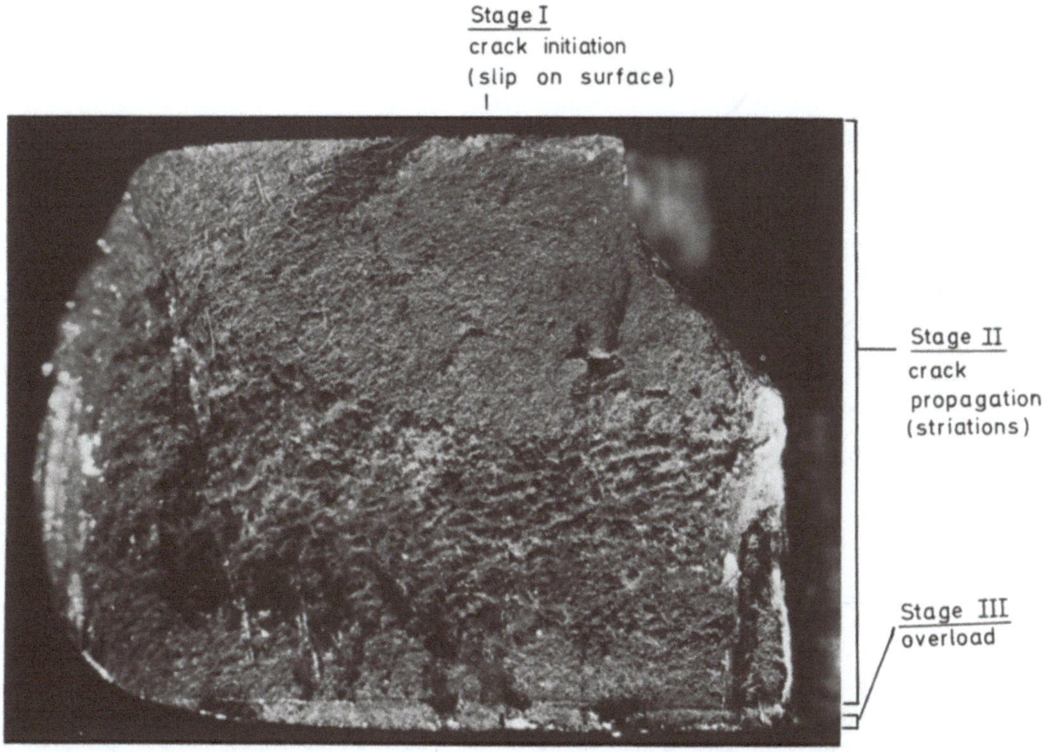

Fig. 3.10. Macroscopic view of fatigue fracture surface of a broken plate. The three main stages of fatigue are indicated

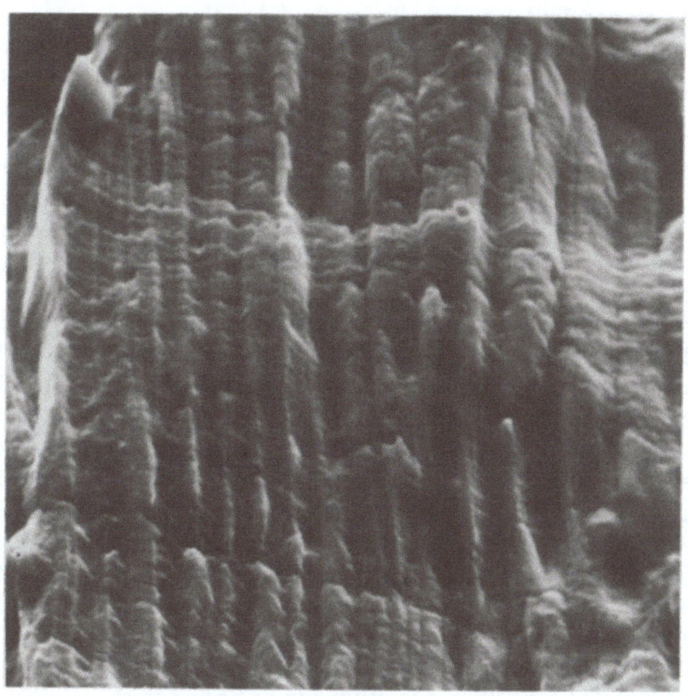

Fig. 3.11. SEM micrograph. Fine parallel horizontal lines show typical fatigue striations caused by single load cycles (propagation stage of Fig. 3.9). ×6000

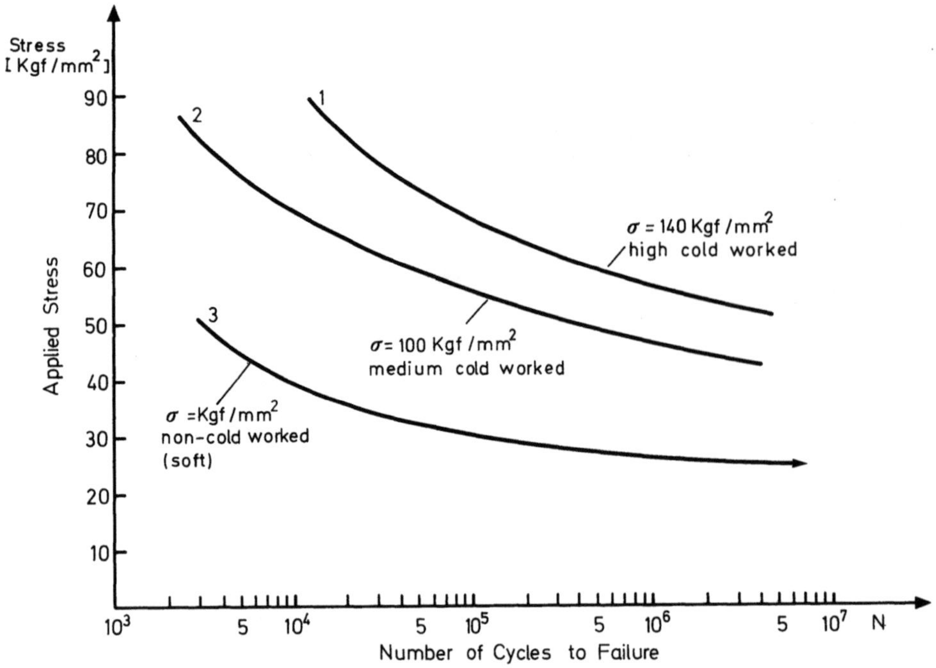

Fig. 3.12. Fatigue curves for stainless steel implant material of varying cold-work degrees generated by rotating-bending beam tests in air. The curves indicate the number of cycles to failure counted under certain applied stresses. The fatigue strength increases with the strength of the material, as seen from *curves 1–3*. *Curve 2* represents the medium cold-worked material used for screws and plates. Interpreted in terms of internal fixation, this curve indicates that no failure will occur when the stresses do not exceed approximately 45 kgf/mm², which is the fatigue limit of the material. For a perfectly rigid internal fixation, the stress concentration would already be below the fatigue limit postoperatively, and no risk of fatigue would exist. However, under severe instability with high stress concentrations assumed in the range of 70 kgf/mm², fatigue failure could occur after about 10 000 load cycles. In cases with smaller instabilities and lower stress concentrations, the bone might heal before the critical number of load cycles was reached, and an implant failure thus be avoided

they are contoured intraoperatively. The fatigue resistance will not be diministhed by this procedure, as can be deduced from the fact that material more cold-worked (curve 1) than the plates (curve 2) has higher fatigue strength. This result has also been verified by fatigue tests on contoured plates. Precise contouring of the plates to fit the bone shape is an important precondition for rigid fixation and should thus be emphasized. However, repeated bending back and forth should be avoided because it leads to loss of ductibility. In addition, contouring in the plate holes is not recommended. Tool marks left on the smallest plate section at a screw hole could serve as stress raisers if the hole became subject to fatigue loading.

The radiographs in Fig. 3.13 show a typical example of a plate that has failed due to fatigue in an unstable internal fixation where bony support was lacking opposite the plate and a considerable fracture gap persisted. The plate broke at a screw hole in the unstable zone, which is characteristic for all clinically broken straight plates. Figure 3.14 illustrates schematically the effect of a fracture gap on a plate hole. When a fracture gap or bony defect is situated beneath or near a plate hole, the uniform stress distribution through the plate is disturbed and the bending stresses which occur under weight-bearing concentrate at this particular screw hole to create a fatigue situation.

In general, analysis of cases with broken implants always revealed an unstable biomechanical situation, and the failure developed by the mechanism decribed above. The instability leading to fatigue can have different sources:

1. Primary instability due to:
   a) Wrong indication, e.g., screw fixation only instead of a neutralization plate fixation
   b) Wrong implant, e.g., implant too weak, plate too short
   c) Missing lag screws
   d) Insufficient reduction and fixation
   e) Missing bony support (becuase of persisting fracture gap or bony defect, lack of a bony buttress opposite the plate)
   f) Lack of bone graft
2. Secondary instability due to:
   a) Delayed healing

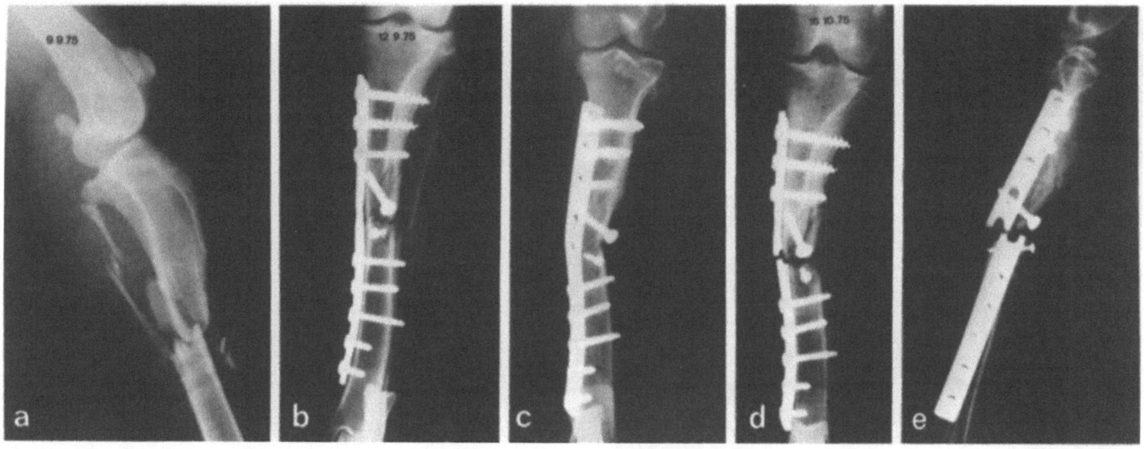

Fig. 3.13a–e. Fatigue failure of a plate in an unstable internal fixation in a dog. **a** Comminuted fracture of tibia and fibula. **b** Three days postoperatively. Although two single lag screws were applied, a wide fracture gap remains. Therefore, medial bony support is lacking and the plate undergoes cyclic bending under load-bearing. **c** Four weeks postoperatively. The fracture gap closes under load and the plate bends. In the fracture zone, the load is only transmitted through the plate without bony support. **d,e** Five weeks postoperatively. Fatigue fracture of the plate. The fracture site of the plate exhibits the typical features of fatigue under high load when examined microscopically

b) Bone resorption
c) Infection
d) Change of biomechanical situation (varization, valgization)
e) Inadequate postoperative treatment, e.g., overloading

In most failures, a number of these characteristics are present at the same time. To avoid complications, the operation should be planned and performed so that optimal stability is achieved. Stability of the internal fixation is necessary not only to prevent implant failure, but also to avoid bone resorption and nonunion. Depending on the type of fracture or orthopedic correction, the achievable degree of stability varies from nearly ideal rigid fixation to highly unstable fixations in which the plate has only a bridging function, as illustrated in Fig. 3.15a–d. With the proper technique, fractures with more than two fragments can be well stabilized (Fig. 3.15c). In fractures with comminuted zones, as depicted in Fig. 3.15b, the stability is practically no better than if a bone segment were missing (Fig. 3.15a). In cases with bony defects and unsecured small fragments, cancellous bonegrafting is an important aid in enhancing bone healing and lowering the risk of complications and implant failure. The postoperative treatment must be adjusted according to the degree of stability of the internal fixation.

3.12 Bone Infection

3.12.1 Introduction

Infection of the bone (osteomyelitis) is defined as inflammation of bone caused by a microorganism. Acute osteomyelitis and chronic osteomyelitis are the same disease, the only difference being the time the disease has been present. Wound infections involve tissues adjacent to the bone, but do not always involve the bone. Osteomyelitis is present only when there is radiographic, microbiological, or histopathologic evidence that the bone is infected. The clinical signs of wound infection include localized swelling and drainage. Wound infection can proceed to osteomyelitis if not properly treated.

Post-traumatic osteomyelitis is the most common type of bone infection in animals. The clinical signs of post-traumatic osteomyelitis include intermittent, localized swelling and drainage. Lameness may or may not be present. Mortality due to post-traumatic osteomyelitis is very low. This disease is reported in all animals that undergo bone surgery or incur trauma.

Hematogenous osteomyelitis is an infection of the bone not associated with trauma or surgery. The source of the bacteria is elsewhere in the body. This is often a systemic disease, and the animal may exhibit the clinical signs of fever and/or anorexia. Compared to the incidence of post-traumatic osteomyelitis, this disease is rare, but the mortality rate is high.

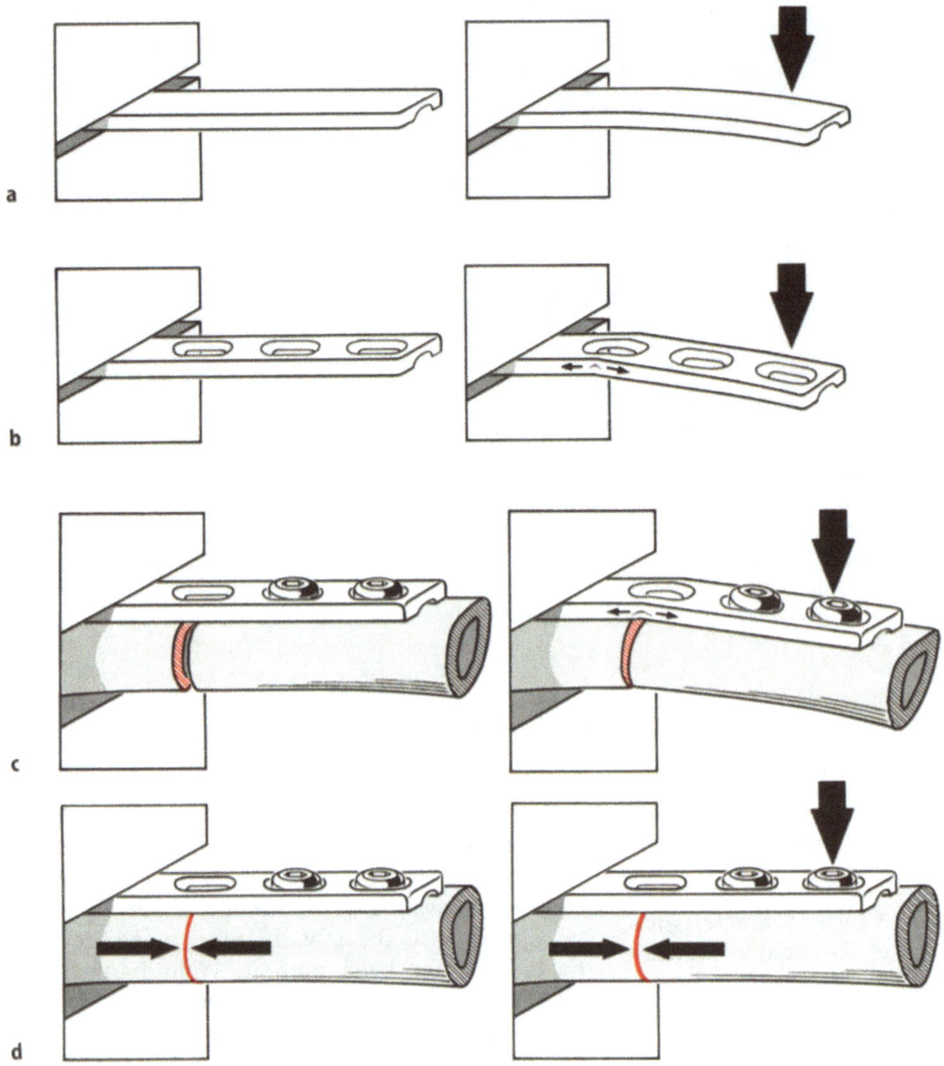

Fig. 3.14a–d. Stress concentration in plate holes. **a** If a plate without holes is bent, stresses are distributed evenly over the plate. **b** If the plate contains a hole, stresses concentrate there, at the smallest cross-section. **c** If, at the same time, the plate is supported, e.g., by a bone, the bending effect on the plate is reduced. However, when support is lacking underneath the plate hole because of a persistent fracture gap, the stresses at the hole are increased, while the rest of the plate is stiffened by the bone. **d** However, if the fracture gap is closed under compression, e.g., tension band plate, the plate is supported continuously and stress concentration in the hole is markedly reduced. If possible, placing a plate hole over a fracture gap should be avoided, as the plate is weakest at this point

3.12.2 Animal Characteristics

Post-traumatic osteomyelitis is not an age-specific disease, nor is there any specific breed predisposition. There is a sex prevalence in post-traumatic osteomyelitis, with males (64%) being represented almost twice as often as females (36%). Due to their behavioral characteristics, males are more likely to suffer trauma than females. *Staphylococcus* spp. are the most common bacteria isolated from dogs with osteomyelitis, followed by *Streptococcus* spp (Table 3.5).

Table 3.5. Bacterial organisms isolated from 67 dogs with osteomyelitis

Organism	Dogs (*n*)	Occurrence (%)
Staphylococcus	50	45
Streptococcus	20	18
Escherichia coli	14	13
Proteus	10	9
Pasteurella	5	5
Micrococcus	4	4
Corynebacterium	2	2
Nocardia	2	2
AerobacterY	2	2

a b c d

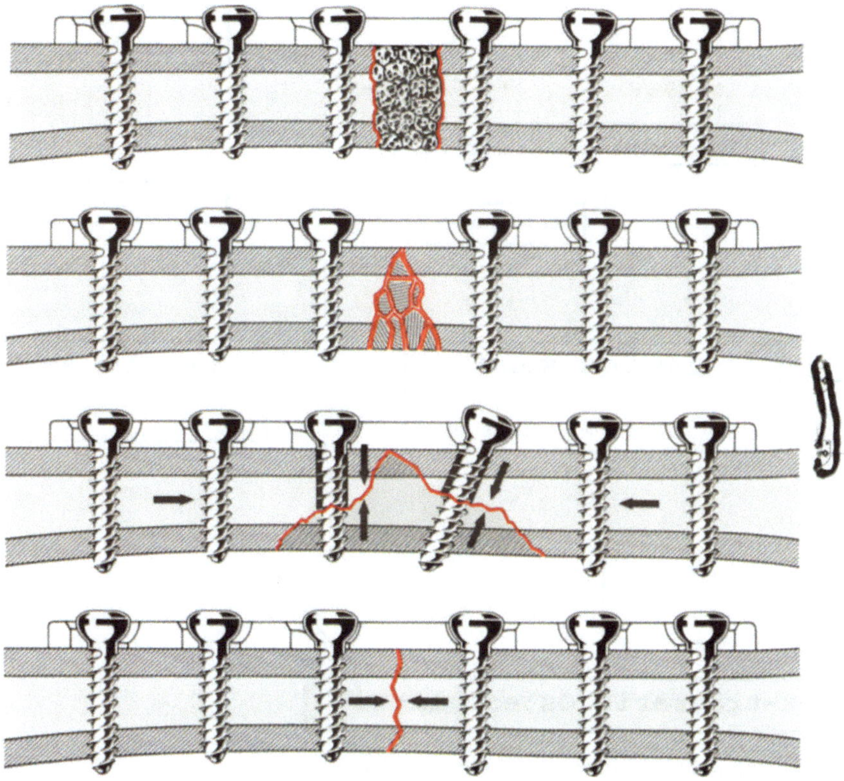

Fig. 3.15a–d. Internal fixations with varying degrees of stability. **a** Wide bony defect, plate has only bridging function – highly unstable situation. **b** No bone support under load because fragments are too small to be fixed – unstable situation. **c** Primary fixation with two lag screws and protection of fixation by neutralization plate. The fragments are in contact and under compression – good stability. **d** Rigid compression fixation with plate under tension and bone under compression – best achievable stability

3.12.3 Pathogenesis

The most common source of bacteria in osteomyelitis is a poor surgical technique. Other sources of infection are the open wound and environmental contamination.

The pathogenesis of osteomyelitis is outlined in Fig. 3.16. Three components are necessary for the creation of post-traumatic osteomyelitis: (1) infected wound, (2) avascular bone, and (3) favorable milieu. If any one of the three components are missing, osteomyelitis is unlikely to develop.

The first component needed to create osteomyelitis is an infected wound. A contaminated wound becomes infected when sufficient bacteria are present to start reproducing ($>10^5$ colony-forming units, CFU) and sufficient time has passed, i.e., lag phase (Fig. 3.17). Traumatic wounds more than 4 h old are considered "dirty wounds," and all traumatic orthopedic wounds older than 4 h are considered contaminated.

Avascular bone is segregated from the body's humoral defenses and systemic antibiotics. In all fractures there will be some dead bone, either separate avascular fragments or the "die-back" zone along fracture lines.

A favorable environment permits bacteria to multiply because they meet their nutritional needs from stagnant blood and/or necrotic soft tissue.

3.12.4 Prevention

3.12.4.1 Prevention of Infected Wound

A wound can be prevented from becoming infected by keeping the bacterial count of the wound at closing below 10^5 CFU per g tissue. Good surgical technique and proper open wound management can keep the CFU below 10^5 per g tissue. Good surgical technique involves aseptic surgery, knowledge of the anatomy of the surgical region, an atraumatic approach, fastidious hemostasis, gentle tissue handling, lavage of soft tissues, anatomic closure, and physiologic postoperative care.

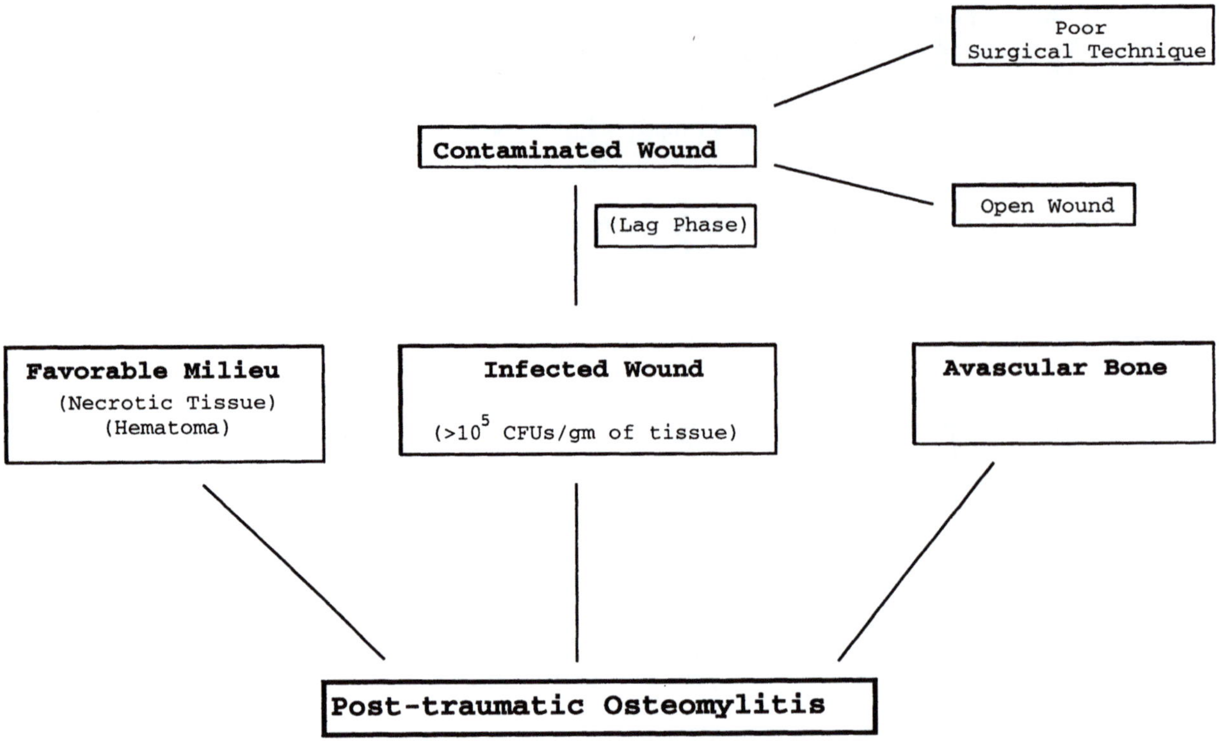

Fig. 3.16. Pathogenesis of post-traumatic osteomyelitis. (*CFU* = colony-forming units)

3.12.4.2 Prevention of Infected Sequestrum

The second component needed to create post-traumatic osteomyelitis is avascular bone. There is always some dead bone present in fractures. Histopathologic sections of fractured bone show a few millimeters of bone along the fracture line with empty lacunae (dead bone). This is caused by vascular damage in the bone. This area of dead bone is the die-back zone. Although this bone is dead, it should not be removed because the bone still supports weight, accepts fixation, and aids in reduction and alignment of the fracture.

Dead bone has vascular channels throughout, i.e., Haversian and Volkmann's canals, which become revascularized during bone healing. Such bone protects new vascularization and allows a slow remodeling process throughout. Bone cells follow the vascular network. The osteoclasts remove dead bone, and osteoblasts invade and mature into osteocytes, which lay down new living bone matrix.

The surgeon can minimize the die-back zone at the fragment end by not damaging the intramedullary arteries or stripping the periosteum and muscular attachments from the bone. The normal blood flow through the cortical bone is from the medullary artery centrifugally to the periosteal venous system. Any break in the flow will result in more dead bone.

Large fragments of bone that have soft tissue attachments must be preserved. If possible, these fragments should be incorporated into the fixation with interfragmentary screws or cerclage wires, without stripping the soft tissue attachments.

If there are avascular fragments in an open fracture too small to be incorporated into the fracture repair with screws or wires, they may be removed from the wound. This is only done in open fractures to minimize the amount of avascular bone where bacteria can isolate themselves from humoral defenses and antibiotic therapy. Small fragments are left in place or packed around the fracture gap in closed fractures. If a significant fracture gap is present, an autogenous cancellous graft can be used because it will not become an infected sequestrum.

3.12.4.3 Prevention of a Favorable Milieu for Bacteria

The third component needed to successfully create post-traumatic osteomyelitis is a favorable milieu. In an environment of stagnant blood and/or necrotic tissue, bacteria can multiply. A wound can rapidly go from a contaminated wound to an infected wound. If the hematoma and necrotic tissue are eliminated from the wound, the favorable milieu is reduced.

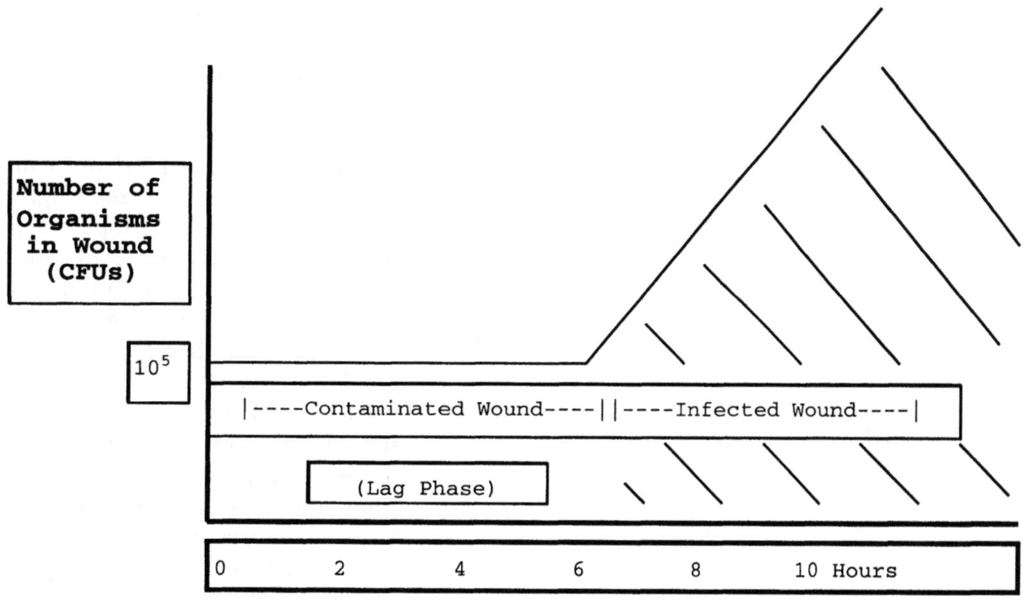

Fig. 3.17. The number of organisms (bacteria) in an open wound versus time. During the lag phase (approximately 6h), the wound is considered contaminated. When the bacteria start to multiply, the infected phase is initiated. *CFU*, colony-forming units

Hematoma is controlled by hemostasis techniques such as ligation or electrocautery. After each layer is closed, the wound should be lavaged and checked for bleeding vessels.

Any necrotic tissue present should be removed by surgical débridement or with microdébridement during open wound management. If there is some possibility that tissue is so traumatized that it may later necrose, the wound is left fully or partially open. Within a few days, the status of the tissue will become obvious. Premature closure of the wound traps necrotic tissue and bacteria inside the surgical site.

The surgeon needs to practise gentle tissue handling and care of the soft tissue. If soft tissues are traumatized during the surgical procedure, necrosis may develop after closure, creating a favorable milieu. Retraction of muscles using atraumatic retractors – and not the hands – is important. The tissues should not be wiped or scraped with sponges, but gently blotted. Tissues must be kept moist. Tissue dries out on exposure to the air and heat of the surgical lights. This can be avoided by lavaging every 10 min.

3.12.5 Diagnosis

Post-traumatic osteomyelitis can be diagnosed by evaluating six different parameters: (1) drainage, (2) soft tissue swelling, (3) periosteal reaction, (4) serial radiographs, (5) microbiology, and (6) histopathology.

3.12.5.1 Drainage

Since wound drainage is not normal after orthopedic surgery, it may indicate infection. Drainage can be intermittent. The infection causes exudate, leading to soft tissue swelling, and exudate pressure eventually results in drainage. As the wound drains, swelling recedes and the draining tract can close. Drainage reoccurs if the exudate pressure increases beyond tissue-holding strength and indicates wound infection and/or osteomyelitis. Infection may be present without drainage.

3.12.5.2 Soft Tissue Swelling

For the first 4 weeks after trauma or surgery, soft tissue swelling cannot be used to diagnose post-traumatic osteomyelitis, because swelling can be normal during that period after surgery or trauma. If swelling is present after 4 weeks, the presence of osteomyelitis should be considered. However, if the lesion is draining, soft tissue swelling is not usually present.

3.12.5.3 Periosteal Reaction

Periosteal reaction is proliferation of the periosteum due to stimulation by the infection. It may be palpable below the elbow or stifle (Fig. 3. 18) and can be seen on radiographs of all infected bones (Fig. 3. 19). Most cases of osteomyelitis show a periosteal reaction. However, osteomyelitis is occasionally very aggressive, lytic, and minimally proliferative.

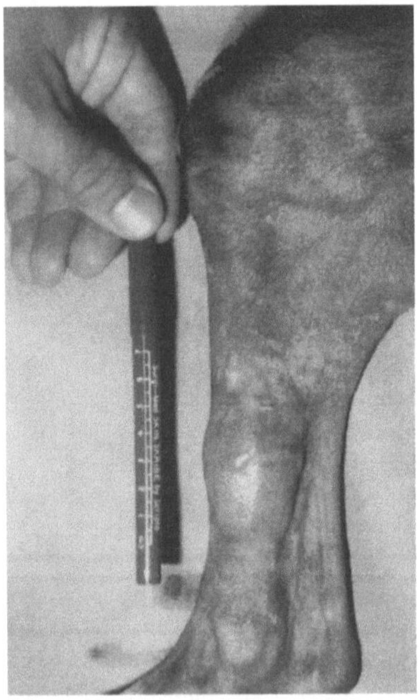

Fig. 3.18. Medial aspect of a tibia of a dog with post-traumatic osteomyelitis. Notice the enlargement (periosteal reaction) in the midtibial region, measuring 7×3.5×2 cm. This periosteal reaction palpates as firm as bone

3.12.5.4 Radiography

The typical radiographic signs of osteomyelitis are proliferative periosteal reaction, soft tissue swelling, increased medullary density, and cortical lysis (Fig. 3.19). Bone sequestrum can be found radiographically in some cases (Fig. 3.19). These signs correlate with the histopathologic changes seen with osteomyelitis (Fig. 3.20). Most of these radiographic signs are similar to the changes seen in secondary bone healing; diagnosing osteomyelitis after a fracture can therefore be difficult. The radiographic signs of secondary bone healing should peak at 6–12 weeks and then proceed into the remodeling stage of healing. If signs are persistent or advancing in extent after 6–12 weeks, post-traumatic osteomyelitis should be suspected. A tentative diagnosis of post-traumatic osteomyelitis can be made sooner if the radiographic signs are present, with soft tissue swelling beyond 4 weeks and drainage.

Serial radiography is a noninvasive parameter used to diagnose osteomyelitis. With serial radiography, two or more different periods are evaluated. Bony lesions develop slowly, and an interval of 3–4 weeks between radiographic evaluation periods is thus recommended. The bone and lesions at the different periods can be compared.

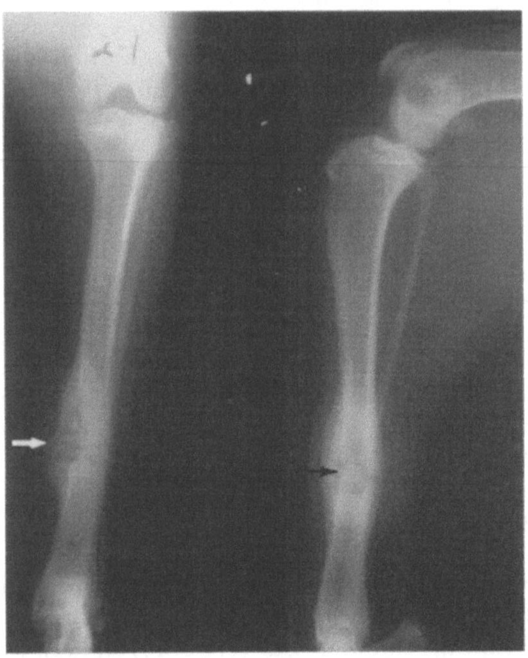

Fig. 3.19. Mediolateral and posteroanterior radiograph of tibia (same dog as in Fig. 3.18). Notice the large amount of periosteal reaction; the cortical lysis, the medullary reaction, and the bone sequestrum (*arrows*)

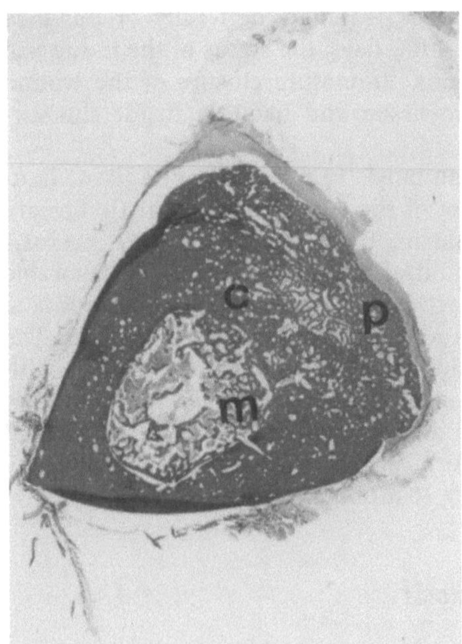

Fig. 3.20. Histologic cross-section of a tibia with osteomyelitis showing the bony changes that are also seen radiographically, such as cortical lysis (*c*), periosteal bone proliferation (*p*), and medullary bone proliferation (*m*)

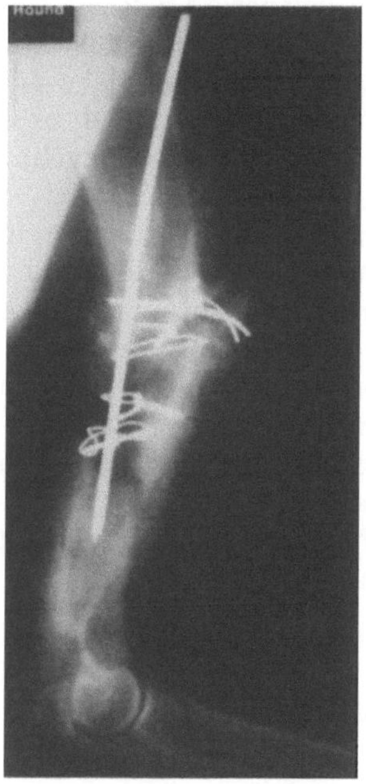

Fig. 3.21. Mediolateral radiograph of a healing humerus with osteomyelitis from an Irish wolfhound

3.12.5.5 Microbiology

Microbiology has the highest sensitivity and specificity in diagnosing post-traumatic osteomyelitis. However, a positive microbiology culture is not 100 % indicative of osteomyelitis, since the wound alone may be infected. Radiology is used to differentiate between osteomyelitis and wound infection.

3.12.5.6 Histopathology

Histopathology can be a useful diagnostic parameter if a significant core of bone can be taken for histologic analysis without further weakening the bone. A core of bone at least 6 mm in diameter is needed. The sample should include the reactive periosteal bone, the cortical or trabecular bone, and contents of the medullary canal from the most pathologic area. If the biopsy is taken through a small incision, two Kirschner guide wires are placed aseptically into the lesion and two radiographic views are taken. With the wires, the most pathologic area can be identified and biopsied.

Histopathologic diagnosis of osteomyelitis is based on the morphologic identification of bacteria in the periosteal reactive tissue, the cortical or trabecular bone, or the medullary canal. Marked myeloid hyperplasia (active marrow) is evident. However, active marrow alone cannot be considered as evidence of osteomyelitis, because hyperplasia of the marrow cells is also present in several other situations, such as healing bone, hematopoiesis, and noninfectious inflammatory conditions of bone.

3.12.5.7 Other Parameters

Other parameters have been used to evaluate osteomyelitis, but these are usually not helpful. Parameters of questionable value include clinical function, local tissue temperature, rectal temperature, pain, complete blood count, serum calcium, serum phosphorus, serum glucose, blood urea nitrogen, uric acid, serum cholesterol, total protein, serum albumin, total bilirubin, alkaline phosphatase, and aspartate transferase. These parameters are of little to no help because they are systemic measurements, and this is a localized disease.

It should be evident that making the diagnosis of post-traumatic osteomyelitis is difficult using only one parameter. The history (trauma, surgery, drainage, lameness), physical examination (soft tissue swelling, periosteal reaction, drainage, lameness), and radiographic and microbiologic findings (and possibly histopathology) need to be evaluated to make this diagnosis.

3.12.6 Treatment

The treatment of osteomyelitis consists of two parts: (1) improving the environment and (2) proper antimicrobial therapy. Of these, the former is by far the most important. The success rate of treating osteomyelitis merely with proper antimicrobial therapy is less than 25 %, while the rate for improving the environment alone is 76 %. When combining both treatments, the success rate is approximately 90 %.

Improving the environment consists in surgically removing the elements from the wound that make the body's defenses and/or systemic antimicrobials ineffective. Post-traumatic osteomyelitis is a surgical disease and should not be treated only medically. One or more of the following is removed surgically: pus, bacteria, necrotic soft tissue, dead bone, unstable implants, and/or foreign bodies. Open wound management is also part of improving the environment.

3.12.6.1 Surgical Management

During the surgical débridement, copious lavage should be done frequently (every 5–10 min) with lactated Ringer's solution. One to 5 l is used, depending on the size of the animal, the size of the wound, and appearance of the wound. The lavage solution should be delivered to the wound via a low-pressure system, such as a bulb syringe or sterile i.v. tubing leading from an overhead container of lactated Ringer's solution. Lavaging combined with suction removes bacteria, debris, and exudate. Large foreign bodies, dead bone, and unstable implants are removed. Any necrotic soft tissue (skin, subcutaneous tissue, fat, or muscle) should be débrided. Fistulous tissue is removed. Once the wound is entirely opened, a swab for aerobic and anaerobic organisms and antimicrobial sensitivity of the tissue that appears most actively infected is performed.

A sequestrum should always be removed. It is usually not connected to other bone, callus, or soft tissue. It is generally yellowish-white, whereas normal bone tends to be white, pink-white, or blue-white. The surface of an infected sequestrum is often pitted, and its size varies but is generally is no smaller than 6 mm. Smaller pieces of bone are generally resorbed or phagocytized.

Typical foreign bodies found in the wound include surgical sponges, wooden twigs, drains, grass, straw, dirt, and gravel or stones. They should be removed. All unstable orthopedic implants should be removed. There are many areas on implants in which the bacteria can be isolated from the body's defense system and systemic antimicrobials.

Stable orthopedic devices should not be removed. Infected bone will heal if it is stably fixed. The implants should stay in place until bony union is evident radiographically. After the bone has healed, all implants should be removed.

After débridement of the infected area, the surgical wound should be treated with open wound management. When the wound is clean and the infection controlled, it can be partially closed. The lowest 1–2 cm of the wound is left open, establishing drainage for exudate or transudate. If the infection is controlled, the 1- to 2-cm wound will heal by second intention.

3.12.6.2 Medical Management

Medical management of osteomyelitis consists in proper antimicrobial therapy. During surgical débridement, a deep microbiological culture of aerobes and anaerobes and antimicrobial sensitivity is taken. Antimicrobial treatment should last for a minimum of 28 days. Cultures should not be taken from draining tracts. Culturing the draining tract generally gives a mixed infection, and in at least 50 % of cases it does not identify the causative bacteria. The patient should not receive antimicrobials for 5–7 days before the culture is taken.

There is usually a 2- to 5-day period between culturing and obtaining the results. During this time period, an empirical antimicrobial should be administered. The bacteriocidal antimicrobial used for this period should be effective in osteomyelitic bone.

Occasionally, an antimicrobial is effective in vitro (petri dish) but seems to have very little to no effect in the animal. One reason for this may be that the bacteria have produced a glycocalyx, i.e., a polysaccharide that forms a protective biofilm. Bacteria produce the glycocalyx in the wound, so an antimicrobial must be able to penetrate the biofilm to be effective. The environment in the petri dish is extremely favorable for the bacteria, so it does not produce the glycocalyx in vitro.

3.13 Gunshot Fractures of Long Bones

3.13.1 Introduction

Fractures and related soft tissue injuries created by a ballistic missile can be more efficiently treated if the surgeon has a basic understanding of the type of missile causing the wound and the pathophysiology related to such injuries. The severity of the destructive effects a missile has on tissues is related to: (a) the action of the missle and its physical properties, including velocity, mass, ballistic shape, design, composition, angle of the missile at impact on the tissue (yaw or tumble), and its course through the tissue and (b) the reaction of the tissues, which depends on their density, elasticity, cohesiveness, and diversion of the bullet path by fascial planes or bone. All of the above factors play a part in the deceleration of the bullet and its release of energy into the tissue.

3.13.2 Definition of Terms

The following definitions are helpful in understanding the pathophysiology of gunshot wounds.

- *Ballistics* is the science of motion of projectiles. Wound ballistics is the effect a moving projectile has on the tissues. Bullet velocity, mass, and the kinetic energy (KE) released in the tissues have major roles in the extent of wounding.
- *Initial velocity* (muzzle velocity) is the speed transferred to the projectile by combustion of the propelling charge. It is measured approximately 5 m from the muzzle of the gun. Wound severity decreases as the distance from the muzzle increases. Gunshot wounds are divided into low-, medium-, and high-velocity wounds. Low

velocity is less than 400 m/s; medium velocity, 400–825 m/s; and high velocity, greater than 825 m/s.

- *Impact velocity* is the bullet's speed as it enters the tissue. With a low impact velocity, the tissue damage is less and there is no explosive effect. With a high impact velocity, the tissue injury is more severe and additional tissue destruction is caused remote to the bullet's path because shock waves are initiated as KE is released.
- *Residual velocity* is the velocity retained by the bullet after it has passed through the tissue. The difference between impact velocity and residual velocity is used to calculate the KE generated in wound production.
- *Kinetic energy* (KE) is the energy resulting from motion of an object. The following formula can be used to calculate the KE of the projectile:

$KE = \frac{1}{2} \times (\text{mass of the projectile} \times \text{velocity of the projectile}^2)$

or

$KE = \frac{1}{2}(mv^2)$

Data is available from the companies who manufacture ammunition listing the KE of the bullet.

3.13.3 Pathophysiology

When a bullet penetrates tissue, KE is released. The tissues offer resistance to the bullet in direct proportion to their density, elasticity, and cohesiveness. The bullet passing through the tissue causes cavitation. Initially, a temporary cavity radiates outward from the bullet's path, forcing tissues apart and sending shock waves through them. The bullet crushes the soft tissue that it contacts directly. In high-velocity injuries, the diameter of the temporary cavity may be up to 30 times the bullet's diameter. The temporary cavity oscillates seven to eight times until dampened, producing pressures which can be thousands of kilograms per square centimeter. The permanent cavity is the space left along the bullet's path after the temporary cavity has come to rest. If the bullet breaks apart, the fragments of the bullet act as secondary missiles, causing further tissue destruction. Fragments of fractured bone can cause further damage to soft tissues. The surgeon should explore beyond the missile tract for injuries.

In high-velocity injuries, the muscle can be pulped and may be blown out through entry and exit sites. Additional muscle damage comes from muscle fiber stretching and tearing and from vascular disruption within the muscle. Larger blood vessels are elastic and, unless hit directly, often remain intact. However, they may thrombose from internal damage. When stretched, the function of large nerves may be impaired. In high-velocity injuries, a long bone can be indirectly fractured without being hit by the bullet due to the kinetic energy released. A bone hit directly by a high-velocity missile is usually severely fragmented, and fragments may be blown out of the entry and exit wounds. Low- and medium-velocity missiles do not have sufficient KE to cause indirect fractures. The healing time for fractures caused by high-velocity missles may be longer than those caused by a low-velocity missile because of more extensive vascular damage.

3.13.4 Infection Associated with Bullet Wounds

Bullets are not sterile. All bullet wounds are contaminated with bacteria. A bullet carries hair, dirt, debris, and bacteria with it into the wound. The negative pressure created by the temporary cavity sucks contaminated material throughout the wound. Contaminated gunshot wounds develop into infected wounds in the same manner as described in Sects. 3.12.3 and 3.12.4. The optimal time for wound débridement and treatment is within 6 h from the time of wounding. If infection becomes established, it is more difficult to treat the soft tissue and the fracture.

3.13.5 Classification

The classification of fractures caused by gunshots is based on the velocity of the bullet:

- *Type I fractures*, caused by low-velocity projectiles, are transverse, oblique, or spiral fractures and have minimal soft tissue damage (Fig. 3.22).
- *Type II fractures* associated with low-velocity projectiles, are comminuted; however, severe cortical bone loss is generally not present (Fig. 3.23) and soft tissue damage is minimal to moderate.
- *Type III fractures* caused by high-velocity projectiles are multifragmented fractures. Extensive cortical defects may be present, and soft tissue damage is severe (Fig. 3. 24).

3.13.6 Initial Treatment

The gunshot fracture patient is treated in the same way as all open fracture patients (see Sect. 3.8). The course of the bullet should be established, as accurately as possible, since body cavities may have been traversed on the bullet's way to the limb. A patient with a high-velocity injury to an extremity may have damage in other body systems caused by

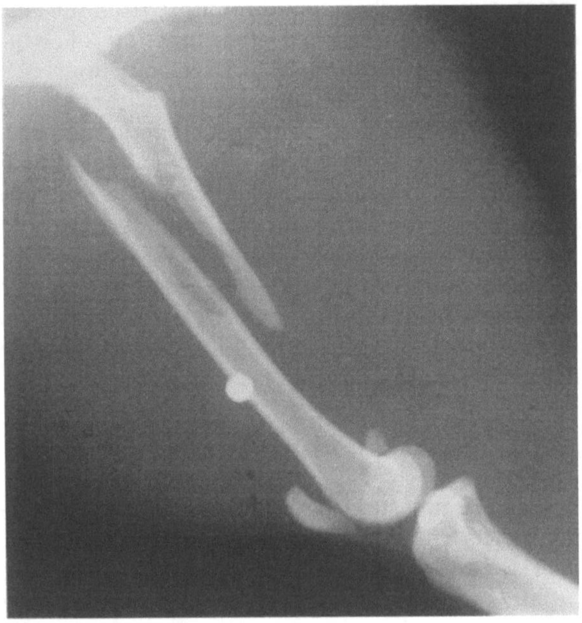

Fig. 3.22. Type I fracture created by a low-velocity projectile

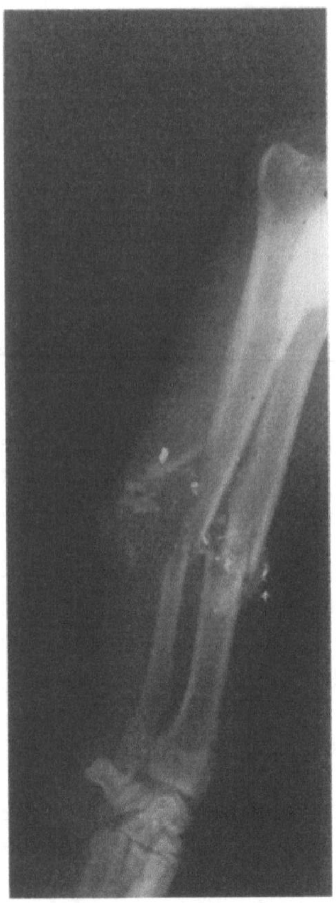

Fig. 3.23. Type II fracture created with a low-velocity projectile. There is more soft and hard tissue damage associated with this type of fracture than with the type I fracture

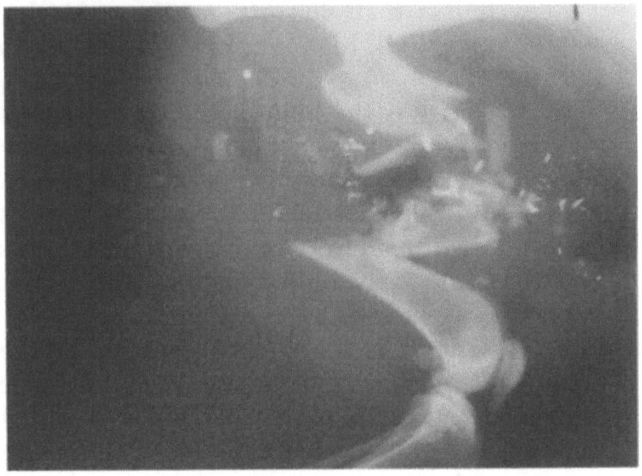

Fig. 3.24. Type III fracture created with a high-velocity projectile. Soft and hard tissue damage is extensive

KE release. The patient's total status must be assessed and treatment instituted as appropriate for the existing conditions.

3.13.7 Fracture Fixation

The methods used for fracture fixation depend on fracture classification, the bone involved, location of the fracture, and the surgeon's preference. Most gunshot fractures are repaired using some type of external fixator or a bone plate. One advantage of using an external fixator for repairing diaphyseal gunshot fractures is that the surgical approach to the involved bone is less extensive than that required for application of a bone plate.

Low-velocity (type I) gunshot fractures involving the humerus, femur, ulna, or tibia may be successfully repaired using an intramedullary pin plus cerclage or hemicerclage wire (Fig. 3.25). Low-velocity fractures of the radius should be repaired using either a bone plate or an external fixator. Medium-velocity (type II) gunshot fractures are generally repaired using a bone plate or an external fixator (Fig. 3.26). Some fractures of this type, involving the humerus or femur, may be repaired using an intramedullary pin and a type I single bar external fixater. High-velocity (type III) gunshot fractures require a bone plate or an external fixator for proper fixation of the fracture (Fig. 3.27).

Autogenous cancellous bone grafts are required in all high-velocity (type III) and most medium-velocity (type II) gunshot fractures. Regardless of the type of fixation that is used for repair of gunshot fractures, it must provide rigid stabilization of the fracture until clinical union of the fracture has been achieved. The entry and exit holes should be left open until any infection that is present is

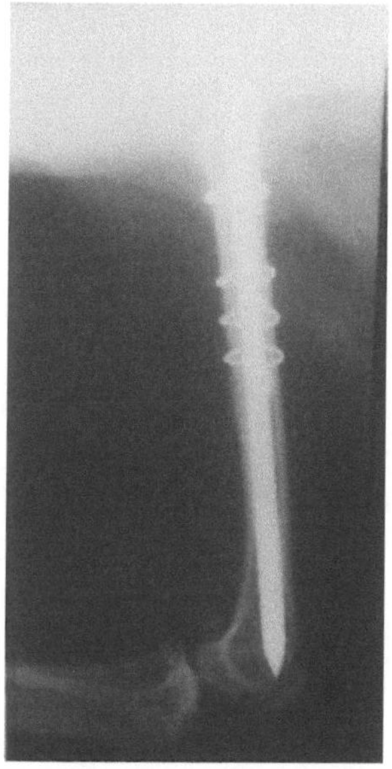

Fig. 3.25. The type I fracture in Fig. 3.22 stabilized with an intramedullary pins and cerclage wire

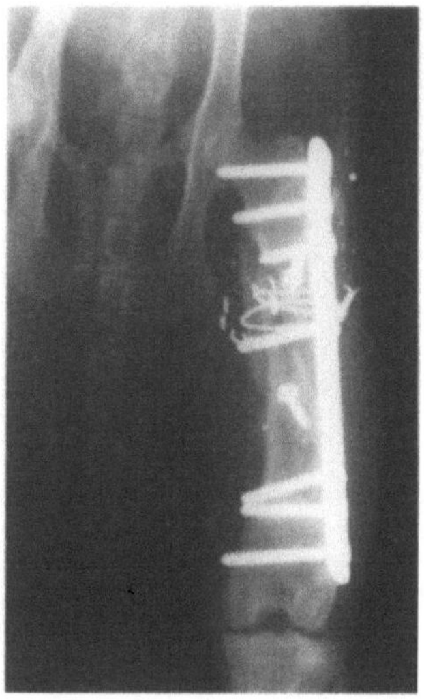

Fig. 3.27. The type III fracture in Fig. 3.24 stabilized with a bone plate, lag screws, and cerclage wires

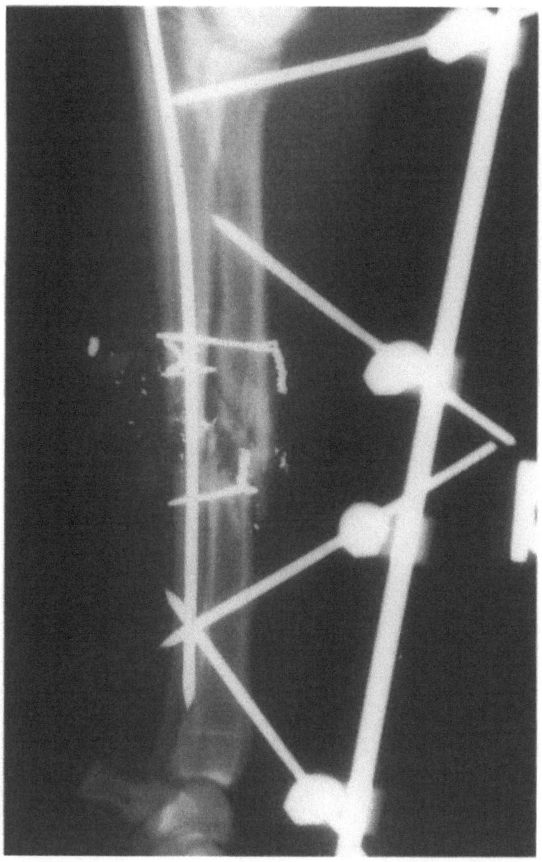

Fig. 3.26. The type II fracture in Fig. 3.23 stabilized with a type I external fixator in the radius and an intramedullary pin in the ulna

brought under control. Because of the severity of skin wound in type III fractures, the skin wound is generally allowed to heal by second intention.

3.13.8 Healing and Complications

In type I and II fractures, delayed bone healing, although possible, is rare. Because of the severe soft tissue, bone, and vascular damage, type III fractures may have a prolonged healing time. Nonunions are unlikely with type I and II fractures, but are a potential risk in type III fractures. Infection is possible in all open fractures. Proper treatment reduces the incidence of infection. Soft tissue complications occur most commonly with type III fractures. Muscle damage may cause limb weakness.

3.13.9 Prognosis

The prognosis for gunshot fractures is directly related to the severity of the classification of the fracture. It is good to excellent in type I, fair to good in type II, and less favorable in type III fractures. Although the soft tissue and bone damage is severe in type III diaphyseal fractures, amputation should not be the first consideration for treating these injuries if the vascular system and nerves are intact.

Part II
Fresh Fractures

This section deals with proven methods of internal fixation for the most common fractures. It has been organized in anatomical sequence. These methods are all based on the principles of internal fixation discussed in Part I and on clinical experience. Where especially important, the most reliable surgical approaches are included along with the surgical techniques and postoperative care. Fractures of immature animals are discussed in a separate section at the end of this chapter.

4.1 Fractures of the Scapula

Fractures of the scapula can be classified into four groups on the basis of the anatomic structures involved:

1. Fractures of the glenoid (articular surface)
2. Fractures of the neck
3. Fractures of the acromion
4. Fractures of the body and spine

A general tendency exists to dismiss scapular fractures as not needing internal fixation and to treat all fracture types by conservative management. However, certain scapular fractures do require accurate reduction and rigid internal fixation in order to maximize return of function of the shoulder joint. This necessity is easily appreciated for those fractures that directly invade the glenoid surface, but may be less apparent in other instances.

Function of the joint is dependent upon factors other than an intact articular surface. A displaced scapular neck fracture will result in mechanical interference with movement of the humeral head, and fracture of the acromion process causes pain due to fragment distraction as a result of contraction of the deltoid muscle. Fractures of the distal half of the body can result in malalignment and may precipitate degenerative joint disease.

The healing potential of the scapula is excellent. Thus truly rigid fixation devices are usually not essential. Multiple Kirschner wires, or simple interfragmentary wiring, are often sufficient, except where muscle tension is strong, as in the case of the supraglenoid tubercle avulsion fracture. Here, and when fractures involve the articular surface, interfragmentary compression with lag screws is ideal.

The only anatomic structure that requires special mention is the suprascapular nerve, which crosses the scapular neck at the base of the acromial region of the spine. This nerve can be intimately involved in the fracture line of a neck fracture and may be difficult to protect during fracture reduction and placement of the fixation device. Open approaches to the region of the joint are complex, and an intimate knowledge of regional anatomy is essential. Several approaches to the body and joint region have been described.

4.1.1 Fractures of the Glenoid

A craniolateral approach with osteotomy of the acromion process and tenotomy of the infraspinous muscle is usually sufficient for reduction of simple fractures. It may be necessary, in multifragment fractures, to osteotomize the greater tubercle of the humerus to allow complete retraction of the supraspinous muscle. Although rarely needed to reduce the fracture, a medial approach is occasionally needed to facilitate placement of the fixation device.

4.1.1.1 Avulsion Fracture of the Supraglenoid Tubercle

Also known as the scapular tuberosity, the supraglenoid tubercle is the point of origin of the powerful biceps brachii muscle, which exerts tension on the fragment. Typically, this fracture occurs in skeletally immature dogs of the larger breeds, such as retrievers. The tubercle is a separate center of ossification from the rest of the glenoid and is subject to avulsion before endochondral ossification is complete (Fig. 4.1a). This avulsion fracture has occasionally been presented bilaterally. The strong distracting tension of the biceps muscle is best neutralized by a lag screw (Fig 4.1b). Although the tension band wiring technique provides good fixation, it is difficult to install in this area, and to do so would require greater surgical exposure. The cranial approach to the shoulder is preferred.

4.1.1.2 Fracture of the Rim of the Glenoid

Fractures involving an articular surface cannot be treated with external coaptation. Malunion of an articular fracture will usually result in progressive osteoarthrosis, and internal fixation provides the best long-term prognosis (Fig. 4.2a). Lag screw fixation of intra-articular fractures is preferable because of the stability afforded. Multiple divergent Kirschner wires are a second possibility, but are advisable only in fragments that are too small for

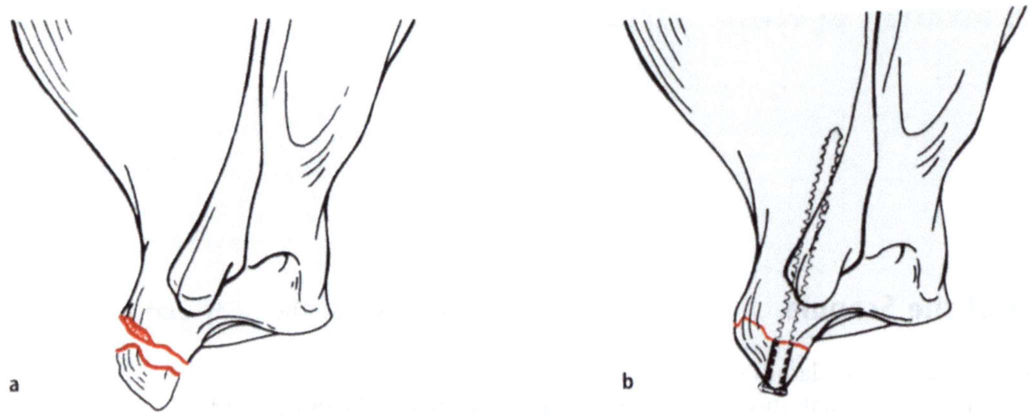

Fig. 4.1. **a** Avulsion fracture of the supraglenoid tubercle (origin of biceps brachii muscle). **b** Interfragmentary lag screw fixation is used to overcome distracting muscle forces

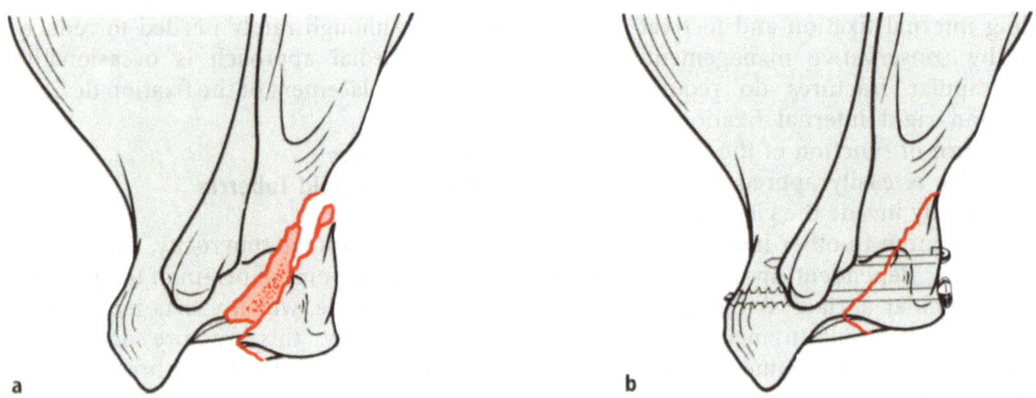

Fig. 4.2. **a** Fracture of the ventral angle of the glenoid. **b** Stabilization by Kirschner wire and interfragmentary lag screw

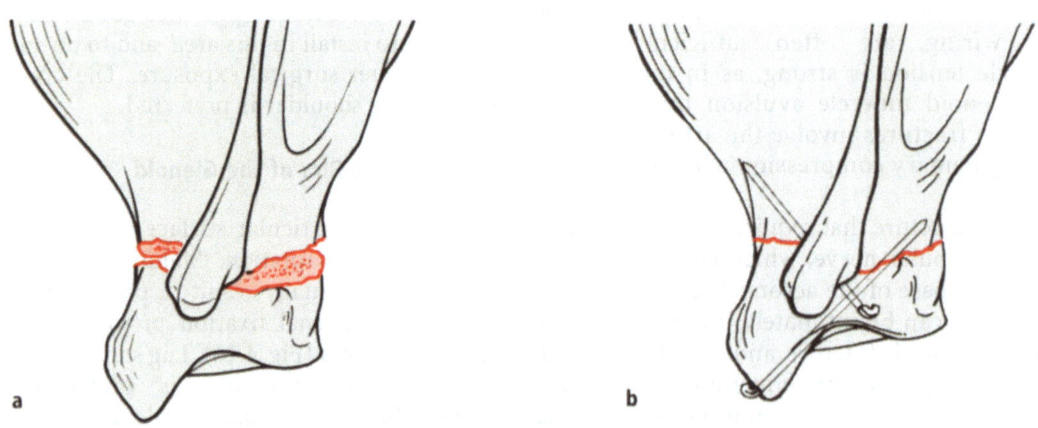

Fig. 4.3. **a** Fracture of the scapular neck. **b** Scapular neck fracture stabilized by Kirschner wires inserted from the dorsal side of the fracture. The L plate in Fig. 4.1 is an alternative implant for this fracture

bone screws. Since the Kirschner wires do not provide interfragmentary compression, they are often useful for holding fragments in position for screw placement if bone-holding forceps are difficult to place (Fig. 4.2b). A foreleg sling bandage for 2 weeks postoperatively may be advisable in very active animals.

4.1.2 Fractures of the Neck

Fractures of the scapular neck are serious injuries (Fig. 4.3a). Although they usually heal if treated by external immobilization, a malunion usually results. This, along with suprascapular nerve damage and the resulting spinous muscle atrophy, leads to malpositioning of the shoulder joint, which in turn affects all the joints of the limb, and degenerative joint disease can be expected, especially in active, large-breed dogs.

For these reasons, internal fixation is the preferred method of treatment. Since these fractures heal quickly, pinning techniques are often sufficient (Fig. 4.3b). In large dogs, the stability afforded by an L or T plate is useful. The neck region is exposed by osteotomy of the acromion process. A sling bandage for 10–14 days is usually indicated.

4.1.3 Fractures of the Glenoid and Neck (T and Y Fractures)

Of greatest concern in fractures of the glenoid and neck (Fig. 4.4a) is accurate reconstruction and rigid fixation of the glenoid fragments. This is achieved with lag screws. The remaining neck fractures can be stabilized with crossed Kirschner wires in small breeds (Fig. 4.4b) or an L or T plate in large breeds (Fig. 4.4c). The crossed wires must be started near the base of the spine and close to the body of the scapula. Care must be taken in placing a bone plate under the suprascapular nerve. The approach of the craniolateral region of the shoulder by osteotomy of the acromion process is the usual choice for exposure. A foreleg sling bandage for 2 weeks is usually advisable, especially if the neck fracture has been stabilized with crossed Kirschner wires.

4.1.4 Fractures of the Acromion

Fractures of the spine that cause detachment and mobility of the acromion and distal spine cause pain and lameness. The deltoid muscle, a major flexor of the shoulder, originates on the acromion and causes motion at the fracture site when the muscle contracts. Although these fractures will heal with immobilization by means of a foreleg sling, internal fixation gives faster and more certain healing. This is especially important in the larger and more athletic breeds. Simple interfragmentary wiring in small breeds and the tension band wire and pin techniques in large breeds both work well (Fig. 4.5). Exposure is by approach to the body of the scapula. A sling bandage for 10–14 days is advisable if simple wiring is used.

4.1.5 Fractures of the Body and Spine

Transverse or oblique fractures through the mid- or proximal areas of the scapula rarely require more than a foreleg sling bandage (Velpeau sling) for healing. The bandage should incorporate cotton padding over the scapula and a generous number of wraps around the trunk, forming a figure-of-eight round the contralateral limb. Conforming gauze

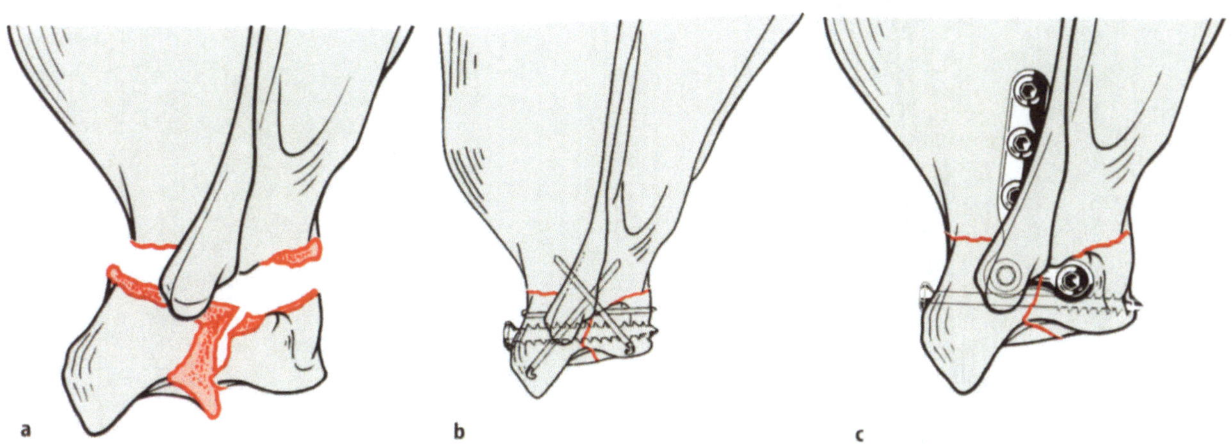

a b c

Fig. 4.4. **a** Fracture of the glenoid and the scapular neck (T fracture). **b** Fixation of T fracture of the glenoid by crossed pins and an interfragmentary lag screw. **c** Fixation of T fracture by an interfragmentary lag screw and L plate

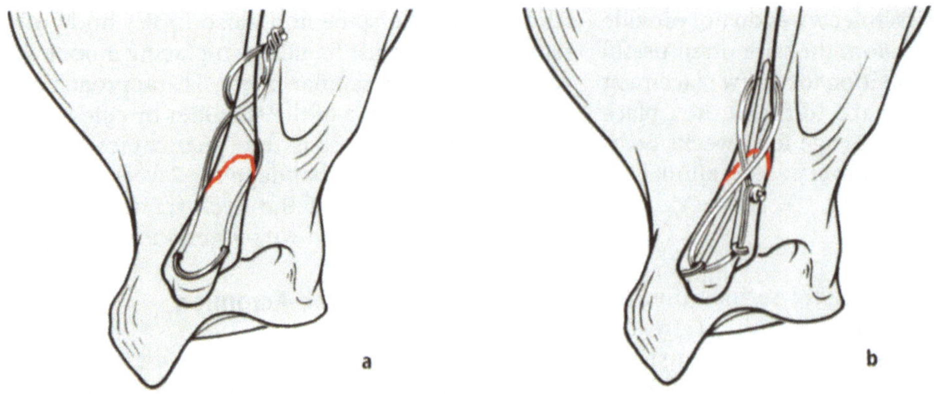

Fig. 4.5. a Fracture of the acromion process with interfragmentary wire fixation as used in small and medium-sized dogs. **b** Fracture of the acromion process with Kirschner wires and tension band wire fixation. Most applicable in giant breeds

covered with wide tape is used. Two to 3 weeks of immobilization is sufficient.

Occasionally, fractures of the body are so severely displaced that they are cosmetically unacceptable (especially in short-haired dogs), or they markedly change the normal position of the glenoid, resulting in degenerative joint disease. Some degree of malfunction of the limb can be anticipated in this situation. Fractures of this type should be treated by open approach and internal fixation.

Minimal internal fixation, combined with external immobilization, as discussed above is often sufficient. Interfragmentary wiring is an efficient

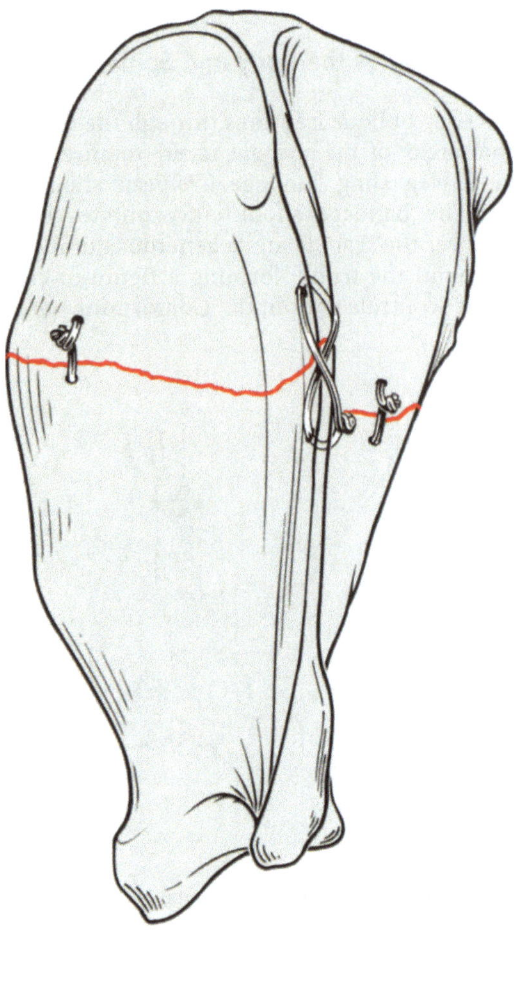

Fig. 4.6. Fracture of the body of the scapula stabilized with two simple interfragmentary wires and a tension band wire

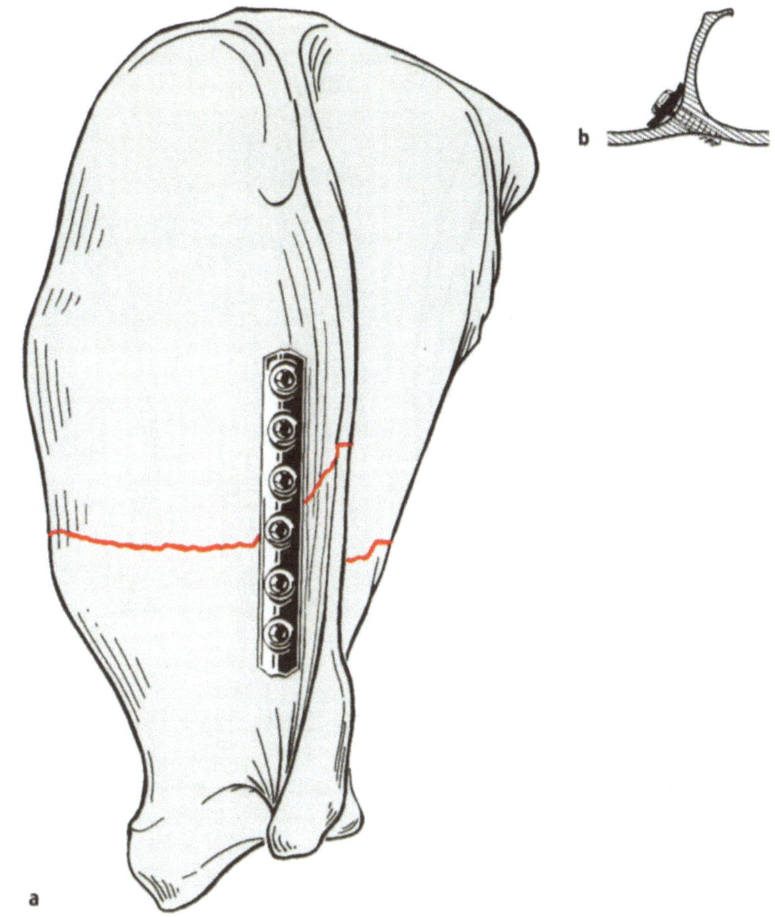

Fig. 4.7. a Fracture of the body of the scapula stabilized with a veterinary cuttable plate inverted at base of the spine. **b** Screws are placed at the angle to take advantage of the thickest bone at the junction of the scapular spine and the body

method in some cases. The wire should not be too heavy or it will cut through the very thin bone of the scapular body. Holes should be drilled through the thickest available bone. Reconstructing the spine with a tension band wire adds a great deal of stability to the repair (Fig. 4.6).

Because of the thinness of the bone, plating is only possible along the base of the spine where screws can be placed in the thickest portion of the bone. The veterinary cuttable plate is the most versatile implant for these fractures. The 1.0-mm plate is used in cats and toy dogs. The 1.5-mm plate attached with either 2.0-mm or 2.7-mm screws is adequate for dogs up to approximately 20 kg. Larger breeds require the 1.5-mm plate to be doubled (stacked) and used with 2.7-mm screws. With other fractures, the major advantage of the cuttable plate is the ability to place more screws per unit of plate length (Fig. 4.7).

Not uncommonly, the scapular spine sometimes remains intact despite marked displacement of the body fragments. The thin cortico-cancellous bone of the spine allows considerable bending before failure. Stabilization of the body fracture can be provided with a cuttable plate applied along the cranial and/or caudal scapular border (Fig. 4.8). An alternative fixation is interfragmentrary wiring. The spine is reattached to the body by a "T" plate (Fig. 4.8). Exposure is by incision directly over the scapular spine with elevation of the spinous muscles. External support is advisable for 10–14 days in most cases.

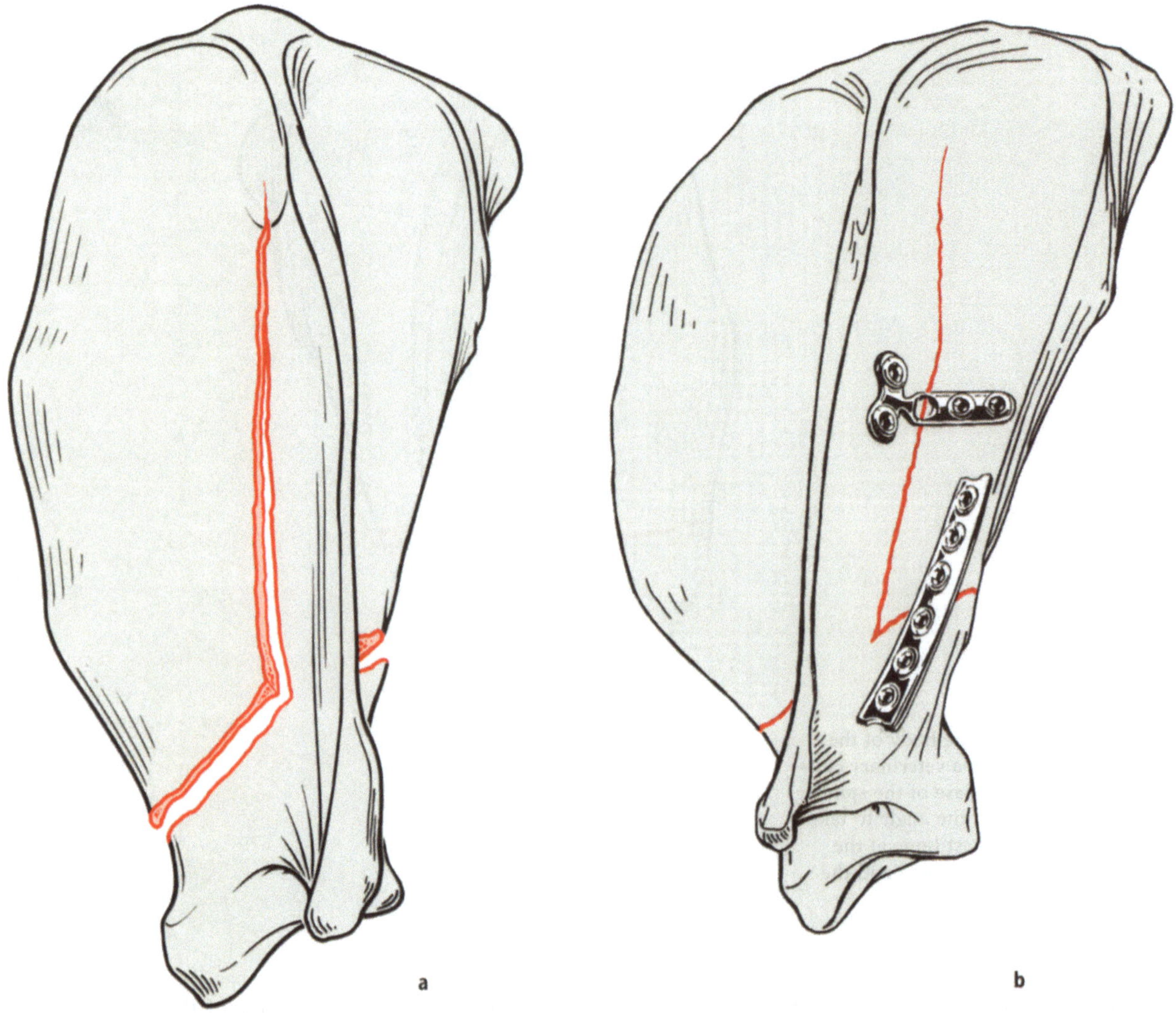

Fig. 4.8. a Craniolateral view of an oblique fracture of the scapular body. The spine remains intact, but partially separated from the body. **b** Caudolateral view of fixation of an oblique body fracture with a plate, and fixation of the spinal fracture with a T plate

4.2 Fractures of the Humerus

The configuration of the humerus is diverse throughout its length. The location of the fracture lines and fragments dictates the approach and the position of implant devices. As all of the surfaces of the humerus may be used for the placement of plates, the fracture position and configuration influence plate position. Occasionally, fractures of this bone involve either the brachial plexus or the radial nerve and, consequently, a thorough presurgical neurological assessment should be performed.

4.2.1 Fractures of the Proximal Humerus

The following fractures occur in the proximal humerus:

- Fractures of the greater tubercle
- Fractures of the humeral head
- Fractures of the proximal third of the diaphyis

The above fractures are approached craniolaterally. Fractures of the greater tubercle may be reduced and then held in temporary stabilization with Kirschner wires, final stabilization being carried out with either one or two lag screws or with pins and a tension band wire (Fig. 4.9). If the bones are soft, metal washers should be placed under the screw heads.

In humeral head fractures, depending upon the course of the fracture line, it may or may not be necessary to perform an acromion osteotomy of the scapula to facilitate reduction. Temporary fixation may again be achieved by means of Kirschner wires; final fixation is usually performed with par-

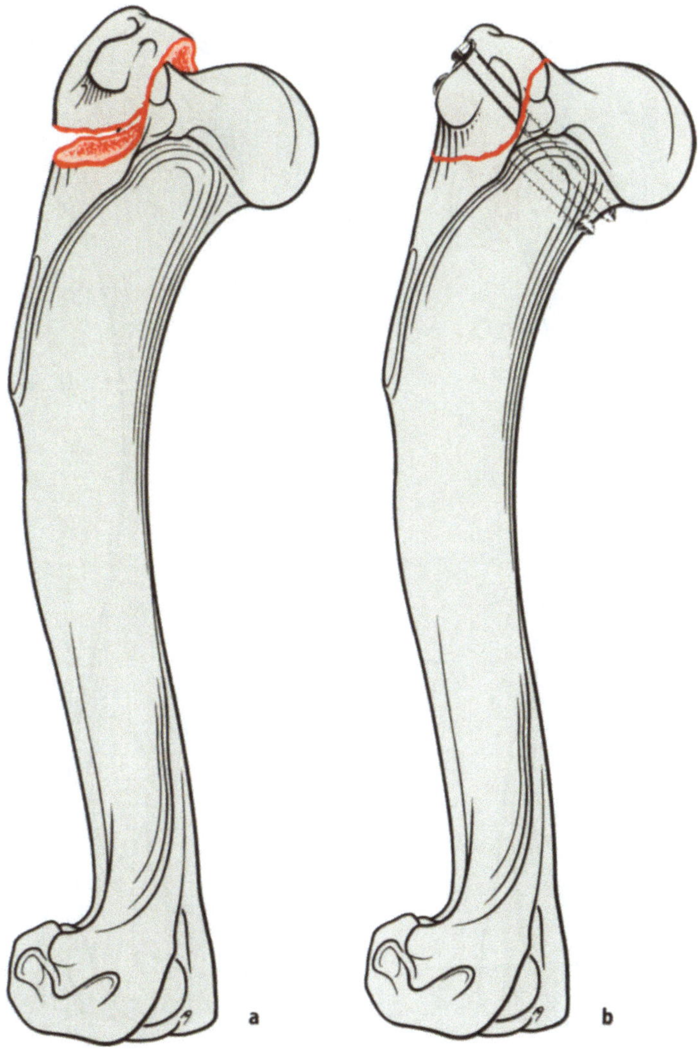

Fig. 4.9. **a** Avulsion fracture of the greater tubrcle. **b** Fixation with two lag screws

tially threaded cancellous screws or cortex screws with lag function (Fig. 4.10). In small patients, where there is insufficient space for two screws, one may be used, in conjunction with a Kirschner wire, to obtain satisfactory stabilization.

4.2.2 Fractures of the Proximal Diaphysis

Fractures of the proximal third may be stabilized by a crainially positioned plate (Fig. 4.11 a–c). In large dogs, when there is insufficient length of bone to permit the insertion of at least two screws, a hook plate gives adequate stabilization.

Fractures of the mid-third of the diaphyis may be stabilized with intramedullary pins, particularly if the fracture ends interdigitate or the fracture is slightly oblique. Excellent stabilization of diaphyseal fractures may be achieved with plating, the implant being placed on the lateral, cranial, or medial surface (Fig. 4.12). The medial surface is flat,

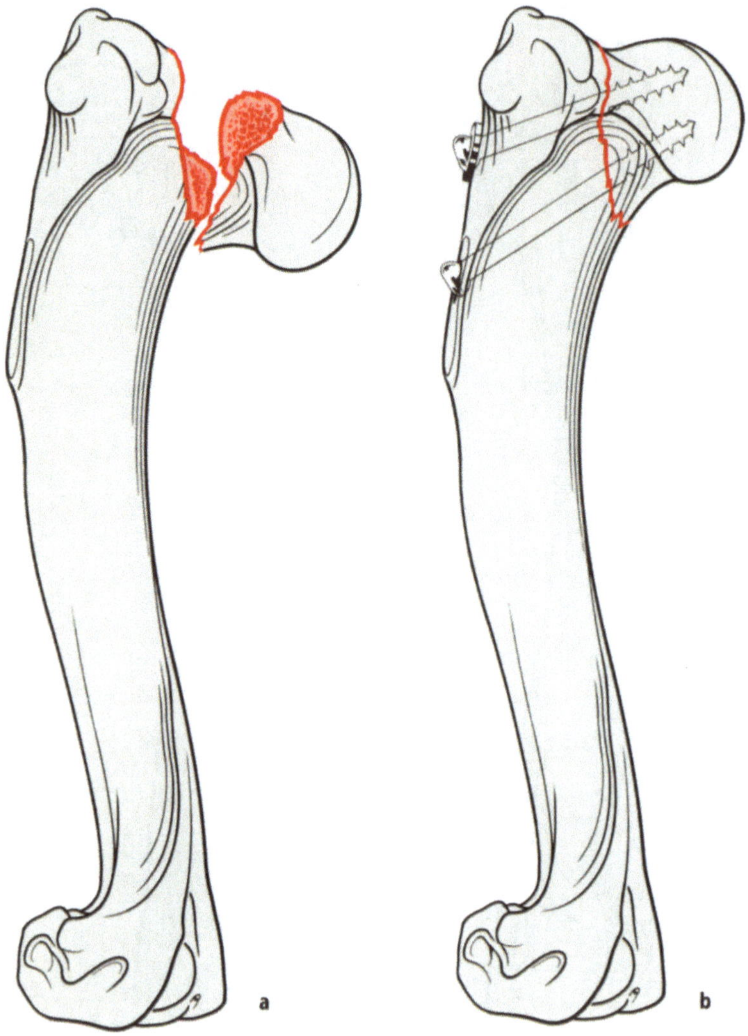

Fig. 4.10. **a** Fracture at the base of the humeral head with a metaphyseal component. **b** Rigid stabilization with two lag screws and a washer, indicating soft bone in this area

but approaching it requires considerable care due to the presence of blood vessels and nerves, where the lateral surface dictates considerable plate contouring (Fig. 4.13).

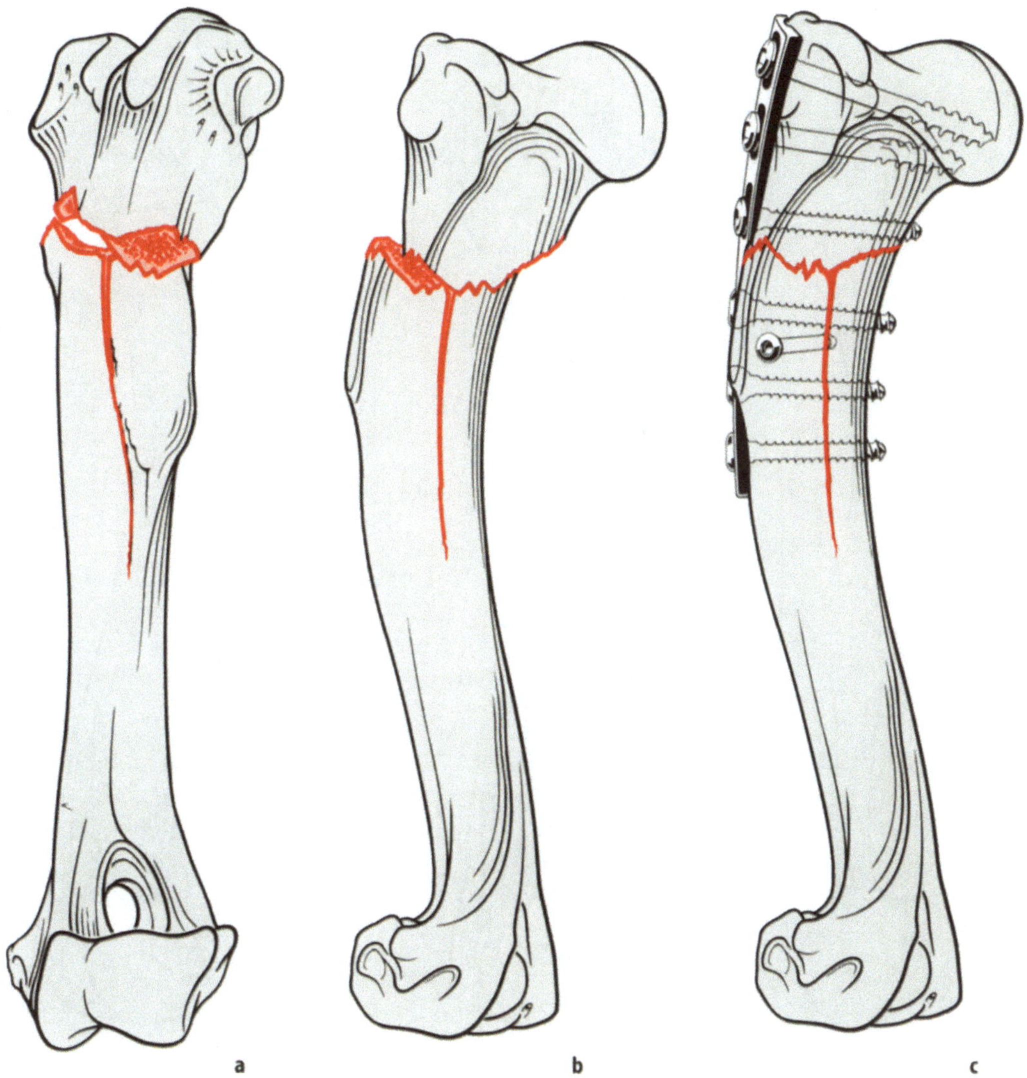

Fig. 4.11. A cranial placed plate is used to stabilize a proximal metaphyseal fracture of the Hunerus

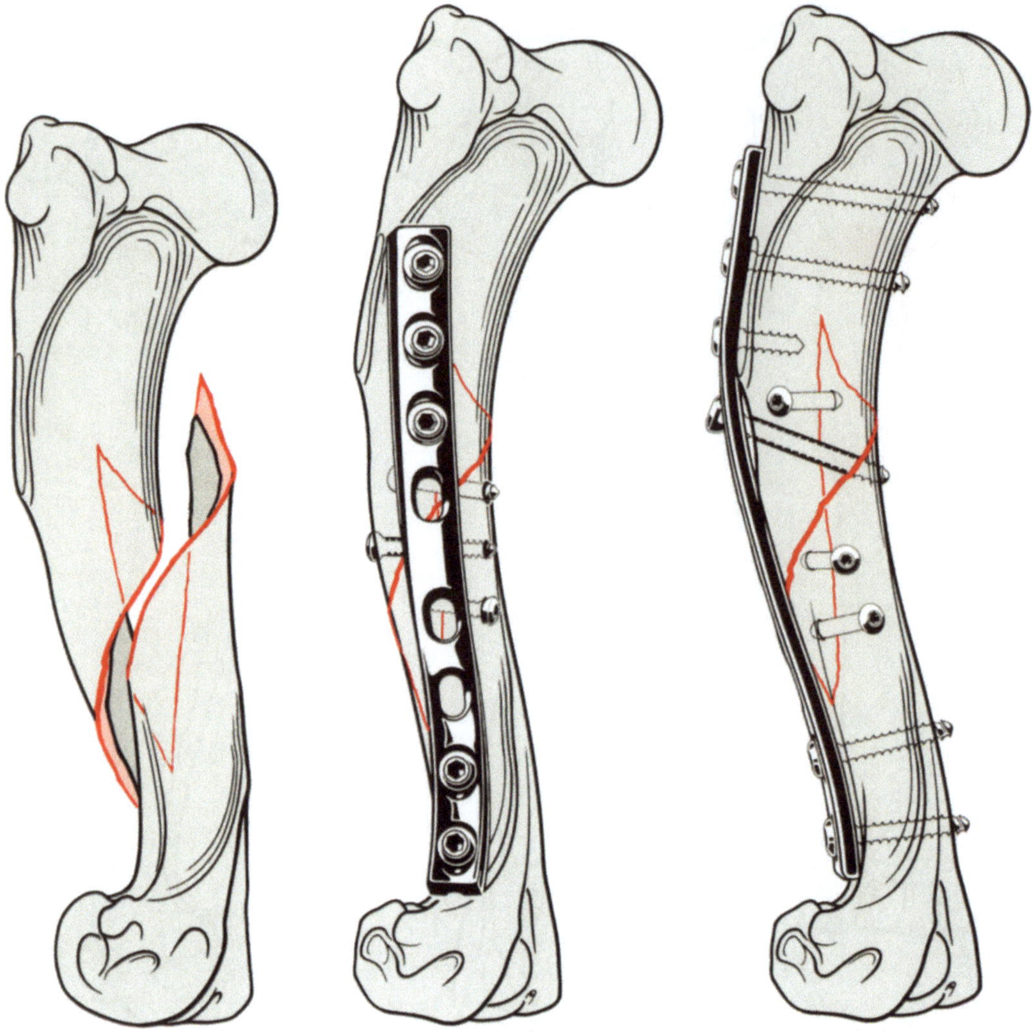

Fig. 4.12. **a** Spiral midshaft fracture of the humerus. **b** Following reduction, three lag screws are inserted in a craniocaudal position. A dynamic compression plate is contoured and applied to the lateral surface. **c** An alternative method of stabilizing this fracture is placement of the plate on either the cranial or medial surface of the bone, with lag screws at a right angle to the plate. In some situations it is possible to insert the lag screws through the plate

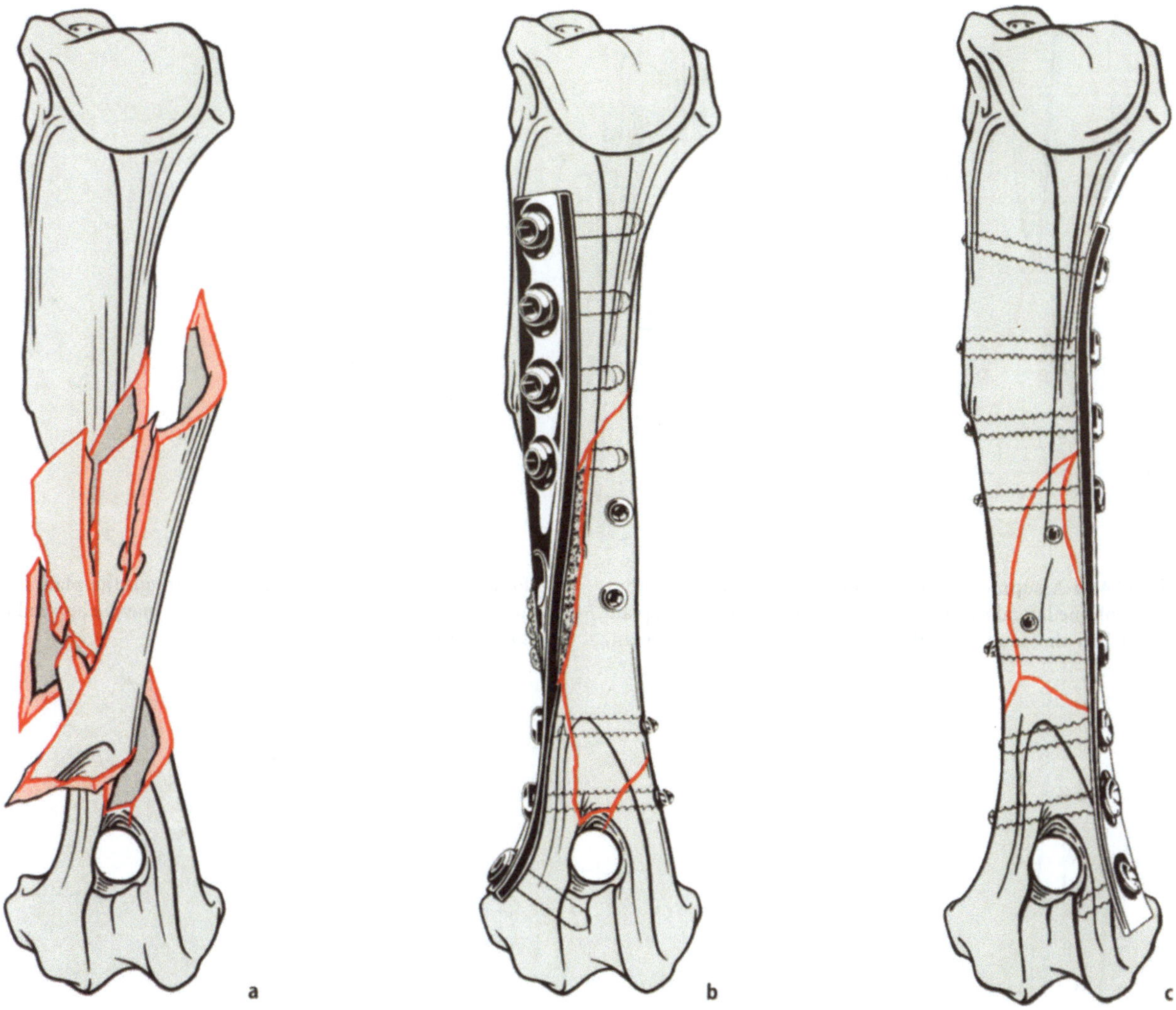

Fig. 4.13. **a** Multiple midshaft fracture with a wedge segment. **b** The wedge segments are first attached using lag screws. The contoured plate is applied laterally and a cancellous bone graft is used to fill defects. **c** Alternatively, the plate may be applied to the medial surface of the bone

4.2.3 Fractures of the Distal Humerus

Supracondylar fracture stabilization, in adult animals, is achieved by means of a plate applied to the medial or caudal surface of the medial portion of the condyle (Fig. 4.14). For similar fractures in immature individuals, see Sect. 4.11. Fractures of the lateral and medial portion of the condyle are stabilized by an intercondylar lag screw and one or more additional fixation devices, e.g., other lag screws and pins (Fig 4.15). Intercondylar fractures (T and Y fractures) may be stabilized by means of a transcondylar lag screw and a plate. The condyles are reduced, one to the other, and then attached to the diaphyis by means of a plate along the caudomedial condylar ridge or, alternatively, the caudal surface of the medial portion of the condyle (Fig. 4.16). In certain multiple fractures in large dogs, it may be advisable to also plate the caudolateral aspect of the condyle.

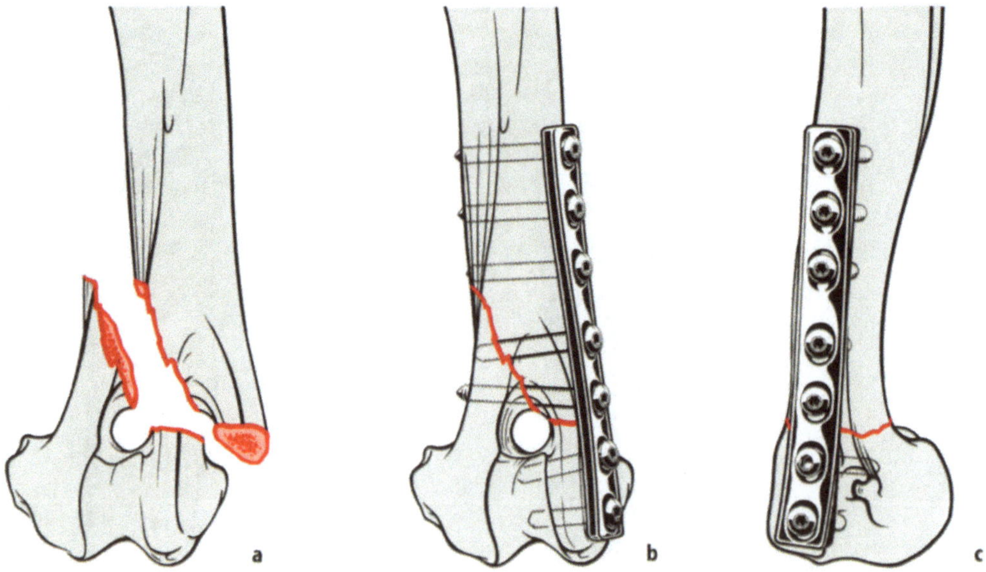

Fig. 4.14. **a** A supracondylar fracture of the humerus with a long oblique lateral portion. **b,c** A dynamic compression plate applied to the caudomedial surface. In the fracture shown, the fourth and fifth screws are lagged through the plate into the lateral segment. Alternatively, the plate may be applied to the caudal surface

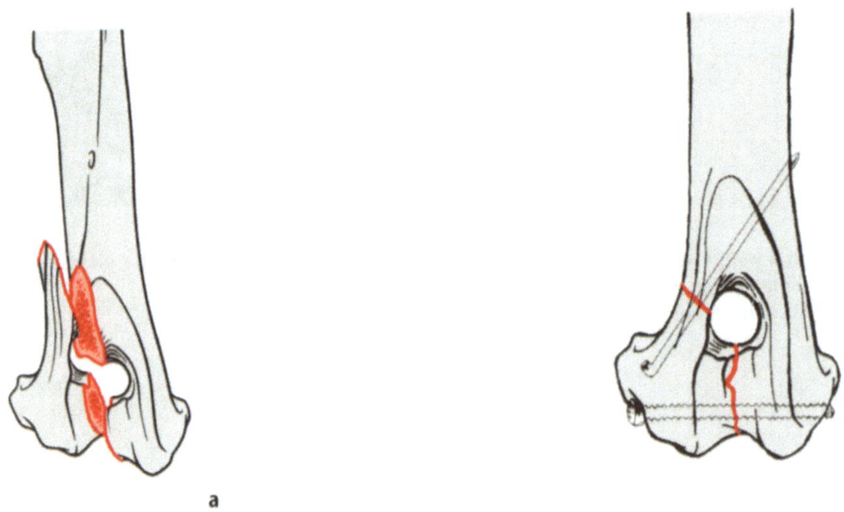

Fig. 4.15. **a** An oblique fracture of the lateral aspect of the humeral condyle. **b** A transcondylar lag screw and a Kirschner wire provide stabilization. Drilling the gliding hole for the transcondylar screw may be performed using either the "inside-outside" or the "outside- inside" methods

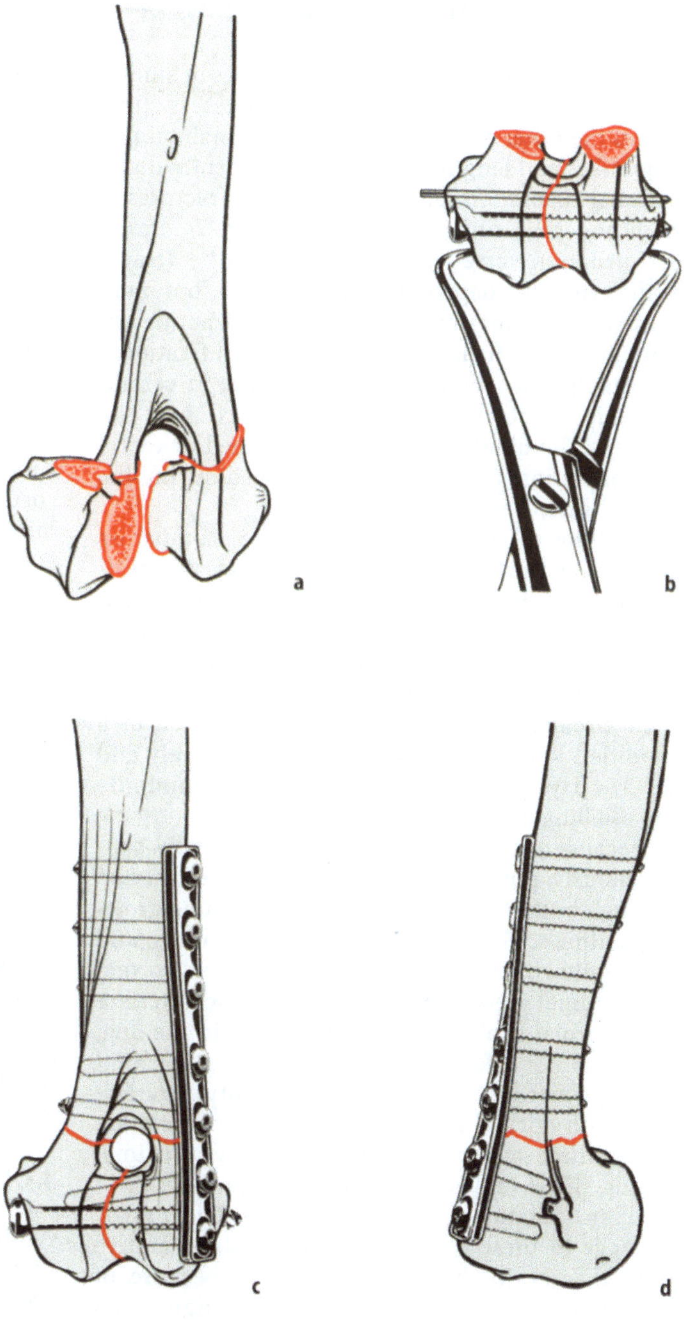

Fig. 4.16. a T fracture of the humeral condyle. **b** The condyle fragments are reduced and temporarily held compressed together with forceps and Kirschner wire while the transcondylar lag screw is inserted. **c** A dynamic compression plate is applied to either side of the metaphysis to fix the condyles to the shaft. **d** Alternatively, the plate may be applied caudally over the medial portion of the condyle

4.3 Fractures of the Radius and Ulna

Since the radius and ulna are paired bones of similar size, when only one of the two bones is fractured, the other acts as a natural splint maintaining alignment and length, permitting treatment with an external coaptation splint or cast. Stable fractures of both bones (incomplete fractures, fissure fractures, serrated transverse fractures) may also be treated with external coaptation. However, for optimum results and fewer complications, most fractures of both bones are treated with rigid internal fixation.

Usually, only the radius is plated, but in certain unstable fractures additional support may be needed. The ulna can be plated or pinned or external coaptation splintage may be applied during the critical early healing period.

Swelling of the foot, which often accompanies open reduction of radial fractures, may be minimized by gentle tissue manipulation, preservation of the cephalic and accessory cephalic veins, anatomical reduction, and stable fixation, which permits early active exercise in order to prevent stagnant circulation and edema. The application of a modified Robert Jones bandage preoperatively and for 3–4 days postoperatively is helpful in minimizing swelling and edema.

Because the radius and ulna do not grow synchronously, pins and screws should not be inserted through both bones during fixation in young growing animals. Synostosis* between the radius and ulna, following fracture, may interfere with normal longitudinal growth. Synostosis may also interfere with normal supination and pronation. In the dog, this does not affect function; however, in cats and some primates it may result in disability. Interference with normal growth or injury to one or more of the three metaphyseal growth plates (proximal radius, distal radius, and distal ulna) may result in angular, rotational, and/or length deformities. Damage to these physes may lead to degenerative joint disease in the elbow or carpus because of malarticulation with the asynchronous longitudinal growth between the radius and ulna. The distal ulnar physis in dogs is particular sensitive to a Salter type-V premature closure as a result of a crushing injury. The proximal ulnar growth plate does not add to the length of the limb below the elbow.

4.3.1 Fractures of the Olecranon Process

Fractures involving the trochlear notch require anatomic reduction in order to restore acceptable function. Malalignment results in the development of degenerative joint disease. A caudal approach is used to expose the fracture site. After exposure and removal of all tissue debris, extending the elbow will facilitate reduction. It may be difficult to see the surface of the trochlear notch, but precise reduction is possible provided all debris is removed.

4.3.1.1 Fixation Using Tension Band Wire

Tension band wire fixation is effective on most transverse or short oblique fractures. The tension band wire is used to counteract tension created by the pull of triceps muscles. Triceps muscle tension results in dynamic compression across the fracture line, when a tension band is correctly applied. Two Kirschner wires are inserted on the caudal proximal corners of the olecranon process extending distally into the ulna, directed somewhat obliquely to engage the cranial cortex of the ulna rather than extending directly down the marrow cavity, since the latter may not achieve rotational stability. A small hole is drilled transversely through the shaft of the ulna distal to the fracture site. The drill hole distance below the fracture site is equal to the fracture site to pin insertion distance. An orthopedic wire (0.8–1.25 mm) is inserted through the hole and the ends wrapped around the Kirschner wires in a figure-of-eight pattern. The projecting ends of the Kirschner wires are bent over, shortened, and then rotated so that they are buried in the triceps tendon if possible (Fig. 4.17). In miniature dogs and in cats, because of the lack of bone stock, the Kirschner wires may be placed one behind the other craniocaudal (anteroposterior) rather than side by side (laterally). In such cases, the tension band wire need only hook behind the caudal Kirschner wire.

4.3.1.2 Fixation Using a Plate

Achievement of stability and dynamic compression using pins and a figure-of-eight tension band wire requires full cortical continuity. A cortical defect or gap results in instability, increased wire cycling, and increased shear forces being applied to the pins. Implant failure and loss of fixation is the usual result. Bone plates are suitable for the fixation of comminuted or unstable olecranon fractures. A 2.7- or 3.5-mm plate is appropriate for most dogs, while the 2.0-mm cuttable plate is best for the cat and toy breeds. Hook plates are useful for the fixation of very proximal fractures; alternatively, a caudal plate can be moulded over the top of the olecranon (Fig. 4.18c). The plate is contoured to the surface of the fractured proximal ulna. Radiographs of the lateral aspect of the normal ulna may serve as a

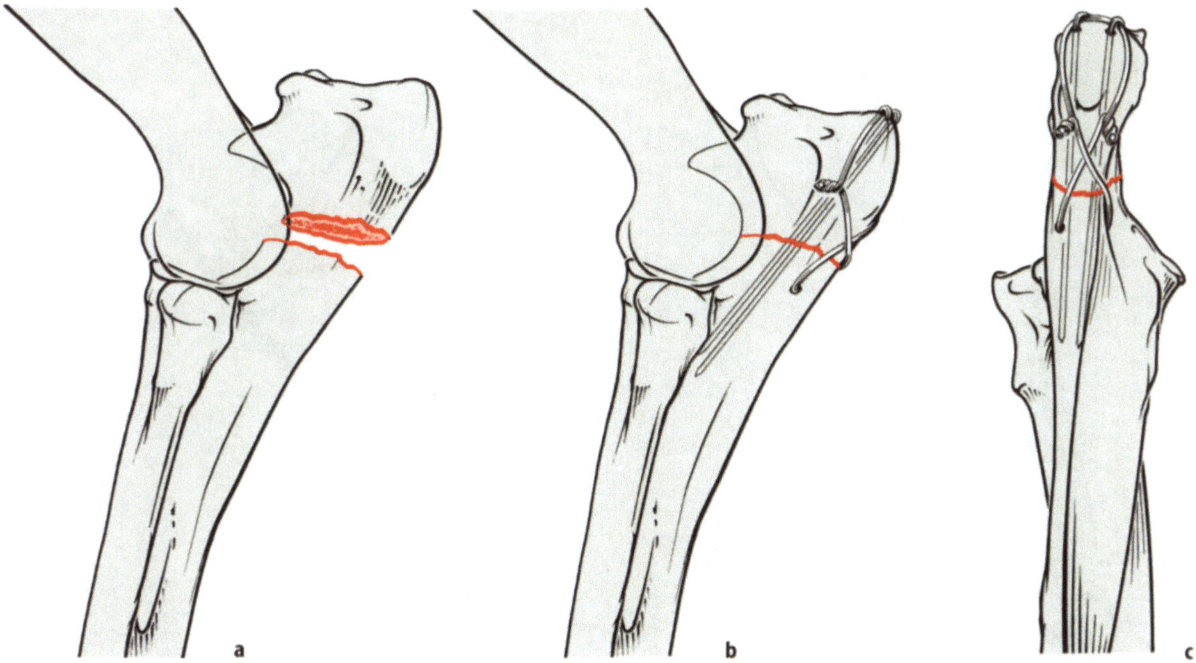

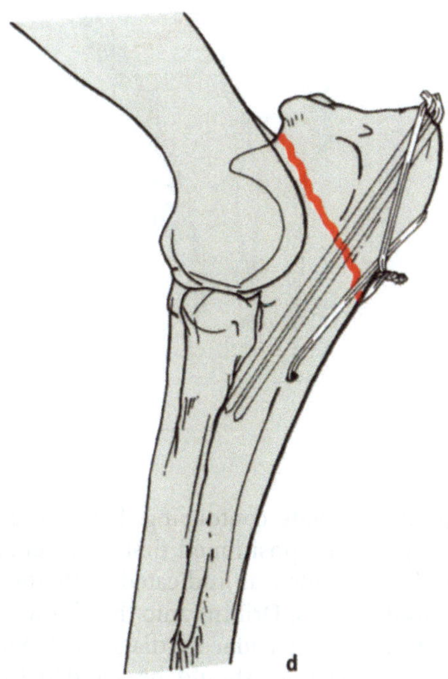

Fig. 4.17. **a** Transverse fracture of the olecranon process, involving the trochlear notch. Fixation using a tension band figure-of-eight wire. **b** Two parallel Kirschner wires are placed from proximal to distal across the fracture site obliquely to engage the cranial cortex of the distal fragment. **c** Two twists have been placed in the tension band wire. A single twist, as shown in **d**, also provides adequate fixation. **d** Oblique fracture stabilized with a tension band wire. This technique is also employed following olecranon osteotomy

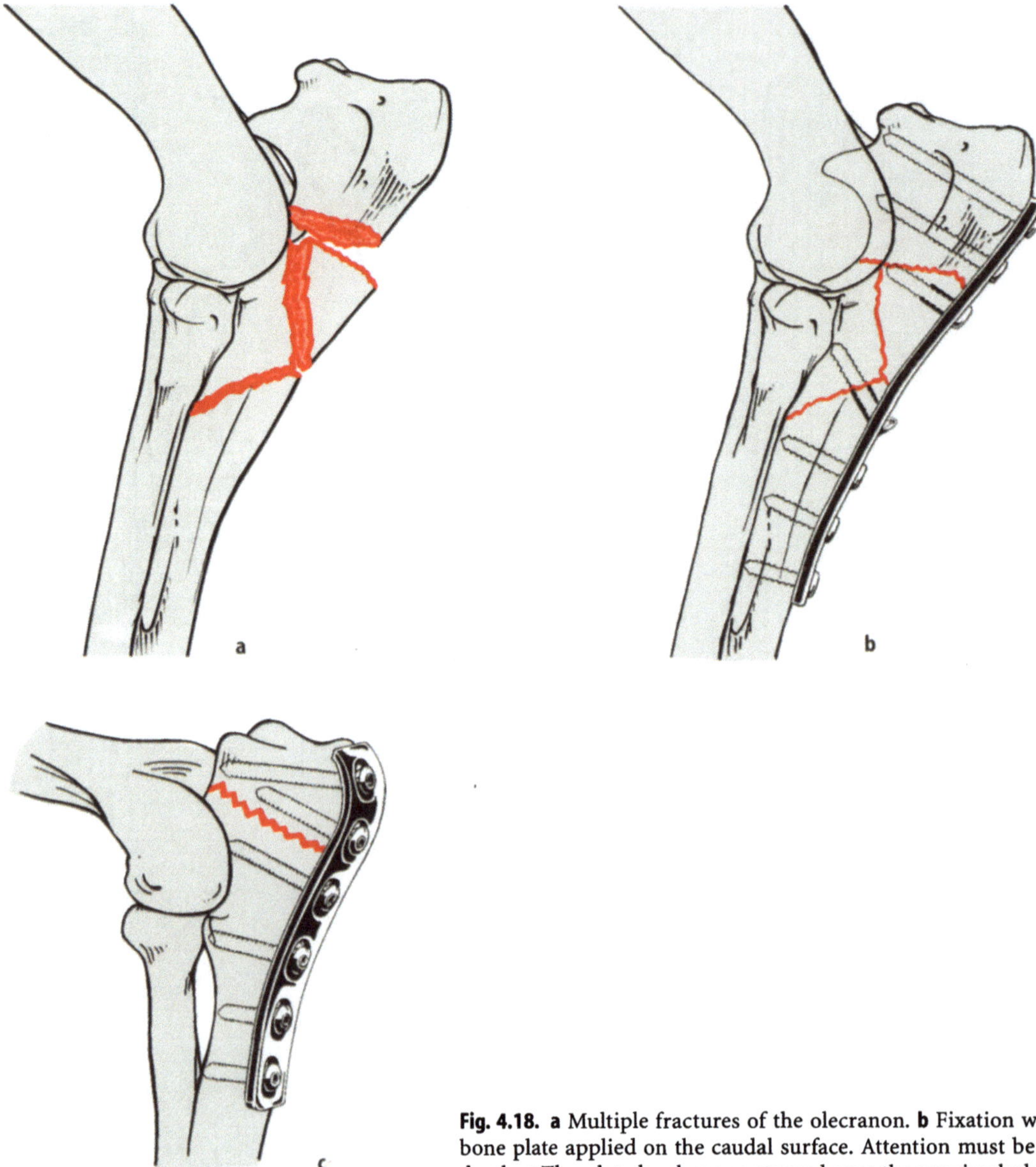

Fig. 4.18. **a** Multiple fractures of the olecranon. **b** Fixation with a contoured bone plate applied on the caudal surface. Attention must be paid to screw depth. **c** The plate has been contoured over the proximal ulna

guide for plate contouring. If lag screws are used, they may be positioned first. The remaining screw holes are filled as indicated with the appropriate length screws. Drilling into the elbow joint and disrupting the articular cartilage or depositing debris within the joint should be avoided by calculating the hole depth from the radiographs. One or two screws may be placed in a load fashion; however, too much compression of the fracture may cause incongruency of the trochlear notch, resulting in a limited range of motion and the development of degenerative joint disease.

4.3.2 Fractures of the Proximal Radius

The radio-humeral joint carries the majority of the load during ambulation and is essential for normal walking. Removal of the radial head usually results in lameness. However, in cases of irreparable fractures, chronic fractures with severe secondary changes, or in the case of congenital lateral luxations in small dogs, radial head removal plus the interposition of fat has been reported. In larger breeds of very athletic dogs, arthrodesis of the elbow should be considered. Fractures of the radial head are rare, owing to the fact that the anatomy of the elbow joint predisposes to fractures of the

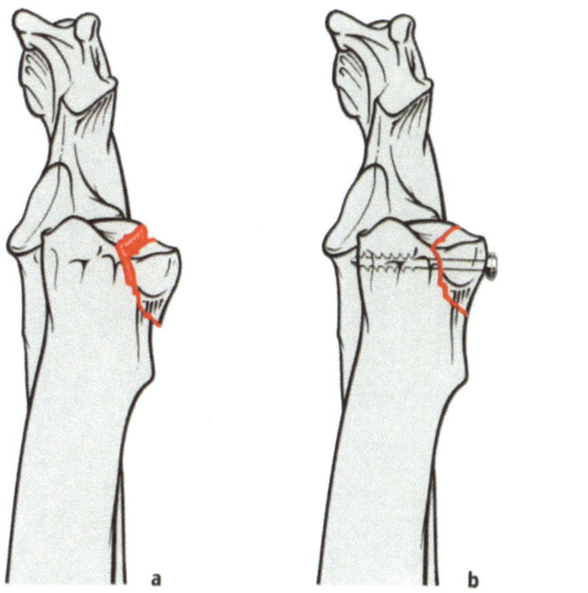

Fig. 4.19. a Longitudinal fracture (slab fracture) of the radial head. **b** Lag screw fixation using one or two screws depending upon the size of the fragment

humeral condyles and not the proximal radius. Most fractures of the radial head involve the articular surface, although immature dogs may suffer a Salter-Harris type I injury. The treatment objectives are to preserve the radial head and to reconstruct the radio-humeral joint (Fig. 4.19). If the radial head is displaced and does not articulate with the humeral capitellum, or if it is unstable, open reduction and internal fixation may be preferred. Transverse and short oblique fractures may be treated with a small plate or with diagonally inserted Kirschner wires (Fig. 4.20). In certain cases, multiple proximal radial and ulnar fractures may be reduced and stabilized by reconstruction and stabilization of the ulna alone.

4.3.3 Monteggia Fractures

Fractures of the proximal half of the ulnar shaft, including the trochlear notch, with separation of the radius and ulna and dislocation of the radial head are known as Monteggia fractures. Chip fractures of the radial head may occur concurrently. In this type of fracture, the annular ligament is usually torn unless the fracture is at the base of the coronoid processes or in the trochlear notch. The ulnar diaphysis may be reduced through a caudal approach and fixed in place with a plate and screws. The radial head and neck can be exposed through a craniolateral approach to remove fracture debris and to explore the annular ligament. The latter can be sutured to maintain stability of the proximal radioulnar articulation. There is a high incidence of reluxation of the radial head if the suturing is not supported with a small screw. In most cases, a position screw is placed through the plate between the

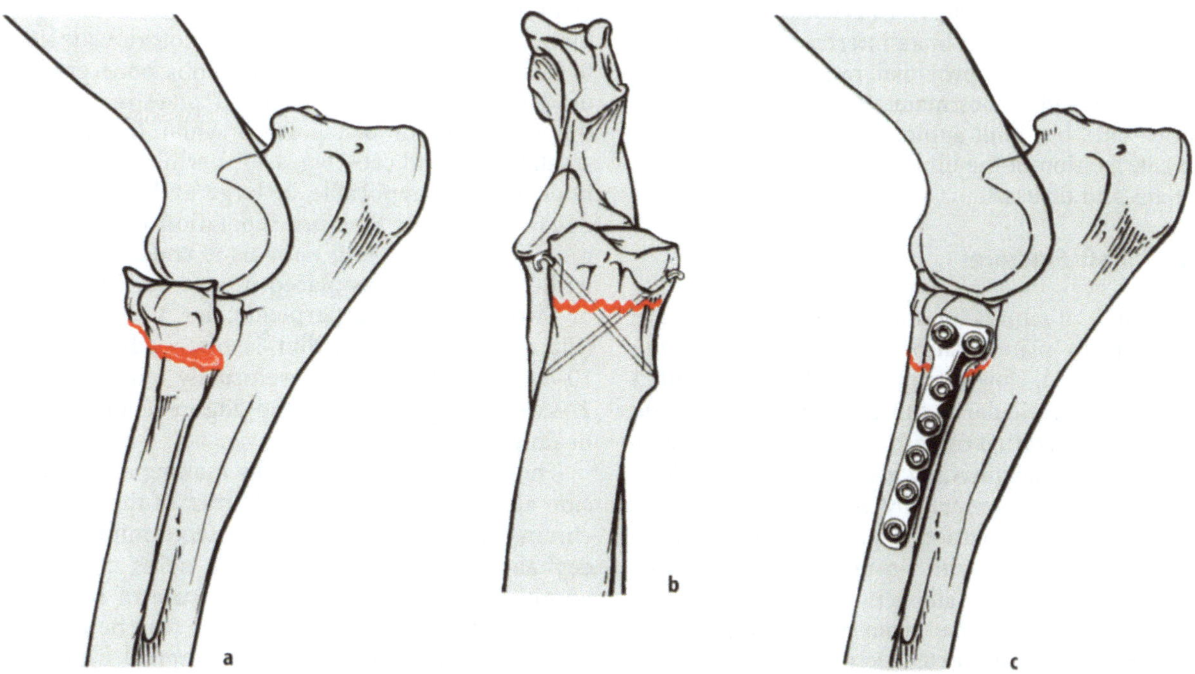

Fig. 4.20. a Transverse fracture of the radial neck. **b** Fixation using crossed Kirschner wires. **c** Fixation with a T plate

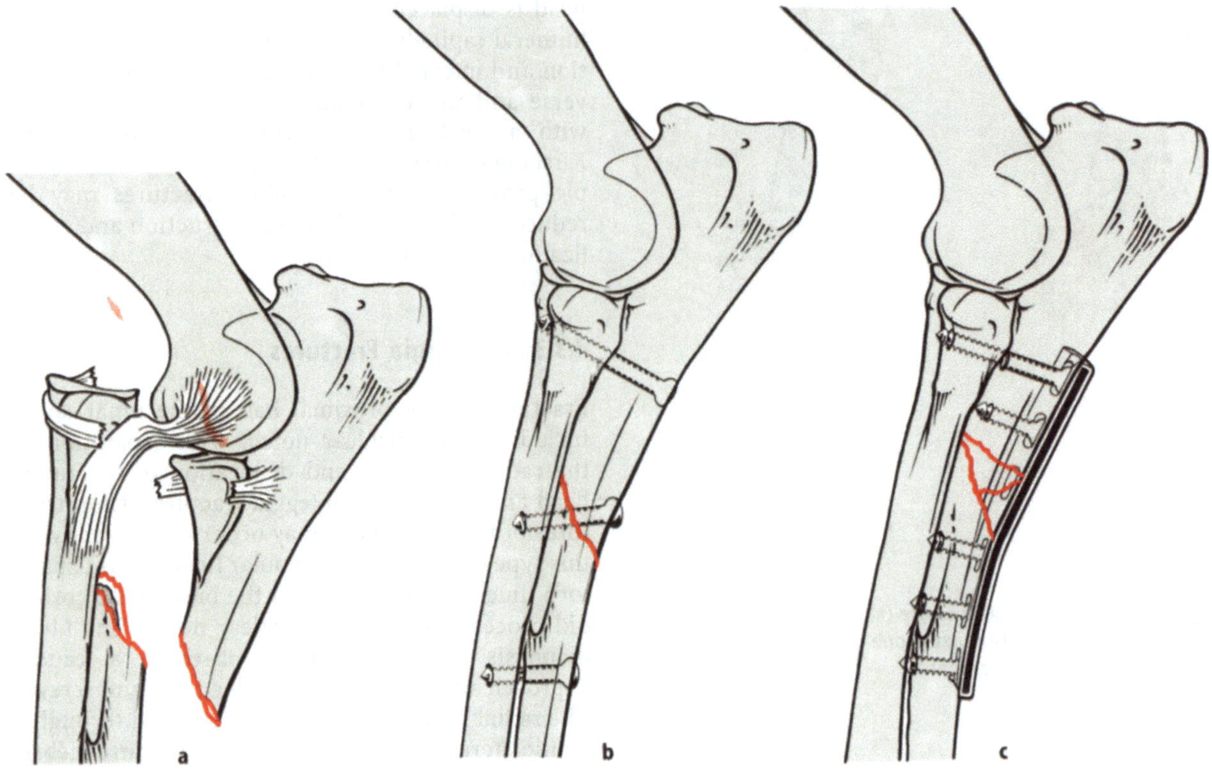

Fig. 4.21. **a** Fracture of the ulna, rupture of the annular ligament with separation of the radius and ulna and dislocation of the radial head (Monteggia fracture). **b** Fixation using three lag screws. **c** Fixation of a multiple ulnar fracture using a plate with proximal screw place in lag fashion into the radius

ulnar and radius (Fig. 4.21). Alternatively, an orthopedic wire can be used in an interfragmentary fashion to stabilize the proximal radioulnar articulation. These techniques maintain articulation of the elbow joint, but limit supination and pronation. In the cat, fixation of the ulna to the radius may result in pain and disuse.

4.3.4 Shaft Fractures

Most shaft fractures of the radius and ulna are amenable to plate fixation. Commonly, only the radius is plated. However, in markedly comminuted cases, and particularly those occurring in large breeds, plate fixation of both the radius and ulna or the use of a 4.5 lengthening plate (4.5 mm) to bridge the fracture gap created by severe comminution may offer a better solution (Fig. 4.22). Defects in the radius associated with comminuted fractures should be filled with autogenous cancellous bone grafts. Care should be taken to minimize plate interference with the extensor tendons. Miniplates using 1.5- or 2.0-mm screws and the 2.0-mm cuttable plate are extremely useful for treating antebrachial fractures in toy breeds. Due to a minimal blood supply, these fractures are notoriously slow to heal, so an autogenous cancellous bone graft is used routinely. The veterinary T plate is ideal for the treatment of distal antebrachial fractures in small breeds and cats (Fig. 4.23b), while the 3.5-mm hook plate is applicable in large and giant breed dogs (Fig. 4.23a). Fracture separation of the distal radial physis in young animals is usually repaired with Kirschner wires placed in a cross-pin pattern or two pins placed perpendicular to the physis (Fig. 4.24). A caudal splint is often advisable for 10–14 days and the pins are usually removed after 2–4 weeks, depending on the dog's age and rate of healing.

The radius is approached by making a skin incision along the craniomedial border of the antebrachium. Care should be taken to avoid injury to the cephalic and accessory cephalic veins. A lateral approach should be used if exposure of both the radius and ulna is required. Plates may be applied on the medial, craniomedial, or cranial aspect of the radius. On the ulna, plates are usually applied on the caudal surface.

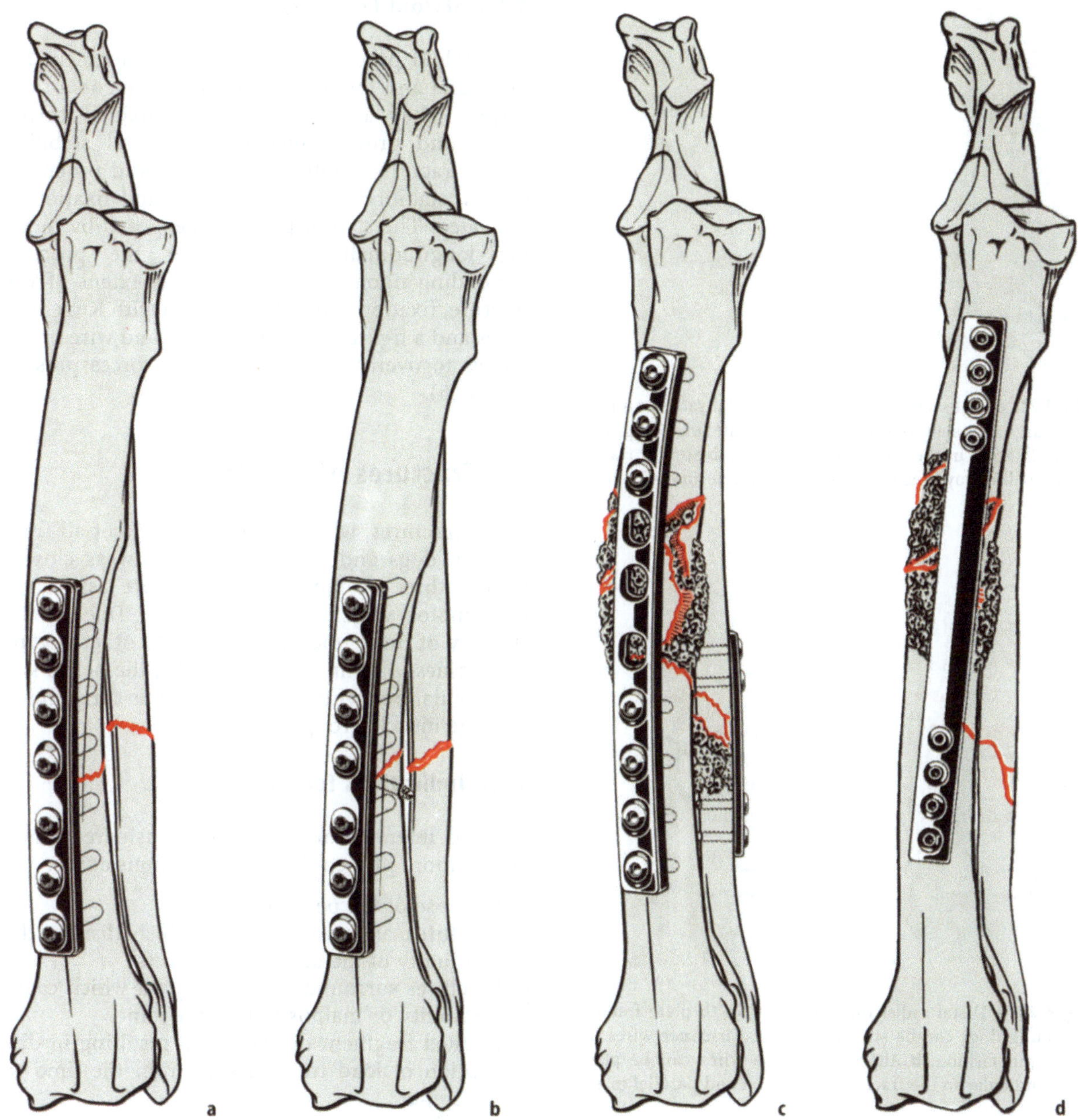

Fig. 4.22. a Transverse fracture of the radius and ulna stabilized with a compression plate applied to the radius. **b** Oblique fracture of the radius and ulna fixed with a lag screw across the radial fracture line and application of a neutralization plate to the cranial aspect of the radius. **c** Multifragmented fracture of the radius and ulna in a large dog fixed with buttress plate on the radius. Fractures sites packed with autogenous cancellous bone graft. **d** Similar fracture in a large dog stabilized using a lengthening plate applied on the cranial aspect of the radius

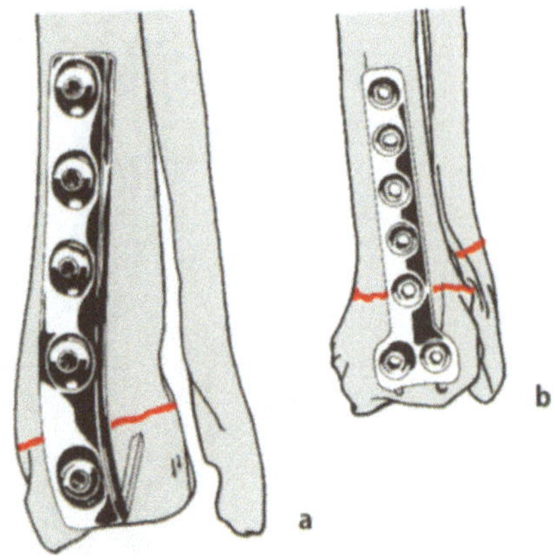

Fig. 4.23. **a** Transverse fracture of the distal radius and ulna in a large dog stabilized using a hook plate providing three-point fixation in the short distal fragment. **b** Similar fracture in a small or toy breed repaired using a veterinary T plate

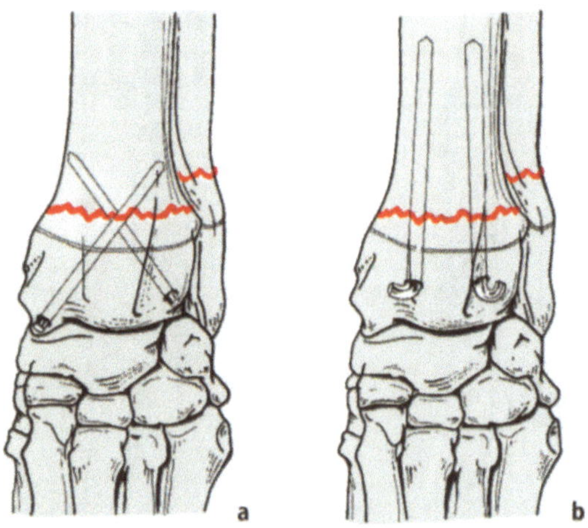

Fig. 4.24. **a** Distal radial metaphyseal growth plate fractures in young dogs can be stabilized using Kirschner wires in a cross-pin fashion. **b** Alternatively, the wires can be placed perpendicular to the fracture separation and parallel to each other

External fixators are useful in the treatment of antebrachial fractures. Type II fixators are more resistant to compressive forces than type I configurations and therefore afford better fixation of unstable fractures. Biplanar type I configurations are useful in treating very proximal or very distal fractures. Intramedullary pinning of radial shaft fractures often results in rotational instability and delay in medullary revascularization and may cause mechanical interference with carpal joint function.

4.3.5 Styloid Fractures

The styloid processes serve as the attachment for the radial and the ulnar collateral ligaments of the carpus. They also buttress the proximal carpal bones and provide medial and lateral stability. When fracture of either or both styloid processes occurs, stability is lost. Reduction and fixation is indicated. The styloid process is exposed by incising longitudinally directly over the process. Depending upon the character and extent of the fracture, fixation is usually achieved with Kirschner wires and a figure-of-eight tension band wire or lag screws to overcome the distractive forces present (Fig. 4.25).

4.4 Fractures of the Pelvis

Pelvic fractures, which total 20%–30% of all fractures in dogs and cats, are almost always closed, involve three or more bones, and are associated with motor vehicle-induced trauma. Due to the etiology of these fractures, trauma to other organs and tissues is common. Structurally, the pelvis is a rectangular box with a center strut. It is surrounded by large muscle groups.

4.4.1 Indications for Surgery

Surgical intervention should be considered when one or more of the following conditions exists:

- Collapse of the pelvic canal
- Fractures of the acetabulum which disrupt the continuity of the articular surface(s)
- Fractures surrounding the hip joint which cause instability or malposition of the joint
- Marked fragment displacement resulting in disruption of load transmission from the limb to the spine
- Significant pain
- Prolonged convalescence would be needed with nonsurgical treatment
- Neurologic compromise

Reduction and fixation are easier if undertaken within 4 days of the original trauma. The three areas of primary surgical concern are as follows:

1. Sacroiliac fracture-luxations
2. Ilial fractures
3. Acetabular fractures

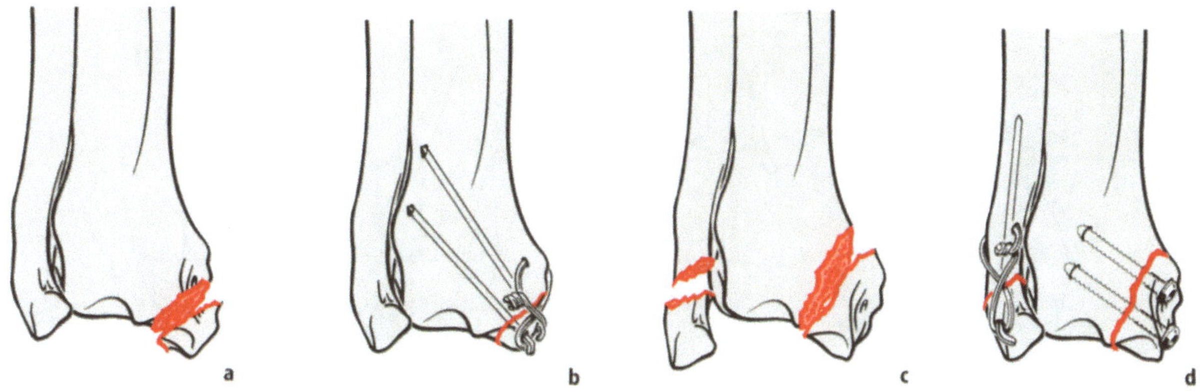

Fig. 4.25. a,b Styloid fractures involving the distal radius and ulna. Repaired using two parallel Kirschner wires and a figure-of-eight tension band wire to counteract the pull of the collateral ligament. **c,d** Fracture of both the radial and ulnar styloid process. Fixation of the radial styloid fracture using two lag screws and of the ulnar styloid fracture with a single Kirschner wire and a figure-of-eight tension band wire

If these areas are properly reduced and stabilized, other fractures generally do not need surgical treatment.

4.4.2 Fracture-Luxation of the Sacroiliac Joint

In sacroiliac fracture-luxations, the ilium is usually displaced cranially and dorsally, but may also displace cranially and ventrally. These fracture-luxations may be unilateral or bilateral and are often associated with fractures of other pelvic bones. Patients treated nonsurgically may exhibit considerable discomfort and lameness for a prolonged period (4–6 weeks) and may have difficulty with limb adduction. Surgical fixation considerably reduces the patient's convalescence time and is most commonly accomplished by using either lag screws or transilial pins or a combination of the two techniques (Fig. 4.26).

4.4.3 Fractures of the Ilium

Ilial fractures are often simple oblique fractures. However, they may have a complex configuration depending on the direction and magnitude of the forces causing them. The caudal segment is usually displaced medially, decreasing the pelvic canal diameter. They are almost always accompanied by fractures of the pubis and ischium.

Fracture reduction is achieved through levering,

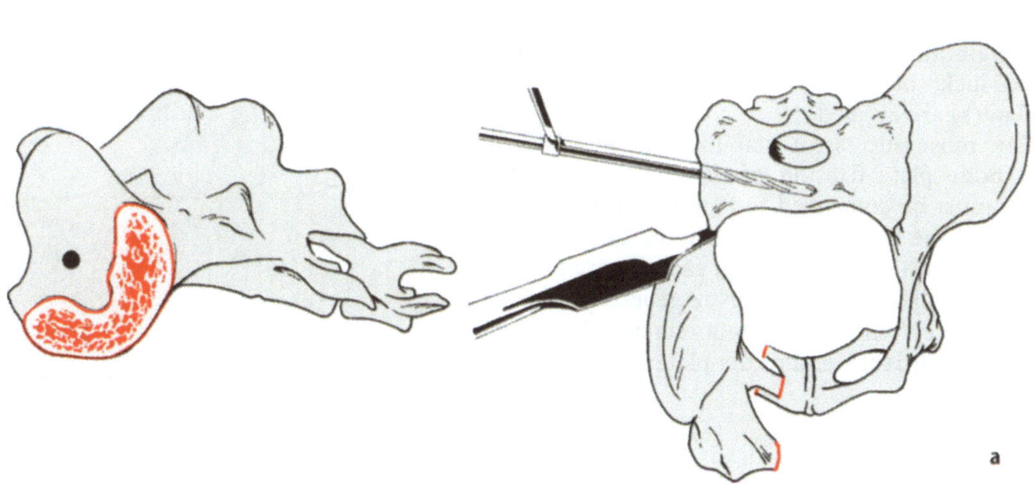

Fig. 4.26a–c. Sacroiliac fracture-luxation. **a** A cortex sc rew is used as a lag screw in the body of the sacrum. From a dorsal approach with the animal straddling sandbags, the lateral surface of the sacrum is exposed. A Hohman retractor placed under the ventral sacrum can be used to displace the illium ventrally. A thread hole is drilled and taped in the center of the exposed sacrum. This hole must be placed ventral to the neural canal.

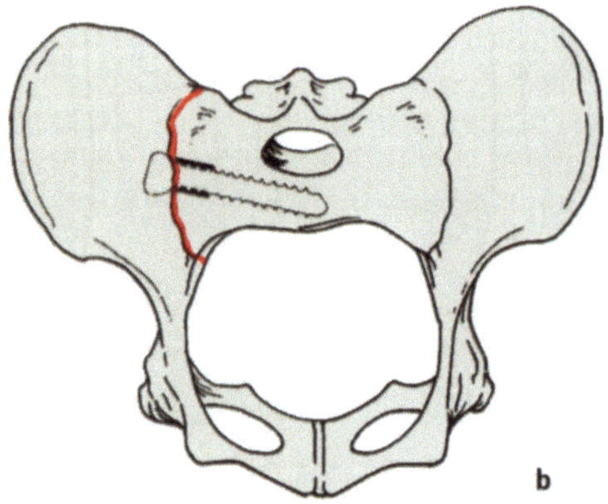

b

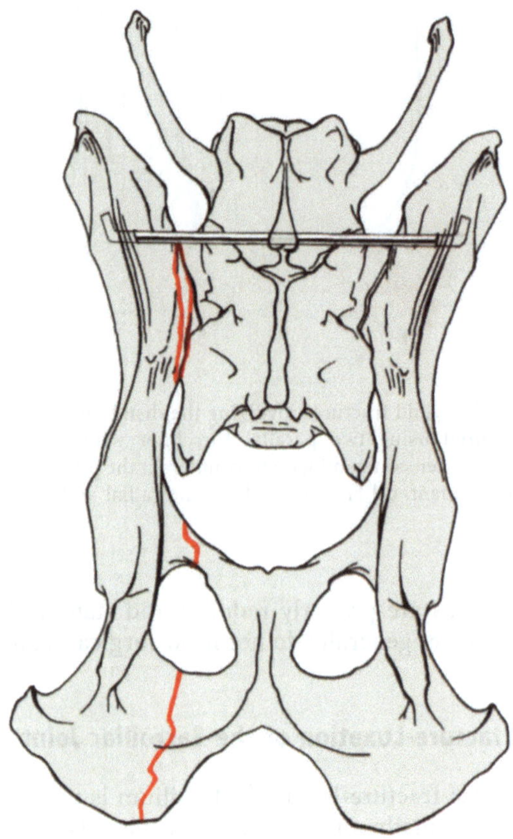

c

Fig. 4.26a–c. Sacroiliac fracture-luxation. **b** A glide hole, centered in the sacroilial articular surface, is drilled in the wing of the ilium. This surface is identified by visualization or palpation of the medial surface of the ilium. The lateral surface of the ilium is exposed and the hole is drilled from lateral to medial. The appropriate cortex screw is passed though the glide hole and its tip is visualized as it is directed into the thread hole. Seating the screw in the thread hole will reduce and stabilize the fracture-luxation. **c** A transilial pin may be used in combination with lag a screw in the sacral body or as primary fixation by itself. This pin should pass through both ilial wings and above the dorsal lamina of the seventh lumbar vertebra. It should be bent at both ends to prevent migration

traction, and rotation of the fragments. The caudal fragment often has to be levered from under the cranial one with a long, flat instrument. Traction and/or rotation can be applied to the caudal fragment by either a bone-holding forceps used to grasp the fragment or by a Steinmann pin inserted through the ischial tuberosity (Fig. 4.27). The reduction of most ilial fractures is maintained by a self-retaining bone forceps (e.g., pointed reduction, speed lock, or self-centering forceps) while the implant(s) are applied.

The most successful stabilization is achieved with bone plate fixation of the ilium (Fig. 4.28). Plates must be contoured to fit the concave lateral surface of the ilium. The plate should be anchored by a minimum of two screws in each fragment. The first screws placed in the plate are generally close to the fracture, with subsequent screw placement moving towards the end of the plate.

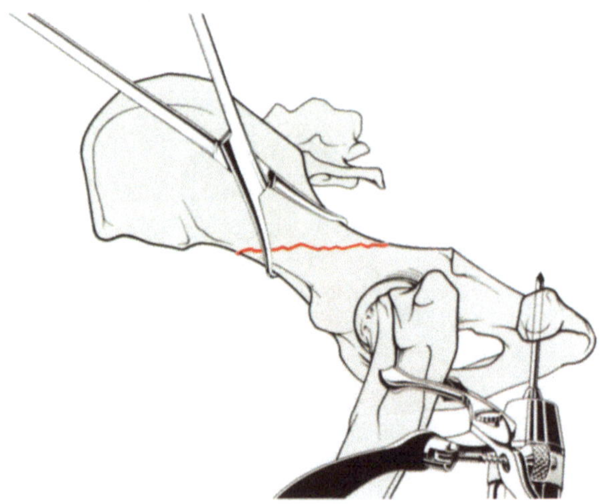

Fig. 4.27. Inserting a Steinmann pin into the ischial tuberosity and grasping the greater trochanter may be helpful in accomplishing reduction. Reduction forceps may be used to maintain temporary reduction while the bone plate is contoured and applied

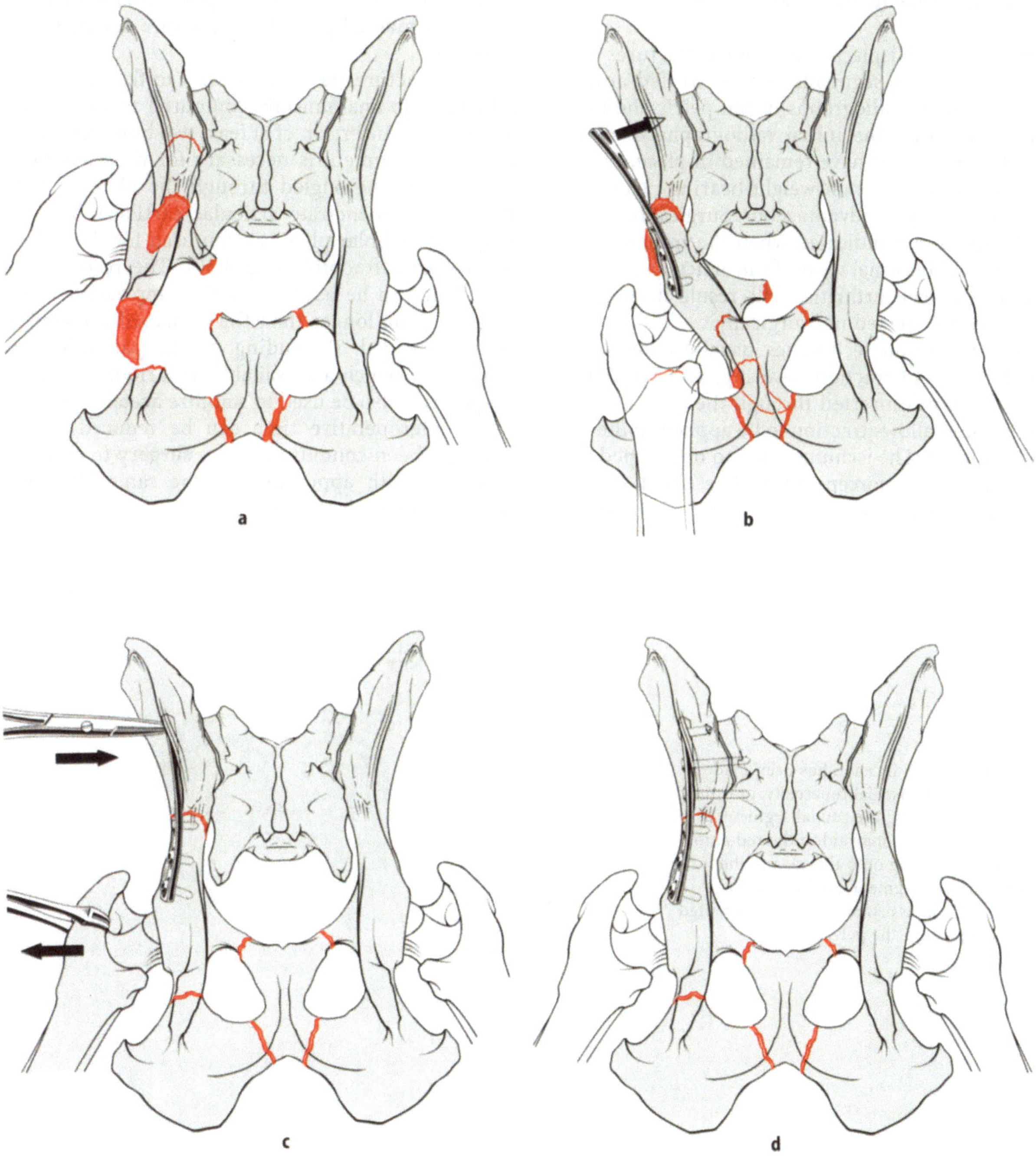

Fig. 4.28. a Oblique fracture of ilium along with fractures of ischium and pubic bones. There is a decrease in the size of the pelvic canal and instability of the rear leg. **b,c** With good reduction and rigid fixation of the ilium, the remaining fractures fall into line and are satisfactorily stabilized. Following open exposure of the ilial fracture area, the caudal segment of the ilium is exteriorized and partly reduced. The ilial plate must be bent concave (slightly more than the opposite normal side). This is essential in order to restore and maintain the normal size of the pelvic canal. The usual procedure in applying the plate is to attach the caudal segment first. An upward lift is exerted on the greater trochanter, with downward pressure on the cranial end of the plate prior to and during insertion of the screws into the cranial segment. This aids in lining up and stabilizing fractures of the ischium and pubic bones. **d** When the sacrum lies immediately under the cranial segment of the ilium, additional fixation is gained by inserting the screw into it

4.4.4 Fractures of the Acetabulum

The rare, nondisplaced acetabular fractures with stabile adjoining segments may be treated nonsurgically. Repeat radiographs of the pelvis should be taken 24 h after the initial radiographs to ensure that the fragments have remained in place. Placing the limb in a non-weight-bearing sling for 1–2 weeks may be advantageous. Surgical reduction and fixation are indicated when the fragments are displaced. Abnormal wear of the articular cartilage, leading to osteoarthritis, will result if displaced fractures are treated nonsurgically.

The reduction techniques usually consist of a combination of traction, levering, and rotation. A Steinmann pin inserted through the skin and caudal ischium allows traction to be applied to the caudal fragment. The ischium can also be grasped with a bone-holding forceps through a short incision over the tuber ischium (Fig. 4.29). To maintain reduction while the plate is applied, it is often necessary to manually hold the fracture segments in position.

Most fractures lend themselves to fixation using a bone plate anatomically contoured to the dorsal acetabulum. Insertion of at least two bone screws in each bone segment is necessary for rigid stability. Screws must be angled through the plate so that they do not penetrate articular cartilage. The C-shaped acetabular plate is often used for the repair of two-piece fractures (Fig. 4.30). The reconstruction plate can be used to repair complex fractures where a plate longer than the C-shaped acetabular plate is needed. Depending on the patient's size, miniplates, which are available in various sizes and shapes, can also be used to stabilize acetabular fractures. Interoperative time can be reduced if the plate has been contoured before surgery to a pelvic specimen with approximately the same size and shape as the patient's pelvis.

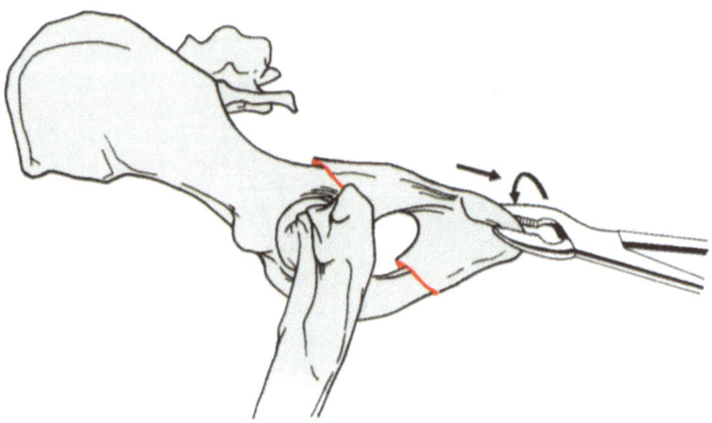

Fig. 4.29. After an incision has been made in the skin over the ischial tuberosity, grasping it and manipulating the caudal segment with a Kern bone clamp may aid in the reduction process. By holding onto this clamp, the caudal fracture segment can be held in reduction by an assistant while the contoured plate is applied to the pelvis

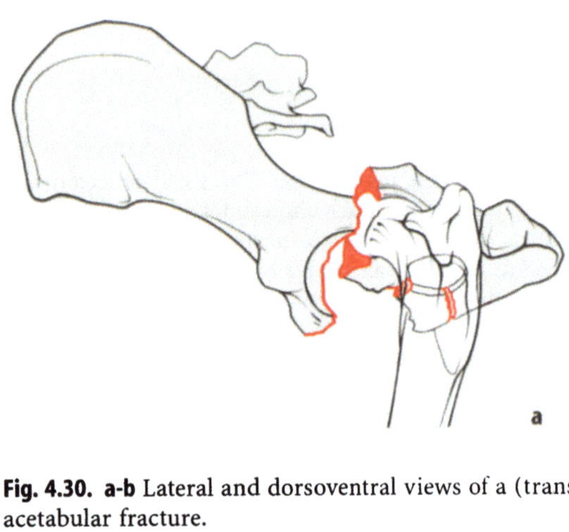

a

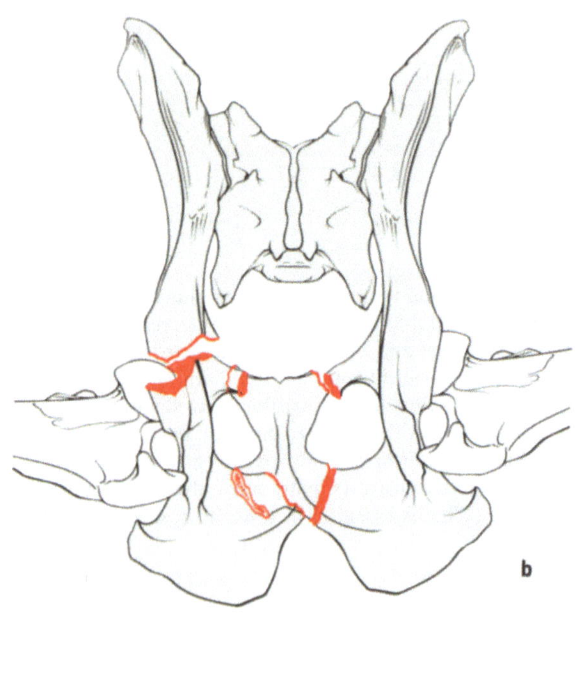

b

Fig. 4.30. a-b Lateral and dorsoventral views of a (transverse) acetabular fracture.

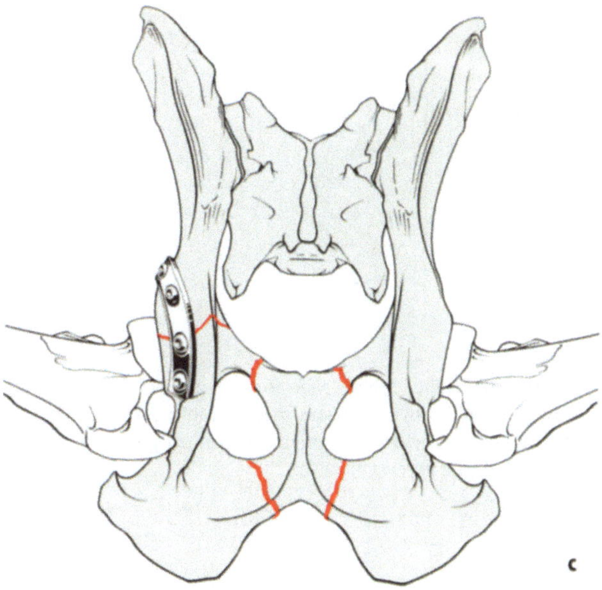

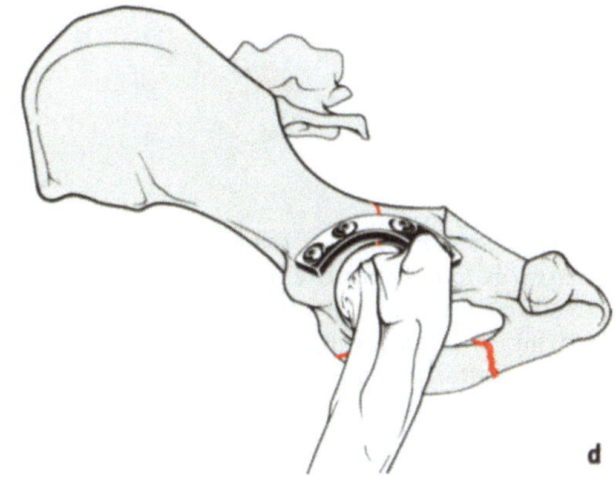

Fig. 4.30. c-d c Dorsoventral view with the acetabular fracture reduced and the contoured acetabular plate in place. Note that reduction and fixation of this area also results in satisfactory reduction and stability of fractures in the pelvic symphysis area. **d** Lateral view with acetabular plate in place. A dynamic compression plate may be helpful in adding compression, particularly in stable fractures

4.4.5 Fractures of the Ischium and Pubis

Most fractures involving the ischium and pubis do not require further treatment if fractures of the iliosacral joint, ilium, and/or acetabulum are stabilized. If an ischial fracture causes significant pain, reduction and fixation with lag screws or intramedullary pins is indicated (Fig. 4.31).

4.4.6 Fractures of the Pelvis Requiring Fixation in Two or More Areas

Many pelvic fractures require fixation of two or more areas. Usually, all areas are stabilized in the same operative session. When fractures of both the ilium and acetabulum exist, the ilial fracture is usually stabilized first (Fig. 4.32).

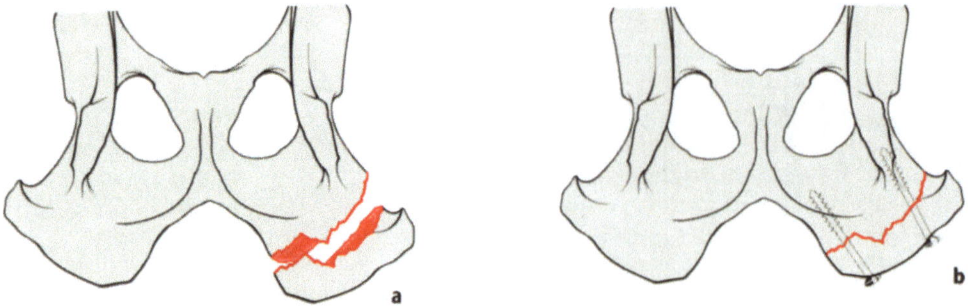

Fig. 4.31. a Most fractures of the ischiatic tuberosity respond satisfactorily to nonoperative treatment. However, in some, a sizable bone segment is fractured and pulled distally by the hamstring muscles, giving rise to considerable discomfort. Surgical treatment is indicated. The ventral surface of the ischiatic tuberosity gives rise to the powerful hamstring group (biceps femoris and semimembranous muscles). **b** The ischiatic tuberosity bone segment is fixed in place using two cancellous bone screws

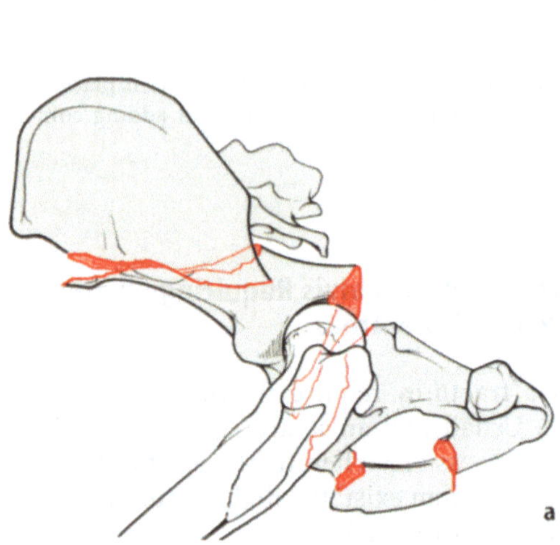

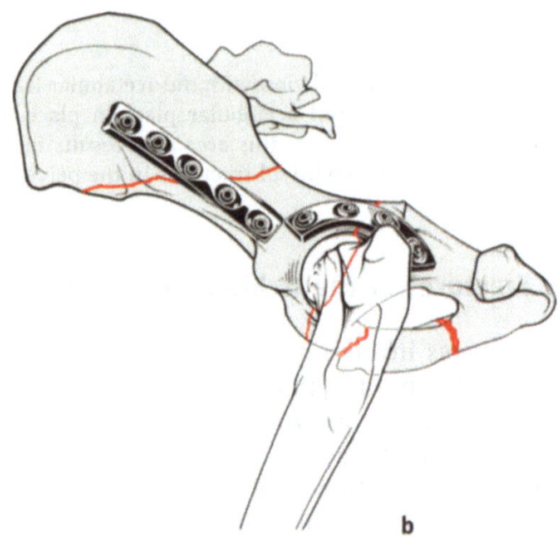

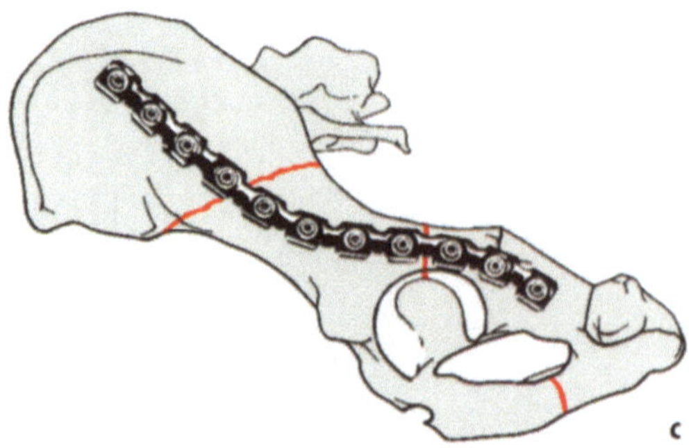

Fig. 4.32. a Oblique fractures of the ilium and transverse fracture of the acetabulum, accompanied by fractures of the pubis. The combined approach is indicated to expose the ilium and acetabulum. Reduction and fixation sequence varies: in some, it is advantageous to reduce both areas approximately and then proceed with fixation; in others, each area is reduced and fixed individually. **b** Lateral view showing fixation in place using two bone plates. **c** A single reconstruction plate can be used to stabilize both fractures. When this is done, the surgical time can be reduced by contouring the plate to a similar-sized pelvis before surgery. The plate is sterilized and minor adjustments in its shape are made on the operating table

4.5 Fractures of the Femur

Fractures of the femur are among the most commonly encountered long-bone fractures in small animals. Most result from trauma, are multifragmented, and involve the diaphysis. Because of their anatomical location, femoral fractures are not easily immobilized with casts or splints, and some form of internal fixation is usually indicated. Temporary stabilization is difficult for the same reasons. Strict confinement and the conscious effort the patient makes to avoid pain are often sufficient to control additional trauma that might be caused by the unstable fracture segments. Repair of femoral fractures should be undertaken as soon as the patient's condition is stabilized.

4.5.1 Fractures of the Femoral Head and Neck

In the mature animal, either capital or neck fractures occur in this area (Fig. 4.33). Capital fractures are intracapsular. Neck fractures may be intracapsular, extracapsular, or both.

4.5.1.1 Blood Supply

The rich blood supply (Fig. 4.34) to the femoral head and neck arises from the lateral circumflex femoral artery, the medial circumflex femoral artery, and to a limited extent from a branch of the caudal gluteal artery. All of these vessels develop into a network within the retinaculum, which penetrates various aspects of the joint capsule supplying blood to the femoral head and neck. It has been observed clinically that, when the fracture is intracapsular, the ventral joint capsule strips from the femoral neck, leaving intact the retinacular blood supply from the medial circumflex femoral artery to the femoral head. The femoral neck also receives some blood supply from the nutrient artery of the femur.

When proper stabilization has been applied to the fracture, avascular necrosis of the femoral head and neck is rarely observed. Some narrowing of the femoral neck is seen in many cases, but this is a sign of rapid revascularization, bone resorption, and remodeling; it is often termed "apple core." The approach used for fracture repair and the time span between injury and surgery does not seem to influence the occurrence of femoral neck narrowing.

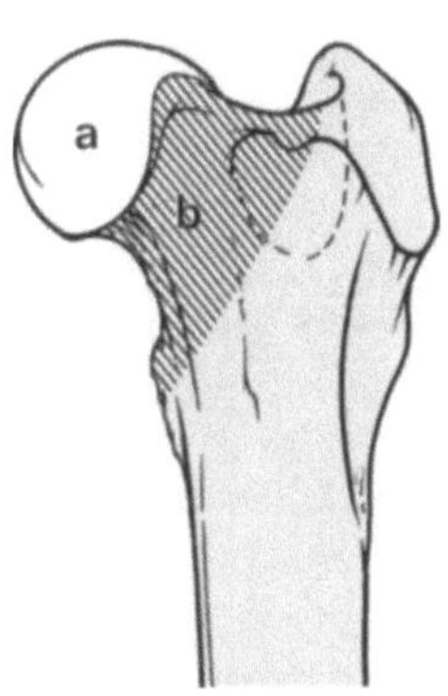

Fig. 4.33. Types of fracture of the femoral head and neck. Capital fracture (*a*) and neck fractures (*b*)

4.5.1.2 Methods of Repair

The proximal femur is usually approached through a modified craniolateral approach or occasionally through a trochanteric osteotomy or gluteal tenotomy. The method of repair is dictated by the location of the fracture and the size of the fragments involved.

4.5.2 Capital Fractures

Capital fractures are usually bony avulsions, involving the insertion of the ligament to the head of the femur, and are associated with coxofemoral dislocations in the mature dog. If the fragment of bone attached to the ligament is too small to accept a screw, the treatment of choice is to remove the avulsed piece of bone during open reduction of the hip. Occasionally, the fracture fragment is large enough for screw fixation (Fig. 4.35).

Early reduction of capital and neck fractures prevents the femoral head or neck from being abrased. When the joint capsule is torn, the femoral head rubs against the craniodorsal rim of the acetabulum. Femoral neck fractures in mature animals carry a favorable prognosis if early surgery, anatomical reduction, rigid internal fixation, and proper postoperative management is provided. Neither the surgical approach used nor the location of

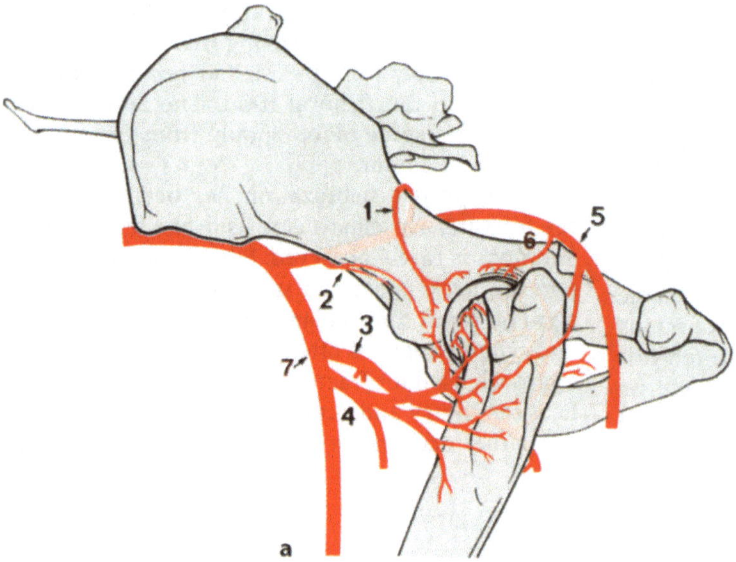

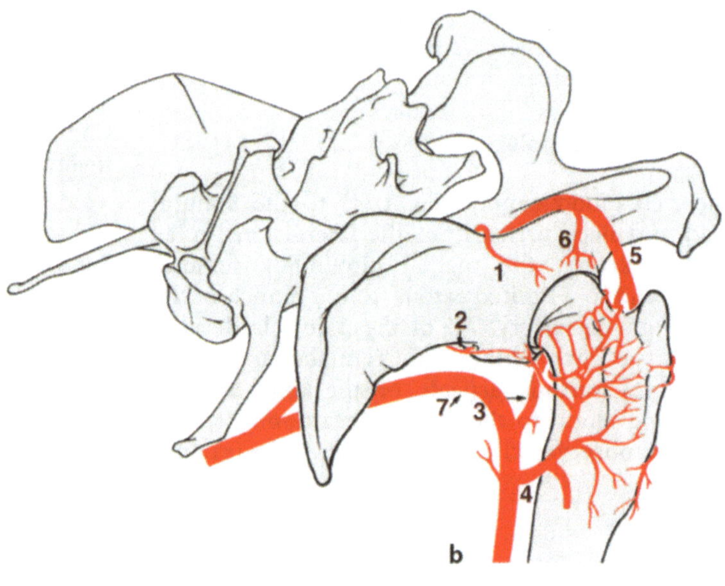

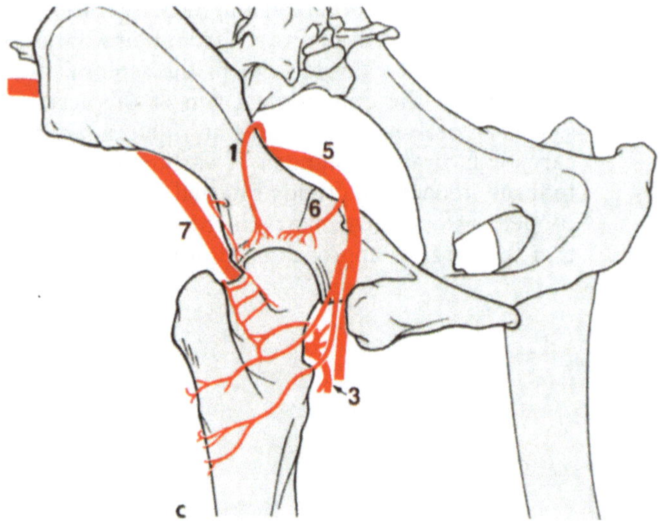

Fig. 4.34a–c. Blood supply to the femoral head and neck. **a** Lateral view. **b** Cranial lateral view. **c** Caudal lateral view. *1*, Cranial gluteal artery; *2*, iliolumbar artery; *3*, medial circumflex femoral artery; *4*, lateral circumflex femoral artery; *5*, caudal gluteal artery; *6*, ventral branch of the caudal gluteal artery; *7*, femoral artery

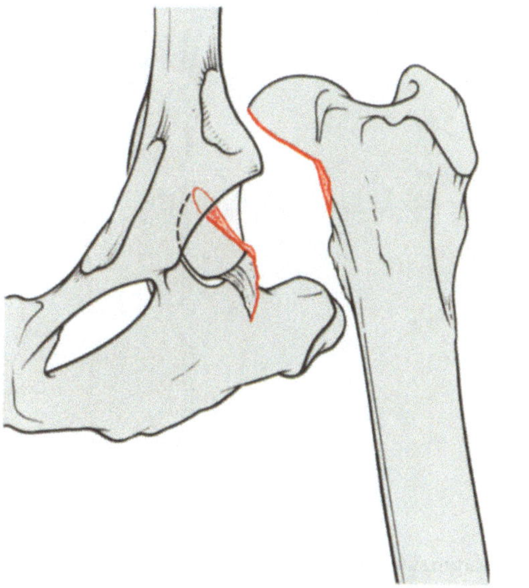

a

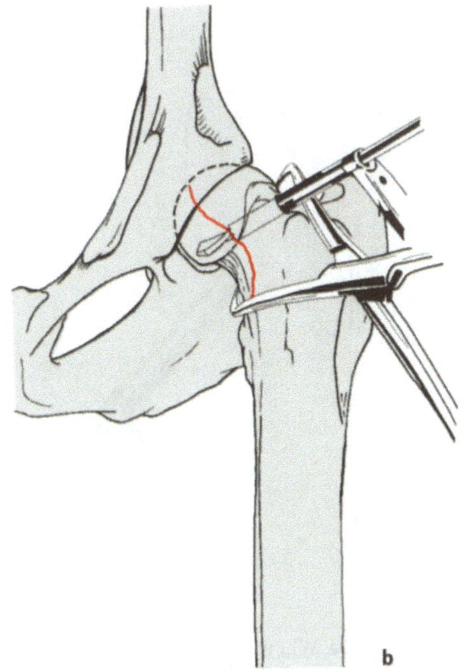

b

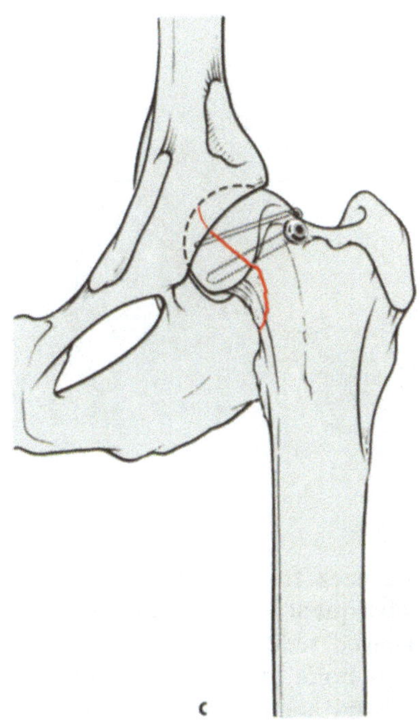

c

Fig. 4.35. **a** If the fragment is large enough, it may be fixed with a lag screw. **b** The gliding hole is drilled before the fragments are reduced. Reduction is maintained with a reduction forceps, while the thread hole is drilled through the drill sleeve. **c** A lag screw is used to compress the fracture, and the Kirschner wire is added for rotational stability

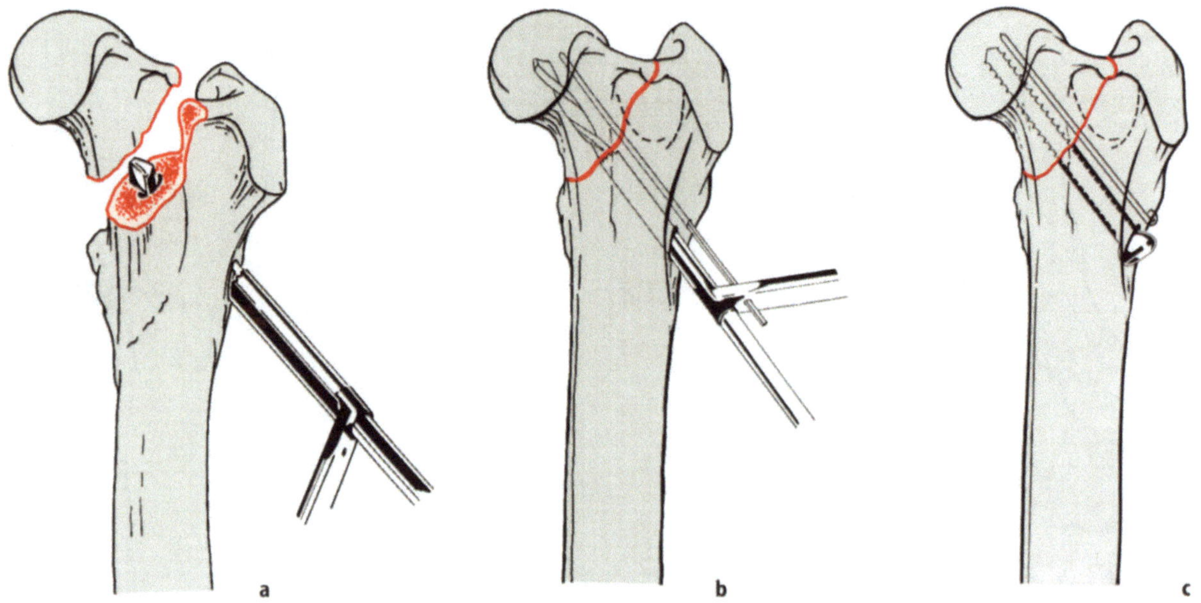

Fig. 4.36a–c. **a** When using a cortex screw, the gliding hole should be drilled through the proximal femur before the segment is reduced, so that this hole is properly placed in the femoral neck. The screw should parallel the long axis of the femoral neck to take advantage of the mechanical forces transmitted up the limb during weight-bearing. Some surgeons prefer to drill the glide hole from proximal to distal. **b** After the fragments have been reduced, they are stabilized by inserting one or two Kirschner wires. These wires should be parallel to the direction of the screw hole and should not penetrate the cartilage surface of the femoral head. The thread hole is drilled through the appropriate insert drill sleeve. **c** After the hole has been measured and tapped, a cortex screw of the appropriate length is seated

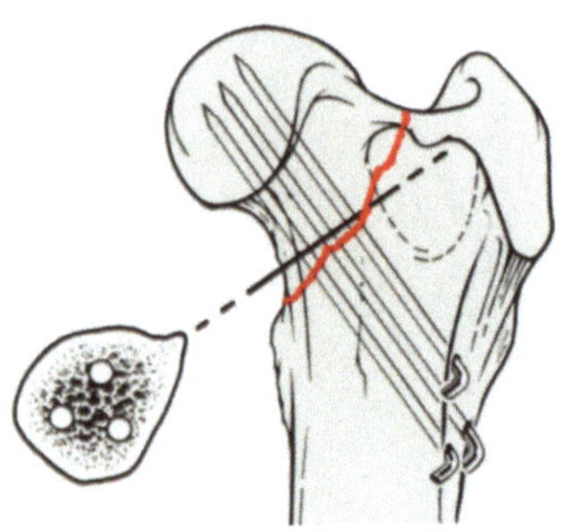

Fig. 4.37. A method of repair referred to as "triangulation" with three Kirschner wires. Ideally, these wires should run parallel to each other in separate locations of the femoral neck. The wires should also be parallel to the long axis of the femoral neck, which means they must start at a point on, or just distal to, the third trochanter and must be inserted until they lodge just underneath the cartilage surface of the femoral head without actually penetrating it. In very small animals, it is usually only possible to use two wires

the neck fractures seems to influence the risk of subsequent degenerative joint disease. However, delayed reduction and fixation is often associated with bone loss from the femoral neck. This may prevent anatomic reduction and increases the risk of subsequent degenerative joint disease. The two commonly used methods of repair are: (1) lag screw fixation combined with a pin for rotational stability (Fig. 4.36) and (2) pinning with two or three Kirschner wires (Fig. 4.37).

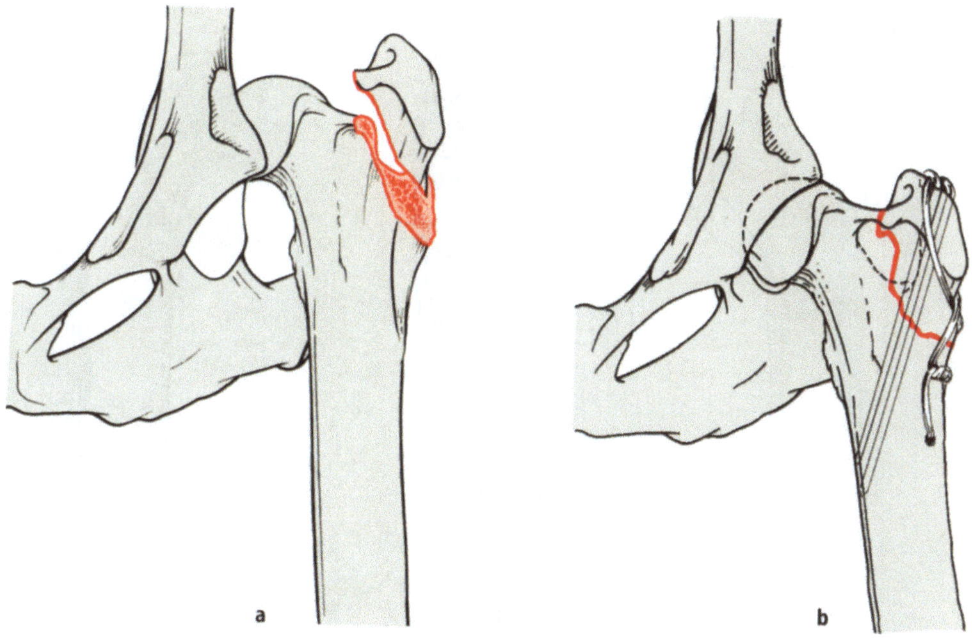

Fig. 4.38. **a** Fracture of the greater trochanter with luxation of the femoral head. **b** After reduction of the femoral head and closure of the joint capsule, the fracture is fixed with a tension band wire. For optimal stability, the pins should be directed medioventrally to engage in the medial cortex

4.5.3 Trochanteric Fractures

Fractures which involve only the trochanter are uncommon in the mature animal and are usually accompanied by hip luxation or femoral neck fractures. Tension band wiring, or lag screw fixation, is the ideal method for repair of these fractures (Fig. 4.38).

4.5.4 Subtrochanteric Fractures

Since the types of fractures encountered in this area are widely diversified, no one standard method of fixation can be applied to all cases. Many of these fractures include a fractured femoral neck (Fig. 4.39). Wherever possible, the bone fragments should be reconstructed and stabilized with the use of lag screws and a plate. Lag screws should be positioned so that they do not conflict directly with the position of the plate (Fig. 4.39) The plate must be contoured precisely so that it fits the lateral surface of the trochanter and shaft to a point where a minimum of three, or preferably four, screws are located distal to the lower fracture line. It is sometimes necessary to flatten the ridge of the third trochanter with a rongeur to facilitate positioning of the plate. The femoral neck fracture can be reduced and fixed with a Kirschner wire and a lag screw, as demonstrated in Fig. 4.36, being sure to keep the wire and screw head sufficiently caudolateral so as not to interfere with the lateral plate placement. In most cases, the femoral neck screw is inserted through the plate just below the level of the third trochanter, paralleling the long axis of the femoral neck (Fig. 4.39c). In certain fractures, it may be advantageous to use the hook plate.

4.5.5 Shaft Fractures

Bone plates provide the most rigid fixation and are the fixation of choice for shaft fractures in large breeds of dogs. The shaft of the femur is approached laterally where the plate is applied to the tension side of the bone. Depending upon the type of fracture present, a plate may function either as a compression plate, a neutralization plate, or a

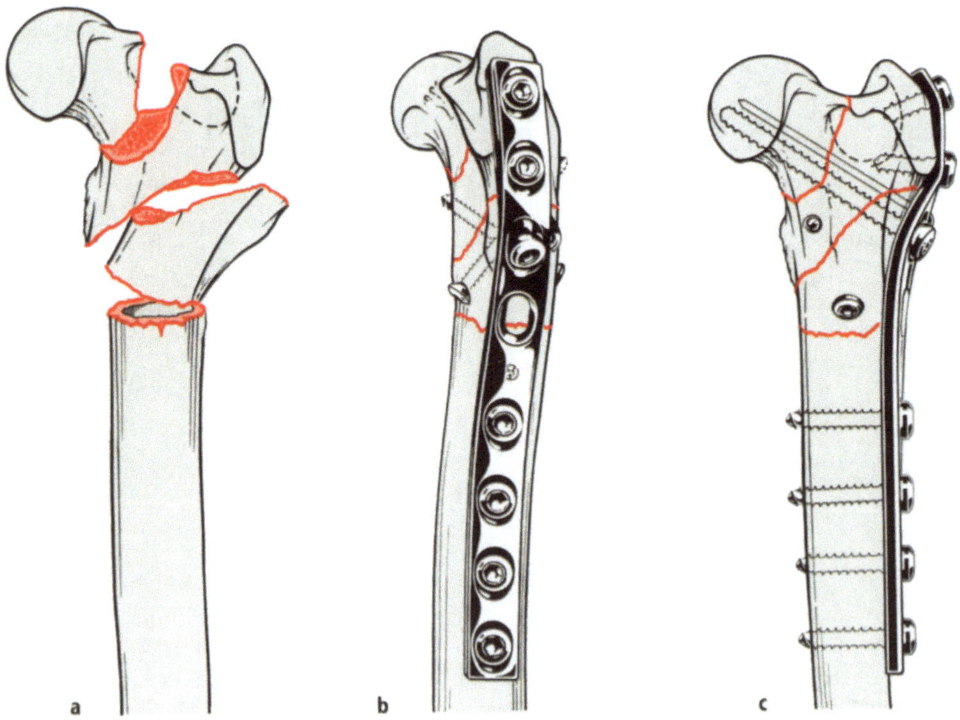

Fig. 4.39. a A comminuted fracture of the proximal femur including a fractured femoral neck. **b, c** Reductiuon and fixation of the butterfly fragment with lag screws. The femoral neck fracture is stabilized with a Kirschner wire and "lag screw". The latter may go through a hole in the plate or be inserted independently caudal to the plate. Many subtrochanteric fracture components are comminuted with a avery short, intact proximal femur in which only two screws can be inserted

buttress plate (Figs. 4.40, 4.41). In the face of severe comminution, anatomic reduction of bone fragments may be neither possible nor desirable. In these cases, the principles of biological osteosynthesis should be respected (Fig. 4.38):

1. The lateral femur should be approached by exposing the bone from the greater trochanter to the distal femoral condyles
2. The actual fracture zone should not be touched and the soft tissue attachments should be preserved in order to protect the remaining blood supply of the main fragments. Fragments should not be removed from the fracture site. The blood clot is left intact.
3. The plate should be selected and contoured based on a craniocaudal radiograph of the opposite femur. In heavy, very active dogs, it may be advantageous to use a bone-lengthening plate.
4. The properly contoured plate should be applied to the proximal femur using at least two screws.
5. The distal femur should be reduced and fixed to the plate using an AO reduction forceps or a similar clamp.
6. Verification of the proper axial and rotational alignment is mandatory. The linea aspera can be used as a landmark for orientation. Proper rotational alignment can also be ensured by checking internal and external rotation of the hip joint. A normal joint allows a 90 ° of internal rotation and 45 °–60 ° of external rotation.
7. If fracture repair is delayed, restoration of length can be carried out by means of the articulated tension device or the AO distractor. Distraction of the proximal and distal femoral fragments allows correct alignment of major fragments by "soft tissue taxis." When the length is regained, the small intermediary fragments may be squeezed and reduced with a dental pick.
8. The plate is fixed to the distal femoral shaft with a minimum of two or three screws. In these severely comminuted fractures, the plate is used as a pure buttress plate. An autogenous cancellous bone graft is recommended to fill architectural defects and to promote fracture healing.

Intramedullary pinning with a Steinman pin is an alternative to stabilize shaft fractures in small breeds of dogs or cats. As the sole form of fixation,

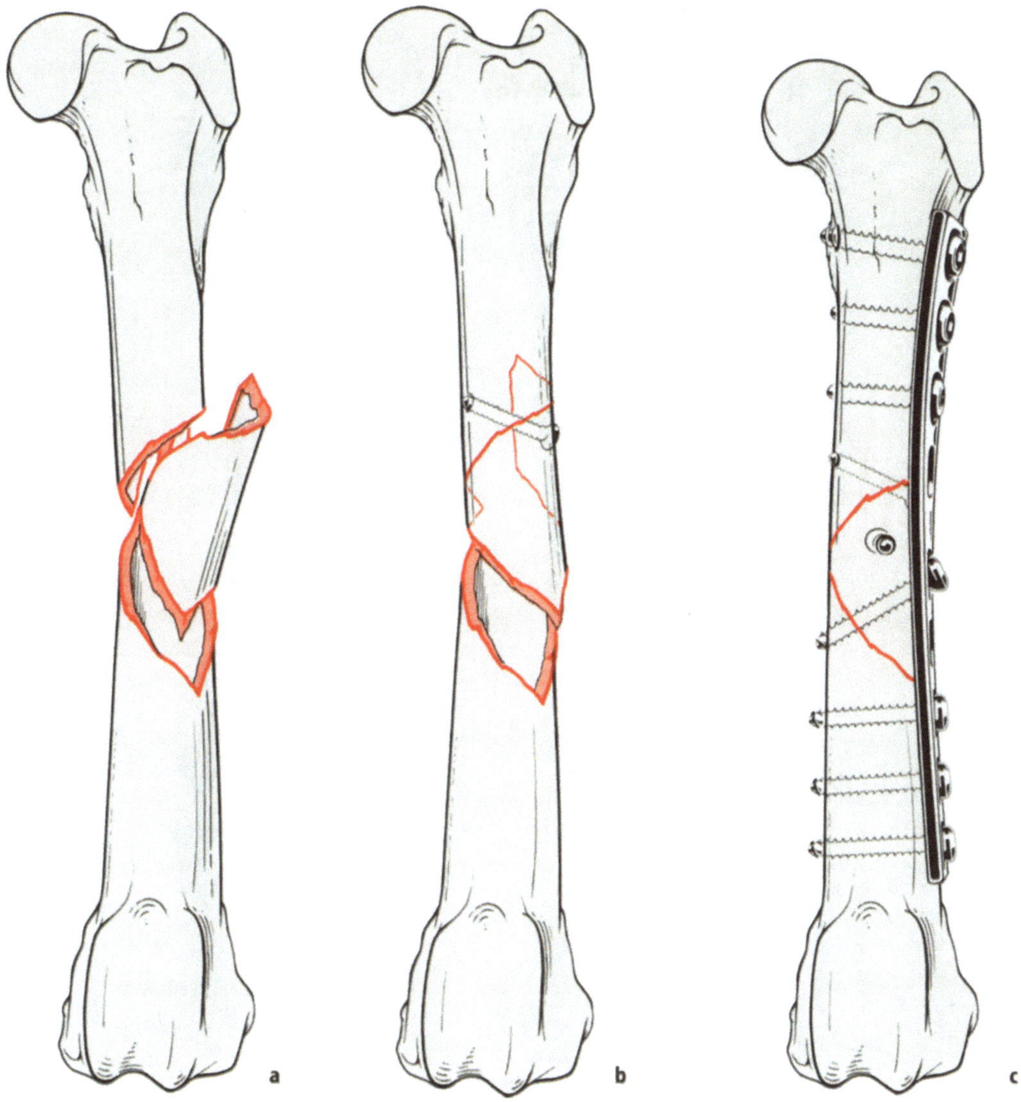

Fig. 4.40a–c. Neutralization plate. **a,b** When comminution is present, the shaft should be reconstructed by laying the fragments in the original position. Starting at one end and working towards the other, it is usually possible to reconstruct the shaft totally or to reduce it to two main segments. **c** A neutralization plate is applied to the tension side of the bone (lateral femur) for final stabilization

Steinman pins are rarely used and are only applied in stable fractures. They are most commonly used with supplementary fixations such as the external fixator, cerclage wires, or stacked pins. Proximal normograde pin placement is the preferred technique of pin insertion in the femur in order to avoid sciatic nerve entrapment or pin placement too close to the femoral head. Transverse fractures should never be fixed with a Steinman pin alone, because the pin does not provide rotational stability. The addition of a type I external fixator eliminates rotation at the fracture site and helps maintaining length (Fig. 4.42).

4.5.6 Supracondylar Fractures

Supracondylar fractures of the femur occur relatively infrequently in adult animals and are seen primarily in the cat and smaller breeds of dogs. Fixation of supracondylar fractures with regular dynamic compression plates (DCP) is difficult, due to the curvature of the distal end of the femur. Two parallel pins, pins and wire, or a pin and external fixator are effective alternatives (Fig. 4.40). Proper alignment of the fracture site is an important factor in determining the outcome of the treatment. If, however, perfect reduction is difficult to achieve, a

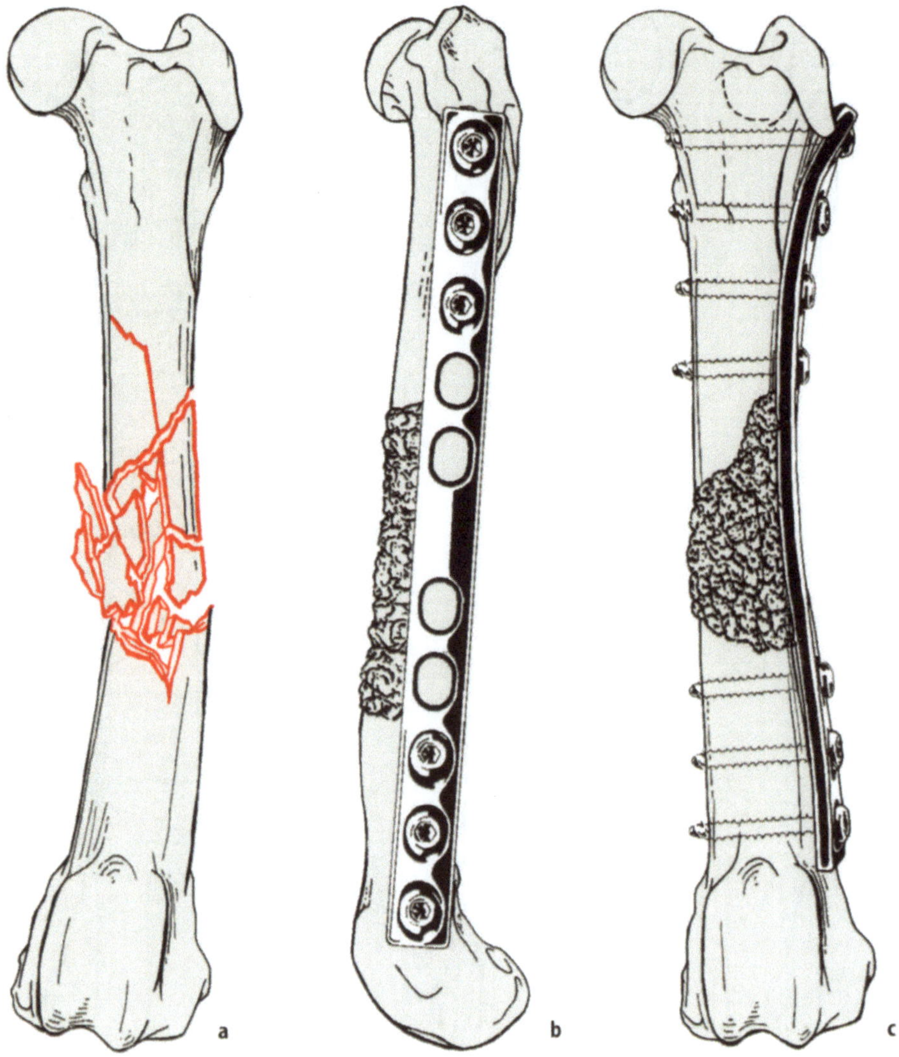

Fig. 4.41 a–c. Buttress plate. **a,b** A severely comminuted fracture of the femur is depicted in which it is not possible to reconstruct the shaft of the bone totally. Those fragments which are large enough to accept screws can be lagged together. Architectural defects in which the fragments are missing or too small to accept screws should be left undisturbed. **c** A buttress plate, in this case a lengthening plate, has been applied to keep the reconstructed bone from collapsing. Whenever possible, a plate performing buttress function in the diaphyseal bone should be large and should extend nearly the entire length of the bone. Cancellous bone graft is added to promote bone healing. If the plate extends to the distal metaphysis, it should be placed as caudally as possible to avoid direct interference with the patella or entrapment of the joint capsule

slight cranial overreduction of the distal fragment prevents patellar impingement during extension of the stifle.

Multiply fragmented fractures may be associated with patellar fractures or straight patellar ligament injury or avulsion. An osteotomy of the tibial crest

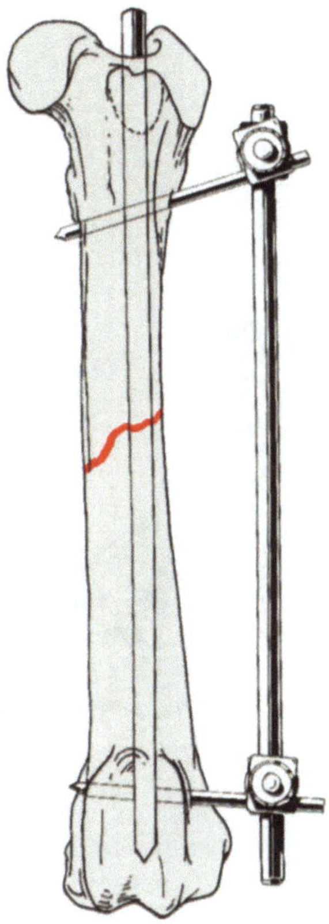

Fig. 4.42. Simple transverse shaft fracture in small breeds of dogs or cats can be stabilized with an intramedullary pin and an external fixator. The latter is important to provide rotational stability

may facilitate reduction of multifragmented fractures and thus fracture fixation. Proper axial and rotational alignment and stable internal fixation are mandatory. The landmarks used for shaft fractures are also used for proper rotational alignment in this area. Reconstruction plates can be used for fixation. The distal extremity of the plate is bent caudally and twisted inwardly (Fig. 4.43d).

4.5.7 Condylar and Intercondylar Y and T Fractures

Condylar fractures are rare. Usually, the medial condyle is affected. In most cases, the caudal cruciate and the medial collateral ligament are attached to the fractured condyle. In rare cases, the fractured condyle is an isolated fragment luxated caudally. Sometimes both condyles are fractured. Most unicondylar fractures are not displaced, and reduction and fixation is easily accomplished. A pointed reduction forceps is used for temporary fixation. A lag screw is inserted diagonally, from the proximal metaphysis into the fractured condyle, or from the condyle into the metaphysis (Fig. 4.44b). In large dogs, two screws may be inserted in a transcondylar fashion. If only the distal part of the medial condyle is fractured and luxated caudally (Fig. 4.44a), reduction may be difficult, especially when the injury is several days old. Reduction is attempted using a hook to pull the condyle cranially. If reduction is impossible, the vertical parapatellar arthrotomy incision is extended by a horizontal capsulotomy. Exposure may be further improved by osteotomy of the origin of the collateral ligament. When the fracture is reduced, complete inspection of the cruciate ligaments and menisci is mandatory. Intercondylar Y or T fractures are usually associated with extensive soft tissue damage and comminution in the supracondylar area. An osteotomy of the tibial tuberosity improves exposure. The fractured condyles are reduced and fixed temporarily using Vulsellum forceps. A transcondylar lag screw is inserted first in order to reconstruct the articular surface. Proper placement of the transcondylar lag screw is important to avoid cruciate ligament or articular surface damage. The supracondylar fracture is stabilized with two cross pins, Kirschner wires, or two screws. If the supracondylar fracture area is comminuted, a reconstruction plate is preferred and is applied as described above (Fig. 4.43c,d).

4.6 Fractures of the Patella

The patella is a large sesamoid bone interposed between the quadriceps tendon and its continuation, the straight patellar ligament. On contraction of the muscle group, the patella is subjected to considerable tensile stress axially and is concurrently compressed against the femoral trochlea. Consequently, fractures of the patella result in distraction and are therefore treated by the tension band technique.

The tension side of the patella is its cranial surface, while the side subjected to compressive stress is the caudal surface that contacts the femoral trochlea. The tension band wire is placed on the cranial surface of the patella. It acts as a tension band preventing avulsive forces of the quadriceps mechanism from distracting thte fracture. As the

Table 4.1. Tension band wire size according to size of dog

Weight (kg)	Wire size (mm)
0–5	0.5
5–15	0.8
15–30	1.0
>30	1.2

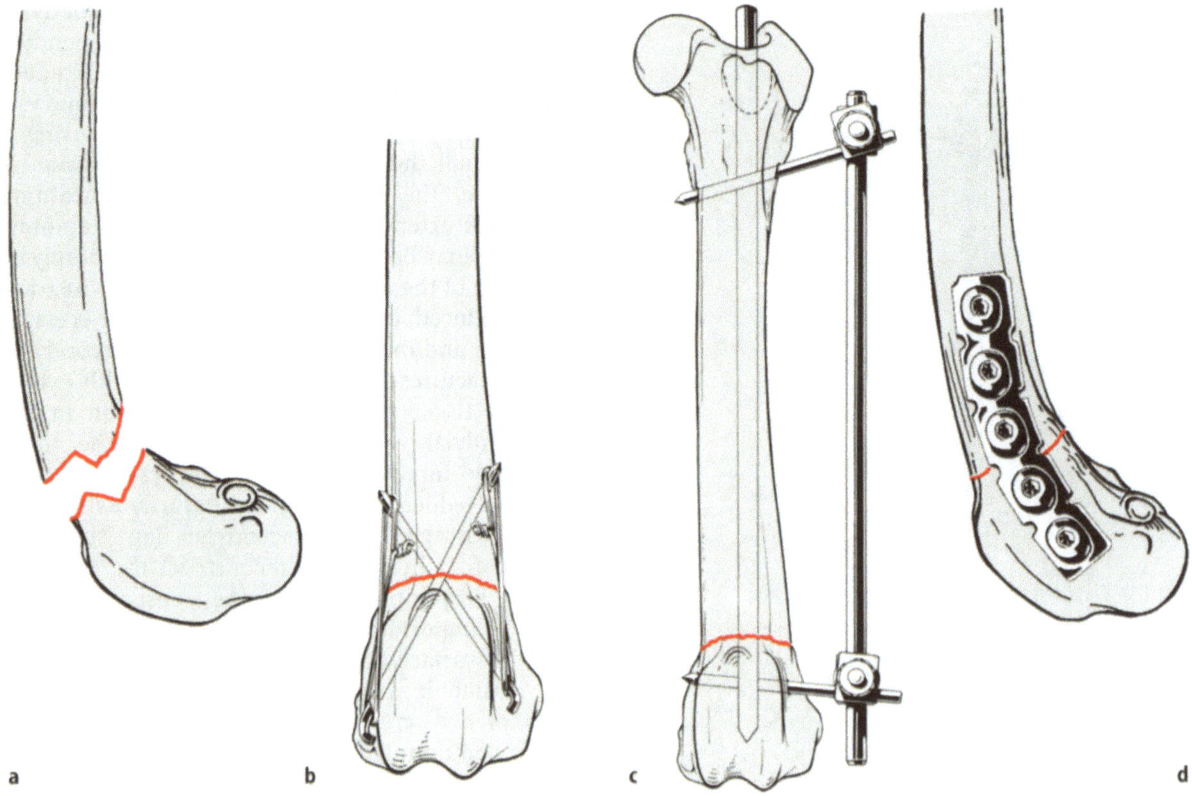

Fig. 4.43a–d. Supracondylar fracture. **a, b** Following reduction, two Kirschner wires or small Steinman pins are inserted in a crossed fashion. The exposed ends of the pins can be secured with tension wires. **c** Fixation using an intramedullary pin and halt-pin splintage. **d** A five hole reconstruction plate is employed to maintain a supracondylar fracture. This is especially useful in femurs, which have marked caudal bowing.

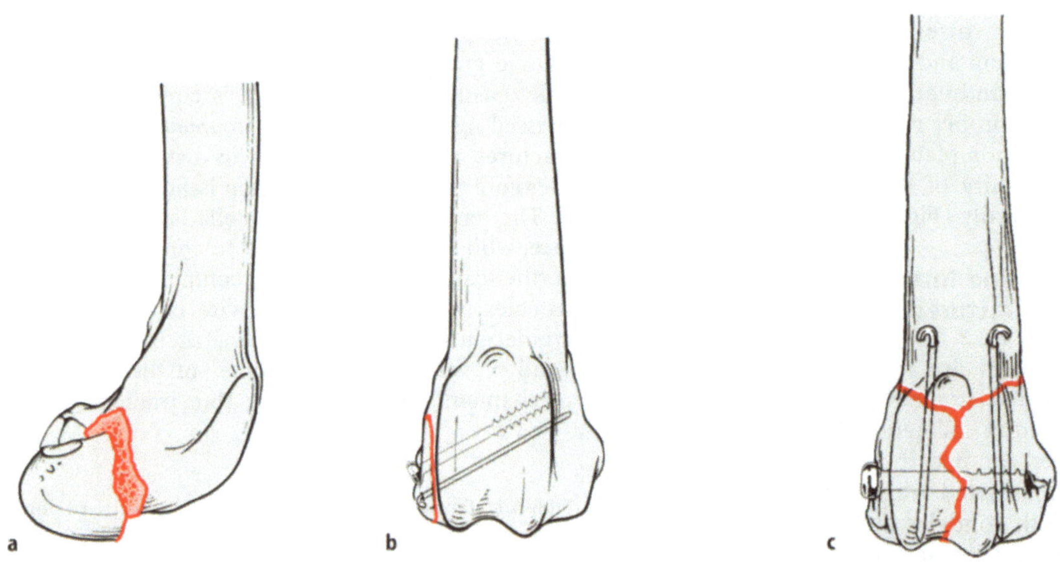

Fig. 4.44.a, b. Condylar fractures may involve only the condyle or they may course through the trochleargroove. Following reduction, one or two lag screws are inserted perpendicular to the fractured plane. Kirschner wires may be inserted in smaller fragments in place of the second screw. **c** Intercondylar Y or T fracture. The intracondylar fracture is reduced and fixed with a transcondylar lag screw. Fixation of the condyles to the femoral shaft may be performed with two parallel pins or similar techniques used to treat supracondylar fractures depending on bone size

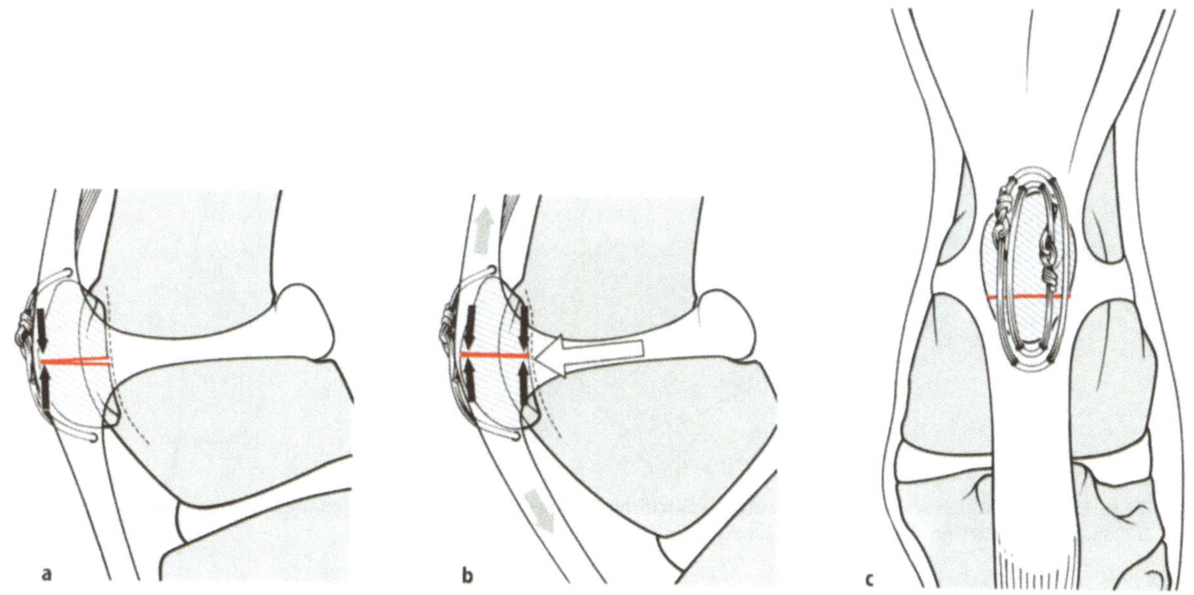

Fig. 4.45a–c. Correct placement of patellar tension band wire. **a** Lateral view with joint extended. **b** Lateral view with flexed joint. When the stifle joint flexes, the force from the femoral trochlea (*white arrow*) will convert the traction forces (*gray arrow*) to compression forces at the fracture site (*black arrows*). **c** In large breeds, the use of two wires may be advisable

caudal surface of the patella contacts the trochlea of the femor during weight-bearing, the avulsive force is converted to compression at the fracture site (Fig. 4.45). Incorrect placement of the wire allows the fracture to open on the tension side (Fig. 4.46).

In order to apply the above principle correctly, some details must be observed. First, the wire must be strong enough (suture wire will not do). A guide to proper size is given in Table 4.1.

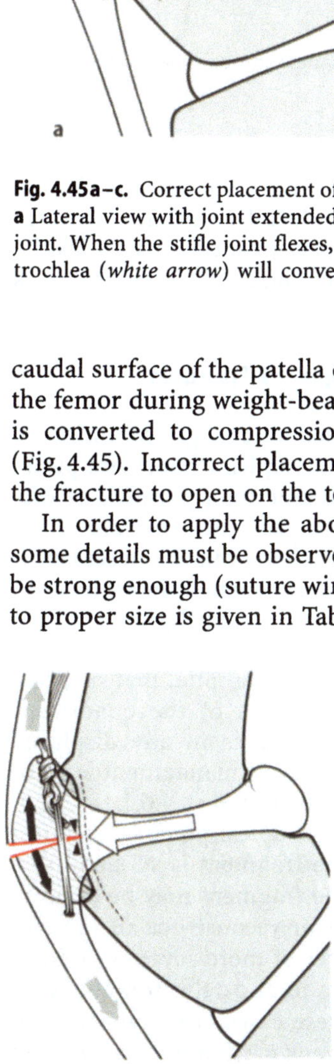

Fig. 4.46. Incorrect placement of patellar tension band wire: the wire is not on the tension side of the patella. When the stifle is flexed, the trochlea of the femur exerts cranial force on the patella (*white arrow*), combining with tractional force of quadriceps mechanism (*gray arrow*). The fracture site pivots about the axis of the incorrectly placed wire and the fracture surface breaks open cranially (*black arrows*)

Second the transverse arms of the wires should be passed just caudal to the quadriceps attachment to the patella and the straight patellar ligament. The proximal to distal arms of the wires must pass superficial to the retinacular tissue overlying the patella on the tension surface (Fig. 4.45). If the proximal to distal arms of the wire are allowed to pass lateral and medial to the patellar surface, respectively, then the repair will invariably fail (Fig. 4.46). Third, the properly placed wire should be tightened until the fracture is slightly overcorrected (Fig. 4.45a). This will cause the fracture fragments to be compressed when the stifle is flexed (Fig. 4.45b).

4.6.1 Types of Fractures

4.6.1.1 Nondisplaced Fractures

In simple transverse or even more comminuted fractures where the quadriceps expansion on either side of the patella has not been injured, the radiograph will reveal little or no displacement of the fracture fragments. These fractures should be repaired by means of the tension band wiring technique. In smaller patients, the tissues will only accommodate one wire. In the larger breeds, two wires should be used (Fig. 4.45).

Intraoperatively, the articular surface must always be inspected for small irreparable chondral

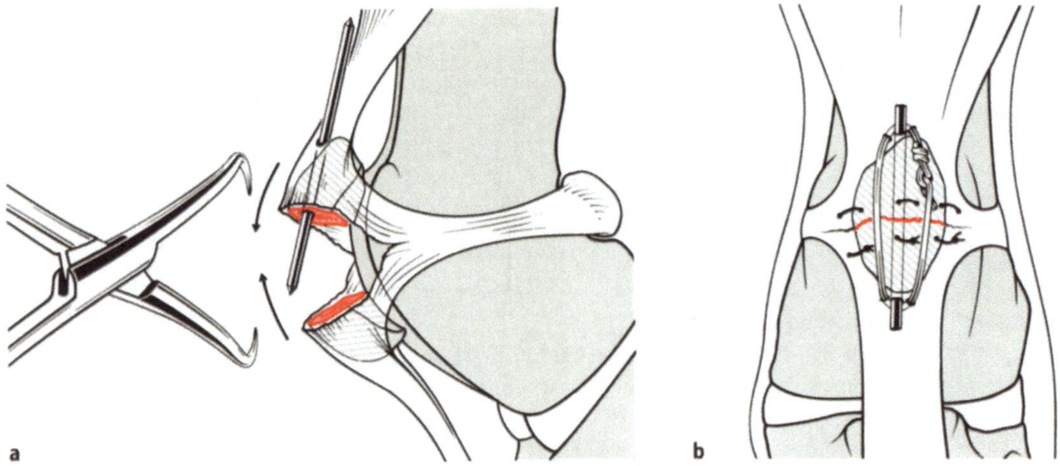

Fig. 4.47a,b. Displaced transverse patellar fracture. **a** insertion of 2-mm Kirschner wire Retrograde through the proximal fragment. **b** Completed reduction. Note the soft tissue repair

or osteochondral fragments. If they are 2–3 mm or less in diameter, they must be removed, since their replacement is impossible. Prior to capsule closure, the articular sufrace should again be inspected to make certain that the placement of the wires has not caused malalignment of the articular surface.

Postoperative care includes a bulky soft dressing for 24–48 h. Activity of the animal should be restricted to leash-walking for the first 2 weeks. If, for some reason, the patient refuses to use the limb within 5 days postoperatively, then passive exercise of the stifle may be initiated. Swimming is also excellent physiotherapy. Gradual increase in activity is encouraged after the second week.

4.6.1.2 Displaced Transverse Fractures

When there is significant displacment of the proximal and distal ends of the patella, this means that the quadriceps expansion on either side of the patella has been completely disrupted. Such fractures are highly unstable and require anatomical realignment of the articular surface prior to the application of the tension band wire. This realignment can be accomplished by the placement of two parallel Kirschner wires longitudinally (one Kirschner wire in the case of smaller breeds). In extremely hard bone, the channel for the Kirschner wire must be predrilled wih a drill bit or corresponding size. The Kirschner wire or wires prevent movement and subsequent malalignment of the fragments as the tension band wires are placed and tightened. In this case, the tension band wires should pass caudal to the Kirschner wires (Fig. 4.47). The reduction of the main fragments as well as the tightening of the wires must be accomplished while the limb is in a hyperextended position. In all cases, the lacerated components of the quadriceps mechanism must be sutured. Postoperative management is the same as for the nondisplaced fractures.

4.6.1.3 Comminuted Displaced Fractures

Kirschner wires are need to realign comminuted displaced fractures. However, Kirschner wire placement may be oblique rather than parallel, as dictated by the direction of the fracture lines (Fig. 4.48). Partial patellectomy may be necessary if the fracture fragments are too small. In such cases, close attention must be paid to the alignment of the articular surfaces to prevent the occurrence of stair-stepping (Fig. 4.49). It is also essential that suturing of the soft tissue components of the quadriceps mechanism be accomplished as in any displaced patellar fracture. Postoperative managment is similar to the regimen described in Sect. 4.6.1.1.

In some extreme distal apical patellar fractures where the distal fracture fragment is so small that repair is not feasible, the fragment may be excised, taking care to preserve or reconstruct all the soft tissue structures. In cases of more severely comminuted patellar fractures, total patellectomy may be the only solution. In these cases, it is important to reconstitute the quadriceps mechanism. In order to do this, the surgeon must judiciously preserve all soft tissues to which the patellar fragments are connected. If this is not done, it is very likely that there will not be enough quadriceps mechanism to accomplish an anastomosis. This latter condition would leave the animal with an ineffective stifle extensor mechanism.

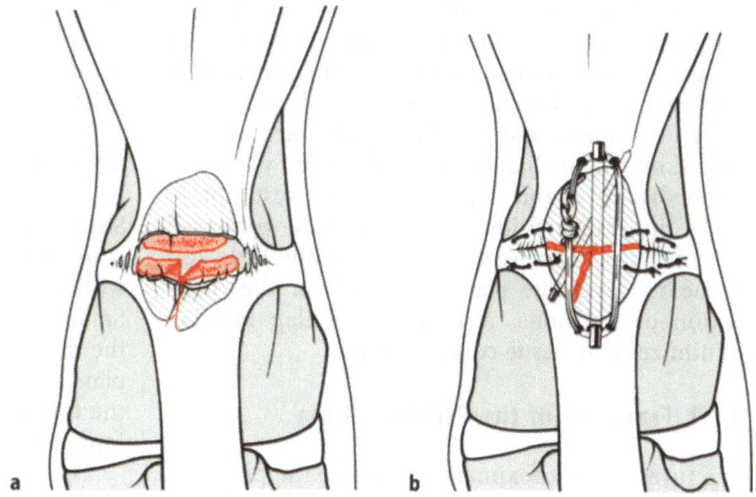

Fig. 4.48a,b. Multiple displaced patellar fracture. **a** Preoperative cranial view. **b** Two Kirschner wires and tension band wire repair of the fracture. Note the soft tissue repair

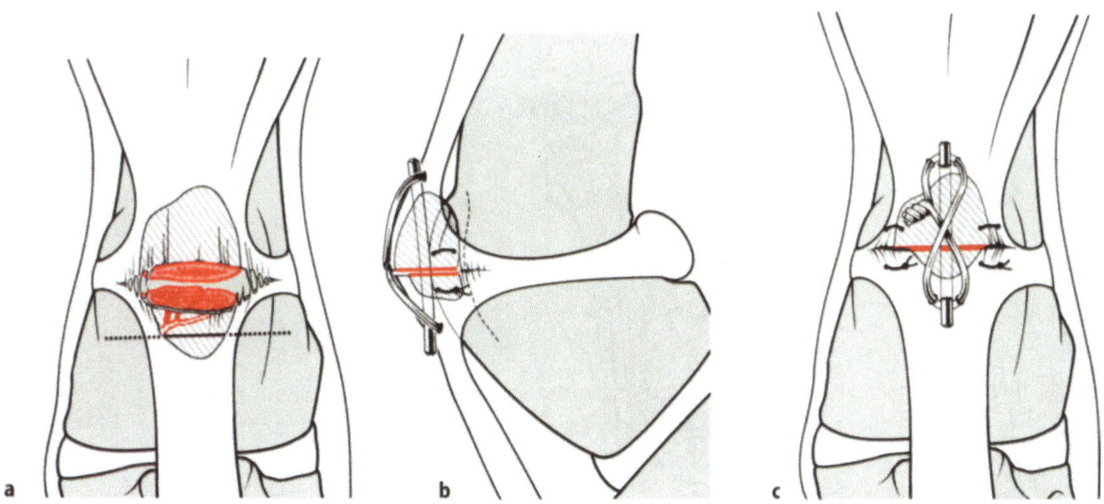

Fig. 4.49a–c. Multiply displaced patellar fracture. **a** Ostectomy of highly comminuted distal portion. All possible soft tissues must be preserved. **b** Lateral view of repair. Note that articular surfaces must be made congruous. **c** Craniocaudal view of repair. Note the soft tissue repair

4.7 Fractures of the Tibia

Numerous methods of repair of tibial fractures have been documented. External coaptation using splints or casts may be adequate for stable shaft fractures, green stick fractures, and fractures in young animals. In some cases, the fibula remains intact and provides a certain degree of stability that can be supplemented by external coaptation.

Generally, rigid internal fixation is the preferred method of treatment. It permits earlier weight-bearing and allows stifle and hock movement during fracture healing.

Intramedullary pins are suitable for transverse or short oblique fractures provided that rotational stability is achieved. Tibial fractures are pinned in an antegrade fashion. Retrograde insertion will result in the pin entering the stifle joint. Intramedullary pinning often requires some form of secondary fixation such as cerclage wires, lag screws, or an external fixator. A unilateral fixator applied medially with either one or two pins proximally and distally provides rotational stability. It should be used until fibrous callus has formed, at which point it can be removed. At this stage, sufficient stability is provided by the intramedullary pin until clinical union is achieved.

External fixators are widely used for the treatment of open fractures, since they provide access for wound management and the pins can be placed away from the contaminated area.

Bone plates can be used to treat most fractures of the proximal end and shaft. They are the method of choice for comminuted or unstable fractures, since they permit rigid stabilization and result in an early return to functional activity. Plates are usually placed on the medial surface of the bone via a craniomedial or cranial approach. It is best not to make the skin incision directly over the proposed site of the plate, since there is frequently little soft tissue to cover the plate, especially in the distal region of the bone. A longitudinal flap incision minimizes soft tissue complications.

4.7.1 Fractures of the Proximal Tibia

Fractures of the proximal end involve the proximal metaphysis and/or diaphysis and are either oblique or comminuted (Figs. 4.50, 4.51). It is essential that the tibial plate be buttressed to assist in alignmant. A T plate is the preferred method of stabilization, if at all possible. Otherwise, a straight plate of appropriate size should be employed.

4.7.2 Shaft Fractures

Shaft fractures are frequently long oblique, spiral, or comminuted fractures. They are best immobilized with lag (or position) screws supported by a plate. Small fissure lines commonly extend distally from the major fracture. Radiographs in at least two planes are required to demonstrate the full extent of the fracture. Failure to identify fracture lines and to immobilize them may result in failure of the repair.

The following methods are some of the ways suggested to achieve rigid fixation using bone plates and screws (Figs. 4.52–4.60).

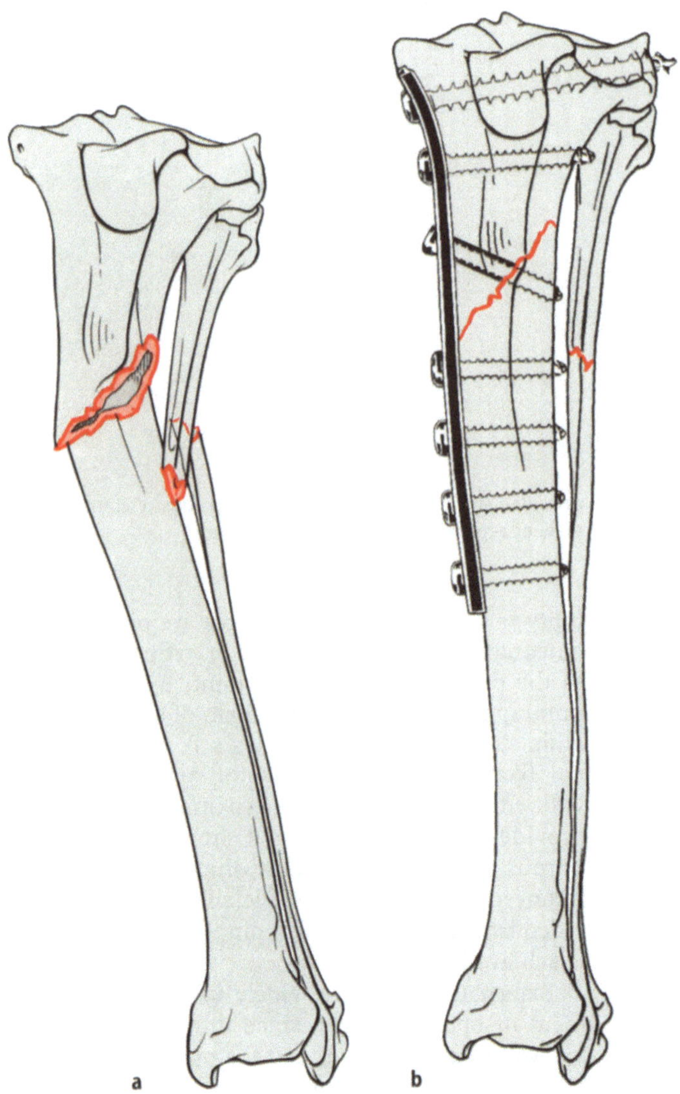

Fig. 4.50. **a** An oblique fracture involving the proximal end of the tibia. **b** Fixation using a dynamic compression plate (DCP) with interfragmentary compression accomplished by use of a lag screw inserted through the plate

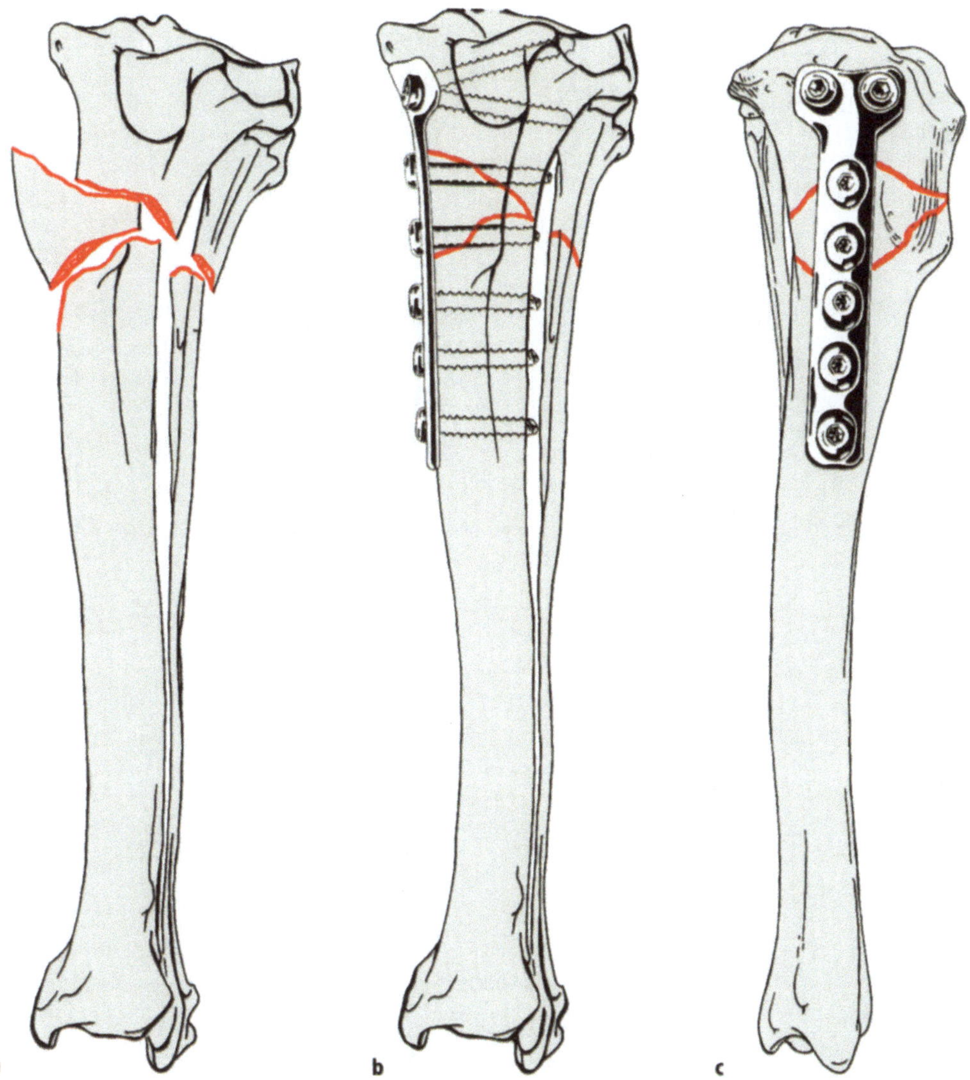
a b c

Fig. 4.51. a A multiple fracture of the proximal end of the tibia with a wedge segment. **b,c** Repair was accomplished using a T plate, which was employed so as to restore length of the bone and the support to the tibial plateau incorrect alignment. Medial view of the proximal tibia, showing the T plate

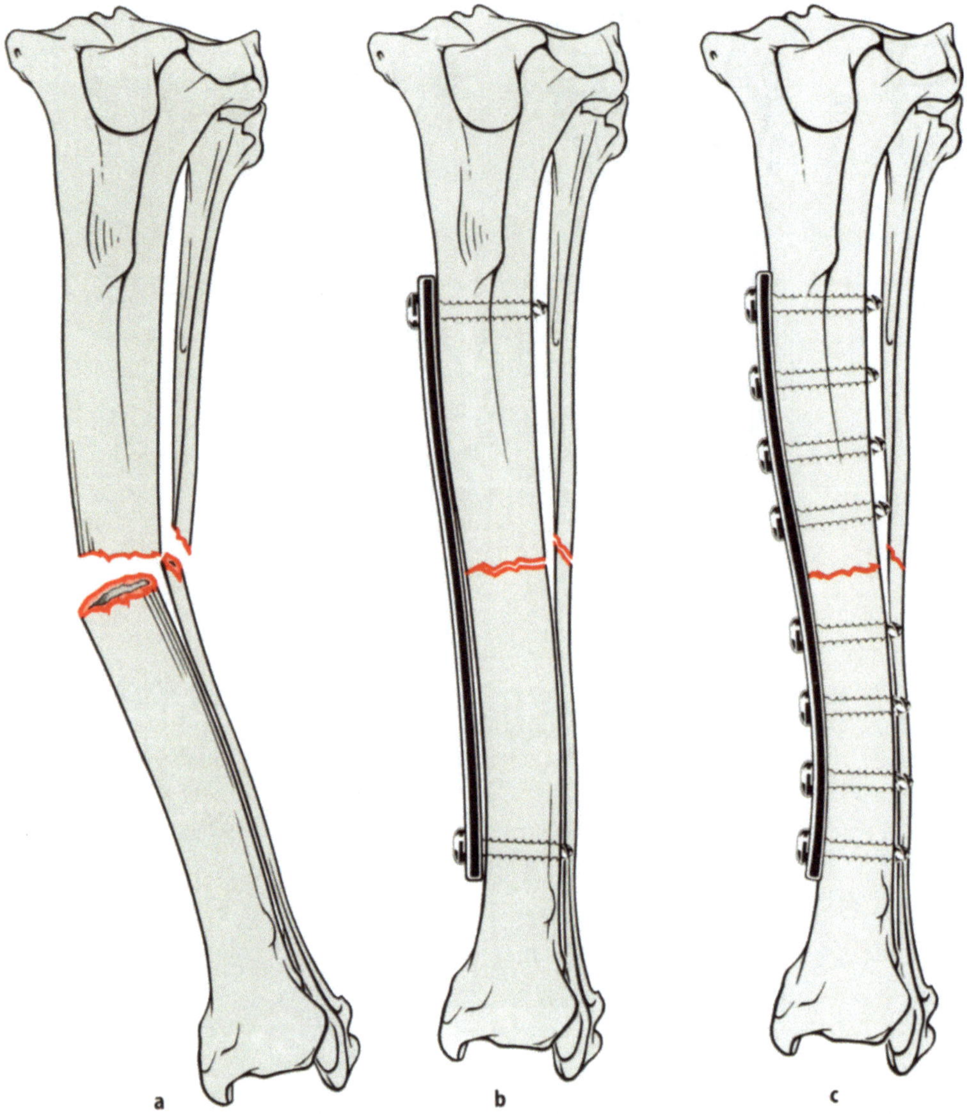

a b c

Fig. 4.52. a A transverse fracture of the mid-diaphyseal area of the tibia. **b** Craniocaudal view of the prestressed dynamic compression plate prior to final seating of the screws. Note the lack of apposition of the far cortex. **c** Final tightening of all screws brings about axial compression and closure of the gap in the cortex on the far side

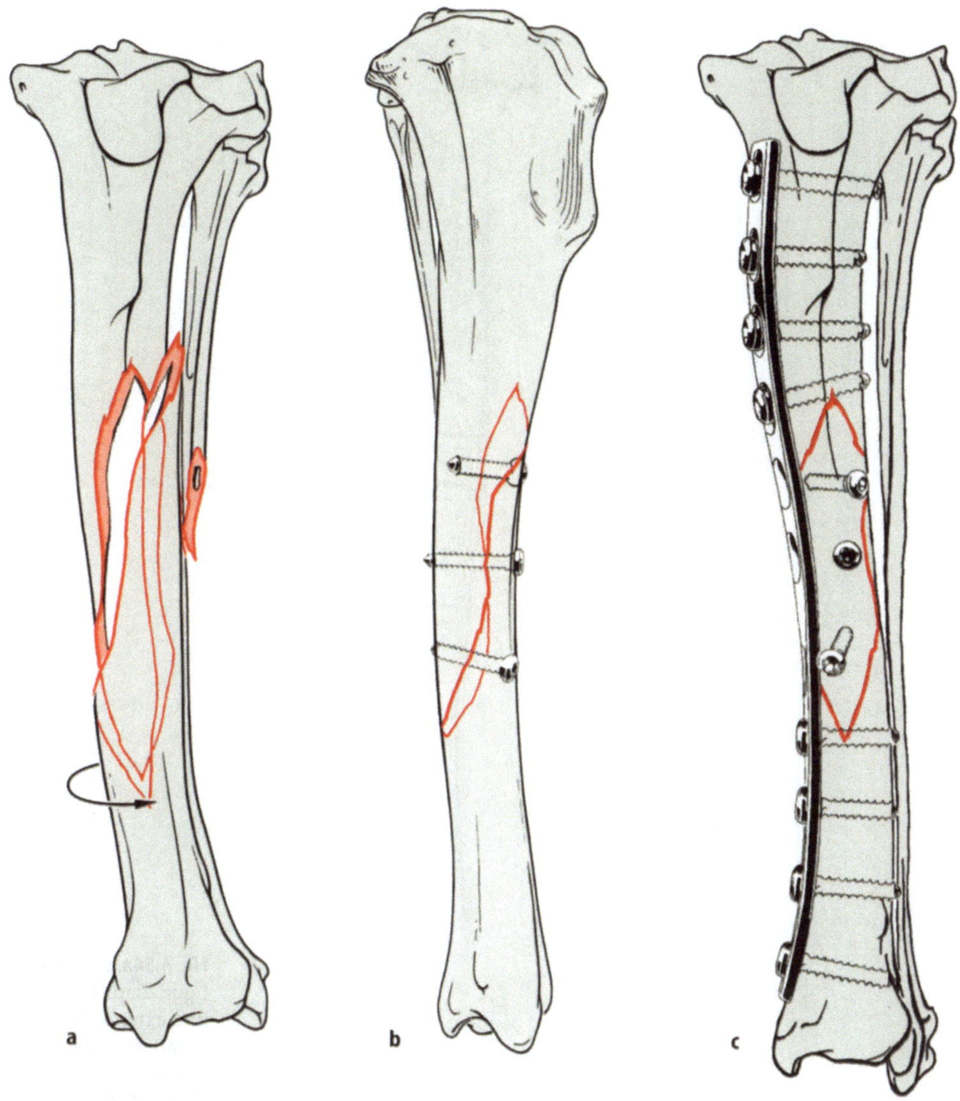

Fig. 4.53. **a** Craniocaudal view of a long oblique fracture, where the fracture line extends from caudal to cranial. **b** Medial view showing reconstruction by use of three lag screws for interfragmentary compression. **c** Craniocaudal view showing final fixation with a neutralization plate

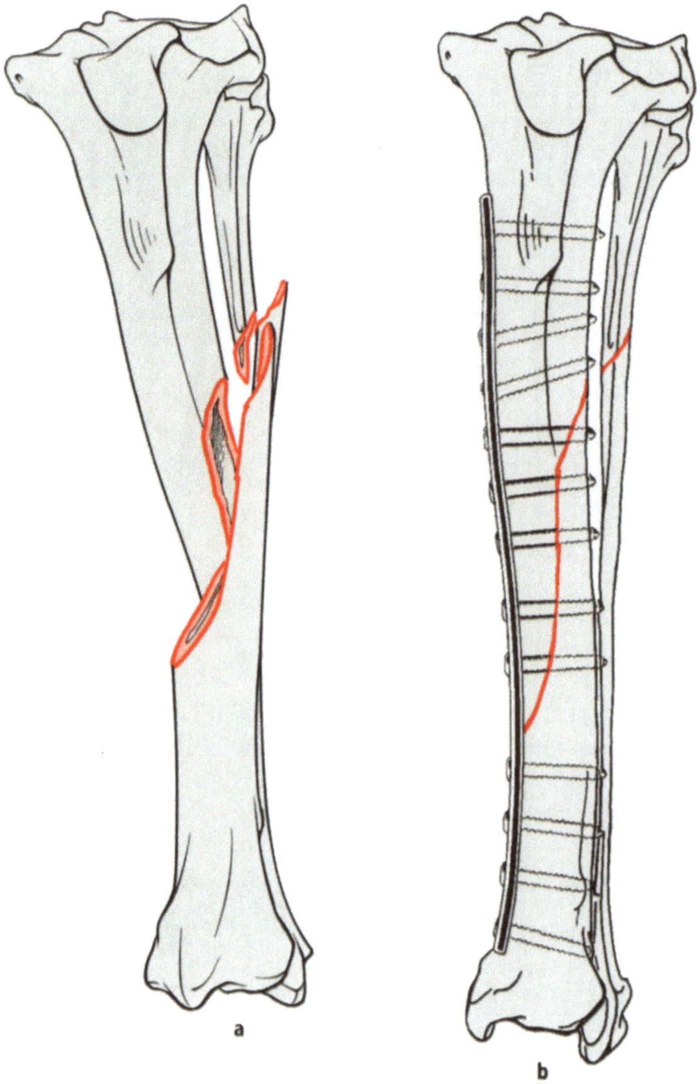

Fig. 4.54a,b. Craniocaudal view of a long oblique diaphyseal fracture, where the fracture line extends from lateral to medial, showing repair by means of lag screws inserted through the neutralization plate to accomplish interfragmentary compression

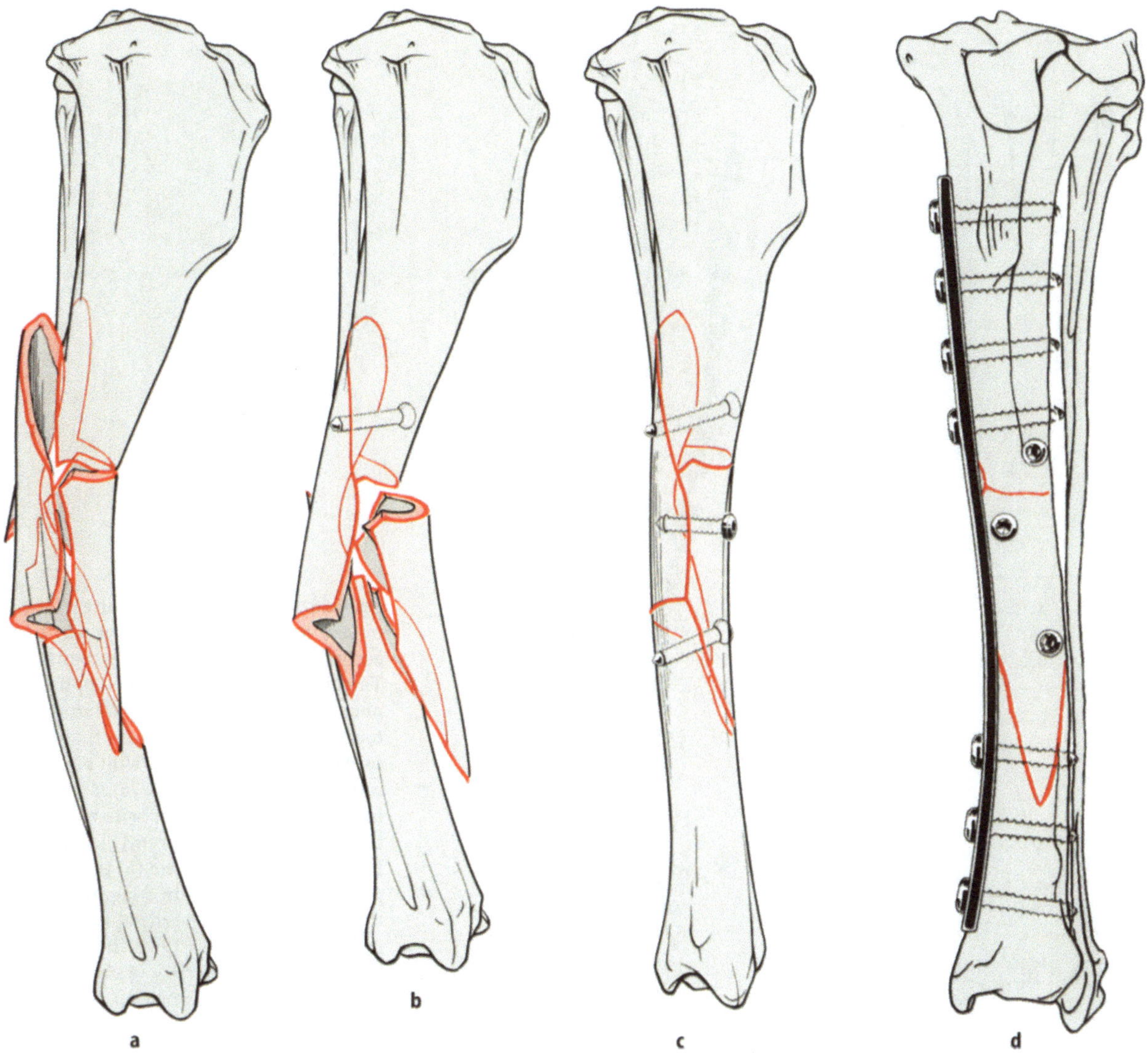

Fig. 4.55. **a** A multiple fracture of the diaphysis with double butterfly segments. **b** The diaphysis is reconstructed by reducing each segment in turn and immobilizing it with a lag screw. Where possible, two small lag screws are preferred to one larger single screw per segment. **c** The reconstructed diaphysis using three lag screws. **d** A long neutralization plate protects fracture reconstruction

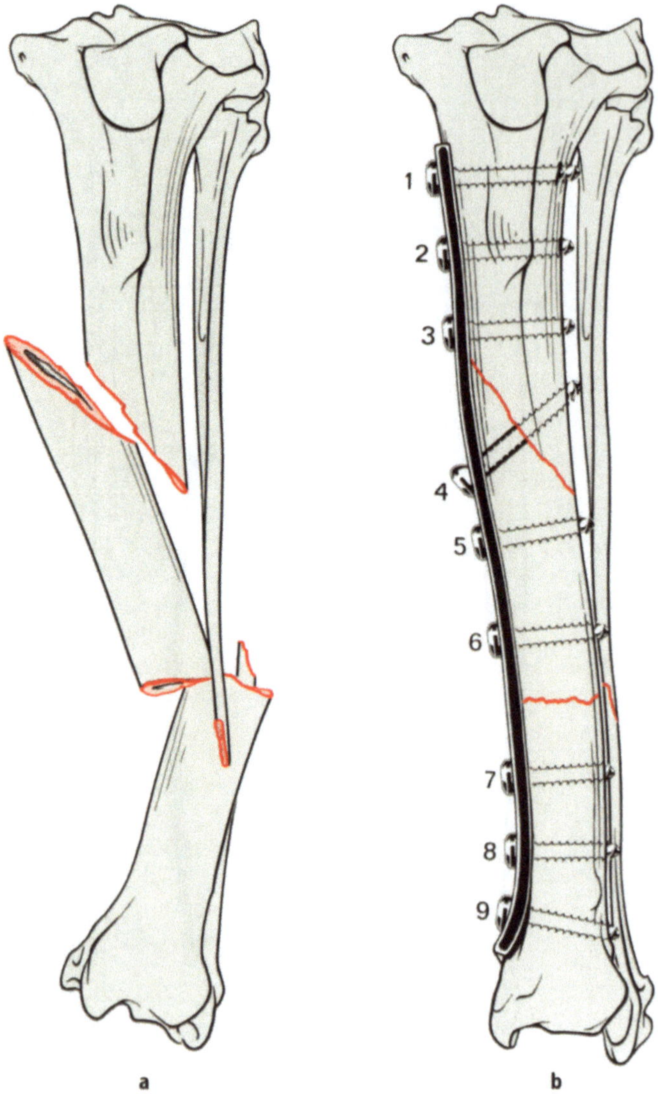

Fig. 4.56. **a** A segmental fracture of the tibia. **b** Reduction and fixation may be accomplished in the following manner: The craniocaudal view of the opposite normal tibia is used as a guide in contouring the plate. The plate is first fixed to the proximal fragment with a plate screw (*1*). The next screw (*6*) is inserted in a loaded position (opposite to the center of the plate). One screw (*2*) is inserted in a loaded position, one (*5*) in a neutral position, and one (*4*) in a lag position through the plate. The distal fragment is reduced, and a screw (*9*) is inserted in a loaded position. A screw (*8*) is also inserted in a loaded position. The remaining screws (3 and 7) are inserted in a neutral position

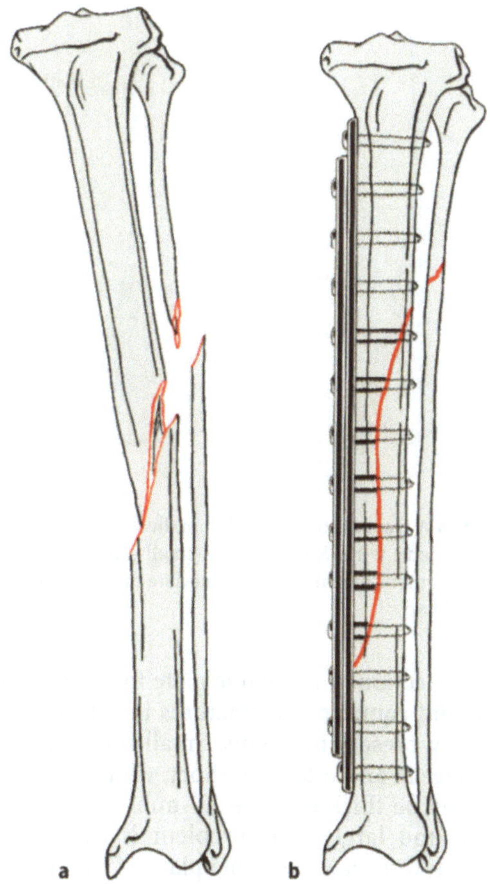

Fig. 4.57. a Craniocaudal view of a long oblique diaphyseal fracture in a cat. The fracture line extends from lateral to medial. **b** Repair with two veterinary cuttable plates sandwiched for increased strength. Lag screws are inserted through the plates to achieve interfragmentary compression

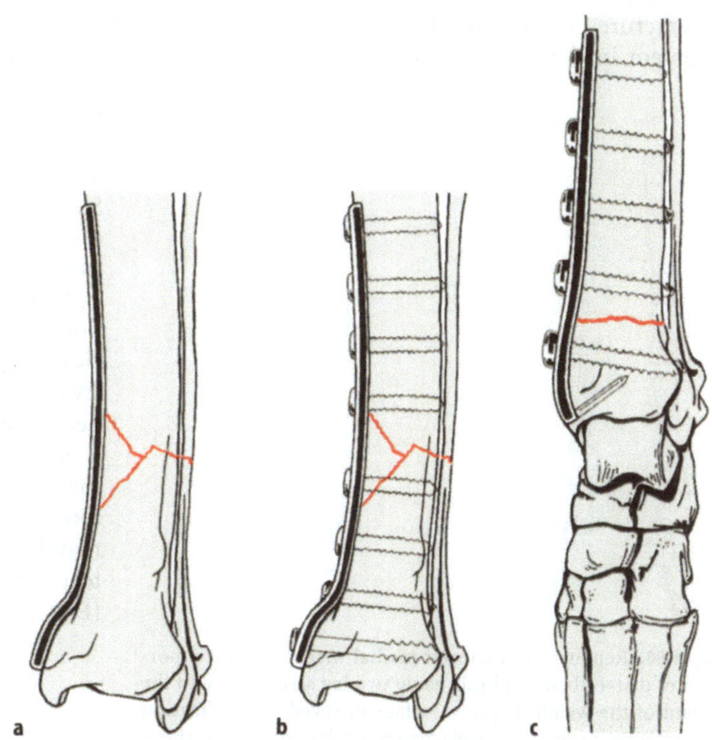

Fig. 4.58. a Distal wedge shaft fracture of the tibia with a contoured plate to permit stabilization and closure of the transcortex.
b The wedge has been lagged to the distal segment through the plate. **c** In extremely distal fractures in large dogs, stabilization may be achieved by means of a hook plate. The two prongs, which may have to be shortened, augment the single screw if there is insufficient room in the epiphysis for two screws

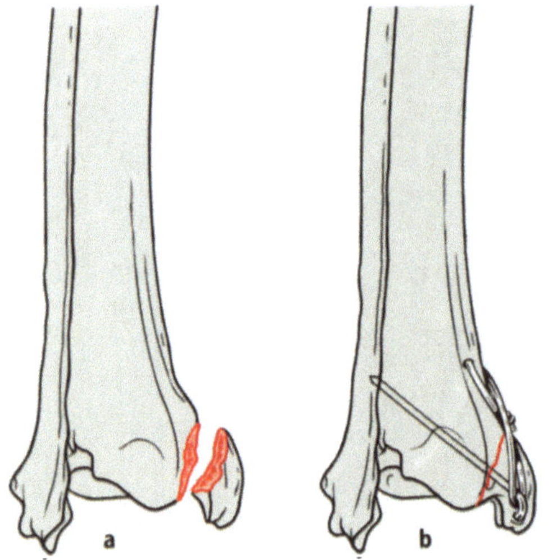

Fig. 4.59. **a** A fracture of the medial malleolus. **b** Repair using a tension band wire. *Note:* In very small animals, the small fracture segment may only accommodate one Kirschner wire instead of two

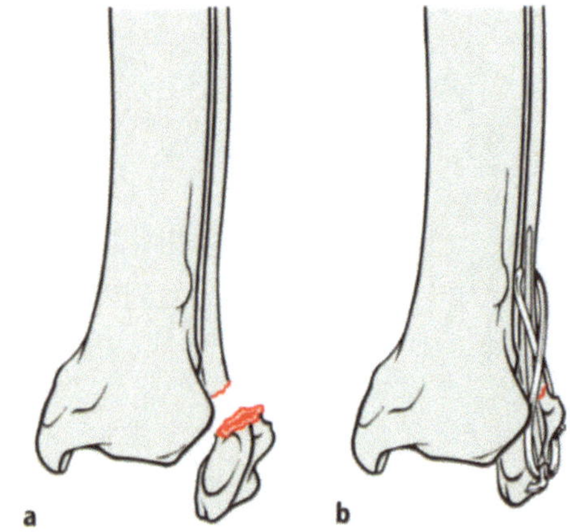

Fig. 4.61a,b. Repair of a fractured lateral malleolus using a tension band wire

The selection of a suitable plate for long oblique, spiral, and comminuted fractures in cats and small dogs may present problems. Small fragment plates are too weak and often too short, while the 2.7-mm DCP may be thick and the 2.7-mm cortical screws may be too large. This problem is overcome by using the veterinary cuttable plate. If the degree of stiffness needs to be increased, the plates can be "sandwiched" by placing one on top of the other (Fig. 4.61).

Fractures of the distal shaft pose a particular problem in that there is little bone for screw purchase in the distal metaphysis. Moreover, the shape of the articular surface of the distal tibia means that distally placed screws must be directed proximally to prevent them from entering the joint. Such fractures may be immobilized with a double hook plate placed with the hooks in the distal metaphysis. It may be necessary to shorten the hooks to prevent them from penetrating the talocrural joint.

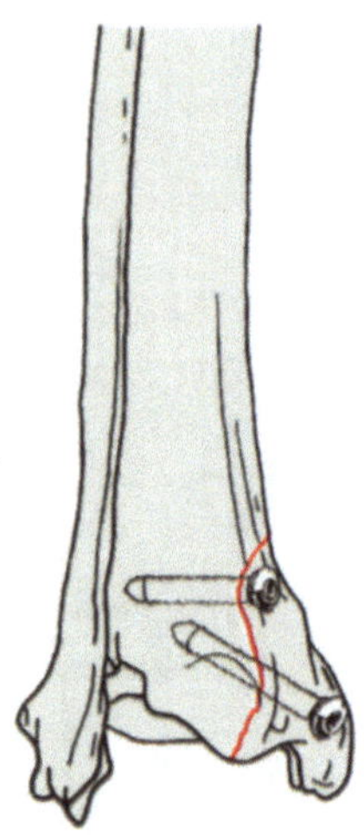

Fig. 4.60. Repair of a fractured medial malleolus and a portion of distal tibial epiphysis using two lag screws. Due to the extent of the weight-bearing surface involved, screw fixation is necessary to prevent displacement of the articular surface

4.7.3 Fractures of the Malleoli

Most malleolar fractures are associated with luxation or subluxation of the talocrural joint. Malleolar fractures may occur singly or as a bimalleolar fracture. Bimalleolar fractures are occasionally seen in association with a caudal triangular fragment. Shearing injuries not infrequently result in hock disruption due to the loss of malleolar bone and associated soft tissue structures.

Since malleolar fractures have an articular component and are accompanied by ligamentous injuries, surgical repair must be precise and internal fixation is mandatory if joint incongruency and degenerative joint disease are to be avoided.

Most malleolar fractures can be repaired using the tension band wire principle or with lag screw fixation. If the fragment is large enough, lag screws may be used. External support is required to protect the repair until healing is confirmed (Figs. 4.62–4.65).

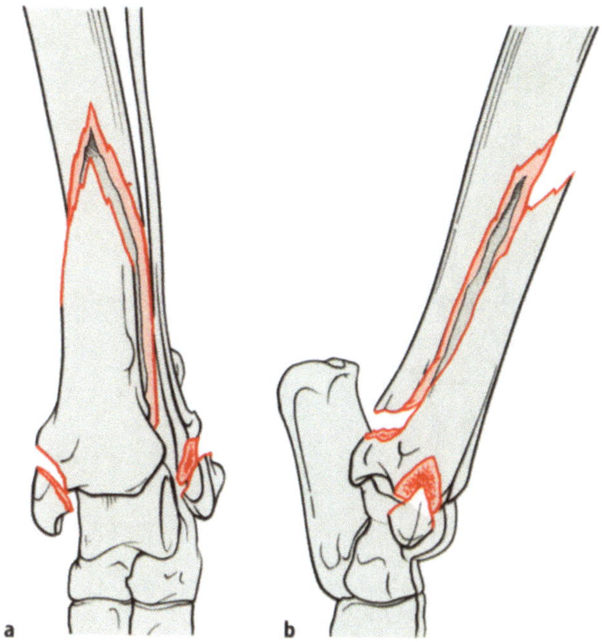

Fig. 4.62a,b. Craniocaudal (**a**) and mediolateral (**b**) views of a long oblique fracture of the distal tibial shaft, with transverse fractures of the medial and lateral malleoli (see Fig. 4.63a,b)

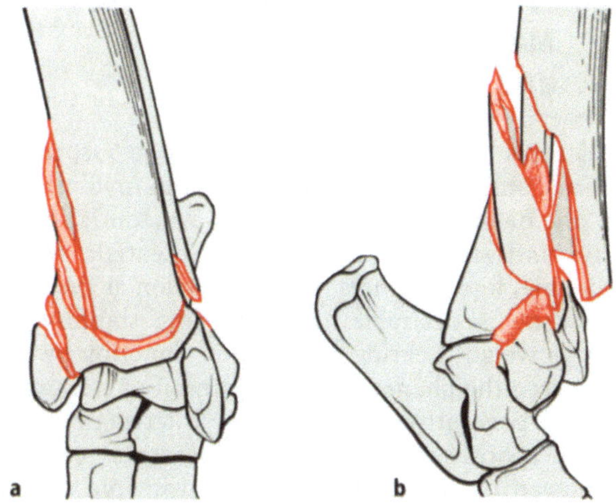

Fig. 4.64a,b. Bimalleolar fracture with a distal caudal triangle fragment and a caudal butterfly fragment (see Fig. 4.65)

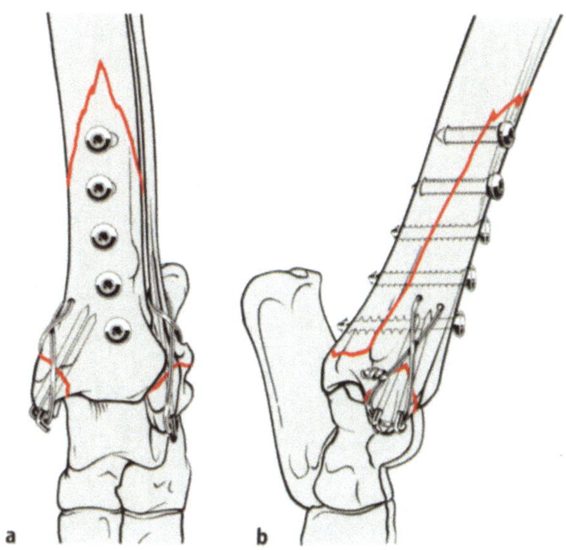

Fig. 4.63a,b. Fixation of the shaft fracture of the distal tibia (see Fig. 4.62a,b) accomplished by using five lag screws. Tension band wires were used on both malleoli. The leg was further supported with a coaptation splint for 2 weeks

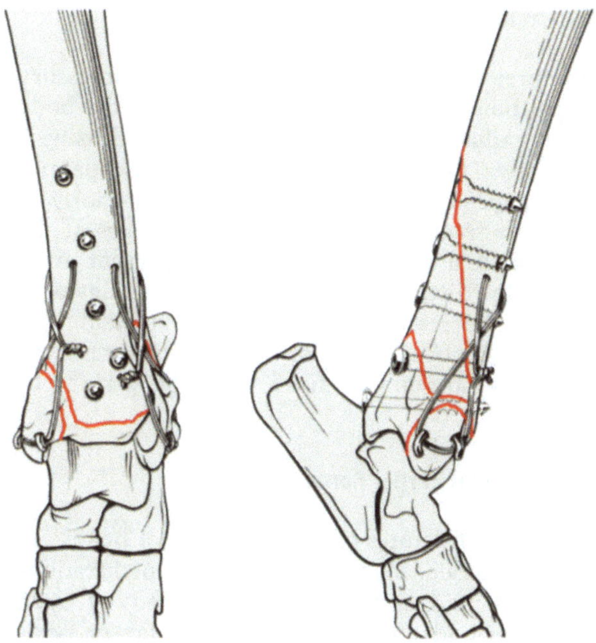

Fig. 4.65. The so-called trimalleolar fracture (see Fig. 4.64) is in reality a bimalleolar fracture with a distal caudal triangle fragment. This case also had a caudal butterfly component. Repair is by interfragmentary compression with lag screws and tension band wires on either side, utiliying a medial and lateral plantar incision (Figs. 4.76, 4.77).

4.8 Fractures of the Carpus, Tarsus, Metacarpus, Metatarsus, and Phalanges

Fractures of the carpus, tarsus, metacarpus, metatarsus, and phalanges usually result in involvement of one or more articular surfaces. Anatomic reduction and fixation are therefore essential. Where possible, interfragmentary compression at the fracture site is desirable, thus ensuring stability for early weight-bearing and joint function while reducing the chance of delayed union or nonunion and degenerative joint disease. Interfragmentary compression between large fragments can be achieved by using the lag screw principle and in avulsion fractures by using the tension band wire technique.

A well-padded temporary coaptation splint should be applied to these fractures prior to surgery to stabilize the fragments, prevent further injury to the adjacent tissue, and reduce swelling of the injured area. For postoperative care a well-padded splint is usually applied for several days up to several weeks, depending on the complexity of the fracture and adequacy of the fixation.

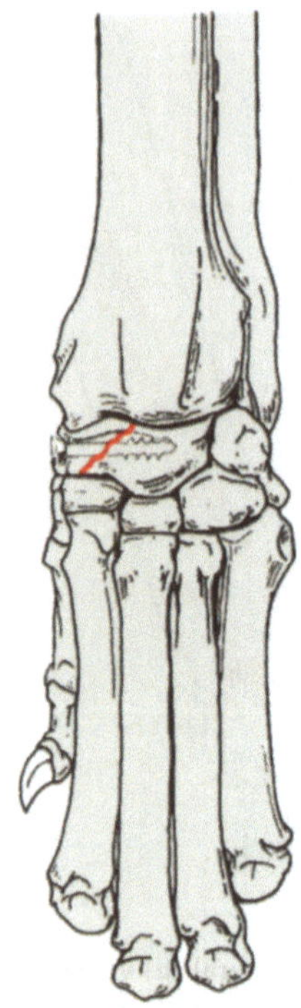

Fig. 4.66. Fracture through the body of the radial carpal bone stabilized with a lag screw (medial)

4.8.1 Fractures of the Carpus

4.8.1.1 Radial and Ulnar Carpal Bones

Fractures involving the radial, ulnar, or accessory carpal bones are rare. Fractures through the body of the radial carpal bone can be stabilized using a lag screw. This screw is placed in the medial palmar prominence and angled laterally and anteriorly to cross the fracture line (Fig. 4.66). Fractures of the distal medial palmar prominence represent avulsion of the distal radial carpal-metacarpal ligament and can be reattached with a tension band wire (Fig. 4.67). Ulnar carpal bone fractures are extremely rare and are fixed using the same technique.

4.8.1.2 Distal Carpal Bones

Small chip fractures of the distal carpal bones are usually excised. Medial slab fractures or luxations of the second carpal bone are treated by open reduction and then maintained by a lag or position screw, respectively, that is, placed medial to lateral. Dorsal slot fractures of the third carpal bone may be exposed by longitudinally splitting the extensor carpi radialis tendon. Repair is by screw fixation. The head should be countersunk.

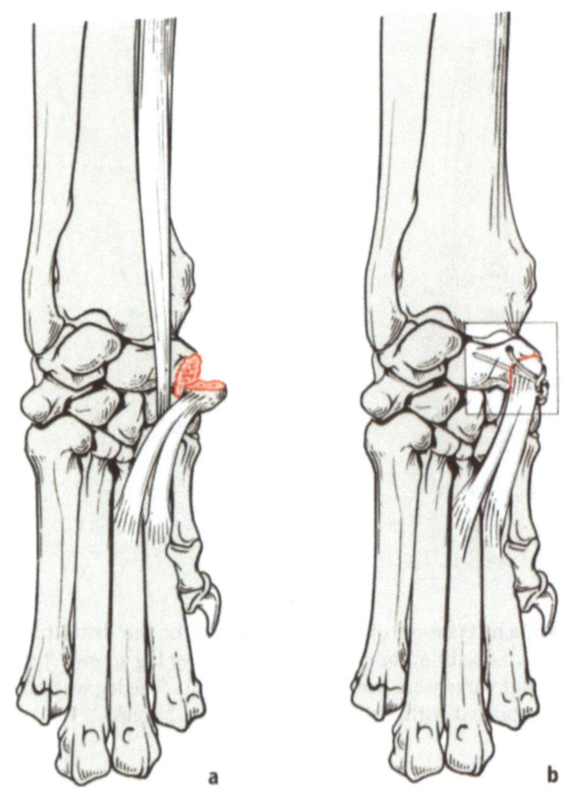

Fig. 4.67. **a** Avulsion fracture of the medial palmar prominence of the radial carpal bone. **b** Fixation with a tension band wire

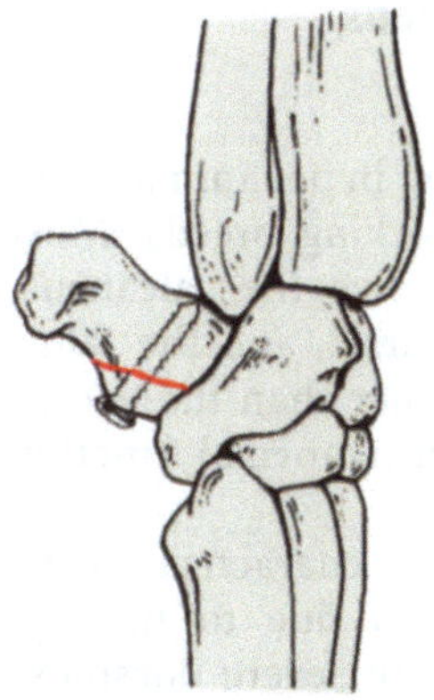

Fig. 4.68. Type 1A fracture of the accessory carpal bone. An intra-articular avulsion fracture of the origin of the accessero-ulvar ligament

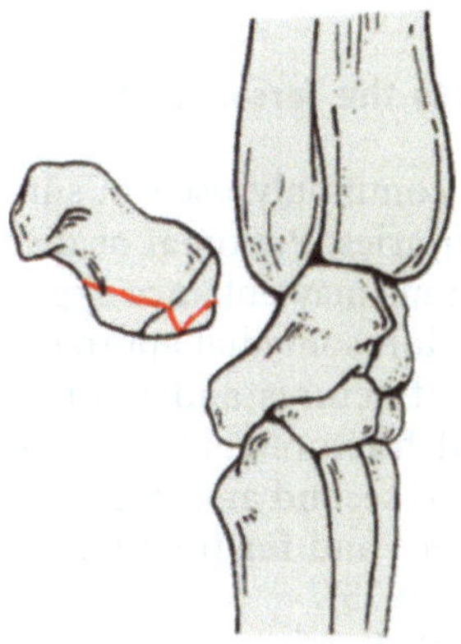

Fig. 4.69. Type 1B fracture of the accessory carpal bone has a medial intra-articular component

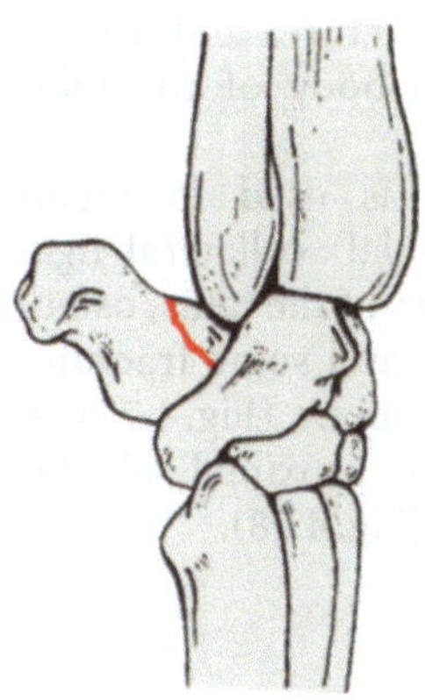

Fig. 4.70. Type II fracture of the accessory carpal bone. An intra-articular fracture of the accessory carpal bone that involves the proximal portion of the base

4.8.1.3 Accessory Carpal Bone

Type IA accessory carpal fractures are intra-articular and should be repaired by either positional or lag screw fixation (Fig. 4.68).

Type IB accessory carpal fractures not only have the classical palmar lateral fragment but also a palmar medial component. These fractures should also be repaired by screw fixation, although the medial component is often small and must be removed (Fig. 4.69). Type II fractures are also intra-articular and must be replaced or removed (Fig. 4.70).

Type III fractures involve an avulsion of the accessory carp-metacarpal ligament and should be repaired by lag screw fixation. The carpus should be supported in flexion postoperatively (Fig. 4.71). Type IV fractures involve the flexor carpi ulnaris. There is either an avulsion of the tendon at its attachment or an avulsion fracture of the tendinous insertion. These are rarely large enough to reattach and are treated by excision of the fragment and

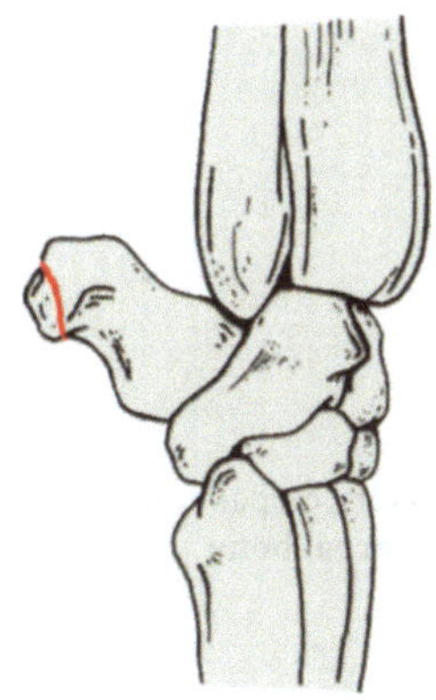

Fig. 4.71. Type III fracture of the accessory carpal bone. An avulsion fracture of the origin of the accessory carpal-metacarpal ligament

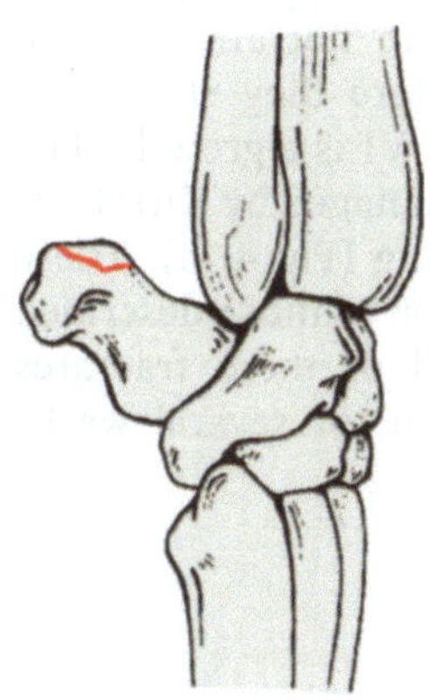

Fig. 4.72. Type IV fracture of the accessory carpal bone. Avulsion of insertion of flexor carpi ulnaris tendon

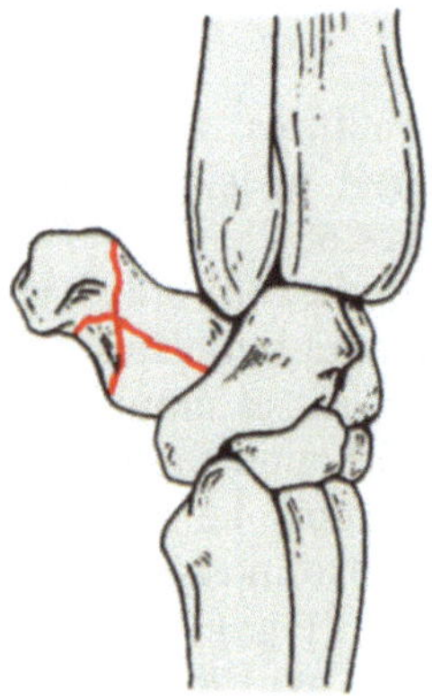

Fig. 4.73. Type V fracture of the accessory carpal bone. A comminuted fracture

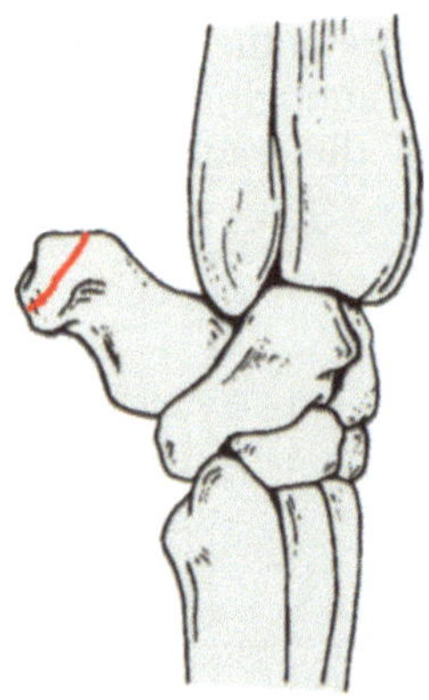

Fig. 4.74. Type VI fracture of the accessory carpal bone. Avulsion of growth plate of the accessory carpal bone

suturing of the tendon (Fig. 4.72). Type V fractures are highly comminuted and are not amenable to surgical reconstruction; therefore they should be cast in flexion (Fig. 4.73). Type VI is a growth plate avulsion and fracture that is managed by Kirschner wire fixation and flexion casting (Fig. 4.74). These classifications are a modification of those described by K. A. Johnson (1988). All of these fractures should be supported in flexion for several weeks following the operation.

4.8.2 Tarsal Fractures, Luxations, and Subluxations

Tarsal fractures are not common in pet animals, but are seen with regularity in working breeds. Most commonly, these fractures involve the calcaneus, the central tarsal, the fourth tarsal, and the talus. Internal fixation is the rule rather than the exception in the dog if a return to near-normal function is to be achieved.

These fractures are usually characterized by being closed, comminuted, and due to indirect trauma. They are associated with severe dorsiflexion, with other tarsal fractures, and with extensive swelling and soft tissue damage. Diagnosis is achieved by palpation, by evaluating the range of motion, and by fine-detail radiographs taken from the anteroposterior, mediolateral, and oblique directions. Additional radiographs may be needed with the joint under load (stress films).

4.8.2.1 Surgical Approaches to the Tarsal Joints

Four primary incisions are commonly used in surgical approaches to tarsal injuries. Proximal or distal extensions of these incisions may enhance exposure in certain instances. A dorosomedial approach is utilized for central tarsal fractures and indirect repair of most fourth tarsal fracture-subluxations. This approach is also used for second and third tarsal fractures and subluxations, and for fractures of the talar head and neck (Fig. 4.75).

A lateral plantar approach is often utilized for calcaneal fractures, lateral malleolar fractures, and for repairs of the lateral collateral ligaments. This approach is occasionally used to stabilize avulsion fractures of the lateral lip of the base of the fifth metatarsal, and to repair tears in the lateral collateral calcaneal insertion of the superficial digital flexor tendon. It is rarely used as partial exposure for repair of some talar neck fractures and for lateral condylar fractures of the body of the talus (Fig. 4.76).

A medial plantar incision is used to repair medial malleolar fractures, (tibial) collateral ligaments, medial condylar fractures of the talus, osteochondrosis lesions of the talus, and some fracture-dislocations of the tibial tarsal bone (Fig. 4.77). A plantar approach is used for proximal plantar tarsal-metatarsal subluxations (Fig. 4.78).

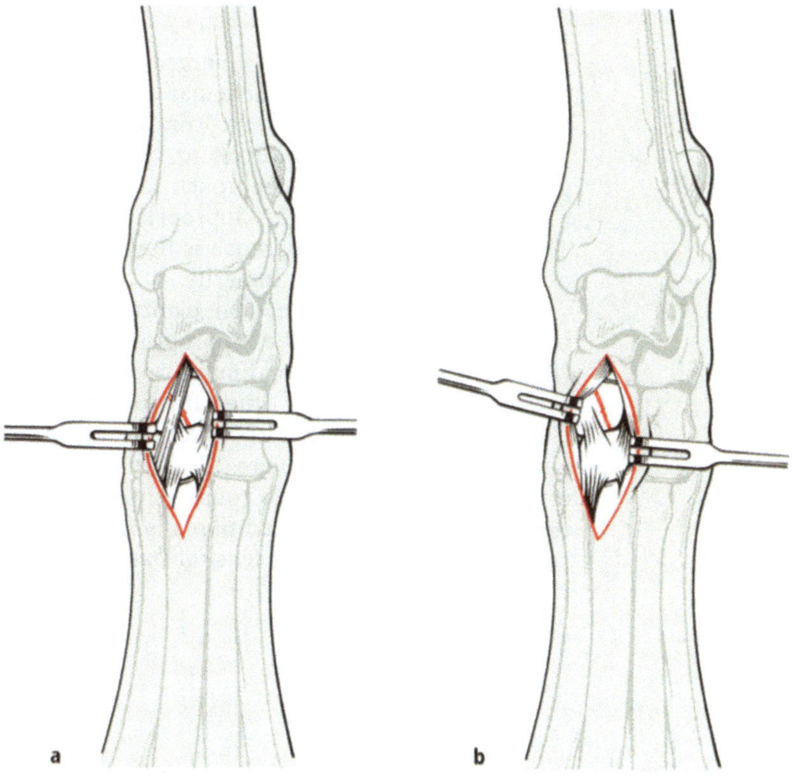

Fig. 4.75a,b. Surgical approaches to the tarsal joints. Dorsomedial approach to the tarsus. **a** Skin incision. Note that the tibialis cranialis tendon obliquely crosses the surgical field. **b** Deep dissection to the ligaments and bone. The tendon is retracted medially

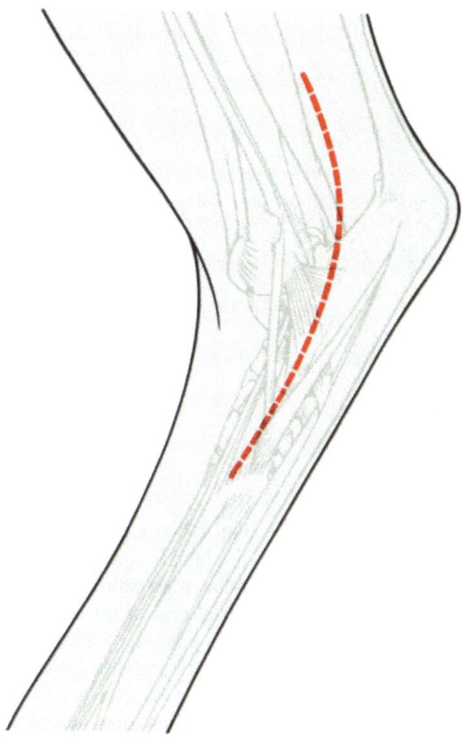

Fig. 4.76. Lateral plantar approach to the tarsus

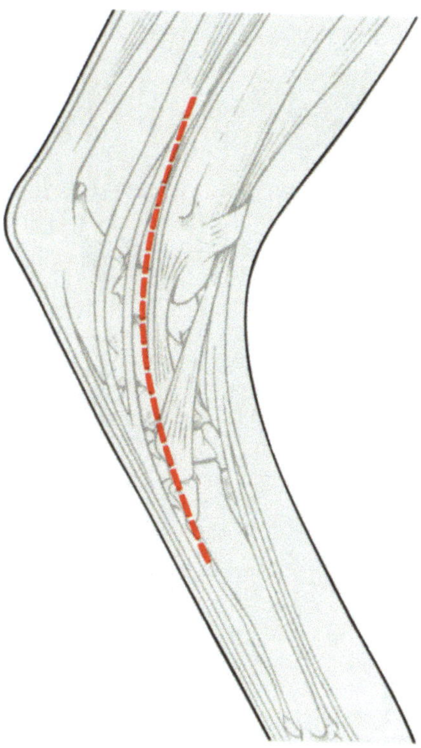

Fig. 4.77. Medial plantar approach to the tarsus

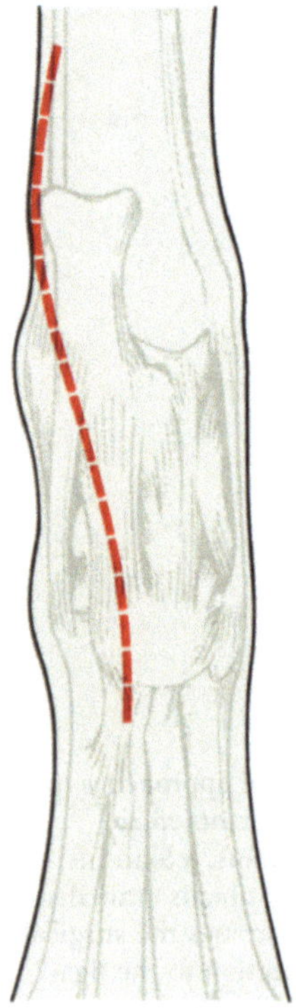

Fig. 4.78. Plantar approach to the tarsus

4.8.2.2 Body of the Talus

The body of the talus is that enlarged proximal portion of the bone with the articular surface termed the trochlea. Fractures of the condyles are quite rare and may be very difficult to visualize radiographically. The surgical approach to the condyles requires osteotomy of the appropriate malleolus. The advantage of this approach is the maintenance of collateral ligamentous integrity.

A lateral plantar or medial plantar incision is utilized to approach the appropriate malleolus (Figs. 4.76, 4.77). The distal fibula and malleolus are osteotomized, exposing the fractured condyle (Fig. 4.79). The fragments are reduced and repaired with multiple Kirschner wires. Since the condyle is articular, it is imperative to countersink the Kirschner wires. The osteotomized fibula is replaced with position screws or by the tension band wire technique (Fig. 4.59b).

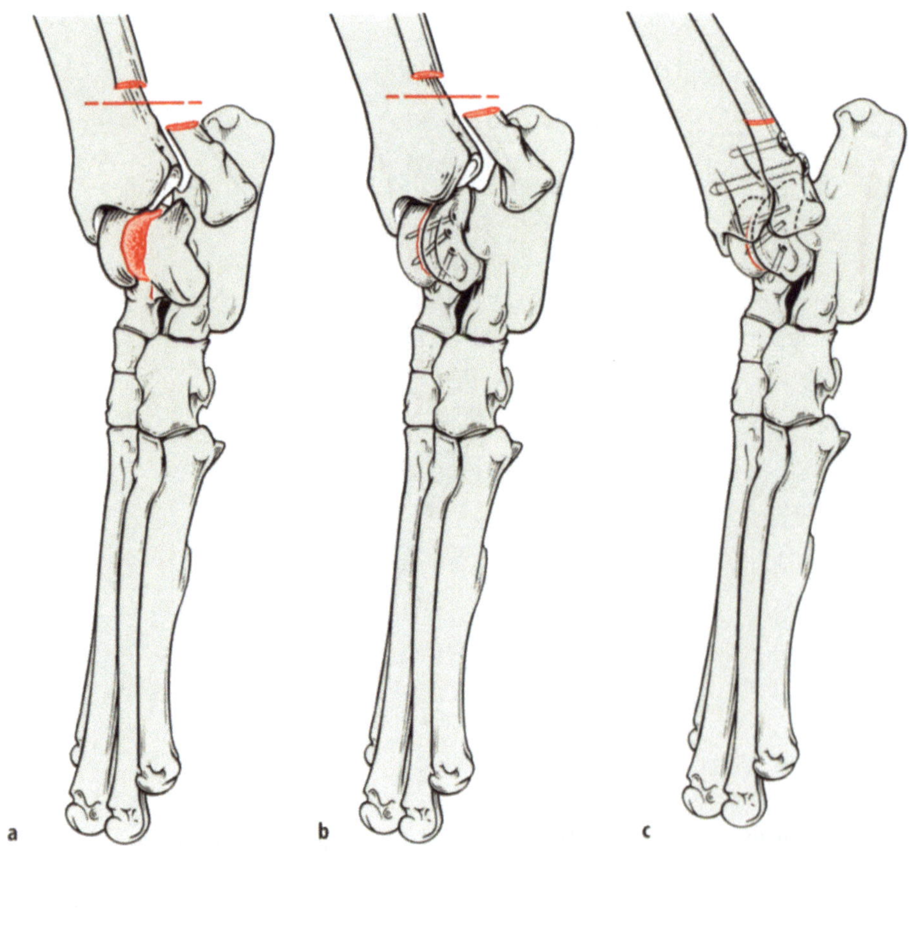

Fig. 4.79a–c. Fracture of the lateral condyle of the talus. **a** Osteotomy of the distal end of the fibula to expose the fractured lateral condyle of the talus. **b** Fixation with three Kirschner wires (countersunk). **c** Repair of the osteotomized distal fibula

4.8.2.3 Neck of the Talus

Fractures of the neck may be managed by one of several methods, depending on fragment size. The area is approached by making an incision on the medial aspect of the tarsus, beginning just dorsal to and above the medial malleolus, curving downward and forward following the normal curvature of the tarsus to end at the dorsomedial side of the distal aspect of the central tarsal bone (Fig. 4.80). The incision is carried through the deeper tissues, splitting the V composed of the tibialis cranialis tendon cranially and the tibial collateral ligament caudally. After reduction, fracture alignment is maintained with self-locking tissue forceps (Vulsellum forceps). On the medial aspect of the neck, distal to the fracture and proximal to the articular surface of the talus, a 4-mm cancellous screw (or lagged cortical screw) is countersunk in an oblique proximal plantar lateral direction into the body of the talus (Fig. 4.81a). Another method involves placement of a screw in the distal fragment in a lateral plantar direction to seat in the base of the calcaneus. This is a positional (noncompression) screw between the two bones (Fig. 4.81b).

Talar neck fractures in small patients, such as cats, may be surgically reduced and stabilized with Kirschner wires, or in some instances simply surgically reduced and coapted.

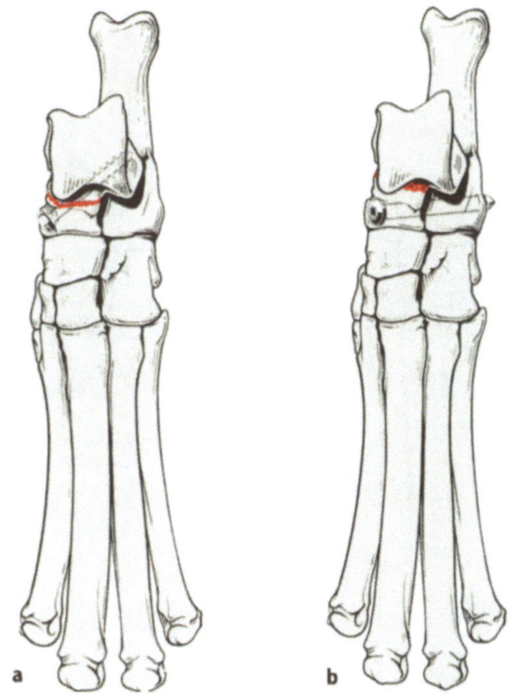

Fig. 4.81 a,b. Fracture of the neck of the talus. **a** Cancellous lag screw obliquely across the fracture line into the body of the talus. **b** Positional screw from the talus into the calcaneus

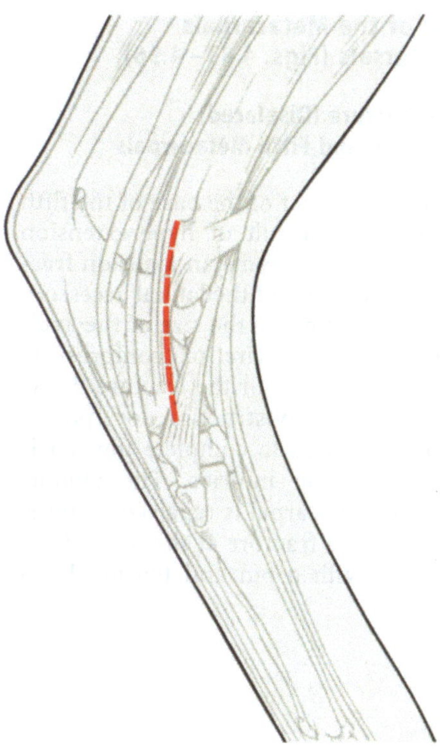

Fig. 4.80. Medial approach to the tarsus

4.8.2.4 Talar Head

Damage to the articular surface of the head of the talus is a frequent finding in central tarsal bone fractures. Occasionally, a dorsal or medial slab fracture of the head of the talus will be found associated with a combination central and fourth tarsal bone fracture (Fig. 4.82a,b)

A dorsomedial approach is utilized as for central tarsal bone fractures, except that the incision will be extended 1–2 cm proximally. Fixation is performed as for a fourth tarsal bone fracture, except that an additional 2.7-mm cortical screw is countersunk and lagged into the dorsal slab fracture of the head of the talus (Fig. 4.82c,d). Fractures of the talar head not amenable to reconstruction and stabilization may be treated by arthrodesis.

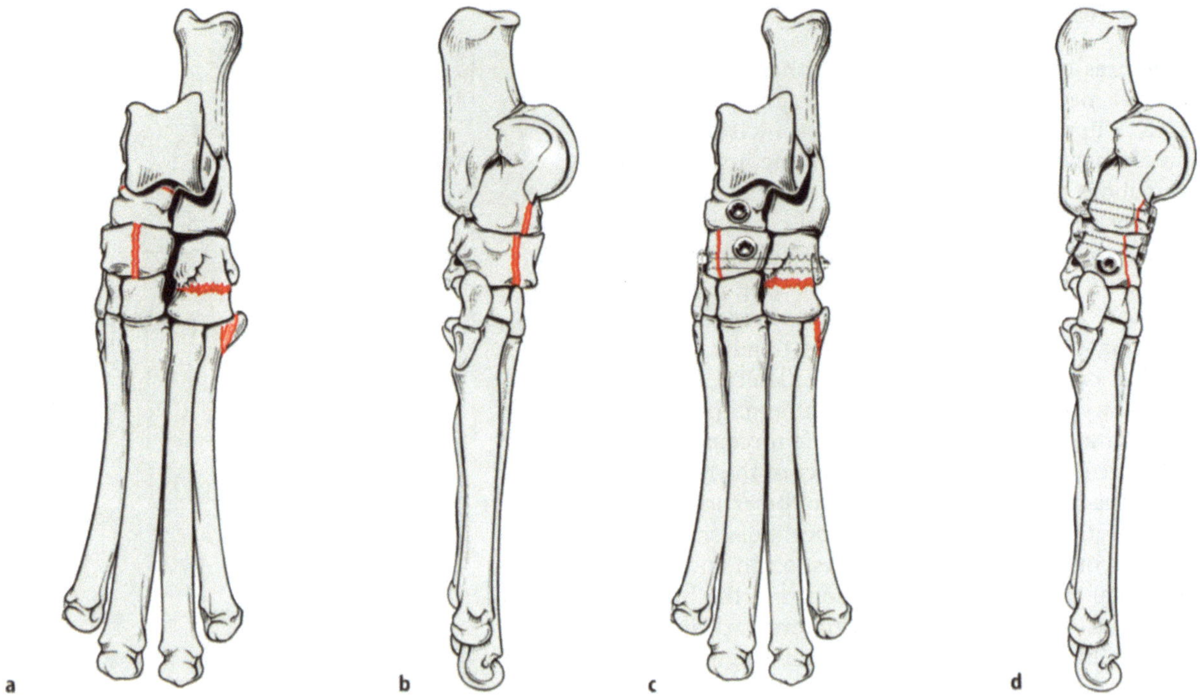

Fig. 4.82a–d. Multiple fractures of the hock. **a** Large medially displaced fragment of the central tarsal bone, compression fracture of the fourth tarsal bone, and an avulsion fracture of the base of the fifth metatarsal. **b** A dorsal slab fracture of the central tarsal bone with displacement and a dorsal slab fracture of the head of the talus with slight displacement. **c, d** Fixation using three lag screws

4.8.2.5 Avulsion Fracture of the Fifth Tarsal (Nondisplaced)

A very small avulsion fracture occurs that is the result of increased tension on the inserting structures and is associated with fracture of the central tarsal bone. Displacement is usually not great and reduction is rarely necessary. Those that are displaced can be managed indirectly by repairing the primary central tarsal fracture, thus relieving the tensile forces of the inserting structures on the base of the fifth metatarsal (Fig. 4.82a).

In selected cases, a figure-of-eight wire may be used for additional support. Because of the small size of the fragment, true tension-wiring with pin fixation is often not feasible.

4.8.3 Fractures of the Metacarpals and Metatarsals (Figs. 4.83–4.96)

4.8.3.1 Avulsion Fracture (Displaced) of the Second and Fifth Metacarpals

Fracture of the lateral aspect of the base of the fifth metacarpal occurs as a result of hyperextension injury to the carpus. It represents an avulsion fracture of the distal attachment of the lateral accessory carpal ligament. Depending on the size of the avulsion, either tension band wire or compression screw fixation is satisfactory for the fracture. However, other ligament reconstruction or panarthrodesis may be indicated to complete the repair for carpal hyperextension injuries. The oblique fracture of the fifth metacarpal is repaired by three lag screws. The avulsion fracture at the base of the second is stabilized with a pin and tension band wire.

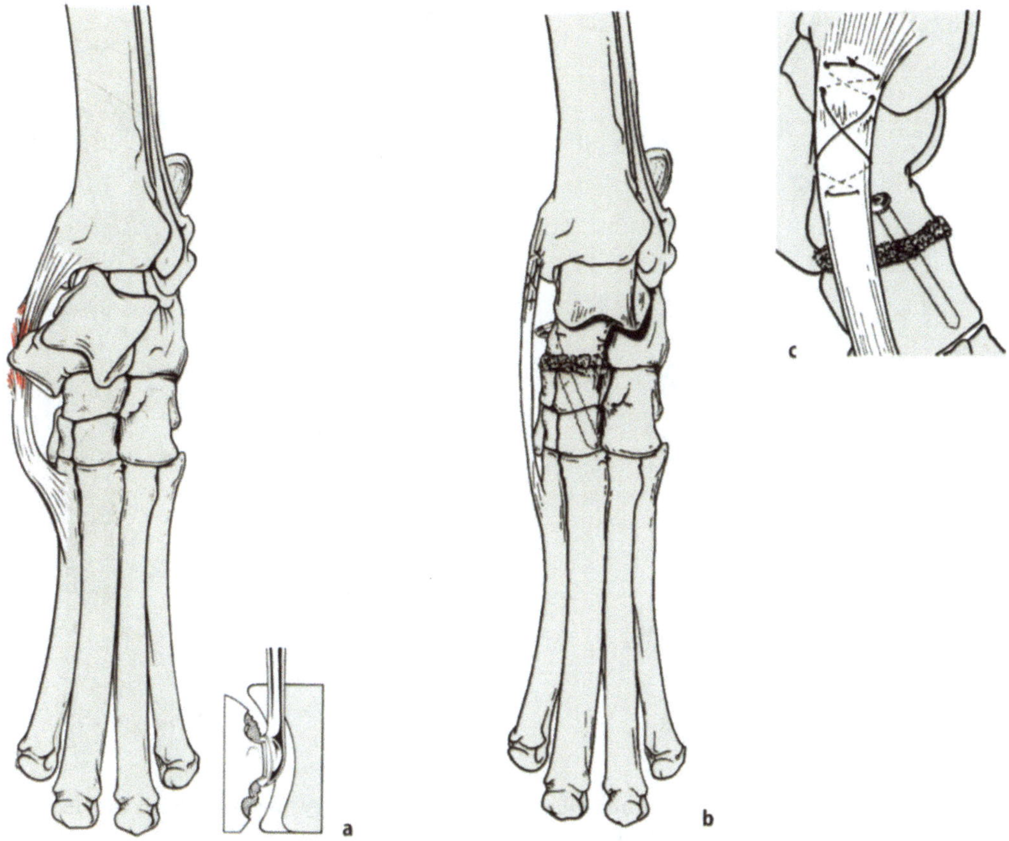

Fig. 4.83a–c. Peritalar dislocation. **a** Peritalar dislocation with rupture of the medial collateral ligament. **b** Anteroposterior view showing screw. **c** Mediolateral view of the talocentral arthrodesis and collateral ligament repair

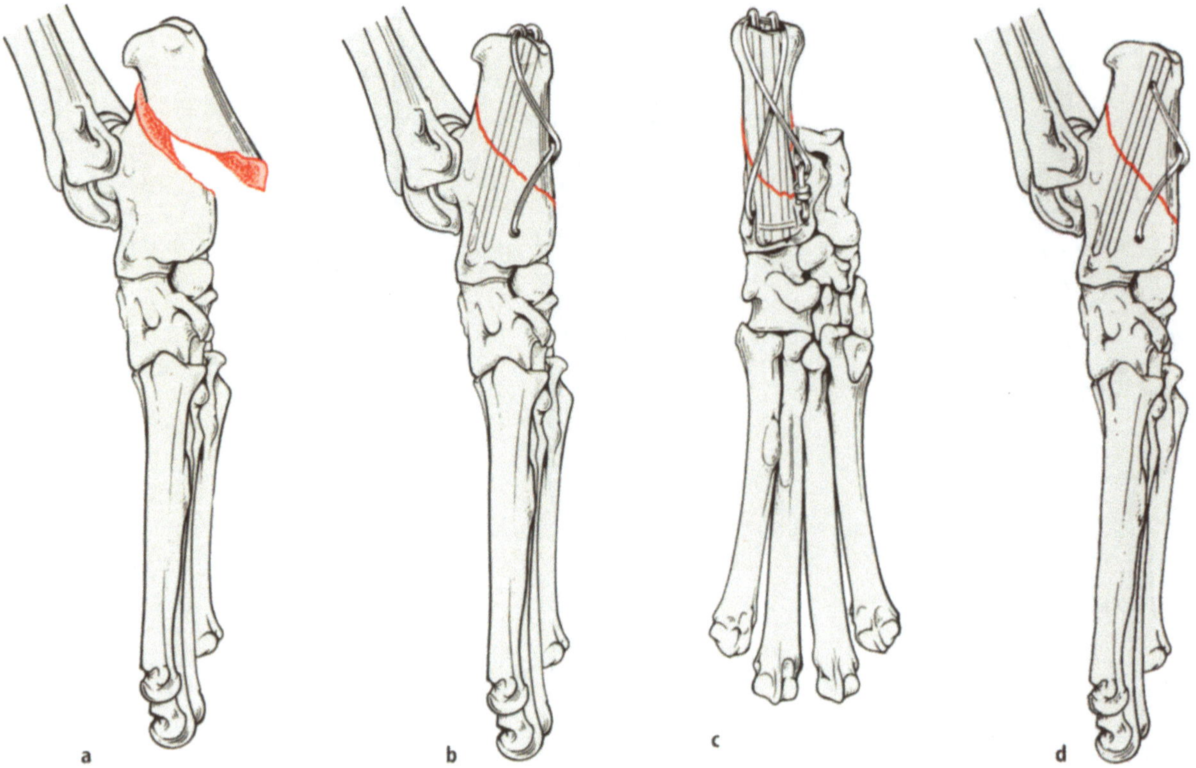

Fig. 4.84a–d. Fracture of the calcaneus. **a** Simple shaft fracture of the calcaneus. **b** Lateral view of tension band wire fixation. **c** Plantar view of the repair. **d** Lateral view with countersunk pins

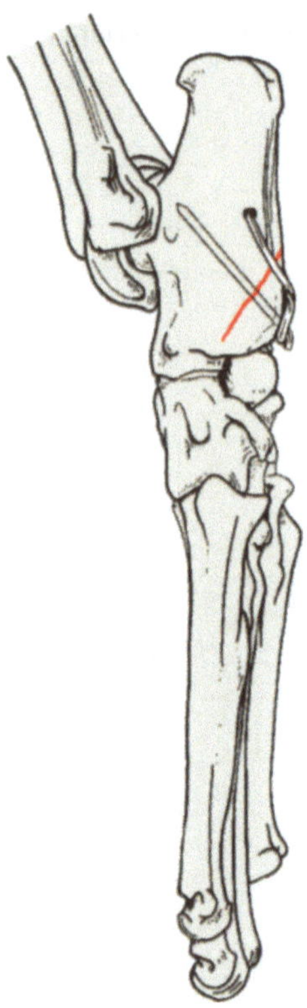

Fig. 4.85. Fracture of base of calcaneus. Lateropalmar view of tension band wire fixation of fractured base

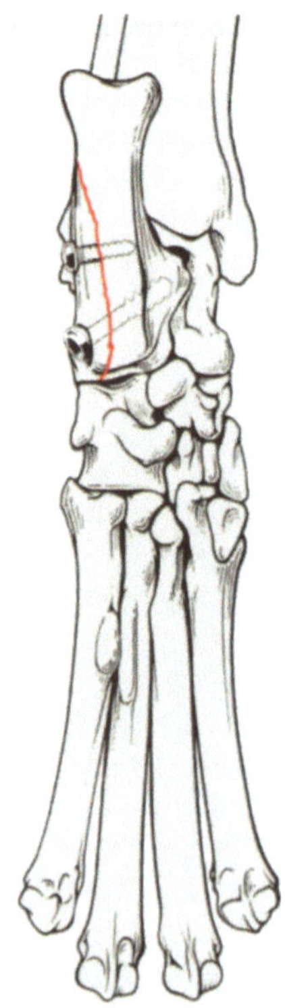

Fig. 4.86. Axial slab fracture of the lateral surface of the calcaneus fixed with two lag screws

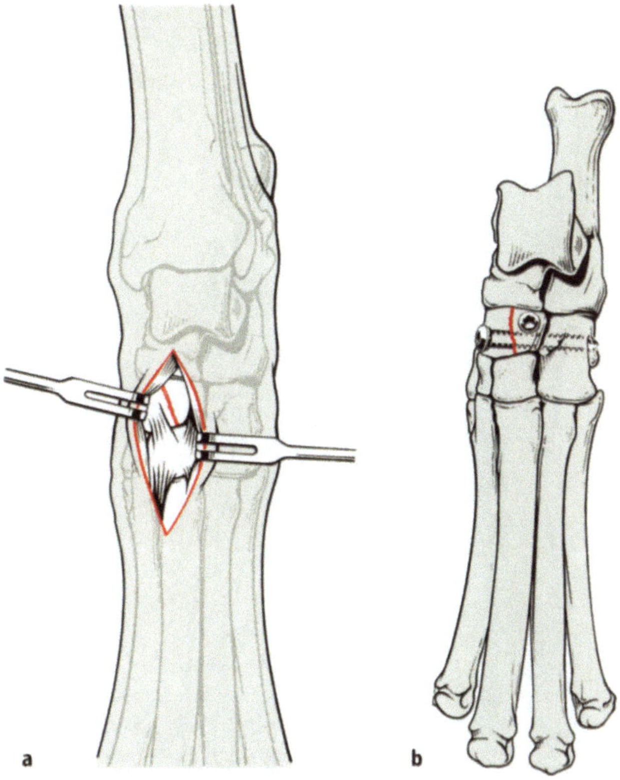

Fig. 4.87a,b. Central tarsal bone fracture. **a** Dorsal exposure. **b** Fixation with two cortical lag screws

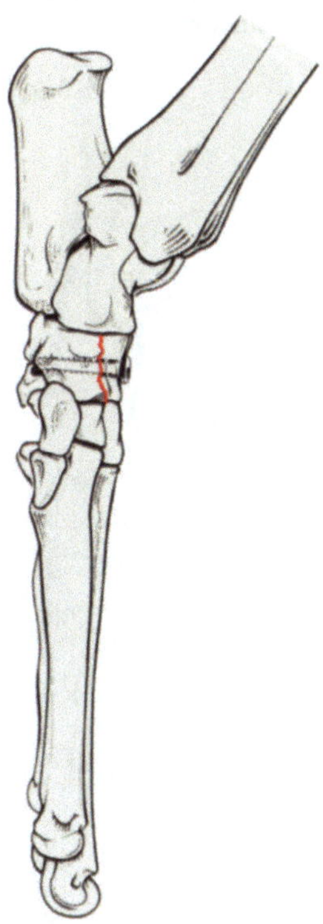

Fig. 4.88. Dorsal slab fracture of the central tarsal bone fixed with a lag screw

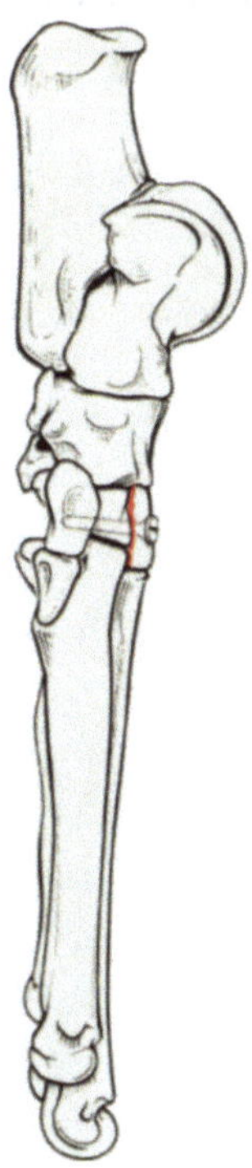

Fig. 4.89. Repair of a dorsal slab fracture of the third tarsal bone

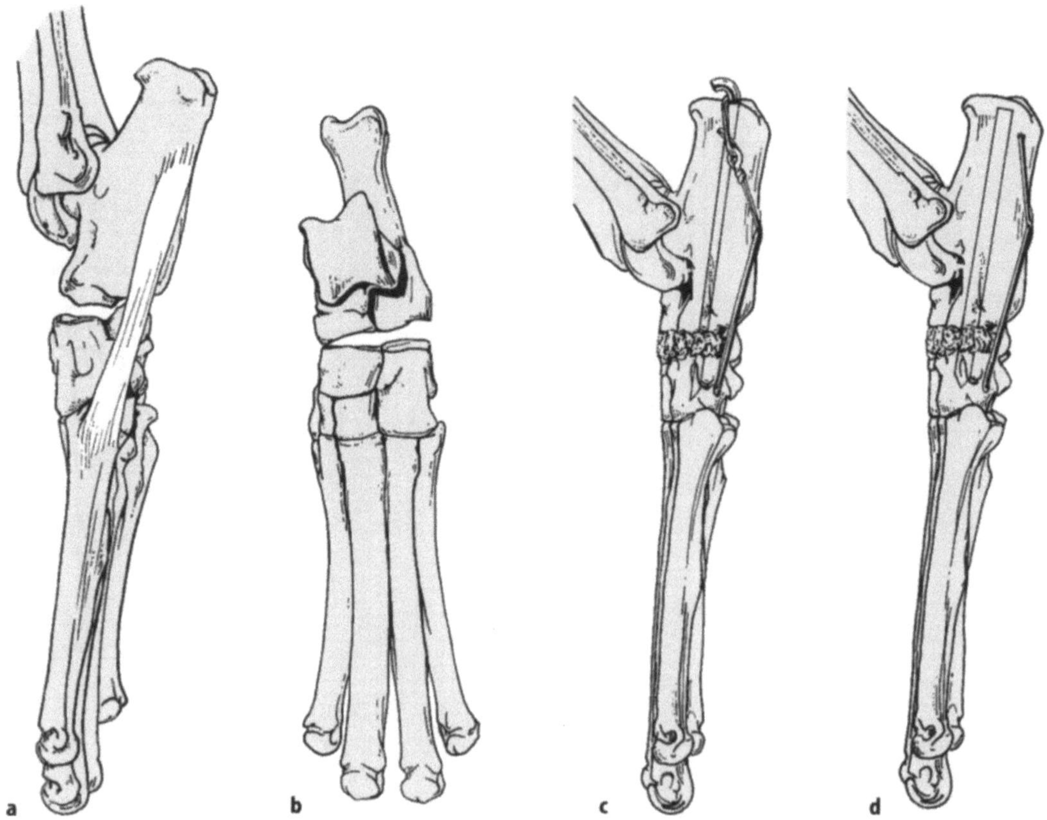

Fig. 4.90. **a** Plantar proximal intertarsal subluxation. **b** Lateral plantar stressed view. **c** Lateral views of the calcaneoquartal joint arthrodesis maintained with a single Steinmann pin and tension band wire. **d** Lateral view with countersunk pin

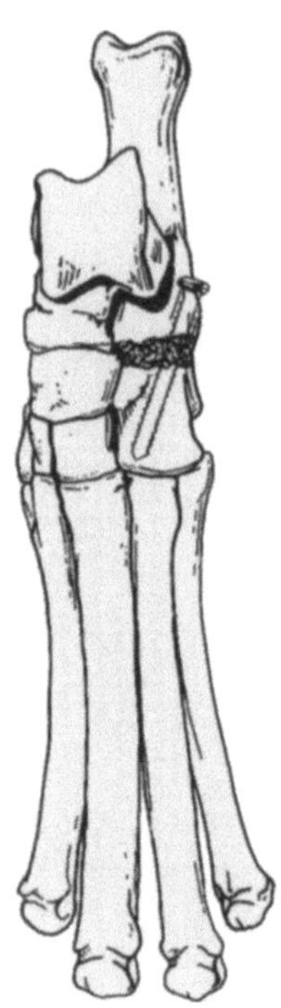

Fig. 4.91. Dorsal view of the calcaneoquartal joint arthrodesis maintained with a single lagged cortical screw

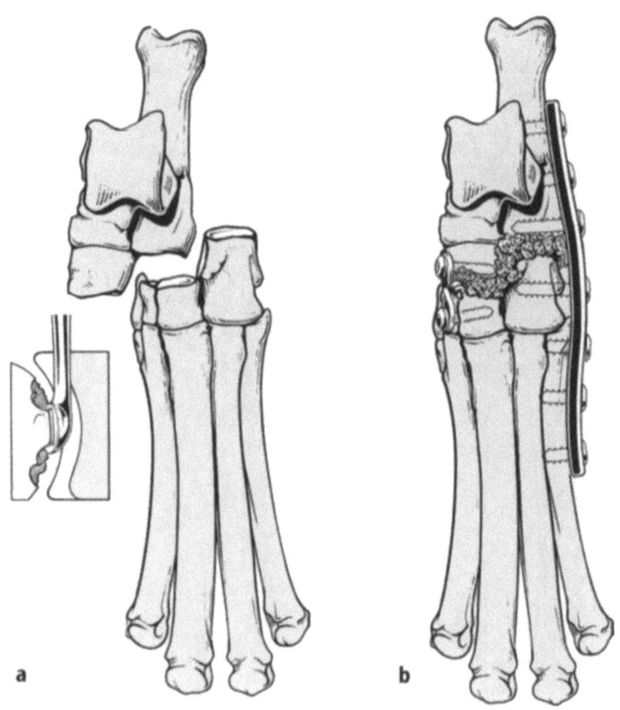

Fig. 4.92a,b. Luxation of the intertarsal joints. **a** Lateral luxation. **b** Arthrodesis of the intertarsal joints maintained with a plate, screws, and figure-of-eight wire

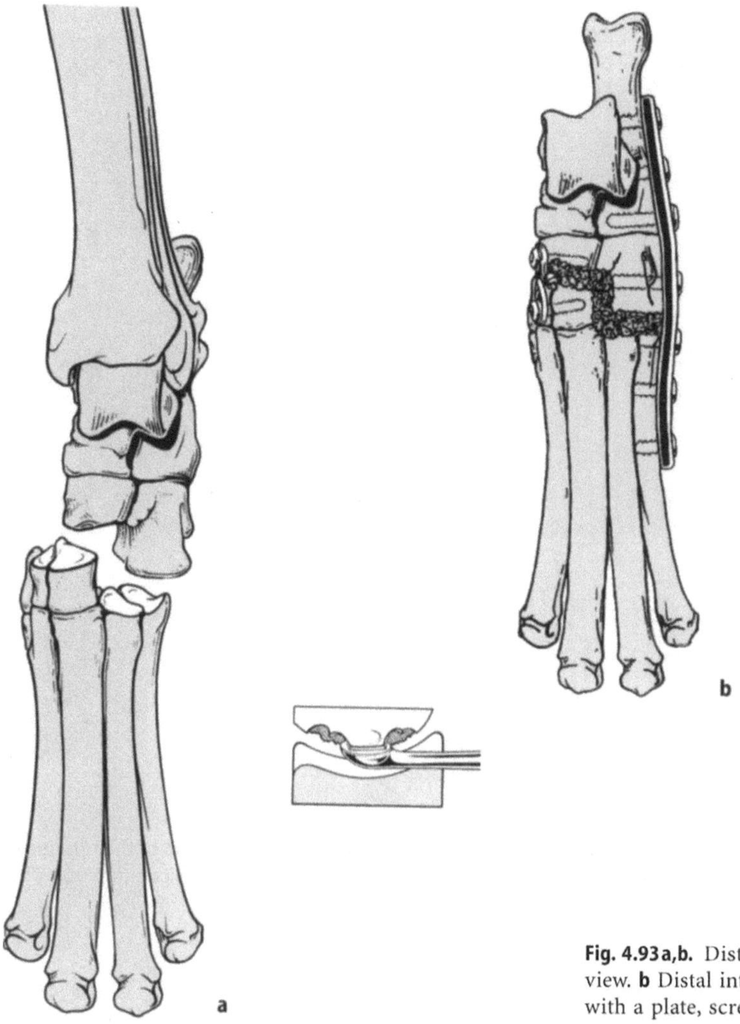

Fig. 4.93a,b. Distal intertarsal-tarsometatsrsal luxation. **a** Dorsal view. **b** Distal intertarsal-tarsometatsrsal arthrodesis stabilized with a plate, screws and figure-of-eight wire

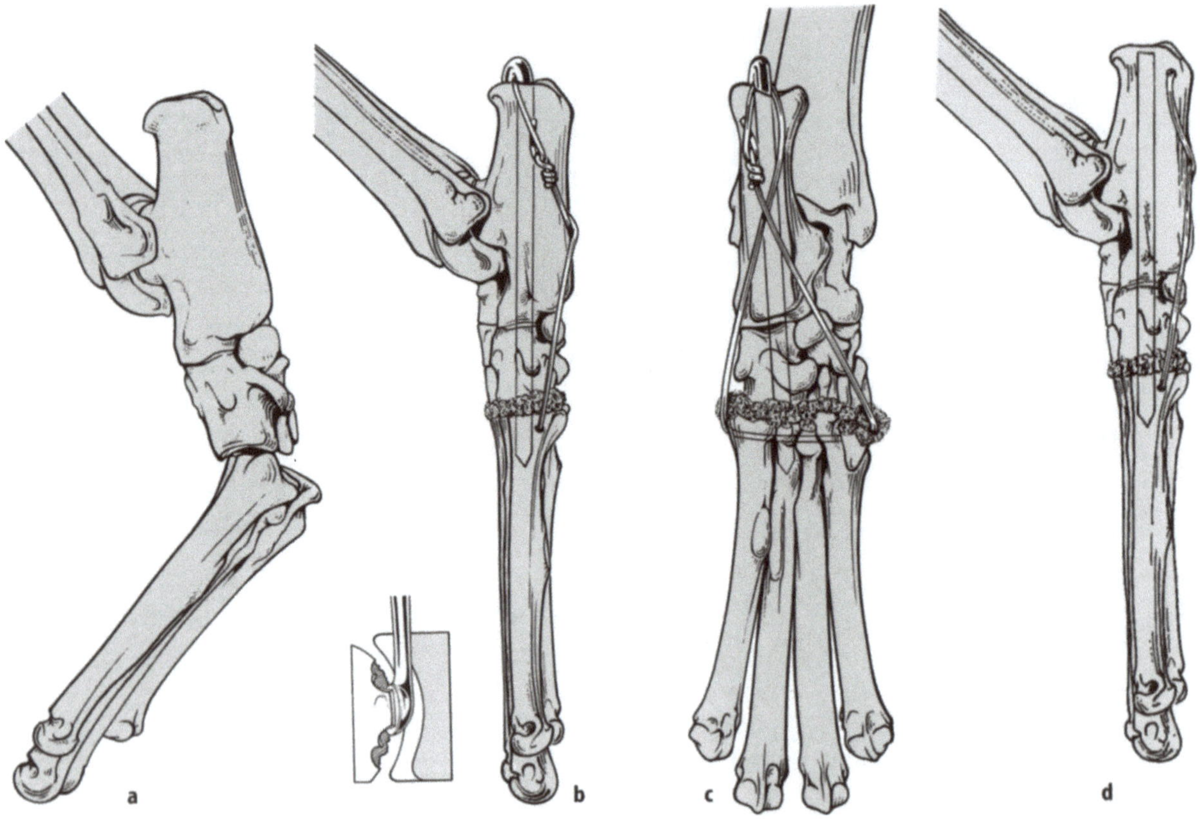

Fig. 4.94a–d. Plantar tarsometatarsal subluxation. **a** Lateral plantar stressed view. **b, c** Lateral and plantar views of the tarsometatarsal joint arthrodesis maintained with a single Steinmann pin and tension band wire. **d** Arthrodesis with countersunk pin fixation

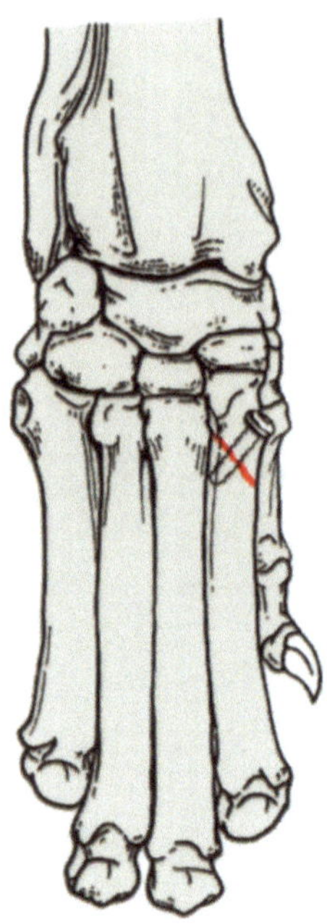

Fig. 4.95. Stress fracture of right metacarpal two repaired with a lag screw

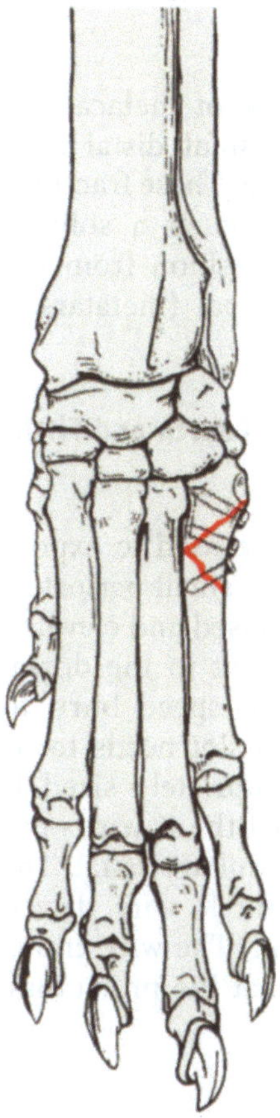

Fig. 4.96. Stress fracture of left metacarpal five repaired with lag screws

4.8.3.2 Avulsion at the Base of the First Metacarpal and Subluxation of the Second Carpal

Avulsion of the base of the first metacarpal and second carpal bone subluxation is an example of hyperextension injury primarily involving bones on the medial aspect of the carpus. The base of the first metacarpal is immobilized by using a positional screw to seat it in the base of the second metacarpal. The fracture in the non-weight-bearing first metacarpal will heal uneventfully. The second carpal is reduced and fixed in position with a positional screw anchored in the third and fourth carpals (Fig. 4.97).

4.8.3.3 Oblique Fractures of the Metacarpals and Metatarsals

Some oblique fractures may be anatomically reduced and stabilized utilizing the lag screw principle in conjunction with coaptation to provide additional support until healing has progressed sufficiently. Two smaller lag screws are preferred to one larger screw (Fig. 4.98a).

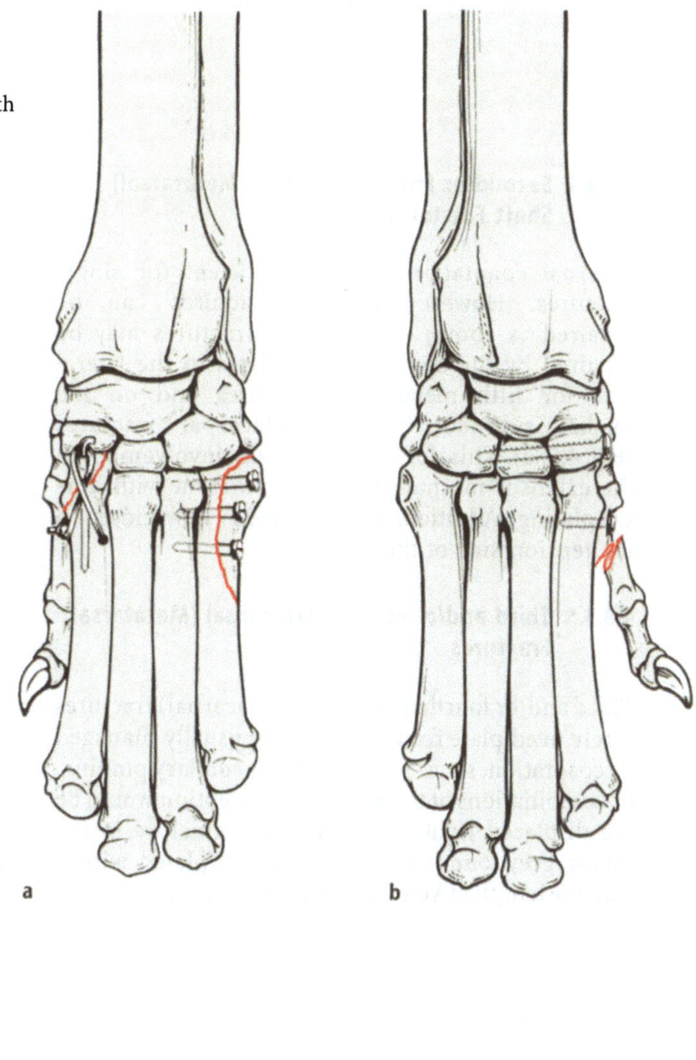

Fig. 4.97. **a** Avulsion fractures of the basis of fifth and second metacarpals repaired with three lag screws and tension band wire technique, respectively (left paw). **b** Avulsion fracture of the base of the first metacarpal and second carpal subluxation repaired with positional screws (right paw). The fracture of MCI is in a non-weight-bearing digit and will heal without fixation

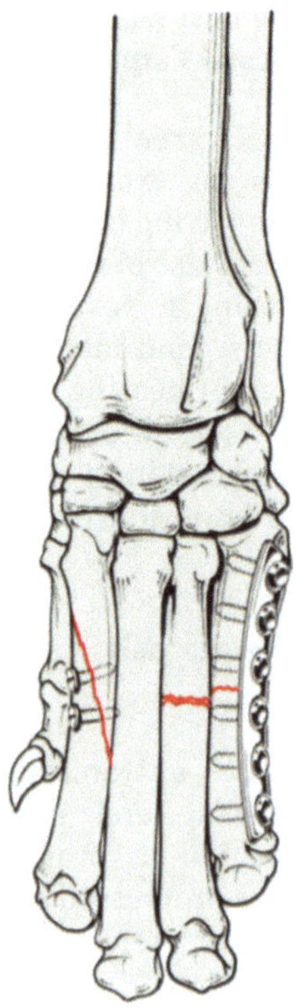

Fig. 4.98. Transverse fractures of fifth and fourth metacarpals (vassal), and oblique fracture of second metacarpal repaired with a plate and lag screws, respectively (left paw)

4.8.3.4 Second or Fifth Metacarpal (Metatarsal) Shaft Fractures

External coaptation is often sufficient for single fractures. However, oblique fractures can be repaired as above, or transverse fractures may be repaired by the application of plates to the lateral side for fifth metacarpal fractures and on the medial side for second metacarpal fractures (Fig. 4.98a). This does away with any involvement to the extensor mechanism that is inherent with dorsal plating. Additionally, the plate is now closer to the tension side of the bone.

4.8.3.5 Third and/or Fourth Metacarpal (Metatarsal) Fractures

Third and/or fourth metatarsal (metacarpal) fractures rarely need plate fixation. They are usually managed by coaptation, screw fixation, intramedullary pinning, or combinations of the above. The exception would be the displaced right metatarsal three fracture in the racing greyhound which is routinely plated with a suitable length of Veterinary Cuttable Plate.

4.8.3.6 Second or Fifth Metacarpal (Metatarsal) Neck Fractures

Fractures in the area of the neck of metacarpals (metatarsals) two or five involve a small distal piece of bone and are inherently unstable. These fractures are best managed by the insertion of a solitary Kirschner wire in a "Rush pin" fashion from the medial or lateral side of metacarpal (metatarsal) two or five, respectively (Fig. 4.99).

4.8.3.7 Fractures of Second, Third, Fourth and Fifth Metacarpals (Metatarsals)

A crescent-shaped incision may be used to expose the fracture area. With the aid of a small periosteal elevator the distal fragment is exposed and elevated into the incision. A slot is then cut in the dorsal aspect of the bone, using a high speed burr, to expose the medullary canal. This slot needs to be wide enough to accept an appropriately sized K wire and also long enough so that the K wire once introduced will remain in the medullary canal. The fracture is now reduced and the K wire driven firmly into the proximal fragment. The wire end is bent dorsally and cut short so that the protruding

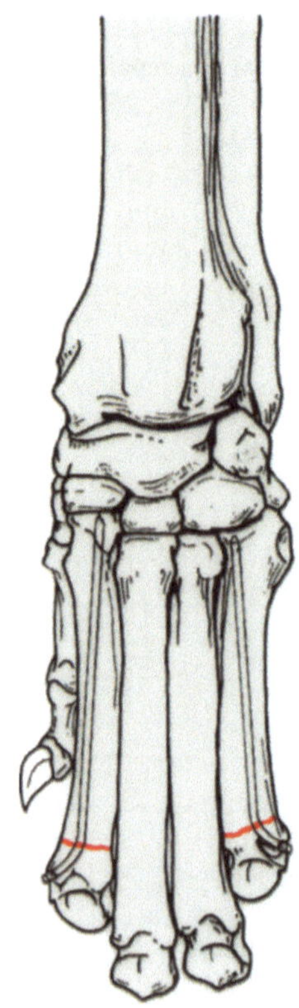

Fig. 4.99. Metacarpal neck fractures managed with Kirschner wires

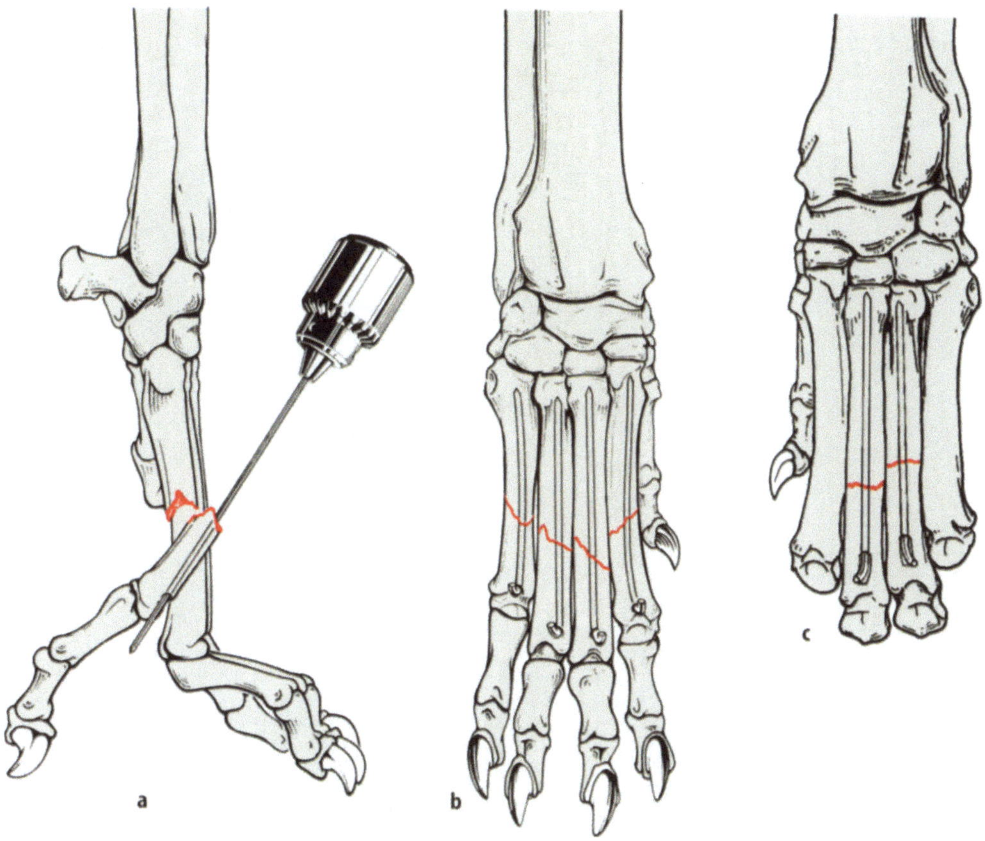

Fig. 4.100. **a** Metacarpal fractures repaired by "slotting" technique. **b** Multiple displaced (metacarpal) metatarsal fractures repaired with Kirschner wires (right forepaw). **c** If there is only minimal displacement of the fractured bones, pinning of the central metacarpal is usually sufficient (left forepaw)

end does not irritate the soft tissues. This procedure is repeated in at least the third and fourth metacarpals and, if necessary, in all four. The foot should be supported in the immediate postoperative period (Fig. 4.100a).

An alternative method of repair is the insertion of pins from the fracture site distally. With the toes flexed, a Kirschner wire of the appropriate diameter is inserted dorsally from proximal to distal through the distal fragment, emerging through the dorsal surface of the metacarpal phalangeal joint (Fig. 4.100b). The fracture is reduced and the wire is seated in the base of the proximal fragment. The protruding wires are not bent in a dorsal and proximal direction before being cut just beneath the skin. A coaptation splint is then applied for approximately 6 weeks (Fig. 4.100c).

4.8.3.8 Fractures of Fourth and Fifth or Second and Third Metacarpals (Metatarsals)

The fracture of the fifth metacarpal is reduced and fixed with a neutralization plate applied to the lateral surface. This affords sufficient support for the fourth metacarpal. The foot is then coapted for approximately 1 month. This illustrates the "vassal rule" (Fig. 4.98a).

4.8.3.9 Phalangeal Fractures

Oblique fractures of the first and second phalanges that are unstable and tend to override may be repaired by lag screw fixation (Fig. 4.101a). Although two small screws are preferable to one larger screw, this is sometimes difficult to achieve, especially in the small patient. The lower limb is coapted postoperatively. Unstable transverse fractures of the first phalanx may sometimes be managed by the application of a small plate (Fig. 4.101b,c). Ideally, a minimum of three cortices on each side of the fracture should be fixed with the plate screws.

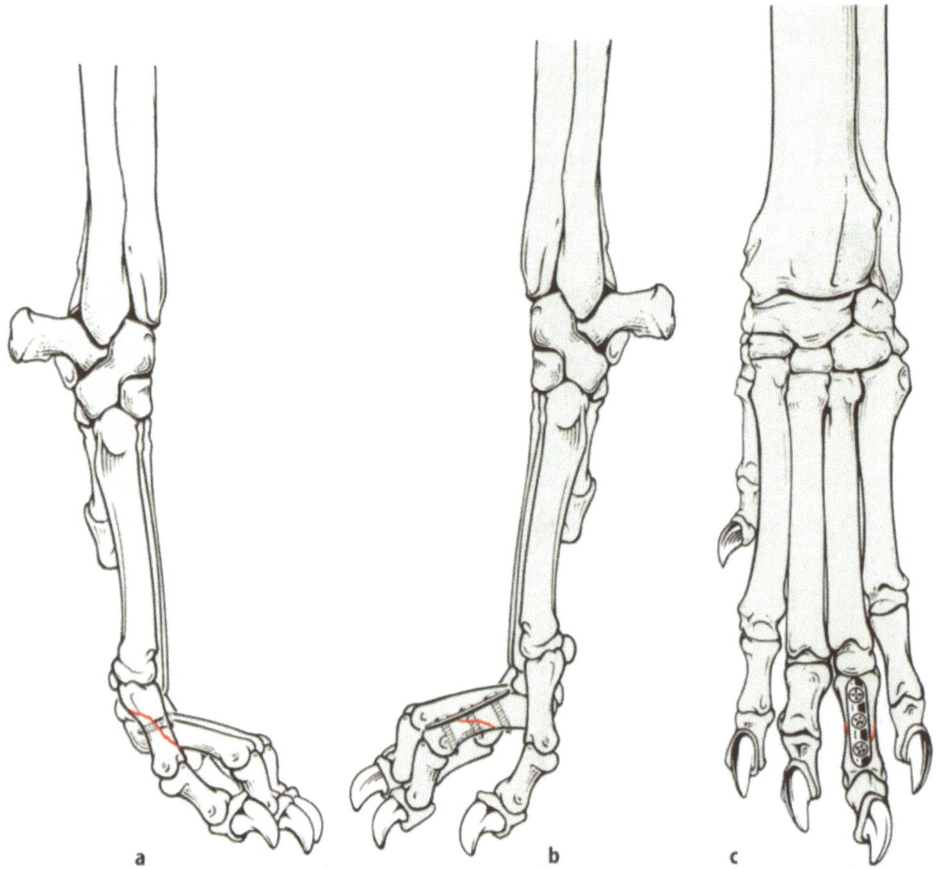

Fig. 4.101. a Fracture of the first phalanx repaired with a lag screw (preferably two screws) (right forepaw). **b, c** Lateral and anteroposterior views of a first phalanx fracture repaired with a plate (left forepaw)

4.8.2.10 Sesamoids

A hyperextension injury resulting in fractures usually involves the second and/or seventh sesamoids. Treatment may be conservative or surgical. Conservative therapy involved the use of support dressings and nonsteroidal anti-inflammatory agents. Surgical therapy consists of surgical excision of either the damaged portion of the offending sesamoid, the whole sesamoid, or both sesamoids on the affected digit.

4.9 Fractures of the Head

4.9.1 Fractures of the Mandible

A vertical fracture of the mandible body will rupture the mandibular canal with the encased mandibular vessels and nerve. The anatomy of the relevant vessels and nerve of the mandible is illustrated in Fig. 4.102.

Most unilateral fractures of the mandible are reducible. They may be treated nonsurgically or stabilized by use of stainless steel wire placed around the base of adjoining teeth (Fig. 4.103). Severely displaced bilateral and multiple fractures should be reduced and stabilized with rigid internal fixation. Following reduction, the vessels recannulize. In affixing screws through the bone, care should be taken to avoid further damage to the canal and its contents, although this may sometimes be unavoidable.

Attainment of satisfactory dental occlusion is of paramount consideration in reduction and stabilization of mandibular fractures. This is best accomplished with the jaws closed and the teeth in normal occlusion during surgery. The airway may be maintained by means of a tracheal tube through a pharyngostomy opening. In describing these fractures, it is assumed that appropriate stabilization of fractures of the opposite mandible or maxilla will also be accomplished.

Fractures of the body are subject to the forces of the muscles of mastication. In humans, the tension

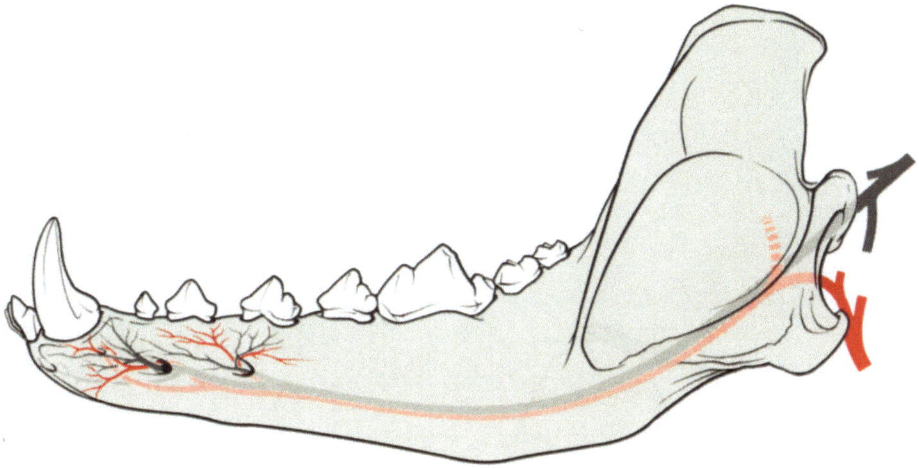

Fig. 4.102. Mandibular vessels and nerves

side of the mandible is the alveolar border, and a plate cannot be placed on that surface. If the plate is fixed on the lower border of the mandible, where the pressure zone lies, it will not be able to neutralize the forces of distraction of the opposite side, neither can these be transformed into forces of pressure. The situation is demonstrated in Fig. 4.104. There is no mechanical evidence that this is the case in animals.

4.9.1.1 Fracture of the Symphysis

Fracture of the mandibular symphysis is a common fracture which precludes normal occlusion and mastication. Fixation may be accomplished by using wires, pins, or screws (Fig. 4.105).

4.9.1.2 Fractures of the Body

Single fractures of the body of the mandible may be stabilized by means of a plate affixed to the ventral border of the bone and by wire fixation around the teeth (Fig. 4.106). The surgical approach and the decision as to the technique to be used will be influenced by the position of the dental roots involved in the site.

The approach to fractures of the body of the mandible may be made through the skin of the ventral aspect of the mandible or intraorally. Incisions made through the skin usually heal well, and sutures are less likely to pull through. Nevertheless, the mucosa within the mouth is noted for its rapid healing.

A ventral approach permits anatomic alignment, and the incision may be continued caudally without the limitations imposed on an intraoral incision by the lip commissures. The incision is made from the level of the canine tooth caudally, as far as necessary for adequate exposure of the fracture site. It should preferably be made slightly lateral to the midline. The subcutaneous tissue and the thin platysma muscle are incised and reflected from the bone exposing the mandible itself. The mental foramina should be identified and the emerging vessels and nerves protected.

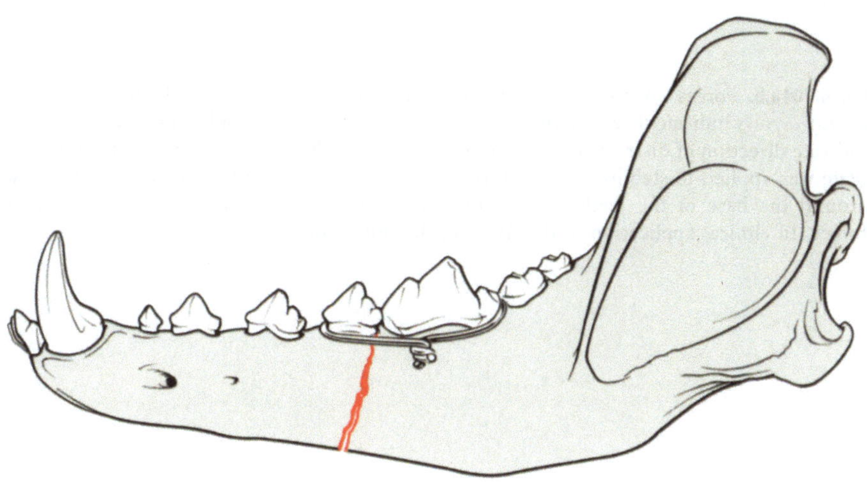

Fig. 4.103. Simple unilateral fracture stabilized with a stainless steel wire around the base of adjoining teeth

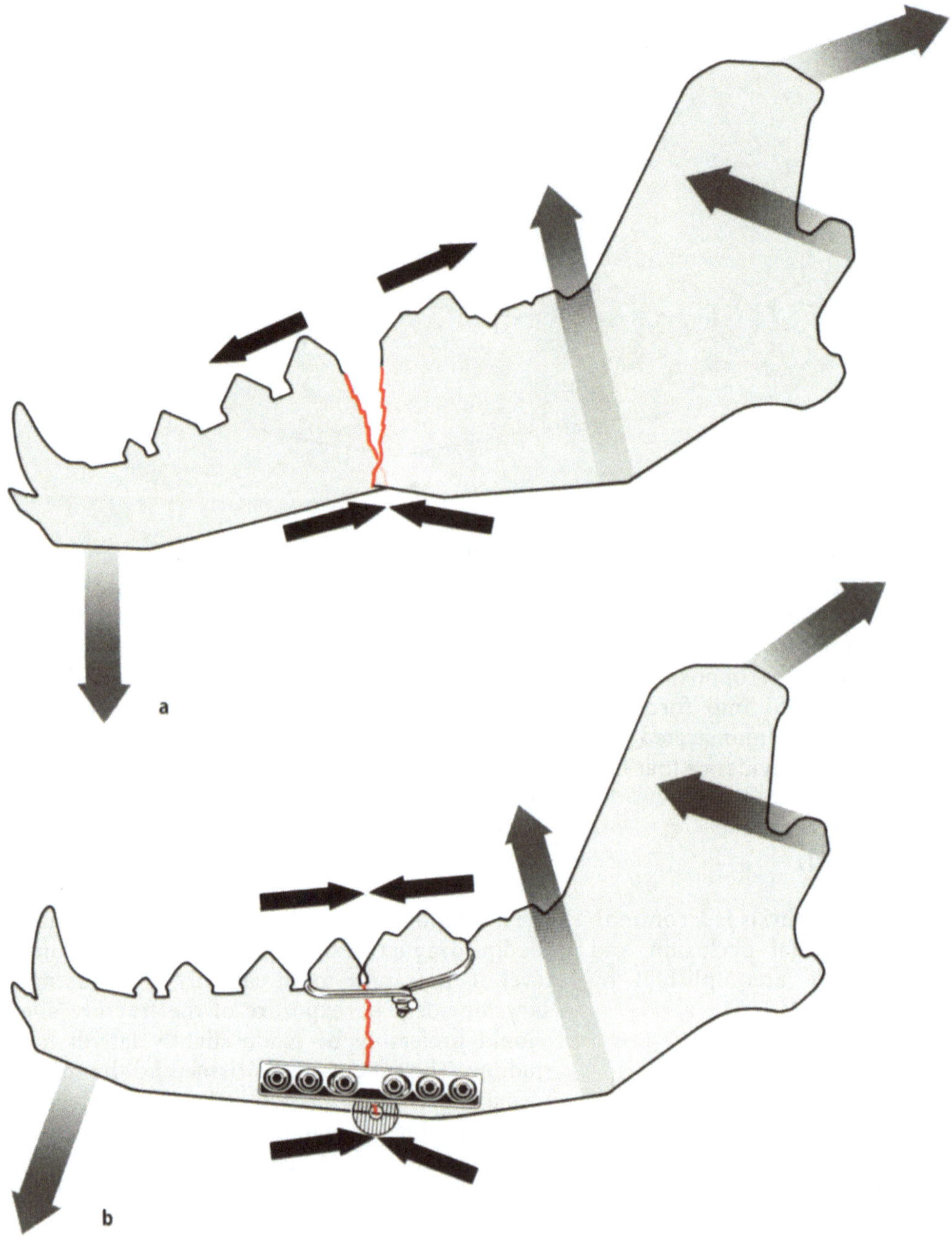

a

b

Fig. 4.104a,b. Forces working on the mandible after fracture. **a** *Gray arrows* indicate direction of muscle pull. *Black arrows* indicate direction of distraction and compression forces. **b** A plate was applied to stabilize the fracture and a wire placed around the base of the teeth to neutralize the distracting forces. In clinical application of the fixation, the holes adjacent to the fracture site are filled first, the second hold being loaded in compression. After the wound is closed, a wire is placed around the base of the adjacent teeth to support the tension surface. For smaller bones, a 2.7-mm dynamic compression plate (DCP) is used

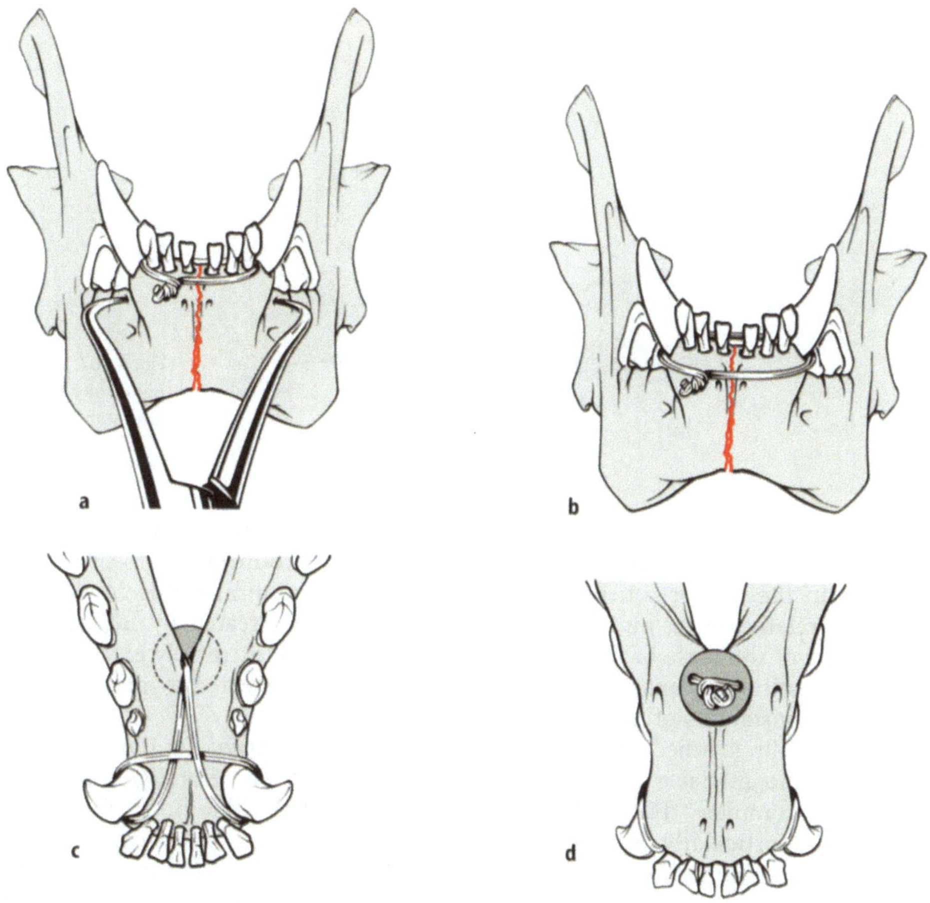

Fig. 4.105a–d. Fracture-separation of the mandibular symphysis. **a** The fracture-separation is reduced and held in place with small reduction forceps. A wire is placed around the base of the incisor teeth for stabilization. **b** In some cases, a wire may be placed around the base of the canine teeth for stabilization. **c,d** Stabilization by placing a wire around the base of the canine teeth and down between the two parts of the mandible, securing it ventrally through a button

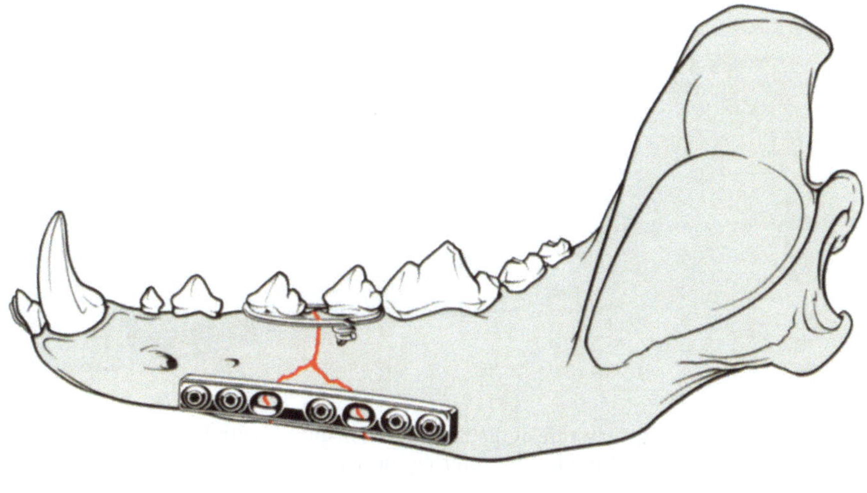

Fig. 4.106. A butterfly fragment fracture following reduction and temporary immobilization with two Kirschner wires. A seven-hole dynamic compression plate (DCP) is contoured and applied. It is necessary to reduce one fragment at a time and to compress as in a segmental fracture

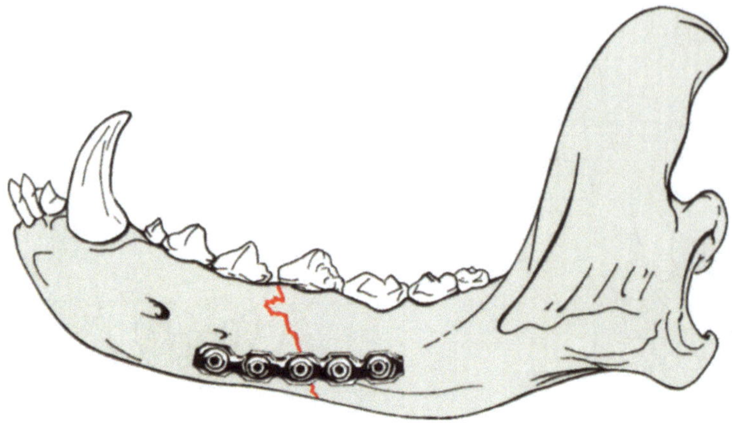

Fig. 4.107. As an alternative, a reconstruction plate may be molded to the mandible body and stabilized with appropriate screws

In humans, teeth are sometimes removed prior to fixation; if at all possible, this is not recommended in the dog or cat, as the roots are much longer in relative terms and occupy a considerable proportion of the mass of the bone. Their removal may well institute collapse of the large alveoli, with consequent instability of the fixation. Sufficient stability is usually attained with a ventral plate, provided that the animal is only given soft food until healing is complete (Figs. 4.106–4.108). In some cases, it is particularly important to withhold all forms of chewable food until radiographic healing is advanced.

There can be no doubt that the use of screws can severely compromise the roots of teeth. It has been shown that such damage can lead to caries, which produces pain. Careful placement of the screws minimizes this complication. Simple fractures may be treated by interdental wiring. Fractures which are extremely extensive and highly fragmented may be treated by plating. (Figs. 4.106–4.108).

External Fixator. Although an external fixator may be successfully employed for some fractures of the mandible body, there is the disadvantage that the patient may catch the frame on a surrounding object, resulting in pain and loosening of the device. However, the method has much to recommend it, provided that great care is taken in placing the pins (Fig. 4.109).

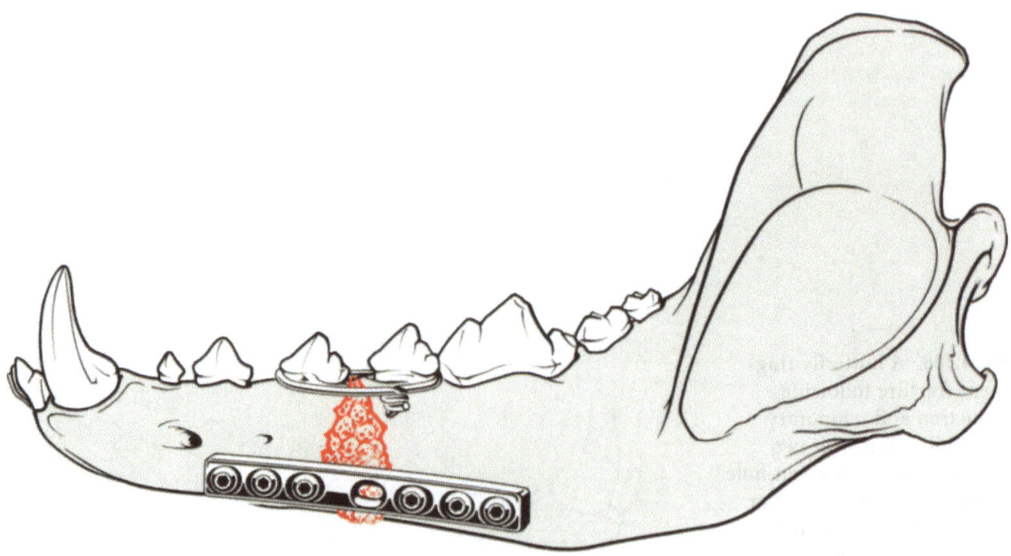

Fig. 4.108. A comminuted fracture of the body of the mandible with bone loss is fixed with a buttress plate. The defect is filled with cancellous bone, held in place by suturing the soft tissues

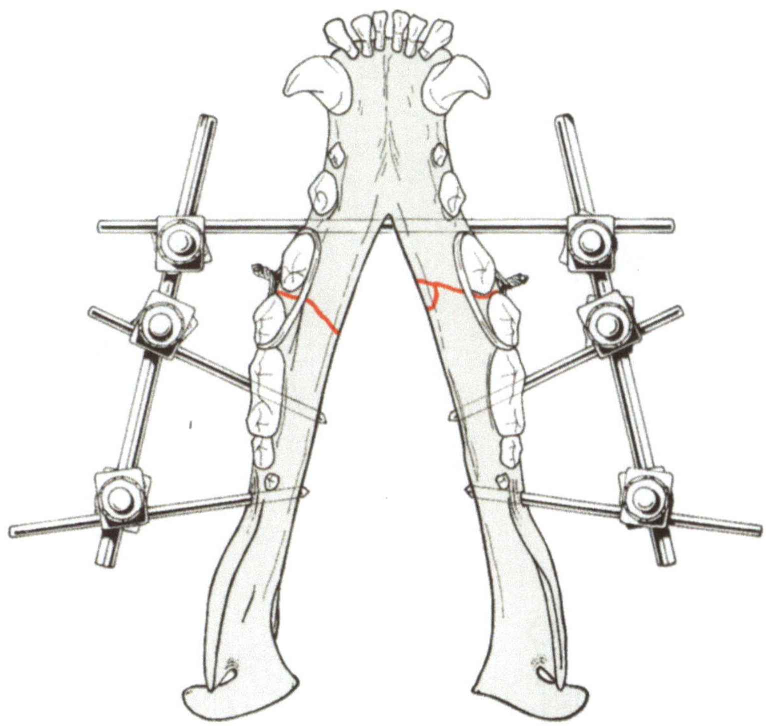

Fig. 4.109. The external fixator may be employed either uni- or bilaterally as the fracture dictates, and interdental wiring may also be used in conjunction with the frame. An example of a bilateral frame, with interdental wiring, is shown

4.9.1.3 Fractures of the Ramus

A ventral approach is made to the ramus. The masseter muscle is subperiosteally reflected. Reduction is obtained and stabilized by a plate of the appropriate size and shape: straight, oblique right angle, or T plate (Fig. 4.110). The advent of reconstruction plates has made available yet another useful series of fixation devices for stabilization of mandibular fractures. The advantage of the plate is that it may be molded in three planes; this is made possible by the scalloped edge of the plate.

4.9.2 Fractures of the Upper Jaw

4.9.2.1 Fractures of the Incisive Bone

Fixation and stabilization of fractures of the incisive bone may be achieved by plates or by the tension band wire principle. This portion of the skull may also be approached through the skin or through the mouth. The intraoral approach usually gives sufficient exposure. The lip is elevated dorsally and an incision made through the buccal mucosa, just below the reflection into the labial surface of the

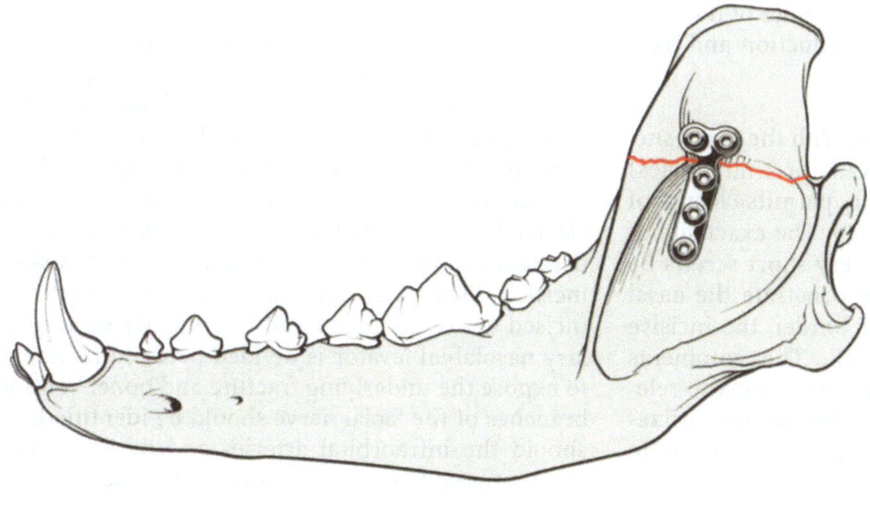

Fig. 4.110. Fracture of vertical ramus stabilized with a T plate

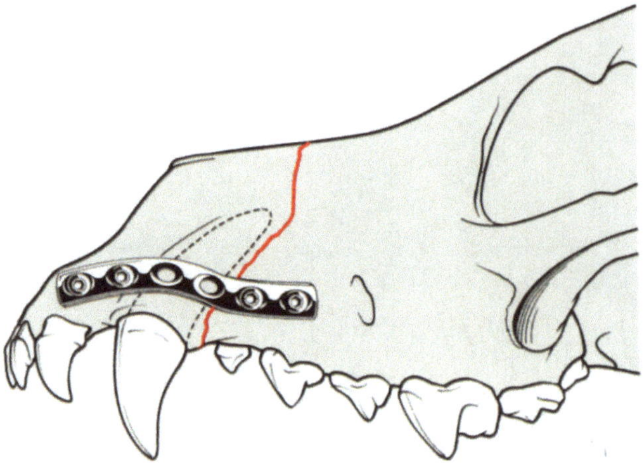

Fig. 4.111. A small fragment plate, or cuttable plate, is fixed to the premaxilla to effect stabilization

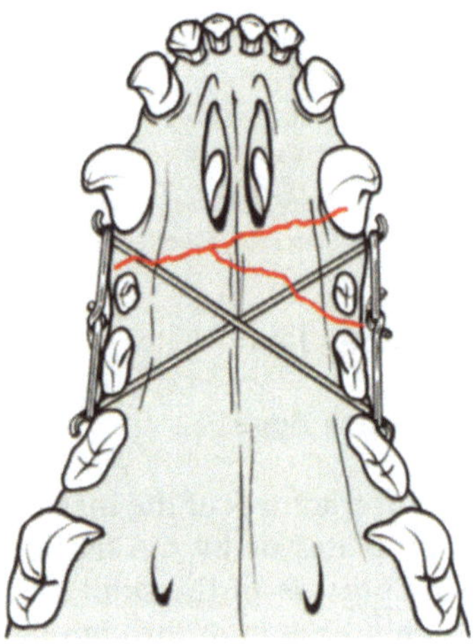

Fig. 4.112. A multiple fracture of the premaxilla is fixed by the tension band wire technique. Following reduction, two Kirschner wires are inserted beneath the buccal mucosa in an X pattern across both premaxillae. The tips of the Kirschner wires are bent away from the fracture site. Tension band wires are connected to the exposed Kirschner wire ends on either side of the jaw

mucosa. With a periosteal elevator, the fibrous tissue of the gum is reflected on both sides of the fracture line, far enough to permit reduction and fixation with the appropriate implant.

The choice of plates will vary with the exact site. Usually, a thin fragment plate (2.7- or 2-mm series) is appropriate, as it more readily permits closure of the soft tissue over it (Fig. 4.111). The exact site of the fracture may require that very short screws be used, as they would otherwise penetrate the nasal cavity. Apart from the inferior border, the incisive bone is only one cortex thick. The comments regarding screws made in Sect. 4.9.1.2 are also relevant here. Some fractures lend themselves to fixation with pins and wires, as is demonstrated in Fig. 4.112.

4.9.2.2 Fractures of the Maxilla

The majority of fractures of the maxilla do not require stabilization. However, butterfly-type fractures may be severely displaced along with the accompanying teeth. The approach to the maxilla is carried out in a similar manner as the approach to the premaxilla. The commissure of the lip is elevated and retracted. However, in some cases it is necessary to approach the mandible through a skin incision. The thin nasolabial levator muscle is incised across its fibers and the underlying maxillary nasolabial levator is divided between its fibers to expose the underlying fracture and bone. Ventral branches of the facial nerve should be identified, as should the infraorbital arteries and nerve, as the latter emerge from the infraorbital foramen.

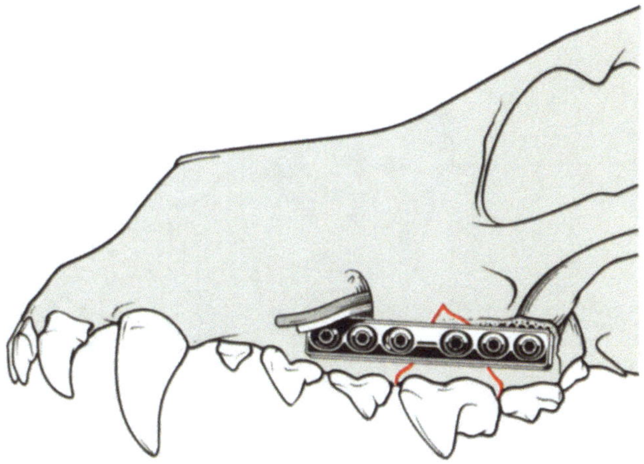

Fig. 4.113. A butterfly fracture of the maxilla including the fourth premolar tooth is stabilized by fixing the small plate first to the caudal segment, then to the butterfly fragment, and then compressed to the rostral portion of the maxilla

In fractures of the maxilla, it is only possible to use very short screws in many areas due to the thinness of the cortical bone. In such cases, the plate should be gently prestressed, and a plate of above-average length should be employed to permit the use of a large number of screws (Fig. 4.113).

4.9.3 Fractures of the Calvarium

Internal fixation is rarely used for fractures of the skull. Small depressed fractures may be treated by decompression and removal of the fragments. If the defect is large, it may be covered with a special plate which is screwed to the surrounding bone. The parietal bone permits use of short, 2- or 2.7-mm screws. The fragments are maintained in position following their elevation by means of small fragment plates fixed to the surrounding stable bone. Areas such as the zygomatic arch on the occiput lend themselves to stabilization by this means.

The necessity and wisdom of surgery in the case of such fractures depends on the underlying trauma to the central nervous system caused by the fracture. If only the frontal sinus is involved, surgical judgment may dictate that the fragments be left to heal or may indicate simple removal of depressed fragments.

4.10 Spinal Fractures and Luxations

Fractures and luxations of the spine (Fig. 4.114–4.125) can involve any level; however, the more mobile regions, particularly the thoracolumbar and the lumbosacral junctions, are involved most frequently. Commonly encountered types of spinal fractures and luxations are illustrated in Fig. 4.114. Thorough neurological and radiological evaluation of the patient must be performed prior to any operative treatment of a spinal injury. Neurologic examination should enable the level of vertebral column injury to be identified and the severity of spinal cord damage to be graded.

4.10.1 Clinical Grading of Spinal Cord Injury

- *Grade 1:* Pain only, without any neurological deficits
- *Grade 2:* Paresis or ataxia
- *Grade 3:* Paraplegia or quadriplegia
- *Grade 4:* Paraplegia or quadriplegia with urinary retention and overflow
- *Grade 5:* Paraplegia or quadriplegia with urinary retention and overflow and absence of conscious pain sensation

Lateral and ventrodorsal radiographs should be taken to evaluate the extent of spinal column injury; however, these will not necessarily show the position of the vertebra at the time of injury. The animal must always be evaluated neurologically along with radiographic evaluation.

Indications for surgical management of spinal trauma and the results of treatment have been reviewed. Animals with grade 1 or 2 dysfunction are usually initially treated conservatively with strict confinement and corticosteroids; external spinal splintage is occasionally needed. Surgery is indicated in these grades if there is a deterioration in neurological status as a result of vertebral instability. Animals with grade 3 or 4 dysfunction are generally classed as surgical emergencies. Prompt reduction and stabilization of the spinal column and decompression of the spinal cord should be undertaken within hours of the accident. Animals with grade 1–3 injuries usually have a good prognosis for recovery, while the prognosis for grade 4 is less favorable. Grade 5 injuries generally carry a poor prognosis.

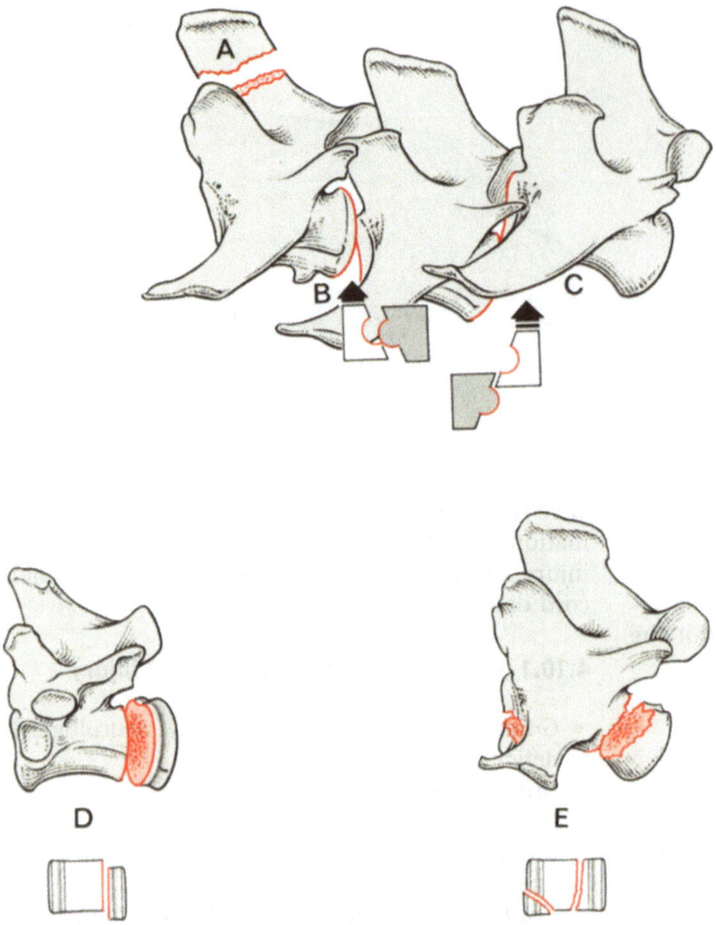

Fig. 4.114A–E. Commonly encountered types of spinal fractures and luxation. **A** Fracture of the dorsal spinal process. **B** Spinal subluxation. **C** Spinal luxation. **D** Epiphyseal fracture of the vertebral body. **E** Simple vertebral body fractures with a large portion of the body intact

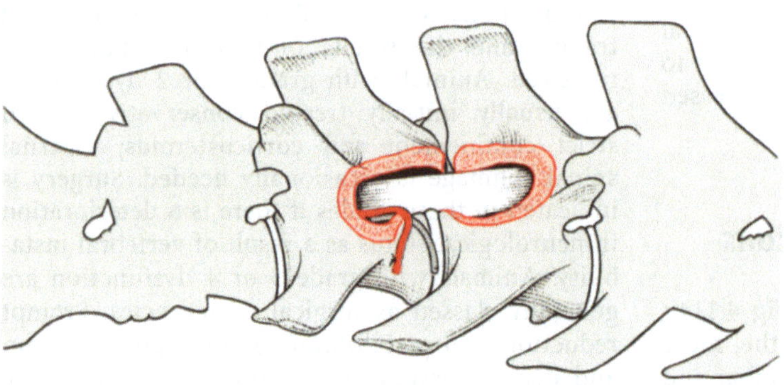

Fig. 4.115. Bone forceps affixed to adjacent dorsal spinous processes can be used to exert traction and countertraction in accomplishing reduction

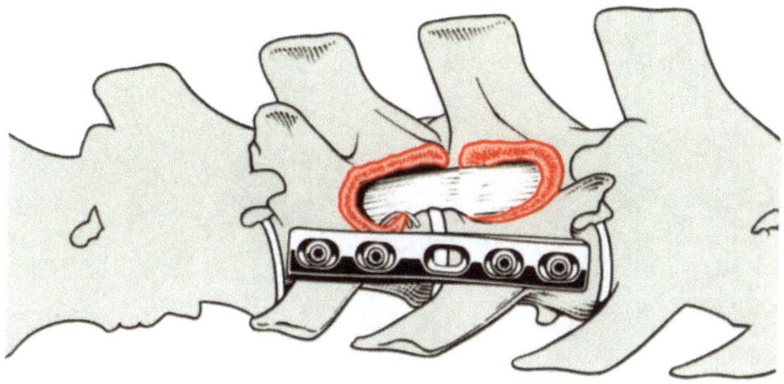

a

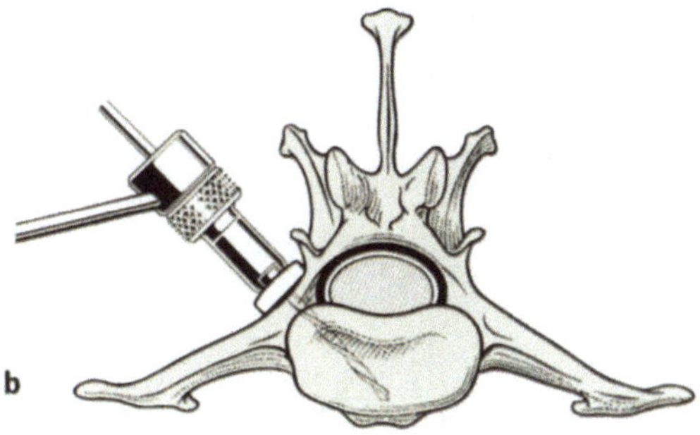

b

Fig. 4.116. **a** Fixation of two lumbar vertebrae using a plate. **b** Direction of insertion of the plate screw

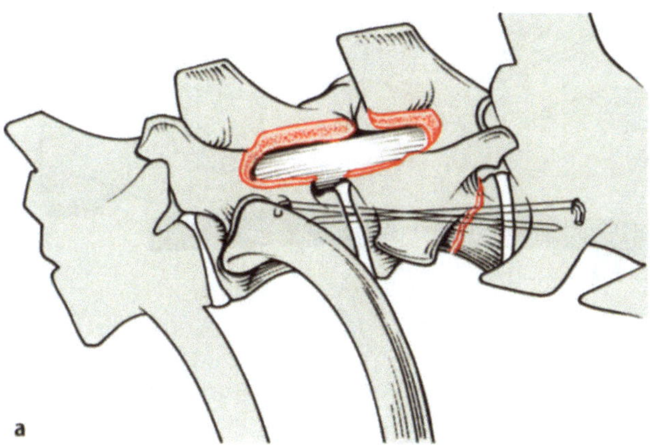

a

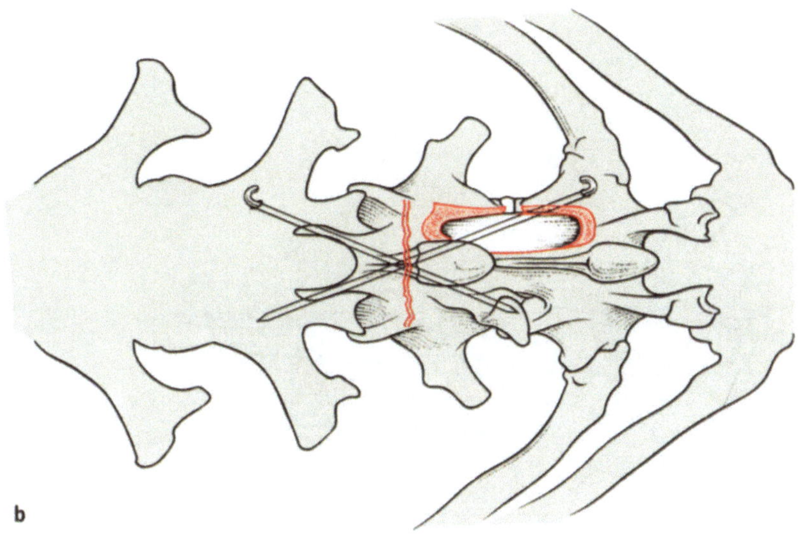

b

Fig. 4.117a,b. Interfragmentary fixation of vertebral body fragments with small pins. **a** Lateral view. **b** Dorsal view. This is usually used in combination with vertebral body plating

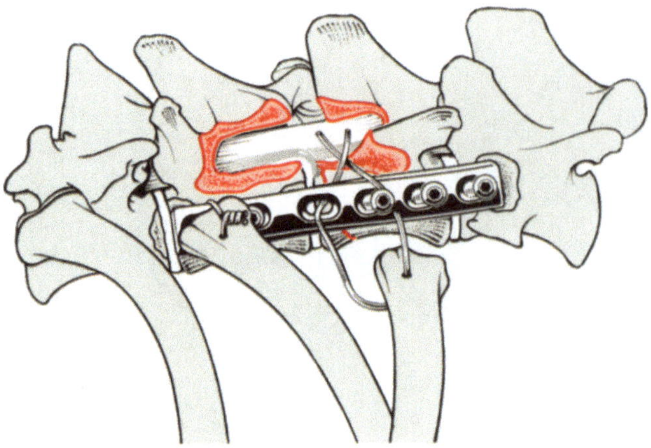

Fig. 4.118. Fixation of two thoracic vertebrae using a plate. The elevated ribs are reattached to the plate with wire

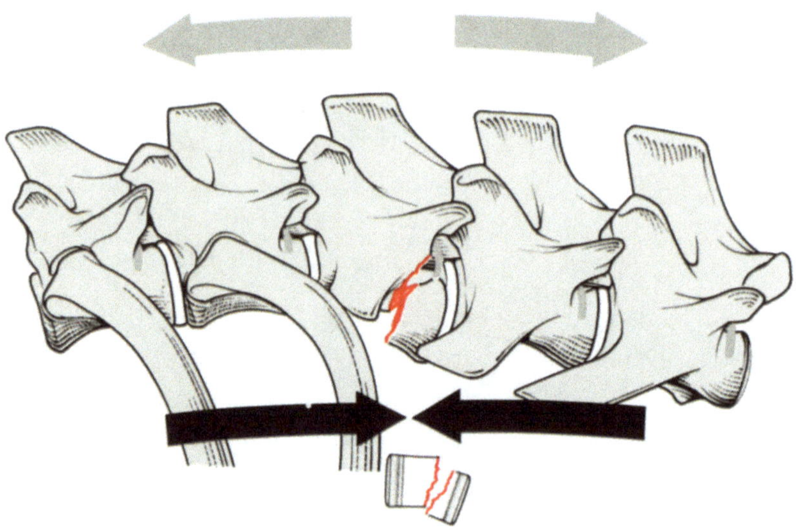

Fig. 4.119. In the thoracolumbar spine, there is a tension side (dorsal, *gray arrows*) and a compression side (ventral, *black arrows*)

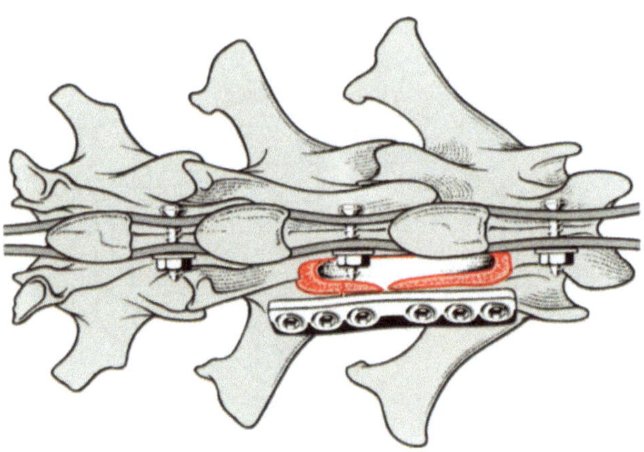

Fig. 4.120. Vertebral body plating used in conjunction with plastic spinal plates

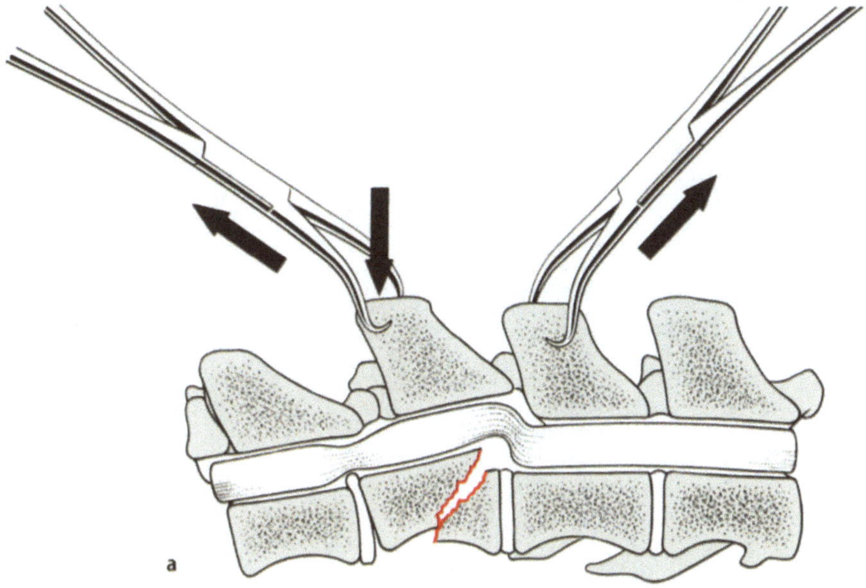

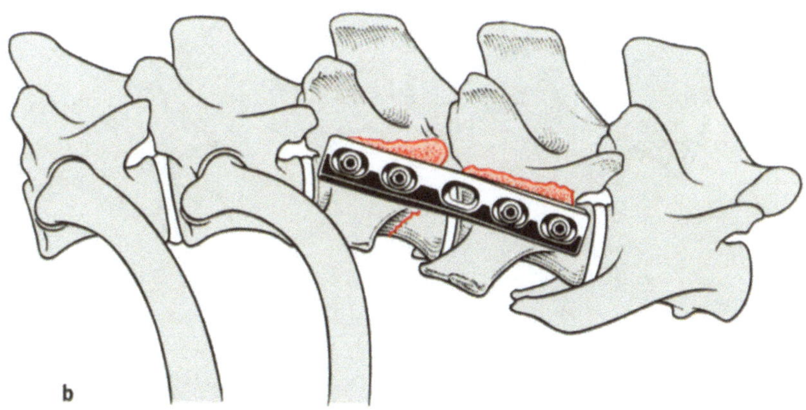

Fig. 4.121. **a** Vertebral body fracture of L1. This is an oblique fracture with a major portion of the vertebral body intact. **b** Fixation utilizing a vertebral body plate

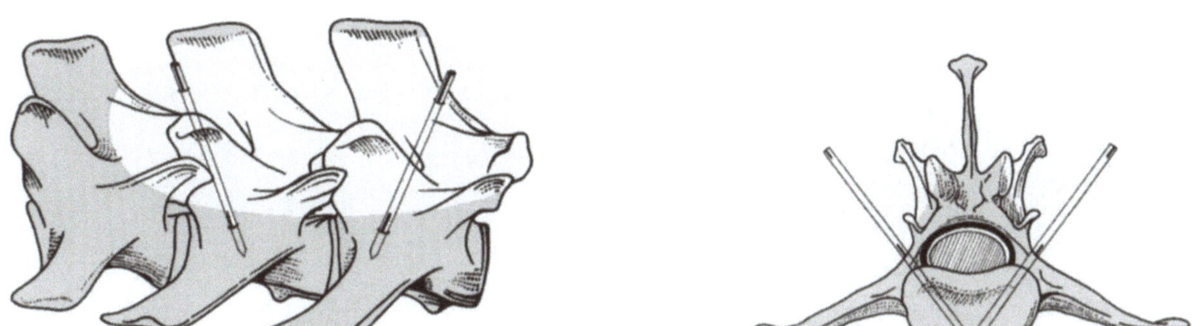

Fig. 4.122a,b. Pins and methylmethacrylate bone cement provides a more versatile method of spinal fixation

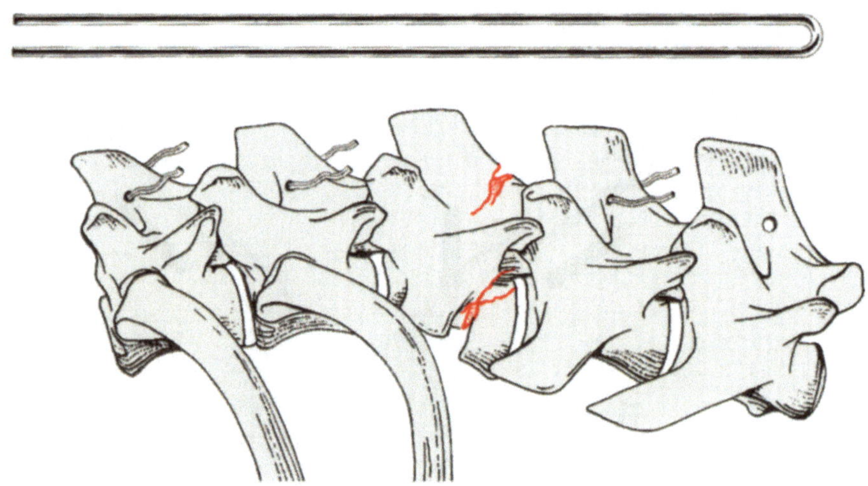

a

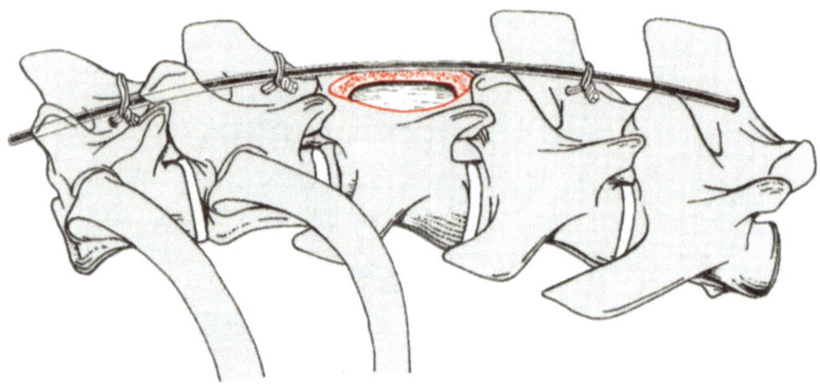

b

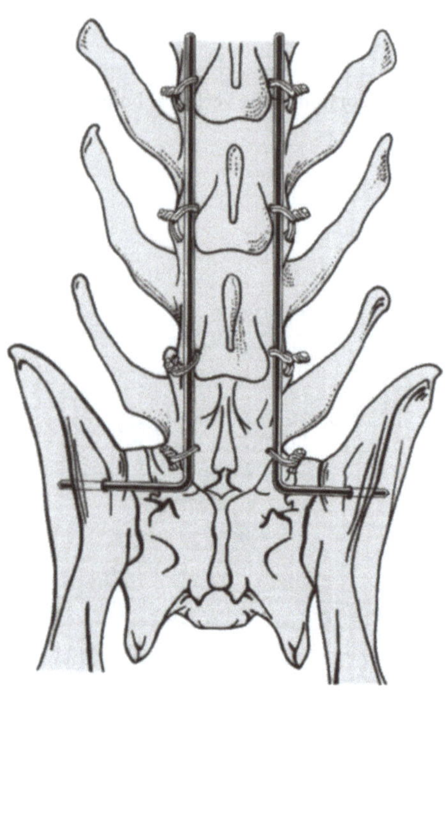

c

Fig. 4.123a–c. U-shaped pin (**a**), wired to the dorsal spinous processes or multiple pins and wires attached to the dorsal spinous process and articular facets (**b**). The wires may penetrate the wings of the ilium in posterior lumbar fractures (**c**)

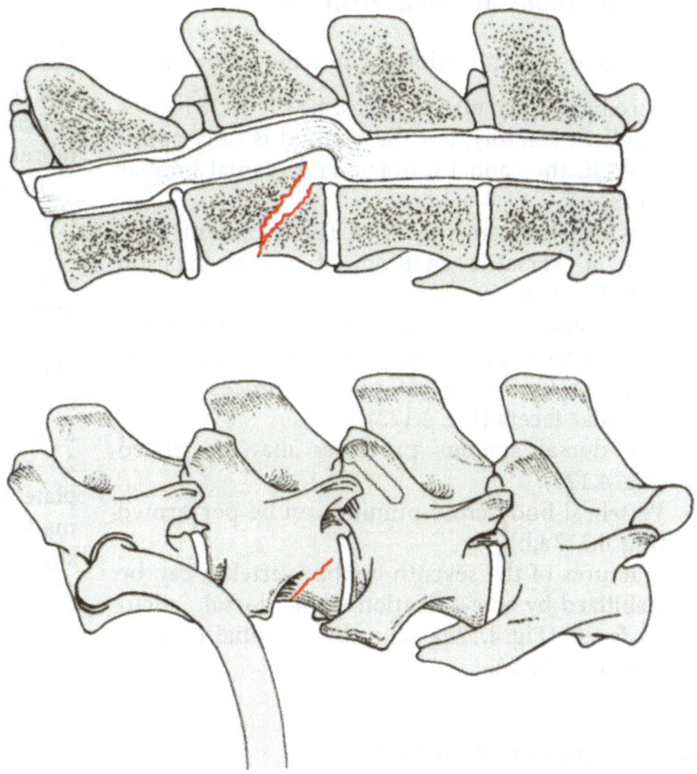

Fig. 4.124a,b. Fracture of the ventral aspect of a lumbar body. Reduction of the articular facets gives simultaneous reduction. Stability of the vertebral bodies is achieved by lag screw fixation of the articular facets

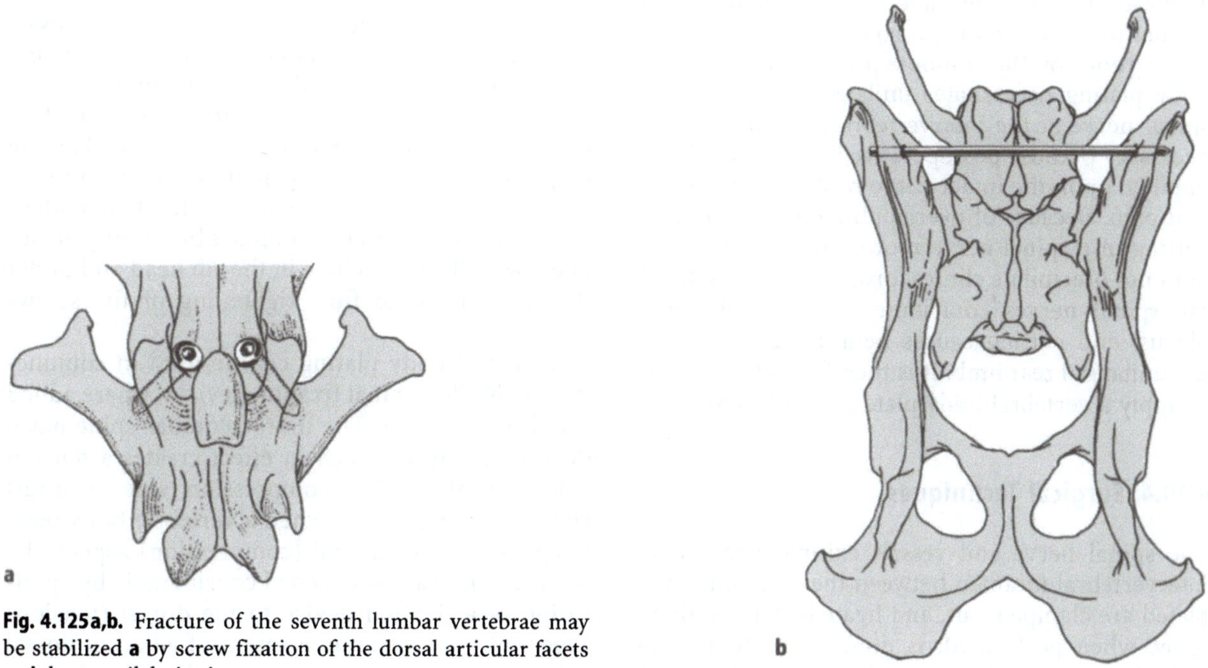

Fig. 4.125a,b. Fracture of the seventh lumbar vertebrae may be stabilized **a** by screw fixation of the dorsal articular facets or **b** by transilal pinning

4.10.2 Methods of Spinal Fixation

Methods of spinal fixation include the following:

1. Vertebral body plating (Figs. 4.115–4.118) gives excellent stability, but the method is only applicable in the caudal thoracic and cranial lumbar areas.
2. Pins and methylmethacrylate (bone cement) provide a versatile method of spinal fixation (Fig. 4.122a,b).
3. A U-shaped pin can be wired to the dorsal spinous processes or multiple pins and wires attached to the dorsal spinous processes and articular facets (Fig. 4.123).
4. The dorsal spinous processes may be plated (Fig. 4.120).
5. Vertebral body cross-pinning can be performed (Fig. 4.117a,b).
6. Fractures of the seventh lumbar vertebra can be stabilized by screw fixation of the dorsal articular facets (Fig. 4.125a–c) or by transilial pinning (Fig. 4.125ba,b).

4.10.3 Vertebral Body Plating

The application of a small bone plate to adjacent vertebral bodies provides excellent fixation for certain spinal injuries. Its usage in the canine patient is limited to the fixation of vertebral bodies T11 through to L3. Cranial to T11, spinal exposure becomes very difficult, and the anatomical structure of the vertebral body does not permit proper application of a bone plate to the vertebral body. Caudal to L3, the problem concerns the important nerve roots of the lumbosacral plexus. Vertebral body plating necessitates unilateral cutting of the spinal nerve at the intervertebral foramen. This is necessary because postoperative bony exostosis can impinge upon the intact nerve root, causing persistent pain. Because of overlapping dermatomes, the cutting of a spinal nerve root between T11 and L3 does not precipitate clinical problems. Caudal to L3, the spinal nerves contribute to the lumbosacral plexus, and cutting causes neurological deficit in the unilateral rear limb. It is therefore advisable not to apply a vertebral body plate caudal to L3.

4.10.4 Surgical Techniques

The spinal nerve and vessels exiting through the intervertebral foramen between the vertebrae to be plated are clamped, cut, and ligated. Hemilaminectomy, when performed, is done by removing the articular processes between adjacent vertebrae with a rongeur. A window is developed using a high-speed drill, rongeur, or trephine. After hemilaminectomy, the injured spinal cord and spinal canal can be visualized. Visualization of the spinal canal aids in the anatomical reduction of the injured vertebrae.

Bone forceps are affixed to adjacent dorsal spinous processes to aid in reduction of the displaced vertebra (Figs. 4.115, 4.121a). A bone plate is selected which fits along the bodies of the two vertebra to be stabilized. It is necessary that at least two screws be placed in each vertebral body. The plate is laid on the dorsolateral aspect of the vertebral bodies, between the transverse process and articular processes of the hemilaminectomy site. A 2.7-mm plate is used for small dogs, and a 3.5-mm plate for dogs weighing over 20 kg. Drill holes are made into vertebral bodies, angling across and slightly ventral. The drilling angle is approximately 45 ° to the horizontal plane of the vertebral bodies. The drill hole in the opposite cortex should be located ventral to the transverse process. The most caudal hole is drilled first, and the screw is inserted in the standard manner. The most cranial hole is then drilled and the screw inserted, and the remaining holes drilled and the screws inserted (Figs. 4.116, 4.121b).

Interfragmentary fixation of vertebral body fragments with small lag screws or small pins can be used to effect anatomical repair. This technique is especially helpful in treatment of vertebral body fractures and is often used in conjunction with vertebral body plating (Fig. 4.117).

When adjacent thoracic vertebral bodies are plated, it is often necessary to expose and disarticulate the rib at the junction with the vertebral body. The vertebral body is then smoothed by removing protruding bone with a rongeur. This provides a smooth surface upon which the plate can be placed. After the bone plate has been positioned and attached, the rib heads are elevated to their normal position and held in place by passing orthopedic wire through a hole in the rib head and under the plate, prior to final tightening of the screws (Fig. 4.118).

Vertebral body plating can be used in conjunction with other spinal fixation devices, where added stability is needed. The thoracolumbar spine has a dorsal curvature, which in effect creates a tension side (dorsal) and a compression side (ventral) (Fig. 4.119). Therefore, when a vertebral body plate is applied to the ventral (compression) aspect, the force upon it can be lessened considerably by application of a fixation device to the dorsal (tension) aspect of the vertebrae. Fixation of adjacent dorsal spinous processes acts to neutralize the tension forces on the vertebral body. Stabilization of the dorsal spinous processes can be accomplished using metal spinal plates or plastic spinal plates. The plates should span two vertebrae cranial and caudal to the point of injury.

Plastic spinal plates utilize a sandwiching technique, affixing spinous processes by bolts through the interspaces between the processes. The entire apparatus is secured by a washer and nut on the screws. The use of two plates, applied to the dorsal spinal processes in conjunction with vertebral body plating, provides a very stable fixation (Fig. 4.120). Incompatibility of implant materials has not been a problem when using this technique for spinal fixation. Closure should include suturing of the lumbodorsal fibrous tunic, fascia, and skin.

4.10.4.1 Pins and Methyl Methacrylate

Multiples vertebral body pins, which are anchored in bone cement, provide a means of stabilizing fractures and luxations at any level of the spinal column. In the thoracic and lumbar regions, a dorsal approach is used to give bilateral exposure of the articular facets and transverse processes. At least two nonthreaded pins are inserted into the vertebral bodies on either side of the fracture or luxation (Fig. 4.122a,b). The pins should penetrate two cortices, and the ends of the pins should be notched or bent to give good fixation in the bone cement. The fracture/luxation is reduced and a cylinder of bone cement is prepared; this is molded to the articular facets and the protruding ends of the pins. As a considerable amount of heat is generated as the bone cement sets, the cord and surrounding tissues should be irrigated with lactated Ringer's solution to prevent thermal damage and necrosis. Implant failure may result if an attempt is made to span too large an area with bone cement.

4.10.4.2 Pins and Wire

Midlumbar and caudal lumbar fractures/luxations can be stabilized using multiple pins wired to the articular facets and/or dorsal spinous processes. For optimal stability and prevention of pin migration, the caudal ends of the pins should be bent and anchored in the wings of the ilia (Fig. 4.123c).

4.10.5 Lumbosacral Fractures and Luxations

In the lumbosacral region, the diameter of the neural canal is large relative to its content, the cauda equina. Considerable displacement of fracture/luxations of the caudal three lumbar vertebrae can be tolerated, without necessarily causing permanent neurological dysfunction. Laminectomy is often unnecessary. The pin and wire method of fixation (Fig. 4.125a,b) is the most useful method of treating fracture luxations in this region. Lag screw fixation of the articular facets is also useful in oblique fractures of the vertebral body of L6 or L7 associated with luxation of the caudal articular facets of the vertebra. Reduction of the articular facets gives simultaneous reduction of the vertebral body fracture. Fixation is achieved by lag screw fixation of the articular facets (Fig. 4.125a). The area should be protected by external splintage for 2–3 weeks following the operation. In fracture luxations of L7/S1, reduction of the articular facets of L7 can be maintained by a transilial pin (Fig. 4.125b) as an alternative to lag screw fixation.

4.10.6 Cervical Fractures and Luxations

The most common site of cervical fracture is C2. Considerable displacement may be noted without severe motor dysfunction, particularly if one of the cranial cervical vertebrae is involved. On admission, the main sign is cervical pain; the prognosis for dogs in this category is good, and most go on to recover with nonsurgical treatment. Animals with nondisplaced fractures are either given cage rest for 4–8 weeks or have their neck immobilized in a reinforced splint or cast for the same amount of time.

Displaced cervical fractures, particularly those associated with motor dysfunction, tend to be managed surgically. Fractures of C2 usually involve the dens and may result in atlantoaxial subluxation. The subluxation is stabilized by lag screw fixation of the articular facets. In fractures which involve the vertebral body, the ventral approach is the easiest. The use of pins and bone cement is the most versatile method of stabilizing the fracture. Ventral application of a plate to the vertebral body can also be used, but implant loosening is a frequent complication.

4.10.7 Postoperative Management

Much of the care needed postoperatively depends upon the neurological status of the patient. Ability to ambulate, urinary and bowel continence, and freedom from decubital ulceration are of primary concern. In general, postoperative care should take into account the following considerations:

1. A body bandage should be worn around the trunk for 14 days.
2. If the animal is not ambulatory, it should be bedded on a soft, absorbent material. Frequent turning helps prevent decubital ulceration.
3. If the animal is ambulatory, it should be encouraged to walk, but activity should be restricted to a controlled environment for 8–12 weeks.
4. The urinary bladder should be emptied four times a day if the patient is not continent. Prophylactic antibiotic therapy helps prevent urinary infection.
5. A program of physical therapy is essential to rehabilitation. Outpatient care, when possible, is preferred.
6. In general, plates and screws used for spinal fixation are not removed. Indications for removal are loosening of screws, pain, infection, and unfavorable patient reaction to the surgical implant.

4.11 Immature Animals

Animals with open growth plates are defined as immature. According to their breed they can be up to 5–11 months of age (see Appendix). As the bones are still growing their structure differs from the bones of adult animals; they contain more collagen fibers, less calcium apatite, and a more extensive blood supply. Cartilaginous growth plates are also evident in all long bones. These factors influence the fracture type and the bone healing pattern. Accordingly, this chapter refers to the special features of growing bones, their clinical significance, and their treatment. In most cases the healing patterns differ from fractures of the same location in adult animals. In young growing bones the following special features are of clinical significance:

1. Young bones withstand greater deformation without fracturing because they are more resilient. Greenstick and fissure-type fractures are relatively common.
2. The periosteum is vascular, thick, and loosely attached; therefore, it easily strips when subjected to trauma. A subperiosteal hematoma develops and induces bone formation, gradually disappearing during the healing stages of reorganization and remodeling.
3. In displaced articular fractures, early anatomical reduction and fixation are essential in order to eliminate or minimize alterations in growth and incongruencies of the joint surface.
4. Fracture or trauma of the growth plate area may arrest or alter growth in that area. The amount of shortening, and/or deformity is proportional to the trauma pattern and the growth potential remaining at the time of injury.
5. Healing is rapid, and although the healing callus may be abundant, remodeling is active and failure to unite is rare.

4.11.1 Diaphyseal Fractures with Minimal Displacement

Fractures with minimal displacement respond very satisfactorily to closed reduction and conservative treatment. In young growing animals the thick periosteal sleeve helps to prevent displacement of fracture fragments. Thus, conservative treatment is often acceptable. Where feasible, external immobilization is the preferred method of treatment. However, fractures of the humerus and femur are not readily immobilized by external methods, and internal fixation affords earlier return of normal function and provides greater stabilization. Shaft fractures in growing animals heal quite rapidly in most cases, with minimal shortening and angulation. However, there is a danger of rotation, a factor which needs to be considered in reduction and fixation. Small deviations of the axis will be corrected by nature if the remaining growing period is long enough. Also it must be understood that limb splintage, during conservative treatment, should not last longer than 8–10 days in very young animals and not longer than 3 weeks in animals in which physeal closure will occur within the next few months. Moreover, limb joints must be fixed in the normal standing position and should never be hyperextended; otherwise fracture disease will occur.

4.11.2 Open Reduction and Internal Fixation in the Young Dog

Primary indications for open reduction and internal fixation are: (a) rotational deformity or excessive shortening, (b) fractures resulting in incongruency of the articular surface, (c) fractures or trauma affecting the growth plate, and (d) anatomical reasons.
The principles to be observed in handling the delicate young tissues are:

1. Tissues should be handled gently in approach and reduction.
2. Early reduction should be carried out – each day of procrastination adds to the difficulty of handling tissues without using excess force. Callus is

formed very early in the young animal, obscuring neurovascular structures and making reduction difficult.
3. Fixation implants must be minimal in size. If the physis is crossed the use of nonthreaded Kirschner wires or Steinmann pins at right angles has little or no detrimental influence on future bone growth.
4. Healing is rapid and the period of immobilization is thus reduced correspondingly.
5. In most cases implants should be removed at clinical union.

4.11.3 Diaphyseal Fractures Resulting in Rotational Deformity or Excessive Shortening

The suggested methods for fixation of shaft fractures are: (a) plate, (b) external fixator, and (c) intramedullary pins.

4.11.3.1 Plates

If plates are used in the young growing animal, they should be minimal in size and removed early (after approximately 4 weeks for the animal 3 months of age or under). Plates should never cross a physis (Fig. 4.126).

The most common type of fracture in the femur and the tibia is long and oblique. The humerus and antebrachium transverse and short oblique fractures are the most common type seen. Multifragment fractures are rare and should be treated according to the rules of biological fracture treatment. The basic rule in such treatment is to avoid any disturbance of the fracture area during reduction and fixation in order to protect residual vascularity. During fragment reduction it is necessary to apply traction to reestablish the anatomical position of both of the main fragments in order to regain normal bone length and to avoid rotational malalign-

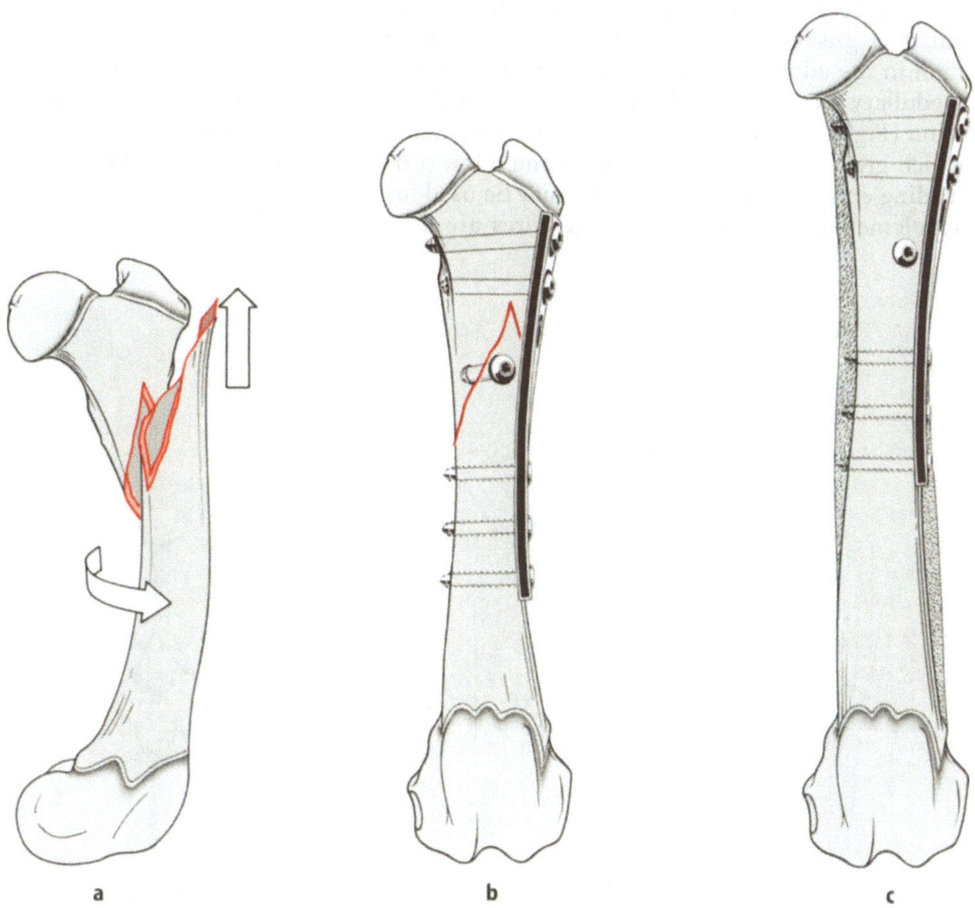

Fig. 4.126. **a** Doberman pinscher, 11 weeks of age; spiral fracture with marked shortening and rotation. **b** Fixation with a lag screw and 3.5-mm bone plate. **c** Clinical union with subperiosteal callus at 4 weeks. The fracture line had totally disappeared. The plate was removed at this time

ment. The intervening fragments are not touched; normally they are brought into nearly anatomic position by traction on the soft tissues during reduction of the main fragments.

Both of the main fragments are then fixed in their anatomic position by a rigid bridging plate or with an external fixator, and the animal is kept in restricted motion for about 4 weeks.

In small and medium sized dogs and cats the use of a VCP (Veterinary Cuttable Plate) is strongly recommended (see Appendix).

4.11.3.2 External Fixator

In most cases, skeletal fixation can be applied without an open approach, but an open approach is not contraindicated. The modified procedure using one connecting bar is followed in the application of fixation (Fig. 4.127).

4.11.3.3 Intramedullary Pins

In the very young animal, cancellous bone is present in a greater percentage of the marrow cavity than in the adult, so that a smaller-diameter intramedullary pin can be used to gain an equivalent fixation (Fig. 4.128) or two pins of a smaller diameter, which give more rotational stability and allow protruding ends to be bent. Lag screws may be used for supplemental fixation, but cerclage wires are usually avoided due to the ensuing growth in diameter and their tendency to become loose and interfere with healing. The use of an external fixator, for additional support, is acceptable when indicated.

4.11.4 Pelvic Fractures

Pelvic fractures occasionally occur in young animals. In most cases the ileum or the physis of the acetabulum is involved. Repair is carried out with a plate as described in Section 4.4.

4.11.5 Growth Plate Separations or Fracture Separations

From the standpoint of location and function, associated growth plate injury may be classified as follows:

1. Traction epiphysis is located at the site of origin or insertion of major muscles or muscle groups and, due to the anchor of strong fibrous tissue distal to the physis, it is subjected to more pressure than traction, e.g., tibial tuberosity, greater trochanter. Injury to a traction epiphysis does not significantly alter future growth (Fig. 4.129).
2. Pressure epiphysis is situated at the end of a long bone and is subjected to pressure transmitted through the joint into which it enters. Injury usually results in abnormal future growth (Fig. 4.130).

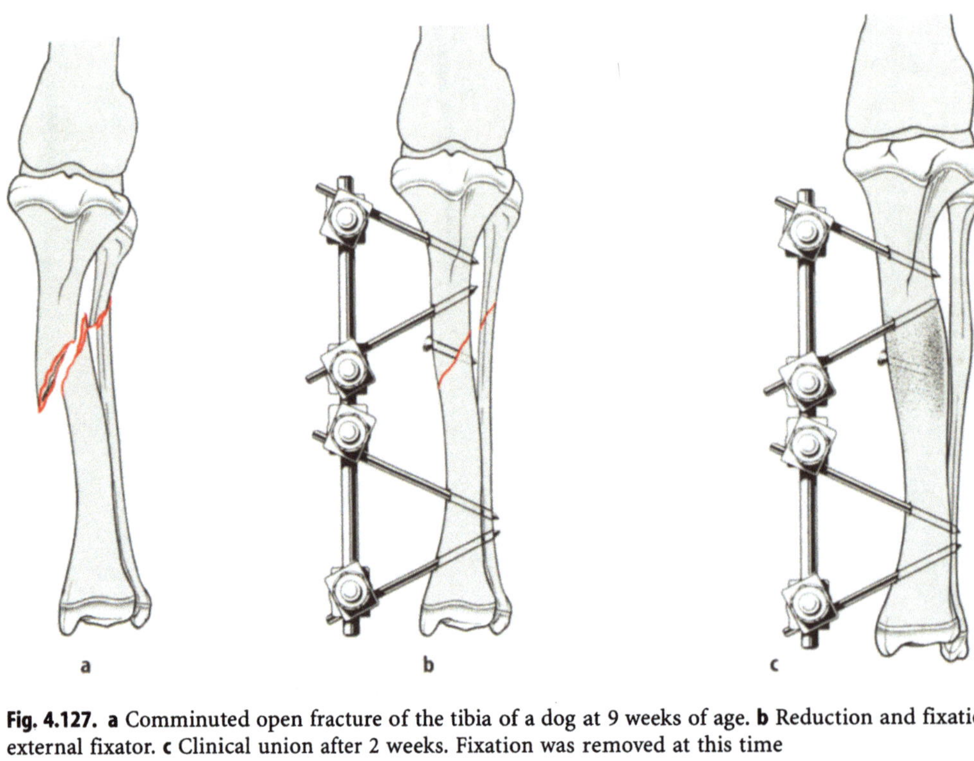

Fig. 4.127. **a** Comminuted open fracture of the tibia of a dog at 9 weeks of age. **b** Reduction and fixation using a lag screw and external fixator. **c** Clinical union after 2 weeks. Fixation was removed at this time

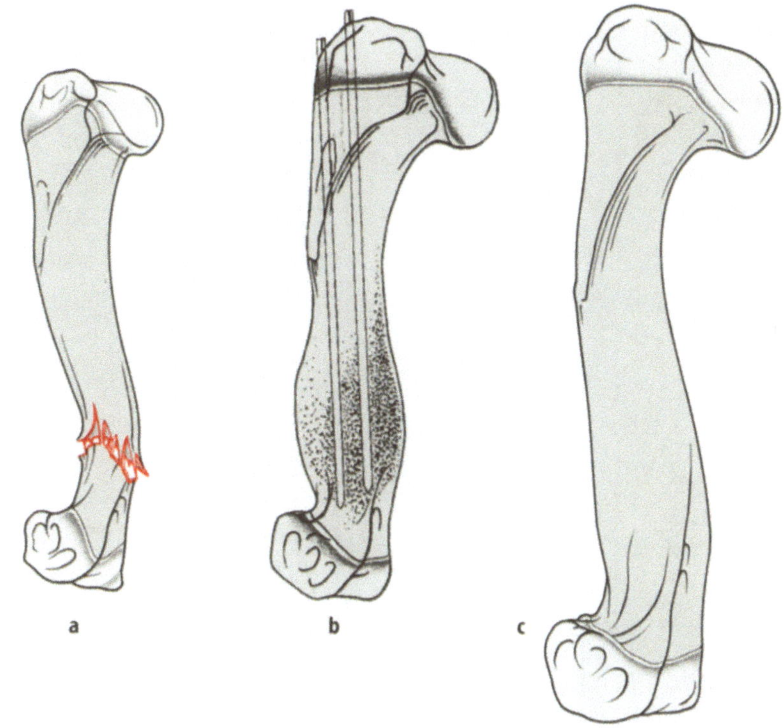

Fig. 4.128. **a** An unstable oblique fracture in a dog 7 weeks of age. **b** An open approach was carried out to accomplish reduction and fixation using two intramedullary pins (small diameter) for better rotational stability. The proximal ends of the pins may, if preferred, be bent over in order to avoid soft tissue trauma and then buried under the skin. Two weeks after treatment clinical union occurred and the pins were removed. **c** Four months after the operation the fracture area was remodeled

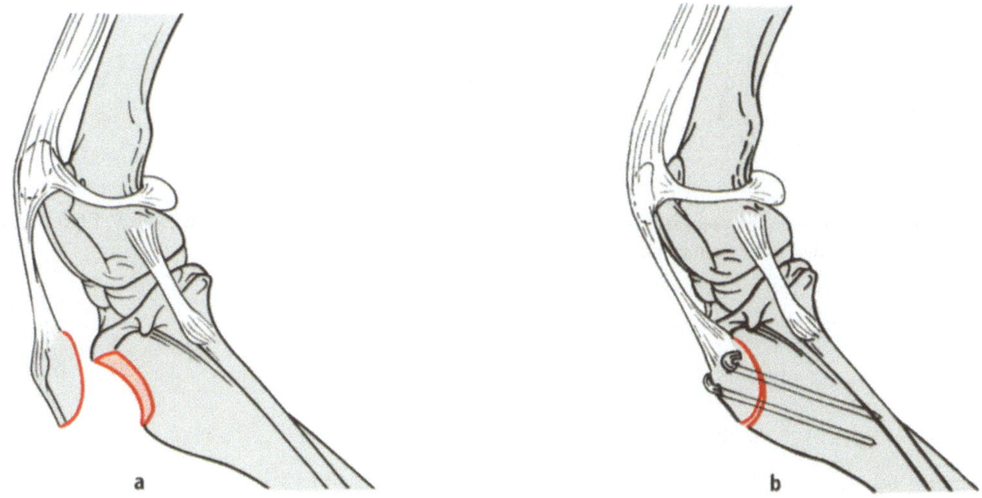

Fig. 4.129. **a** Type I avulsion separation of tibial tubercle. Since it is the insertion of the powerful group of quadriceps muscles, reduction and fixation must be carried out immediately. **b** In the young growing animal, fixation with two parallel Kirschner wires is sufficient. **c** In heavyweight dogs, just before physeal closure a tension band wire fixation is necessary, but it should be removed at the time of clinical union. An immobilization bandage is to be indicated for 2 weeks

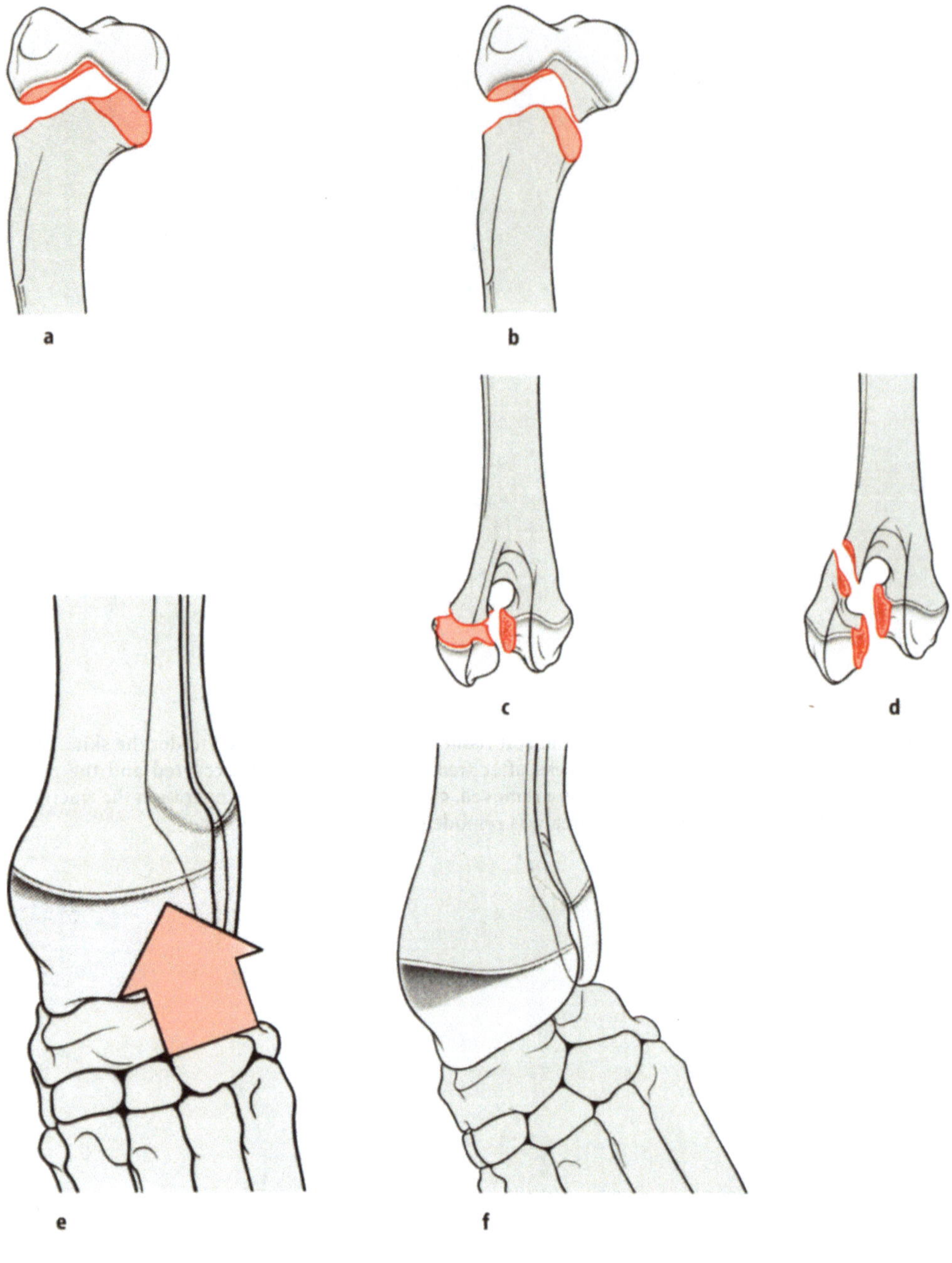

Fig. 4.130a–f. Examples of physeal injuries. **a** Type I. **b** Type II. **c** Type III. **d** Type IV. **e** Type V. **f** Growth alteration at 1 month posttrauma. (Classified after Salter and Harris)

Separations or fracture-separations of the physis from the metaphysis are relatively common in the immature animal. This can be accounted for by the fact that the ligaments and joint capsule linking two adjacent bones are several times stronger than the growth plate attachment between the epiphysis and metaphysis.

4.11.5.1 Classification of Separations or Fracture-Separations Involving the Physis

The classification of these separations or fracture-separations is based on their pathoanatomy and prognosis (Table 4.2, Fig. 4.130).

4.11.5.2 Treatment of Separations or Fracture-Separations Involving the Growth Plate

Open reduction and rigid internal fixation of fractures involving the joints is mandatory in order to obtain and maintain a congruent articular surface. The severity of these manifestations is proportional to: (a) the degree and pattern of injury, (b) the growth potential remaining at the time of injury, and (c) the particular growth plates affected. The decision to operate on the various separations or fracture-separations involving the articular surfaces must be made early, as growth and remodeling changes take place very rapidly. The open approach to expose the various areas is usually the same as for the adult animal except that the exposure should be kept to a minimum. Nonthreaded Kirschner wire transfixation is an excellent means of internal fixation and can be used safely, but these wires should be removed at clinical union, which is usually 2–4 weeks later.

Lag screw fixation can be used if more purchase is indicated, but should not cross the growth plate). Incomplete fracture between the two condyles must also be repaired with a lag screw; otherwise the fracture gap remains (Figs. 4.131–4.143).

Table 4.2. Classification of fractures involving the physis according to Salter and Harris

Type	Description	Prognosis
I	Separation at physeal line	Good
II	Separation of a portion of the physeal and metaphyseal fragment	Good with anatomical reduction and stabilization
III	Partial separation of the physis and fracture through the epiphysis	Good with anatomical reduction and stable fixation, otherwise poor
IV	Fracture through the epiphysis and metaphysis	Good with anatomical reduction and stable fixation, otherwise poor
V	Compression damage to all or a portion of the physis	Poor. Many make a satisfactory response after early corrective surgery (see Sect. 4.11.5)

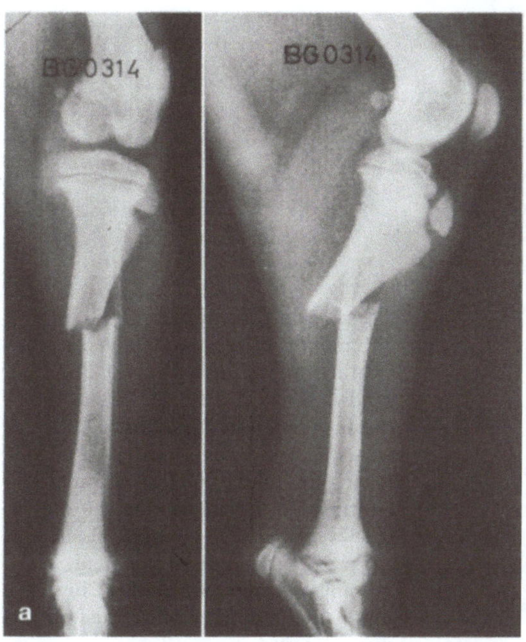

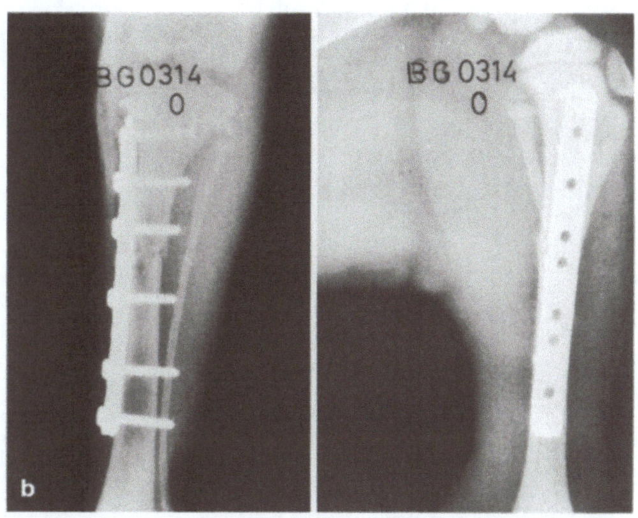

Fig. 4.131. **a** Collie, 3 months old, 8-kg bodyweight, with a short oblique tibial shaft fracture. **b** Fixation with two 2.0/2.7 VCP, fully sandwiched (1/1 sandwich), using 2.7-mm screws.

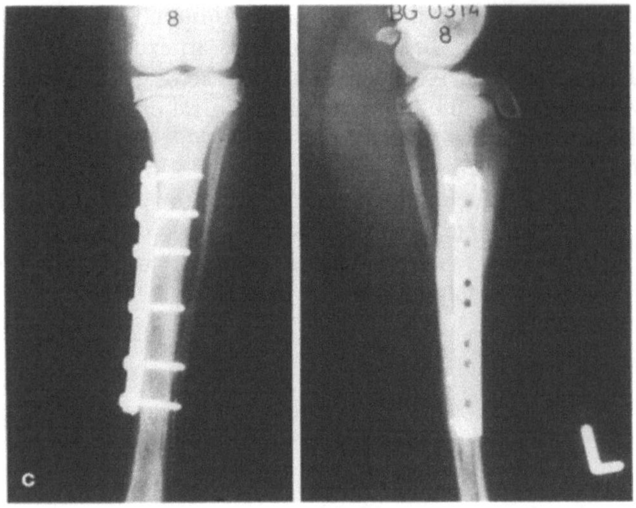

Fig. 4.131.c At 8 weeks healing had occurred and the plate was removed

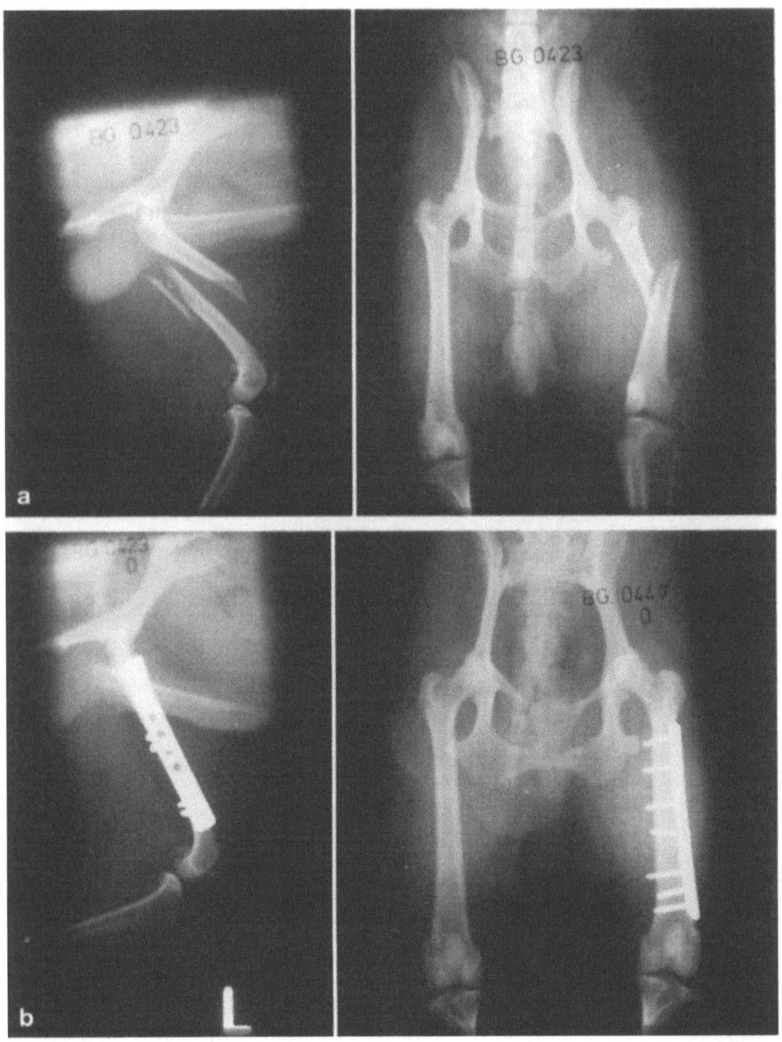

Fig. 4.132. **a** Yorkshire terrier, $7^{1}/_{2}$ months of age, comminuted femur fracture. **b** Fixation with a 2.0/2.7 VCP sandwiched with a 1.5/2.0 VCP at two thirds of length (2/3 sandwich 2.0/ 2.7–1.5/2.0 VCP) as a buttress plate following the rules of biological fracture treatment. For plate fixation, 2.0-mm screws are used. To compress fissures in the proximal and distal fragment, 1.5 mm lag-screws are used. **c** Clinical union after 6 months, when the implants were removed

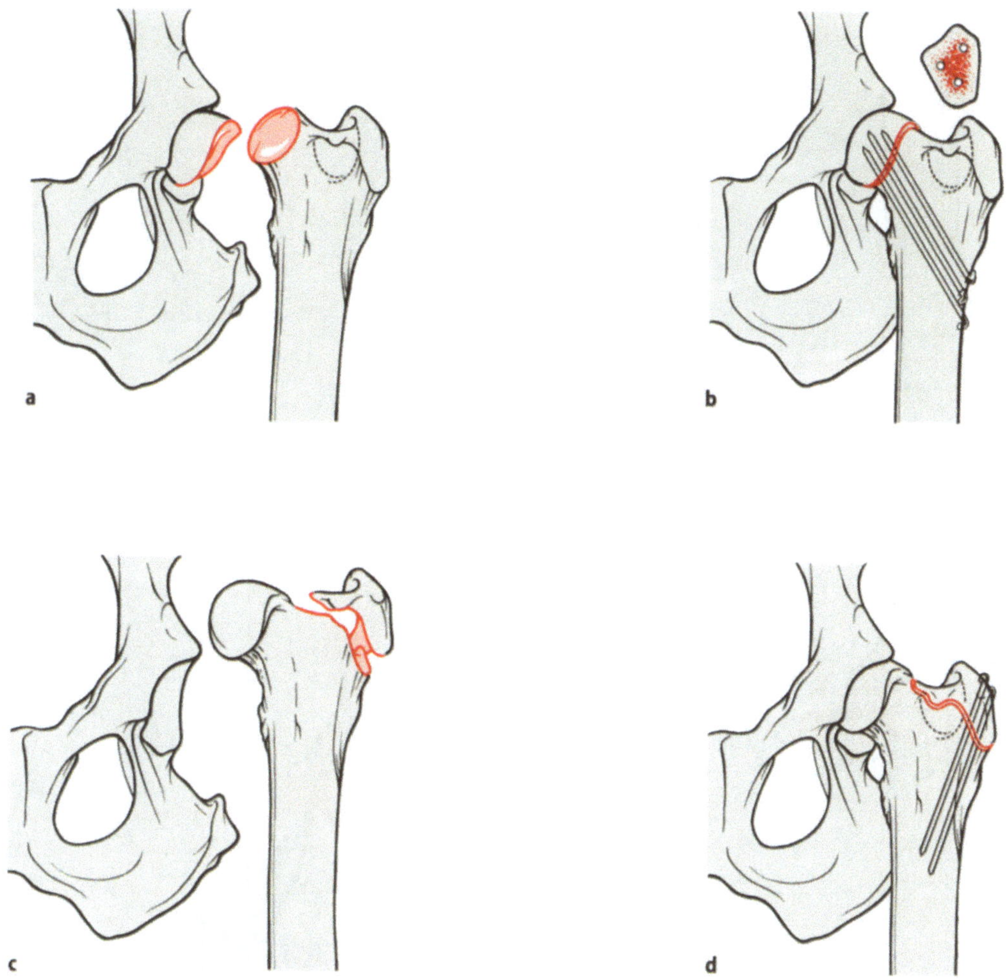

Fig. 4.133a–d. Examples and suggested methods of internal fixation for some of the commonly encountered fracture-separations of the femur. **a** Type I separation of proximal femoral epiphysis. **b** Fixation using multiple smooth Kirschner wires. **c** Type I separation of greater trochanter with dislocation of femoral head. **d** After reduction of the femoral head, the greater trochanter is fixed in place using two Kirschner wires. In heavy dogs an additional tension band wire fixation may be necessary close to the physeal closure. Postoperative excessive loading of the limb has to be avoided by marked restriction of activity for 3–4 weeks

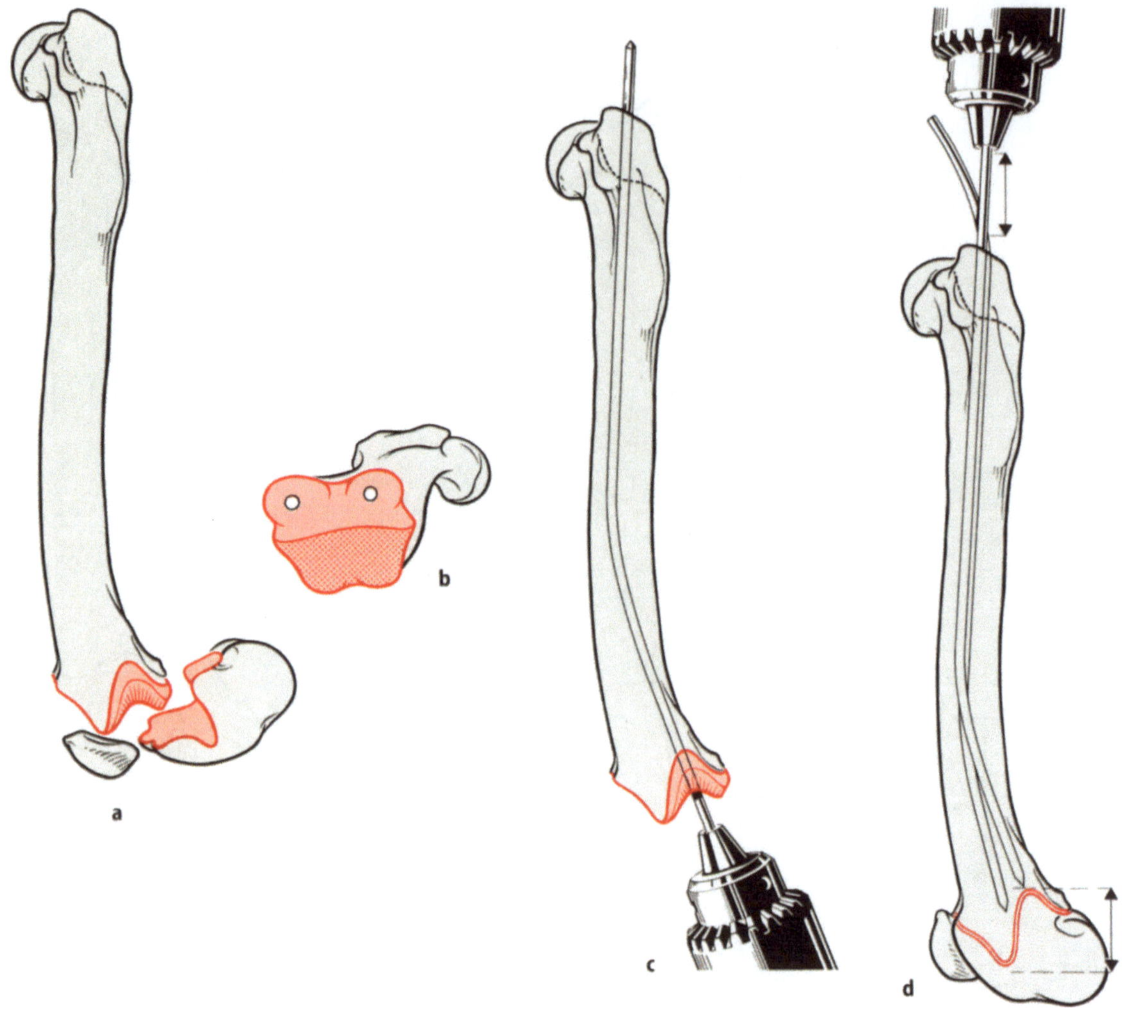

Fig. 4.134. **a** Type I separation of distal femoral epiphysis. **b** Two Kirschner wires are inserted retrograde, entering the distal end of the proximal segment, one near the caudomedial border and one near the caudolateral border. **c** Small-diameter wires were used so that they could bend according the curvature of the bone when inserted retrogradely. **d** The fracture is then reduced and the leg is held in marked extension of the stifle joint (this compresses the fracture gap and maintains reduction during insertion of the pins).

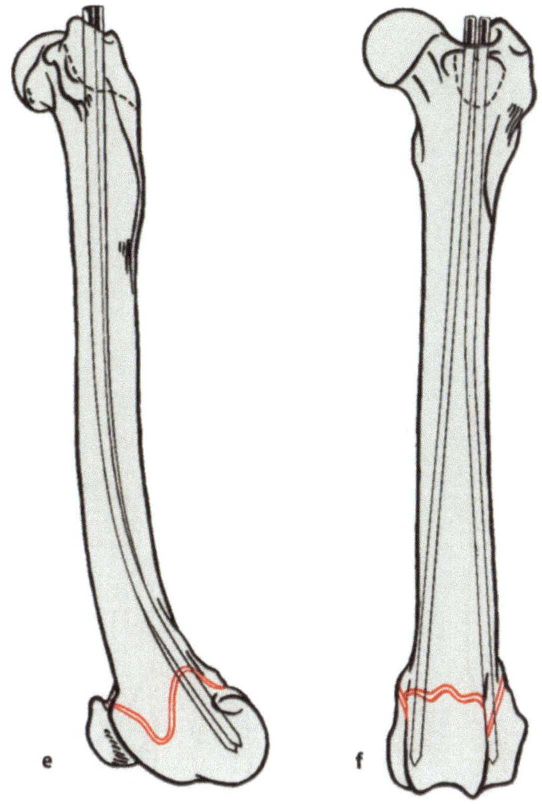

Fig. 4.134. e, f The pin chuck is fixed to the proximal end of the wire at a distance from the skin (1') equal to the thickness of the epiphysis (1") and the pins are inserted. Their points should just touch the subchondral bone. Two pins will combat rotation, and the combination of weight-bearing and muscle traction will compress the fracture line

4.11.6 Trauma Affecting the Growth Plate

Developmental deformities following arrested or altered bone growth are manifested by shortening, incongruency of the articular surfaces when paired bones are involved, angular deformity, or any combination of these. Indications for treatment are as follows:

1. Angular deformity of the lower extremity in the nearly mature or mature animal. Corrective osteotomy is usually indicated (see Chap. 6).
2. Premature closure of the distal or proximal radial physis (short radius syndrome). Osteotomy of the radius and lengthening to restore congruency of the elbow joint is required. It is preferable to use a lengthening apparatus. In animals over $5^1/_2$ months of age, one lengthening procedure will usually be sufficient. Those under this age may need a repeat procedure in 6–8 weeks to restore length and congruency again.
3. Premature closure of the distal ulnar physis. Growth cessation (short ulna syndrome) of the ulna has a bowstring effect on the radius, resulting in valgus deformity and outward rotation of the foot, and incongruency of the elbow joint. Removal of a 2- to 4-cm section of the distal ulna is necessary to remove the bowstring effect. To prevent early union of the ostectomy, the periosteum is stripped from the ostectomy area and either sutured over the bone segments or completely resected. Corrective osteotomy of the radius is usually carried out at the same time. An external fixator or a bone plate is used for the fixation of the radius (see Chap. 6).
4. Partial or complete premature closure of the distal radial and ulnar physis. Corrective osteotomy to restore congruency to the elbow joint and to realign the foot are the objectives. Treatment varies with individual cases. Since the traumatized leg is already shorter than the opposite leg, the surgical procedure should include lengthening or at least avoid further shortening.

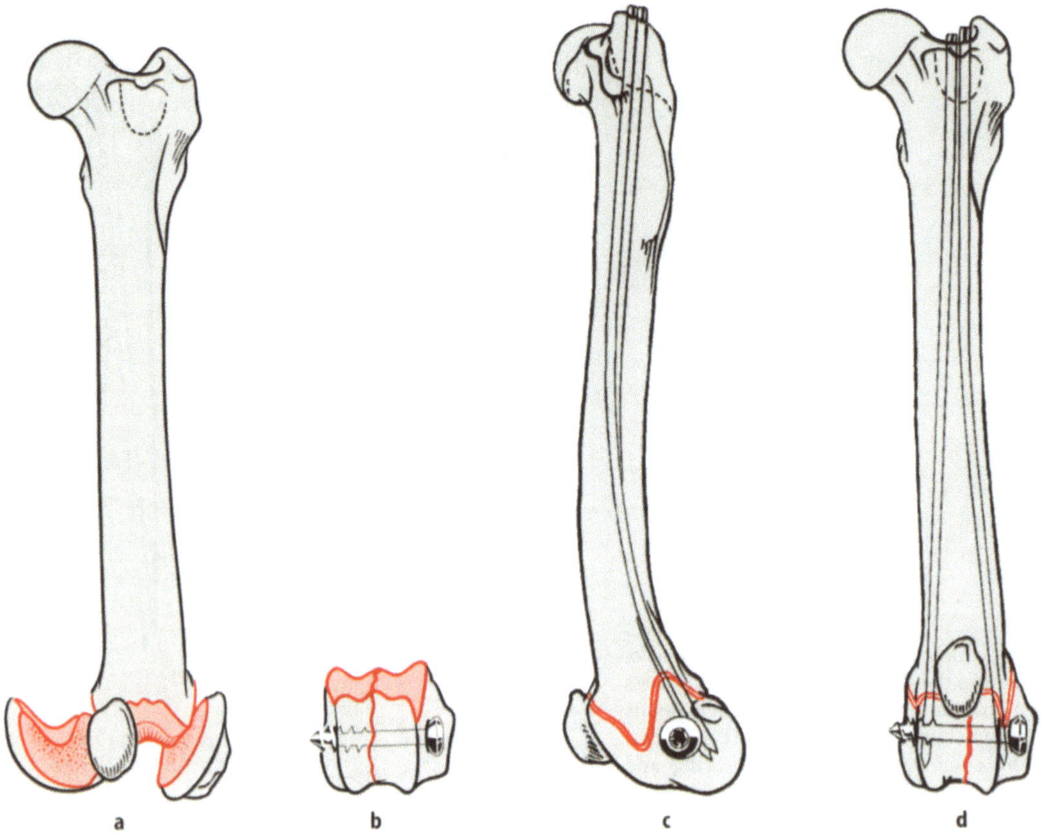

Fig. 4.135. **a** Type III fracture of the distal femoral epiphysis. **b** Both condyles are first reduced and then fixed with a transcondylar lag screw. **c, d** The condyles are attached to the shaft using two intramedullary pins. Supportive external immobilization is indicated for the first 10–14 days in most cases

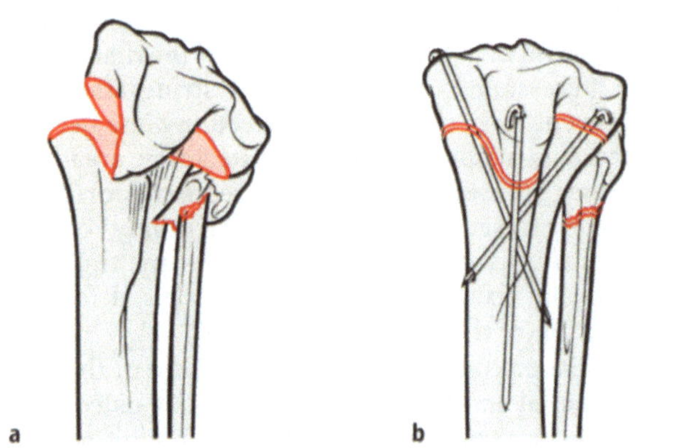

Fig. 4.136a,b. Examples and suggested methods of internal fixation for some of the commonly encountered fracture-separations of the tibia. **a** Type I separation of proximal tibial epiphysis. **b** Fixation with three Kirschner wires. Limb immobilization by bandage is usually indicated for 1–2 weeks

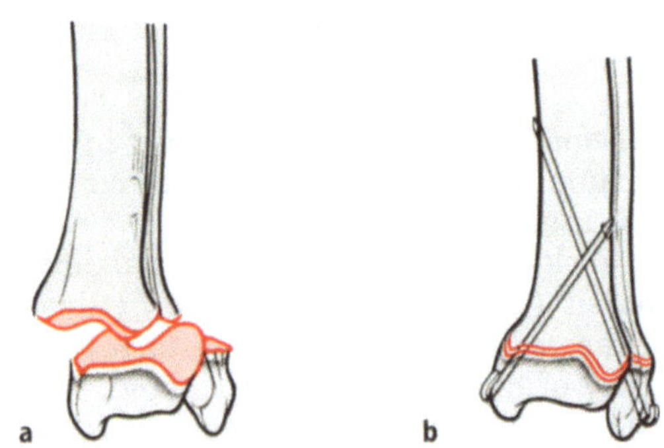

Fig. 4.137. **a** Fracture-separation of distal tibial epiphysis and fracture of fibula. **b** Fixation by two obliquely inserted Kirschner wires. The leg is also immobilized for about 2 weeks

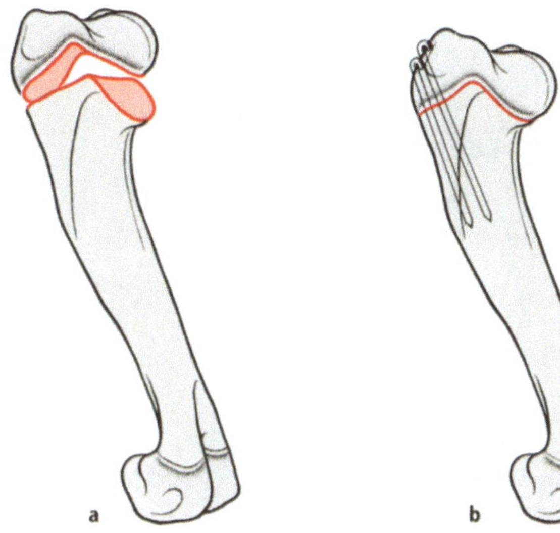

Fig. 4.138a,b. Examples and suggested methods of internal fixation for some of the commonly encountered fracture-separations of the humerus. **a** Type I separation of the proximal humeral epiphysis. **b** Fixation by inserting two pins into the ridge of the greater tubercle

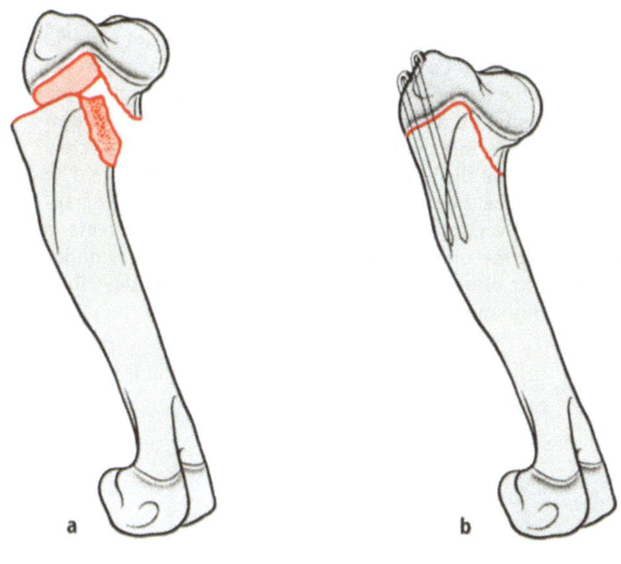

Fig. 4.139. **a** Type II fracture-separation of proximal humeral epiphysis. **b** Fixation by inserting two pins into the ridge of the greater tubercle. Activity should be restricted for 10–14 days

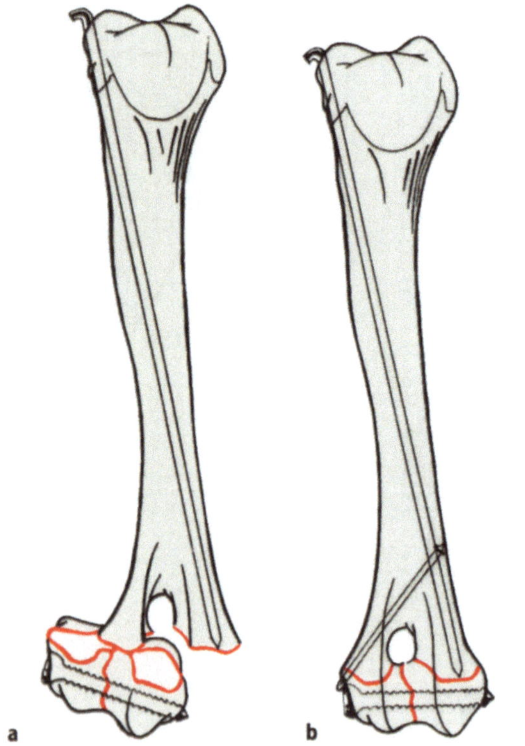

Fig. 4.140. **a** Type III (T type) fracture-separation of condyle of the humerus. **b** Fixation with a transcondylar lag screw, an intramedullary pin inserted into the medial portion of the condyle, and with a diagonal pin through the lateral portion of the condyle and shaft. A washer is fitted under the screw head to prevent the head from sinking into the soft bone. The screw size must be selected according to the size of the fragments; an oversized screw must be avoided. The screw is removed at the time of clinical union if the animal is under 4–5 months of age. The technique is the same as described for the adult animal (see Sect. 4.2.3)

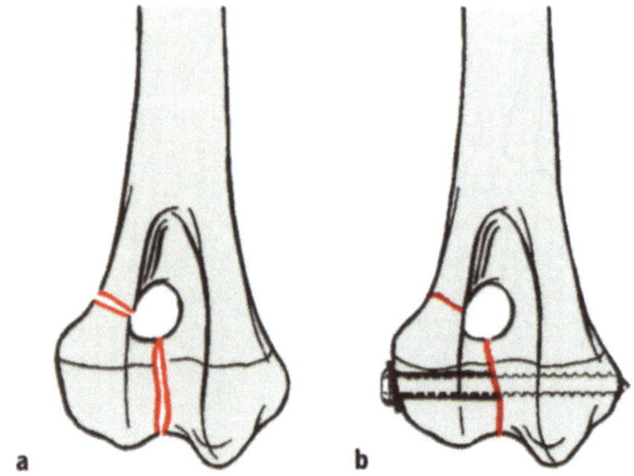

Fig. 4.141. **a** Type III (T type) fracture-separation of distal humeral condyle. **b** Fixation using a transcondylar lag screw and one or two Kirschner wires on both sides to fix the distal fragments to the shaft. In larger animals and those approaching maturity, the condyle is attached to the shaft by means of a plate

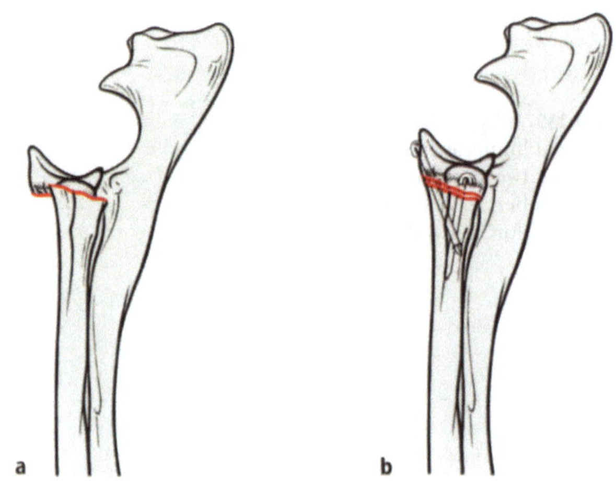

Fig. 4.142a,b. Examples and suggested methods of fixation for some of the fracture-separations involving the radius and ulna. **a** Type I separation of proximal radial epiphysis. **b** After reduction, stabilization is accomplished by inserting two or three Kirschner wires

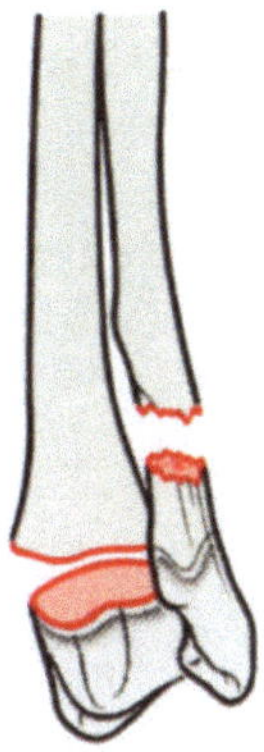

a

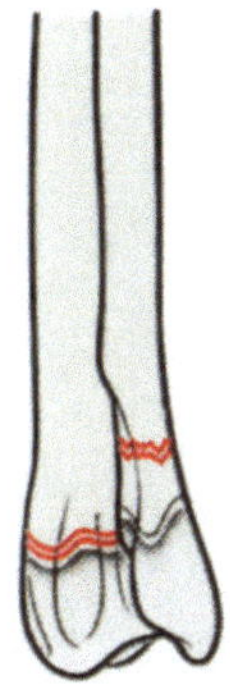

b

Fig. 4.143. **a** Type I separation of the distal radial epiphysis and fractured ulna. **b** In most cases these are reduced closed. They are stable and lend themselves to stabilization using a coaptation splint or cast. Most cases heal in 3–4 weeks. If unstable, they are pinned as in Fig. 1.133

Part III
Reconstructive Bone Surgery

5 Delayed Union and Nonunion

No surgeon embarks on an operation to repair a fracture expecting it to fail. However, despite this optimistic approach, fracture repairs may have some form of complication, with the incidence of delayed union and nonunion of fractures being approximately 4 %.

5.1 Delayed Union

A delayed union is defined as a fracture which has failed to heal within an anticipated period. The normal time it takes for a fracture to heal will naturally vary for any given bone, type of fracture, fracture location, age of the animal, and type of fixation. Shaft fractures, where the bone is primarily cortical with a minimal loss of bone substance and no complications, should heal in the times given in Table 5.1.

Fractures rigidly stabilized by a plate and screws may take longer to reach clinical union than those stabilized with less rigid methods. Direct cortical union, commonly observed with plate stabilization, is not supported by periosteal callus, but this does not inhibit function. The time it takes to achieve clinical union may be increased in the face of extensive comminution and/or bone loss or other complications such as infection. Metaphyseal and epiphyseal fractures unite more rapidly than cortical fractures because of the more abundant vascular supply to the cancellous bone. Serial radiographs are helpful in evaluating fracture union (Fig. 5.1).

5.1.1 Causes

The main causes of delayed union are:

1. Inadequate or inappropriate stabilization, usually as a result of a technical failure or inadequate preoperative and/or operative evaluation
2. A gap between the fragments due to bone loss, distraction, malpositioning, or soft tissue interposition
3. Vascular damage from the original trauma and/or surgery
4. Infection
5. Systemic or local tissue disease

Table 5.1. Times taken to reach clinical union

Age of animal	External skeletal and intramedullary pin fixation	Fixation with plates
Under 3 months	2–3 weeks	4 weeks
3–6 months	4–6 weeks	2–3 months
6–12 months	5–8 weeks	3–4 months
Over 1 year	7–12 weeks	5–8 months

5.1.2 Diagnosis

In many cases, the distinction between a delayed union and a nonunion is a matter of judgement. The time period since the fracture was repaired has to be considered against the clinical evaluation of the patient and the radiographic appearance of the fracture. Typically, a radiograph of a delayed union shows a persistent fracture line, evidence of nonbridging and sometimes profuse periosteal callus, an open marrow cavity, and no significant sclerosis.

5.1.3 Treatment

Appropriate treatment of a delayed union is determined by first identifying the underlying cause or causes. In many cases, this consists of continued and increased stabilization, combined with restriction of the animal's activity, until union occurs (Fig. 5.1a–e). Fractures initially immobilized by limb splintage may need rigid internal stabilization. Inadequate intramedullary fixation may require additional skeletal support with an external fixator or replacing a pin with plate and screws. Loose cerclage wires will need removal and replacement with tight loops or an alternative method, such as lag screw fixation.

When a delayed union is evident in fractures stabilized by a plate and screws, it is possible that the implants may have loosened, permitting movement at the fracture site. Loose screws may need to be replaced either by a larger size or redirected for better holding. The plate may have to be replaced by a longer one to regain rigid stabilization. In addition, cancellous bone grafts are indicated if there is an

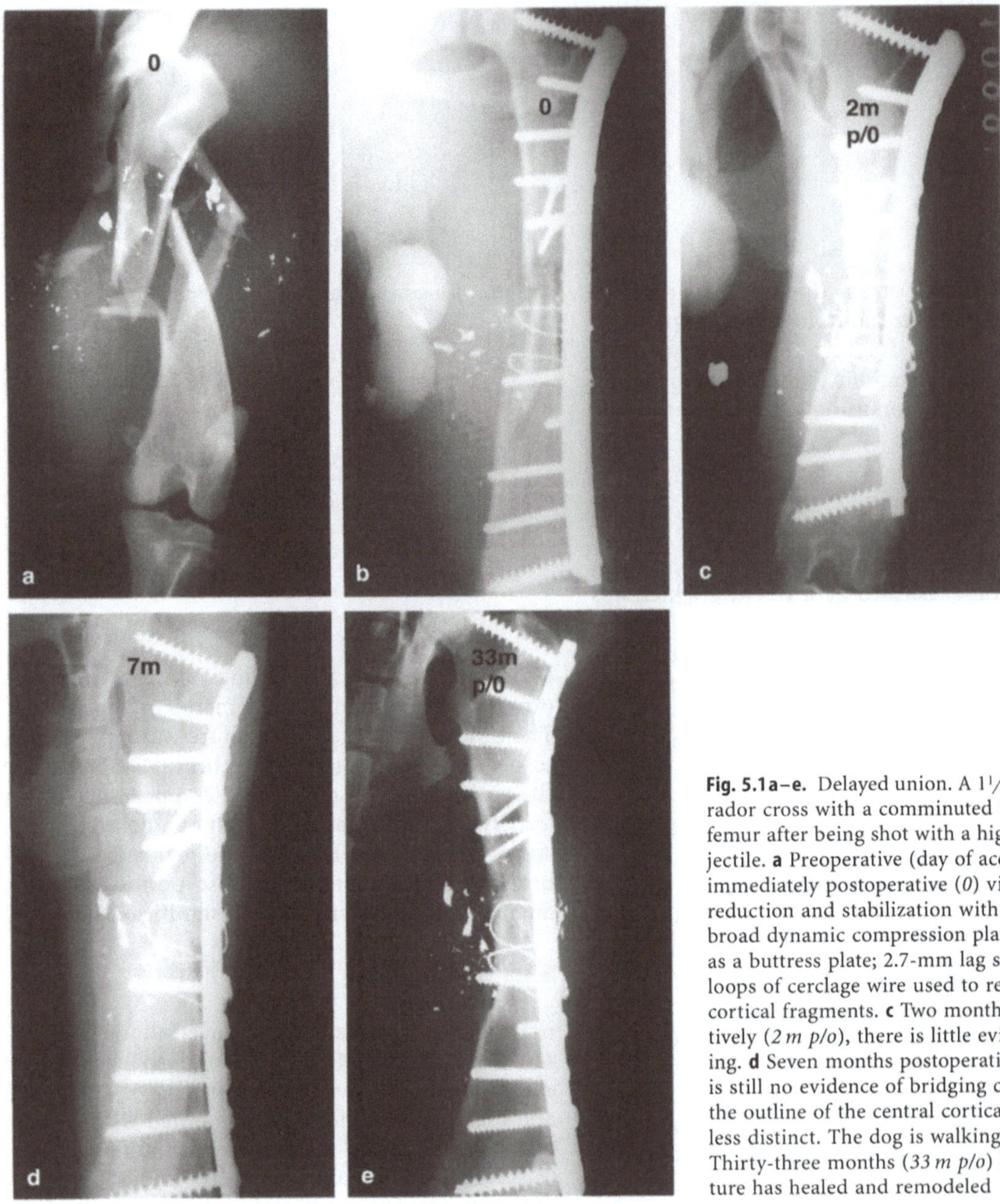

Fig. 5.1a–e. Delayed union. A 1½-year-old Labrador cross with a comminuted fracture of the femur after being shot with a high-velocity projectile. **a** Preoperative (day of accident, *0*) and **b** immediately postoperative (*0*) views following reduction and stabilization with a 4.5-mm broad dynamic compression plate (DCP) used as a buttress plate; 2.7-mm lag screws and two loops of cerclage wire used to retain two large cortical fragments. **c** Two months postoperatively (*2 m p/o*), there is little evidence of healing. **d** Seven months postoperatively (*7m*) there is still no evidence of bridging callus, although the outline of the central cortical fragments is less distinct. The dog is walking normally. **e** Thirty-three months (*33 m p/o*) later the fracture has healed and remodeled

insufficient buttress of cortical bone opposite the plate or necrosis of bone fragments. Delayed unions of periarticular and intra-articular fractures usually require additional internal fixation to achieve rigid stability of the fracture. Joint motion may promote loosening of the inadequately secured implants.

5.2 Nonunion

A nonunion fracture is defined as a fracture which has failed to heal and the process fracture healing has ceased. The fracture gap is filled with fibrocartilaginous tissue or a false joint (pseudarthrosis). Operative intervention is necessary to promote fracture union. Prevention of nonunion is often possible if the surgeon recognizes, at an earlier stage, that delay in union is taking place and thus implements steps to assist healing of the fracture (see Sect. 5.2.5).

An expected timetable for bone-healing in small animals is given in Table 5.1. Differentiation of a delayed union from a nonunion is based not only on time, but more specifically on serial radio-

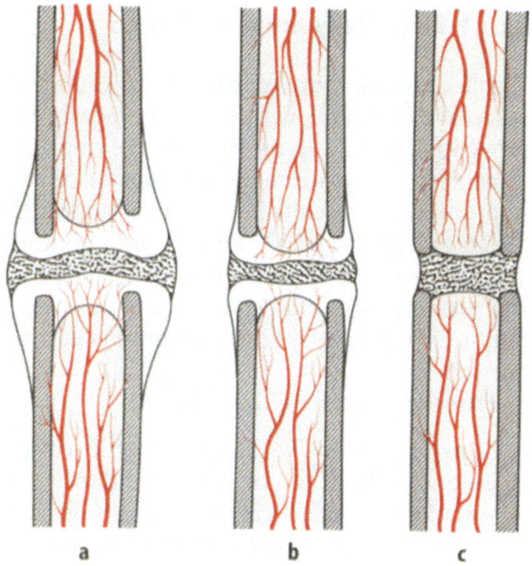

Fig. 5.2a–c. Biologically active nonunions. **a** Hypertrophic callus. **b** Minimal callus. **c** No visible callus

graphs. Except in young, growing dogs, it is unusual to diagnose a nonunion before 2 months after fracture. Nonunions occur less frequently in cats than in dogs.

5.2.1 Classification

A simple classification based on four factors is preferred:

1. Fracture site
2. Displacement of fragments
3. Presence or absence of infection
4. Biological activity

Although the fracture site (whether diaphyseal, metaphyseal, or epiphyseal) and the position of the fragments (whether displaced or in alignment) is of practical importance, the presence or absence of infection and the biological activity of the fracture, based on viability and osteogenic potential (which relates directly to the vascularity), is of greater clinical importance.

Weber and Cech (1976) classified nonunions as biologically active, with good vascularity and varying degrees of callus formation, or as nonviable and inactive, with little or without callus formation and inadequate vascularity. These two groups can be further subdivided based on the radiographic findings (Figs. 5.2, 5.3).

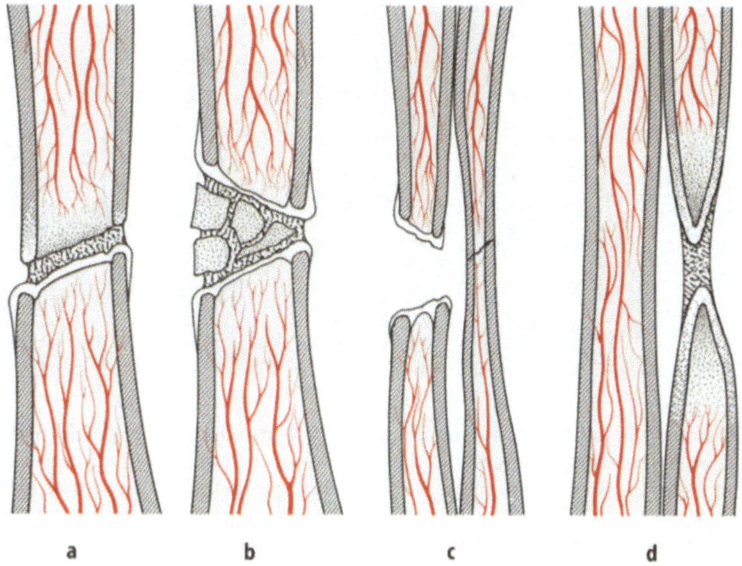

Fig. 5.3a–d. Biologically inactive nonuions. **a** Dystrophic. **b** Necrotic. **c** Defect. **d** Atrophic

5.2.1.1 Biologically Active Nonunions

Viable nonunions are typified by an abundant, well-vascularized callus, with fibrocartilage in the fracture gap (Fig. 5.2). In most cases, the cause is failure to achieve adequate reduction and stability of the fracture, which results in excessive motion between the fragments (Fig. 5.4). This form of nonunion has a much better prognosis than the nonviable type and usually responds well to stabilization of the fracture, particularly if the fragments can be compressed.

Three subtypes are described:

1. *Hypertrophic callus.* Hypertrophic callus nonunion is typified by an abundance of well-vascularized wide callus with fibrocartilage in the fracture gap. This response is usually associated with insufficient stabilization and is typically seen when an intramedullary pin is used as the sole method of fixation of a rotationally unstable fracture (Fig. 5.5).
2. *Slightly hypertrophic callus.* This type of nonunion is characterized by a "narrow" callus and is a variation of the previous type. It is usually associated with continued slight motion at the fracture site following inadequate internal fixation with a plate and screws.
3. *Oligotrophic callus.* These nonunions have no evidence of callus and can easily be mistaken for the biologically inactive nonunion. They may be associated with gross displacement of the fracture fragments. The ends of the fragments may take on a rounded and demineralized appearance (Fig. 5.6). The viability can be verified either by techniques designed to appraise the regional blood supply or by the clinical response to reduction and stabilization of the fracture. This type of nonunion may be encountered with untreated avulsion fractures.

5.2.1.2 Biologically Inactive Nonunions

Nonviable nonunions are typified by an absence of callus, lack of blood supply, necrotic bone fragments, and bone atrophy (Fig. 5.3). The bone ends may have a rounded, osteoporotic appearance with a sealed medullary canal. Four subgroups are recognized, and they all have a poor potential for healing. The incidence of nonviable nonunion is much lower than that of the biologically active type.

Four subtypes have been described:

1. *Dystrophic nonunion.* This type is associated with comminuted fractures in which an intermediate fragment is poorly vascularized and

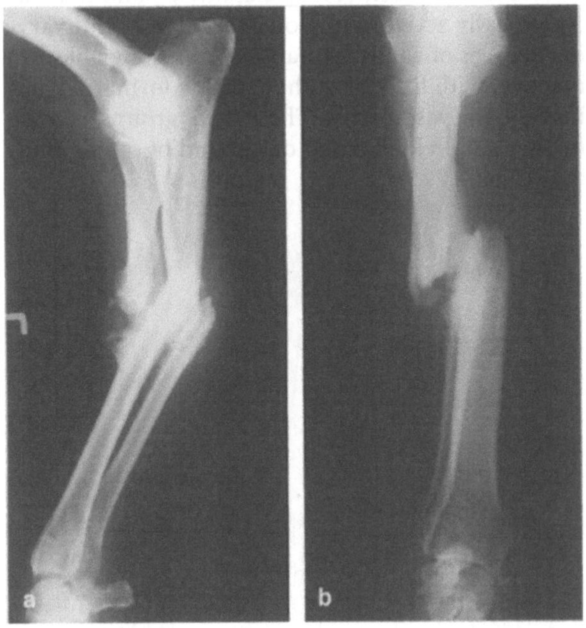

Fig. 5.4a,b. Biologically active nonunion. Three-year-old Australian Kelpie with a nonunion of the midshaft of the radius and ulna. The limb had been cast for 2 months and then the dog confined for a further month. **a** Lateral and **b** craniocaudal views of the fracture. There is a false joint present and evidence of periosteal callus formation

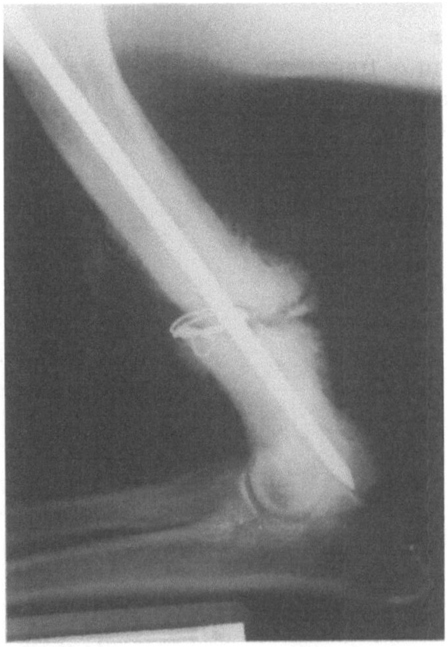

Fig. 5.5. Biologically active nonunion, hypertrophic callus. Two-year-old Bull Terrier with nonunion of a short oblique midshaft humeral fracture 3 months after treatment with an intramedullary pin and cerclage wire. This combination of implants is inadequate to neutralize the rotational forces present at the fracture site

necrotic. This interferes with callus formation and fracture repair (Fig. 5.7).

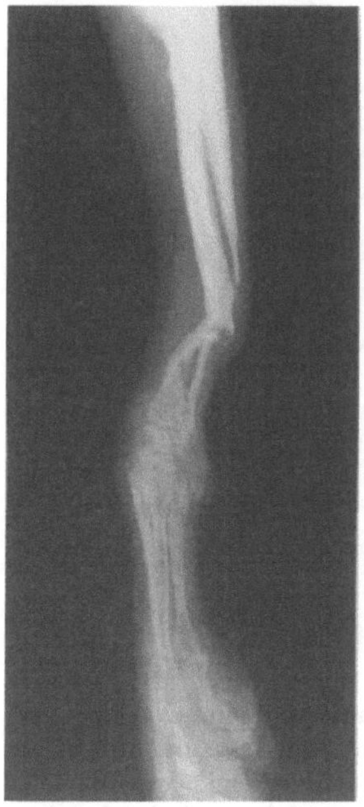

Fig. 5.6. Biologically active nonunion, oligotrophic callus. Two-year-old Poodle with a nonunion of the distal shaft of the radius and ulna after the fracture was immobilized in a cast for 12 months. This fracture appears radiographically to be very similar to an atrophic nonunion, but in fact the fracture healed 2 months after internal reduction, cancellous bone grafting, and external fixation with a type-2 external fixator

2. *Necrotic nonunion.* This type is associated with comminuted and/or infected fractures where there is extensive loss of vascularity to the fragments. Serial radiographs reveal that the fragments are not taking part in the healing process.
3. *Defect nonunion.* In this type, bone loss due to the injury, surgical intervention, or infection has resulted in a large defect, which is filled with inactive soft tissue (Fig. 5.8).

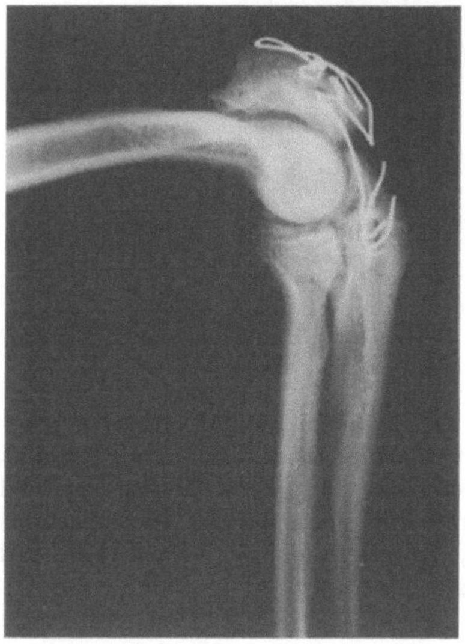

Fig. 5.8. Biologically inactive nonunion, defect type. Ten-year-old Poodle with a 4-year history of nonunion of the olecranon. There is not any evidence of union despite bone grafts and repeated attempts at internal fixation

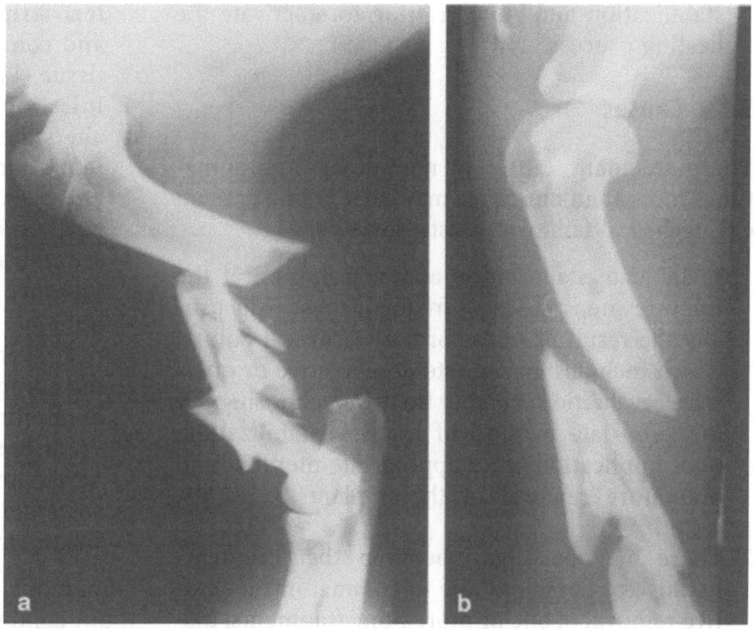

Fig. 5.7a,b. Biologically inactive nonunions, dystrophic type. Two-year-old male cat with a highly comminuted fracture of the humeral shaft which was treated by closed reduction and stabilization with a type-1 external fixator. **a** Preoperative appearance. **b** Three months later following loosening of the fixator. The distal fragments have united, but there is an inactive nonunion at the proximal end of the shaft fracture

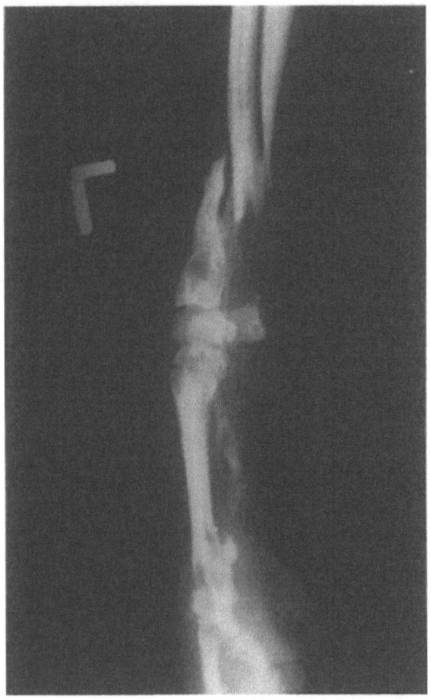

Fig. 5.9. Biologically inactive nonunion, atrophic type. Two-year-old Poodle with a fracture of the distal radius and ulna following a fall. Nonunion is present despite repeated attempts at stabilization with pins and a cast. These fractures are better treated by internal fixation with small plates and screws from the outset

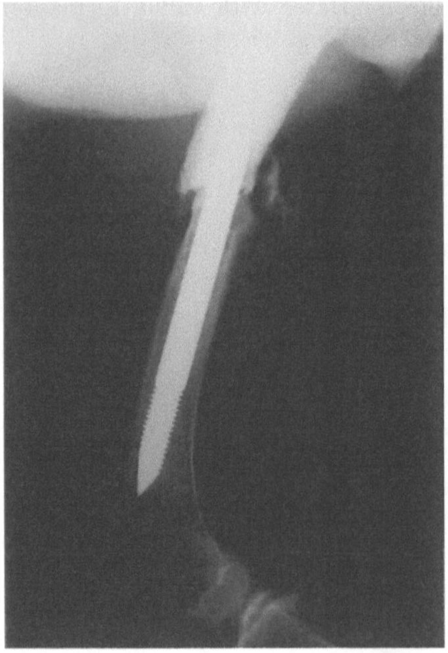

Fig. 5.10. Technical failure as cause of nonunion. Four-year-old Irish Setter with a midshaft transverse fracture of the femur 3 months after treatment with a single large-diameter intramedullary pin. The wrong method of fixation was selected in this case; the pin does nothing to prevent rotational forces at the fracture site

4. *Atrophic nonunion.* The bone ends are atrophied, rounded, and sealed, and the surrounding bone is osteoporotic. This type of nonunion occurs most frequently in fractures of the extremities of adult toy breeds of dog, particularly fractures of the distal radius and ulna that have been treated with a cast (Fig. 5.9). These cases require both stabilization and bone grafting to reactivate the healing process.

5.2.2 Causes

There are many causes of nonunions, and sometimes more than one cause may exist in one patient, e.g., technical failure and osteomyelitis:

1. Inadequate stabilization allowing motion at the fracture site is the most frequent cause. It is usually the result of some form of technical failure, which includes inadequate preoperative or operative evaluation of the fracture, choosing an inappropriate method of fracture stabilization, poor application of an appropriate method, and premature removal of the implants (Figs. 5.9, 5.10).
2. There may be a gap between the fragments because of bone loss due to trauma, intraoperative removal of one or more bone fragments, distraction by muscular forces or implants, malpositioning, or soft tissue interposition. This gap allows for fibrous and/or cartilaginous ingrowth rather than bone formation (Fig. 5.8).
3. Loss of blood supply to bone may result from the trauma of a high-velocity impact or from intraoperative trauma. This includes excessive periosteal stripping, damage to the nutrient vessels, and comminution or crushing of bone and soft tissue (Fig. 5.11).
4. Infection results in lowered local pH, which alters the local calcium homeostasis. In addition, infarction of the local blood supply leads to dead and sclerotic bone at the fracture site. Devitalized and infected cortical fragments may sequestrate. However, fractures will heal in the presence of infection, provided the fixation remains stable. Implants tend to loosen more readily in infected bone. Motion appears to be the common denominator in perpetuating both nonunion and infection (Fig. 5.12).
5. Predisposing factors which may contribute to the development of nonunions include old age, corticosteroid or anticoagulant therapy, radiation treatment, burns, and cachexia.

Nonunions are best avoided by providing the optimum conditions for fracture healing from the out-

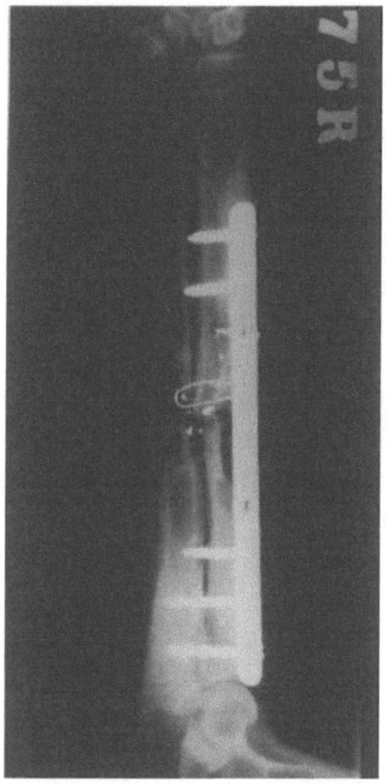

Fig. 5.11. Loss of blood supply as cause of nonunion. Three-year-old Labrador that sustained a midshaft fracture of the radius and ulna after being shot with a .22-caliber bullet. The fracture has been stabilized with a bone plate and screws. The fracture has failed to unite due to loss of blood supply, caused by the combination of operative interference and damage to the soft tissues by the impact of the bullet

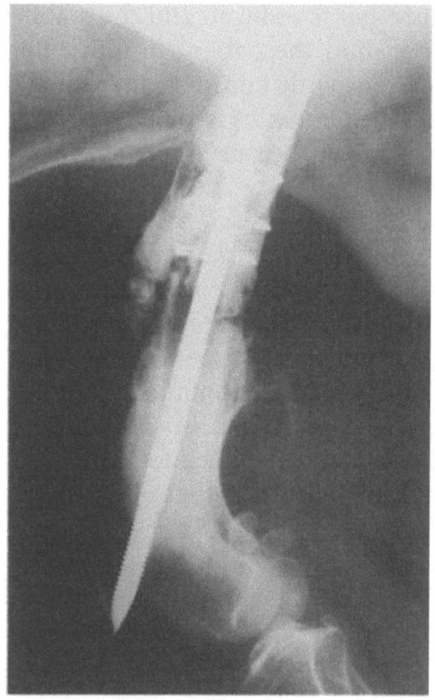

Fig. 5.12. Infection as cause of nonunion. One-year-old Poodle with a comminuted midshaft femoral fracture, 5 months following treatment by repeated attempts at intramedullary pin fixation and cerclage wiring. The pin penetrated the cranial cortex of the femur and entered the stifle joint. Pus was pouring from the wound and dead bone was present at the fracture site. A resistant *Escherichia coli* was cultured from the fracture. The nonunion is the result of infection and technical failure

set and taking early action if a delayed union is apparent.

5.2.3 Clinical Diagnosis

The diagnosis of a nonunion is based on an evaluation of the history, the clinical signs, and the radiographs. Repeated examinations may be needed to determine whether the process of fracture healing is progressing normally. Enlargement of the fracture area, pain on palpation of the fracture site, and lameness are the main clinical findings. However, the amount of pain and lameness varies considerably between individuals and is not a reliable guideline. Pronounced disuse of the limb will result in muscle atrophy, joint stiffness, and osteoporosis. Deformity of the limb is associated with hypertrophic callus formation and/or malalignment of the fragments. These changes are manifestations of fracture disease.

Instability at the fracture site is a clear indication of nonunion, but the amount and type of instability (e.g., angular or rotational) may be quite subtle and difficult to detect, especially if the fracture is adjacent to a joint. Stressed radiographs can be helpful in evaluating subtle degrees of instability.

5.2.4 Radiographic Diagnosis

Signs vary according to the type of nonunion, as noted above (see Sect. 5.2.1). Sclerosis at the fracture site with a gap between the fragments, a sealed marrow cavity, and smooth fracture surfaces may be evident, with demineralization and/or atrophy of bone distal to the fracture. Osteomedullography can be used to differentiate between a delayed union and a nonunion. Under general anesthesia and using an aseptic technique, a small amount (3–5 ml) of iodized contrast is injected into the medullary canal of the distal fragment using a bone marrow biopsy needle. Pressure is applied to the surrounding soft tissues to prevent leakage. In normal fracture repair, the contrast will flow across the fracture gap after about 3 weeks; failure of the contrast to flow indicates that a nonunion exists.

5.2.5 Treatment

If possible, it is important to identify the cause of nonunion so that the correct treatment can be implemented. In many cases, treatment involves compression of the nonunion to achieve rigid stabilization. The fracture gap is reduced and the stability of the fracture enables the patient to move the limb and to bear weight with minimal discomfort, thus preventing further muscle atrophy, fibrosis, and joint stiffness, while at the same time stimulating the circulation.

Under the influence of compression and stability, vascular pseudarthrotic fibrous tissue and cartilage will be replaced by bone. In these circumstances, it is not necessary to remove the interposed tissue, unless it is interfering with realignment of the fracture fragments. Nondisplaced nonunions should therefore be compressed and fixed in situ with as little bone exposure and disturbance to the blood supply as possible. Normally, only the callus which interferes with the application of the plate is removed; the rest is left, as it will heal and remodel once effective stabilization is provided. Resected callus can be retained and used as a bone graft (Fig. 5.13).

In displaced nonunions, the pseudarthrotic tissue is excised, partially or totally, to achieve reduction (Fig. 5.14). The medullary canal is opened and the fragment ends are cut, if possible, in a stepwise fashion to convert shear forces into axial compression. Stabilization will promote union even in the presence of infection. Cancellous bone grafts are always used when there is a defect and biologically inactive and nonviable bone.

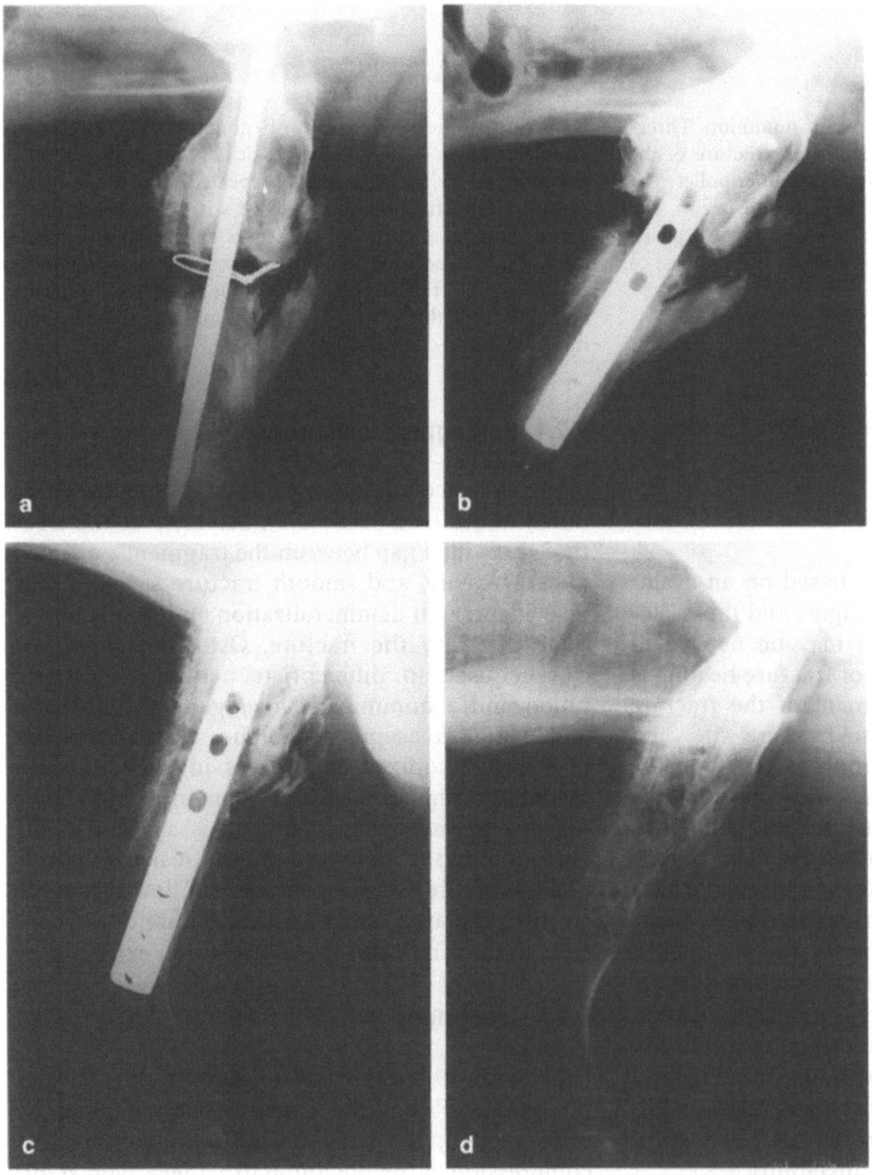

Fig. 5.13a–d. 1½-year-old Briard with a nonunion of a midshaft femoral fracture. **a** Three months after internal fixation with an intramedullary pin and a single cerclage wire. **b** Immediately following implant removal and stabilization with compression using a 3.5-mm broad dynamic compression plate (DCP). Only the periosteal callus necessary to insert the plate was removed. Despite the fact that the fracture was compressed, a large gap was apparent on the radiograph. **c** Three months later, the fracture had healed and the periosteal callus appeared less active. **d** Four months after surgery, the implants were removed

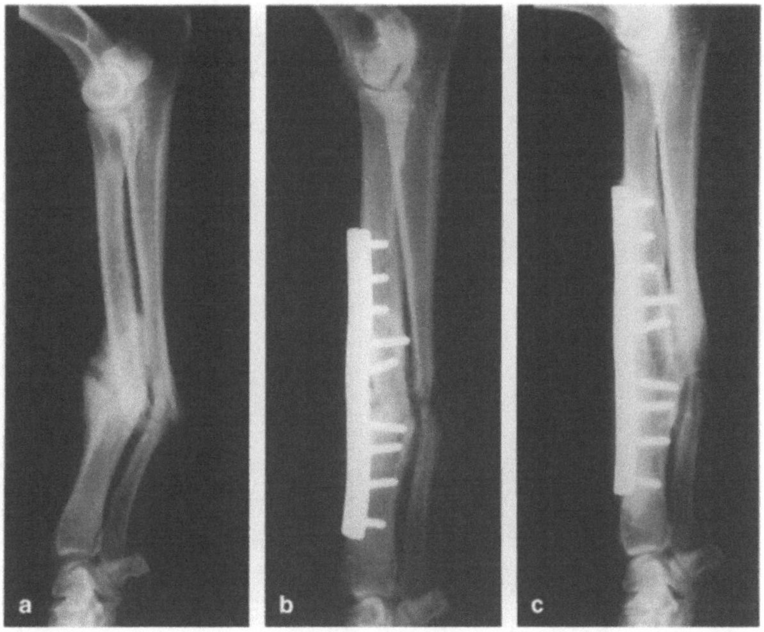

Fig. 5.14a–c. Two-year-old Rhodesian Ridgeback with a displaced midshaft nonunion of the radius and ulna. **a** Three months after treatment with a cast. **b** Immediately following open reduction, partial resection of the pseudoarthrosis, and stabilization with compression using a 3.5-mm broad dynamic compression plate (DCP). Callus has been used as a bone graft in the radius. **c** Six months later, the fracture has united and remodeled. A synostosis is present between the radius and ulna

5.2.5.1 Diaphyseal (Noninfected) Nonunions

Treatment of nondisplaced nonunions with a compression plate is preferable to other methods because of the greater stability achieved (Figs. 5.13, 5.14). Standard surgical approaches are utilized to expose the nonunion. All previously placed implants that are unstable are removed, and only the bone surface where the plate is to be placed is exposed. Compression, using the 3.5-mm or 4.5-mm dynamic compression plate (DCP) principle, is adequate provided the fracture gap is less than 4.0 mm (3.2 mm for the 2.7-mm plate). With wider gaps, the tension device should be used to gain maximum compression of the pseudarthrotic tissue and to regain stability. The tension device can only be used with the 4.5-mm plating system. Removal of excess callus where the plate is to be applied may be necessary to ensure that the plate is contoured correctly for normal shaft and joint alignment. At least a six-hole plate should be utilized, but a longer one is preferred wherever bone length allows. In nonunions with very osteoporotic bone, fully threaded cancellous screws may be necessary for secure fixation in cortical bone. Drill holes may also be filled with bone cement for better screw anchorage. Interfragmentary compression may be used in oblique nonunion fractures.

An alternative approach for nonunions with large bone defects is to use a technique first described by Ilizarov to move an osteotomized segment of the diaphysis from one side of a nonunion to the other, using an external fixator with threaded bars. Fine wires placed transcutaneously into the fracture fragments are attached to clamps, which in turn are attached to the threaded external bars. The clamps can then be used to gradually transport a segment of bone (about 1 mm per day) which has been osteotomized from one end of the fracture gap across to the other end. This technique relies on the formation of new bone within the ever-lengthening osteotomy site and is called distraction osteosynthesis. When contact between the transported segment of bone and the site of the nonunion is established, a cancellous bone graft is performed and the external fixator is modified to provide sufficient rigidity to prevent bone motion during weight bearing (Figs. 5.15–5.17). In displaced nonunions, the procedure differs only in that greater exposure is required. More soft tissue and callus is removed at the nonunion site in order to achieve correct axial alignment. All interposing pseudarthrotic tissue should be removed and the marrow cavity opened to allow for more rapid revascularization. This compensates somewhat for the surrounding vascular impairment caused by the realignment process. The addition of a cancellous bone graft is indicted in these cases.

The wound is closed in layers and a compressive dressing applied for 2–3 days postoperatively. Drains are used if tissue pockets are present. They should be removed as soon as drainage has ceased, usually by 48 h. Active but controlled (leash) exercise is advocated. Eventual removal of the plates is in accordance with the described technique.

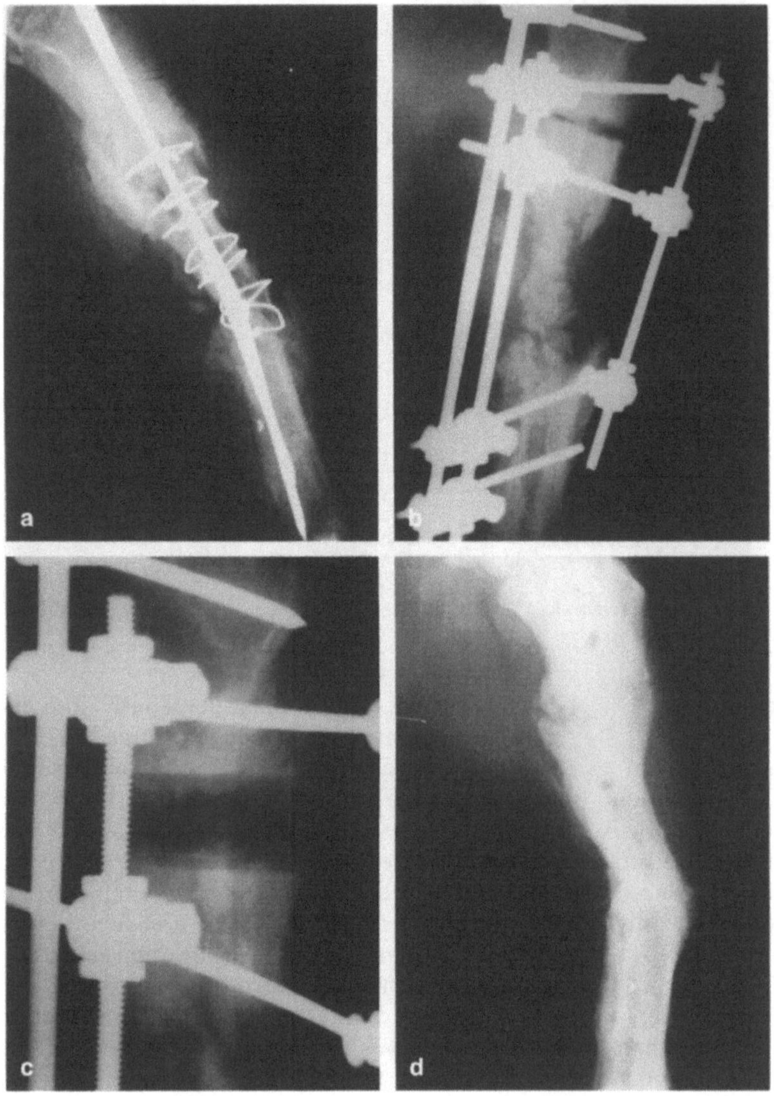

Fig. 5.15a–d. Distraction osteosynthesis in a dog. (Courtesy of A. Lesser). **a** A long oblique tibial fracture fixed with two intramedullary pins failed after 9 weeks. An infected, atrophic nonunion with a 7-cm mid-diaphyseal sequestrum was present. **b** The sequestrum was excised, the bed grafted, and a free bone segment created in the proximal tibia via an osteotomy of the proximal fragment. A bilateral external fixator was constructed with two threaded bars to allow the controlled distraction of the free bone segment. **c** At 3 weeks, calcification of the distracted callus is visible emanating from both edges and lining up along the lines of distraction. A 4-mm fibrous interzone (radiolucent area) persists, denoting active distraction. **d** At 15 weeks, the graft has hypertrophied to full cortical thickness along with the area of distracted new callus, and the apparatus was removed

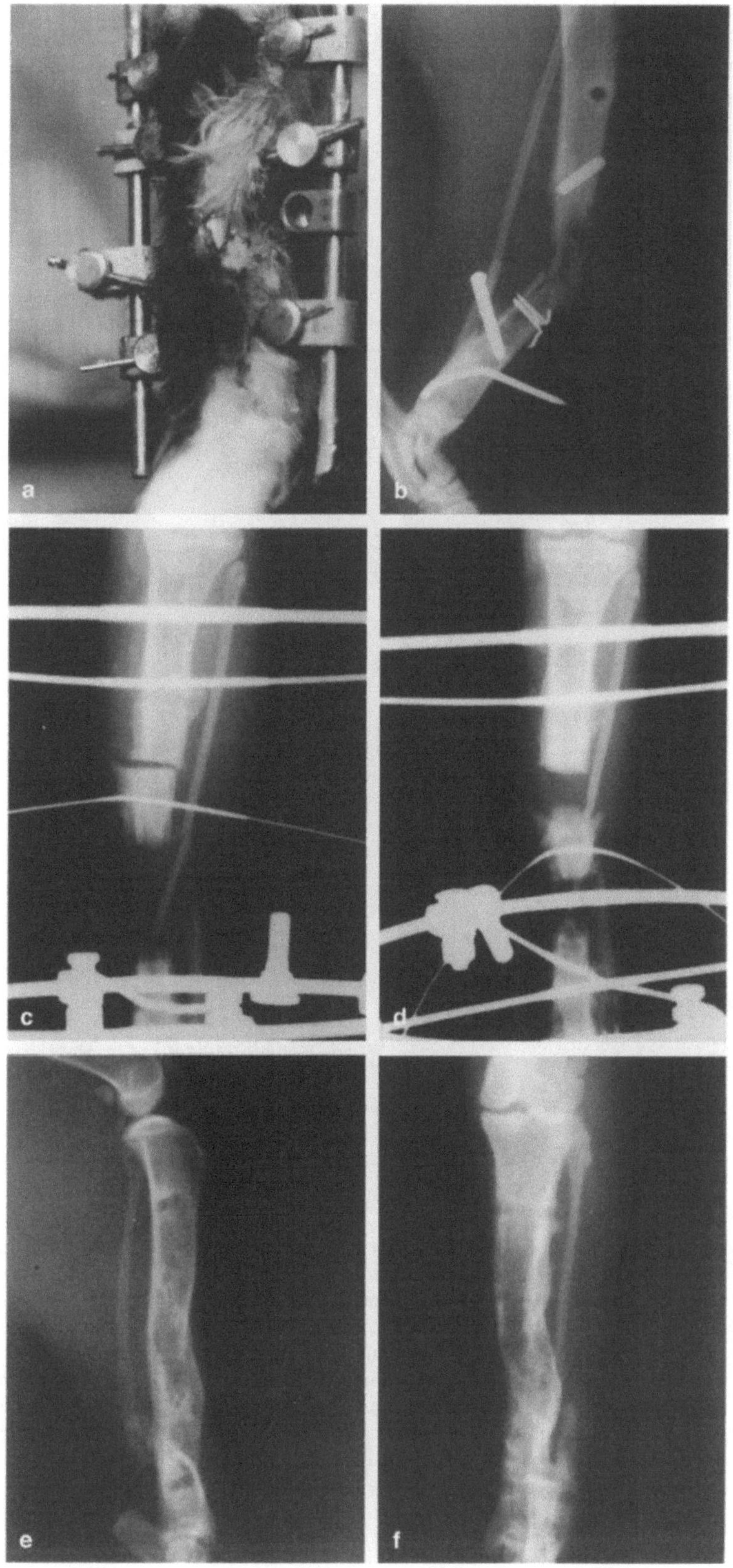

Fig. 5.16a–f. Distraction osteosyntheses in a cat. (Courtesy of A. Lesser.) **a** A cat presented with an open, infected nonunion of the right tibia. Dead bone is visible. **b** Radiograph of the leg showing devitalized bone at the ends of both fragments. **c** A 2-cm gap was created after the dead bone had been excised, and a free bone segment was created in the proximal fragment with an osteotomy. **d** The bone segment has been advanced toward the distal fragment 1 cm in the first week. **e** Lateral and **f** craniocaudal view at 11 months; the gap is filled with mature bone

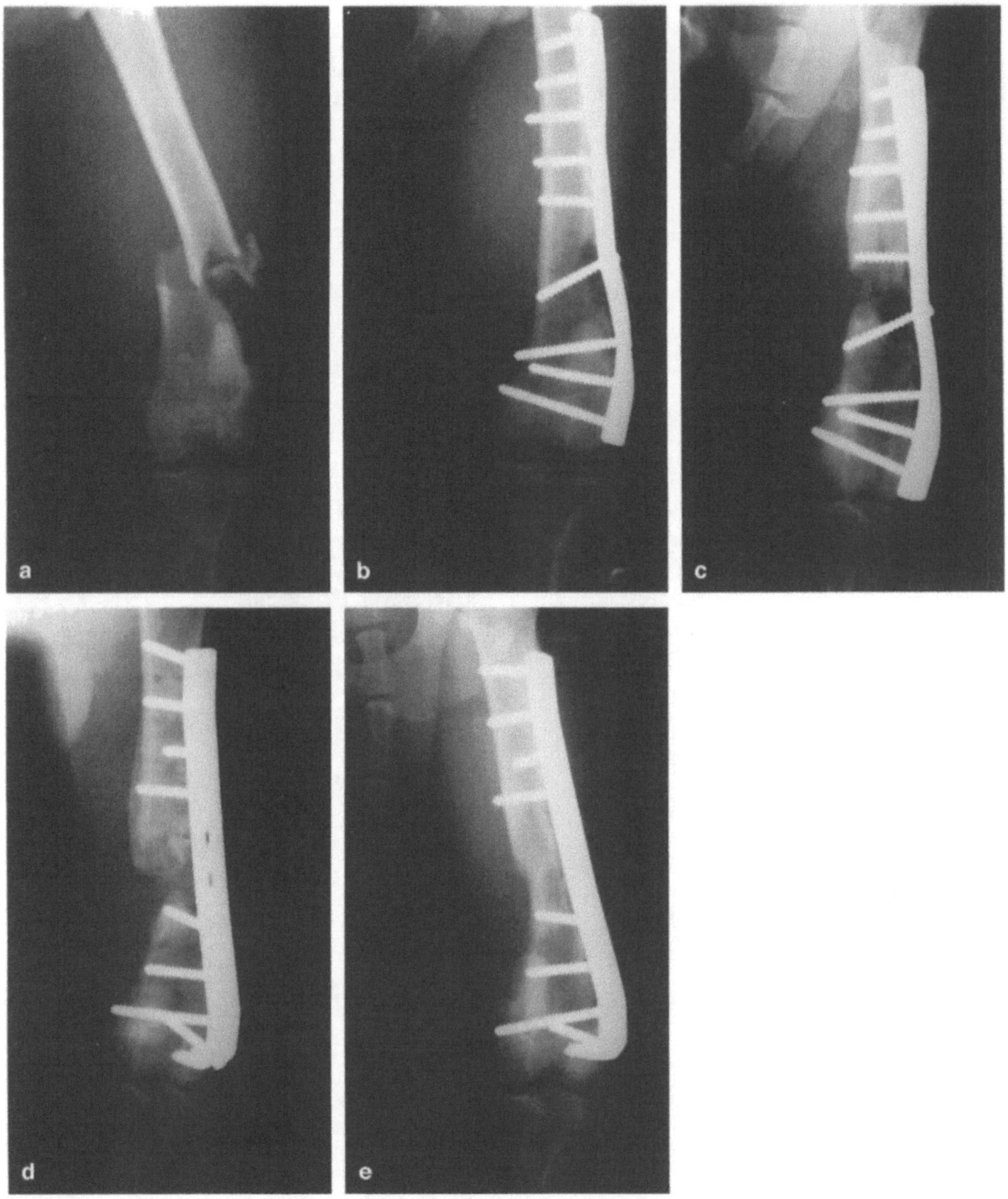

Fig. 5.17a–e. Two-year-old Bull Terrier that was hit by a car and sustained midshaft humeral and femoral fractures. **a** Preoperative view of the distal femoral fracture. **b** Immediately following internal fixation with a 3.5-mm broad dynamic compression plate (DCP). During reduction of the fracture, some of the smaller fragments were removed. A suction drain was inserted for the first 24 h. **c** Two months later, the fracture gap has widened, some of the implants are loosening, and the dog is reluctant to bear weight on the limb. A nonunion was diagnosed with the possibility of osteomyelitis. **d** Immediately following a second operation in which the original implants were replaced by a customized hook plate fashioned from a 3.5-mm broad DCP used as a buttress plate. The hook plate was selected to insure that the plate had adequate fixation in the short distal metaphyseal fragment. A cancellous bone graft was inserted. A culture revealed *Staphylococcus intermedius* infection. **e** Three months following the second surgery, the fracture had united and the dog was walking normally

5.2.5.2 Metaphyseal and Epiphyseal (Noninfected) Nonunions

Metaphyseal and epiphyseal nonunions are often more difficult to treat because of concurrent joint stiffness, loss of cancellous bone substance, and the unequal length of the fracture fragments. Stiff joints should be mobilized by open joint capsulotomy or capsulectomy and resection of hypertrophic synovial membrane and adhesions. Free bone fragments and restrictive hypertrophic bone should be removed. If the articular surface is involved, the fragments should be accurately aligned and maintained temporarily with Kirschner wires to facilitate interfragmentary compression with one or more lag screws. Fixation of the reconstructed metaphyseal-epiphyseal fragment to the diaphysis with special compression plates, such as the T,Y, or L plate, reconstruction plate, or hook plate, is preferable (Fig. 5.18). In some cases, the size and shape of the bone fragments may dictate the use of an external fixator or one or more Kirschner wires instead.

Apart from the very effective use of the technique of tension band wiring in the treatment of distracted nonunions, there is very little indication for the use of intramedullary pins and cerclage wires in the management of nonunions. Cancellous bone grafts are rarely indicated except where there are gaps. Early, active motion is essential in order for normal joint motion to return.

5.2.5.3 Atrophic Nonunions

Atrophic nonunions require not only stabilization, usually with plates and screws, but also aggressive débridement and bone grafting to stimulate osteogenesis. The medullary canal should be opened by reaming, usually with a small drill or an intramedullary pin, and the intervening callus resected. Elevation of the surrounding periosteum with the flakes of cortical bone attached (shingling or decortication) is frequently practiced in human orthopedic patients, but in very small animals it is difficult to perform and impractical. Autogenous cancellous bone grafts should be incorporated in the treatment of all biologically inactive nonunions, especially where there are necrotic fragments or bone loss. Bone grafts act as a stimulus to reactivate the dormant fracture-healing process in these biologically inactive nonunions. In large defects, autogenous corticocancellous bone may be necessary in addition to cancellous bone. A frozen allograft may be substituted if autogenous bone is not available, but this is not as effective.

In some cases of atrophic nonunion, satisfactory fracture union is never achieved; instead, the animals walk on the limb supported entirely by the implant. It is also important to recognize that in certain circumstances it may not be appropriate to offer any treatment other than amputation. Animals with severe soft tissue contraction, peripheral nerve injuries, severe osteoarthritis adjacent to the nonunion, and severe osteoporosis may fall into this category.

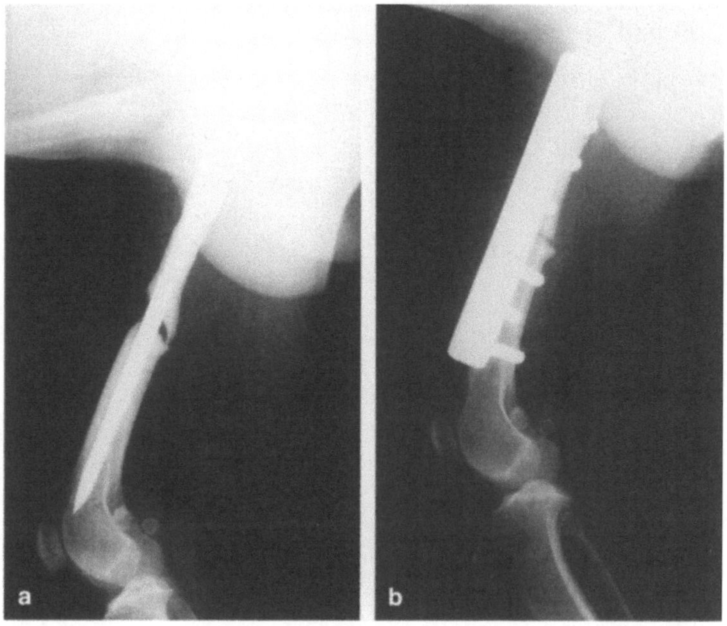

Fig. 5.18a,b. Three-year-old Poodle with a midshaft femoral fracture. **a** Four months following internal fixation with an intramedullary pin, there was not any evidence of fracture union and there was minimal periosteal activity. The dog was non-weight bearing and the fracture was palpably unstable. **b** Immediately following internal fixation with compression using a 2.7-mm dynamic compression plate (DCP). The fracture ends were resected and a cancellous graft, taken from the proximal tibia, inserted into the fracture site

5.2.6 Infected Nonunions

Osteomyelitis is defined as inflammation of a bone and the accompanying soft tissue elements of the marrow, endosteum, periosteum, Volkmann's canals, and haversian spaces. It is usually caused by an aerobic and/or anaerobic bacterial infection. The organisms most commonly cultured are *Staphylococcus* (45 %–75 %), *Escherichia coli*, *Pseudomonas*, *Proteus*, and various anaerobes, including *Actinomyces* and *Clostridium*.

It is of great concern that about 60 % of osteomyelitis cases result from intraoperative, iatrogenic contamination of closed fractures that have undergone open reduction and internal fixation. Many of these orthopedic disasters could be avoided by applying the principles of aseptic and atraumatic surgery. The presence of bacteria alone is not sufficient to cause osteomyelitis. Other factors, including instability of the fracture, vascular stasis, dead bone, and foreign bodies such as surgical implants, render the surrounding tissues susceptible to bacterial infection.

For details on the treatment of acute and chronic osteomyelitis, see Sect. 3.12.

6 Osteotomy

Osteotomy is an elective surgical procedure in which the bone is cut, realigned, and stabilized until union occurs. The usual purpose of osteotomy is correction of bone deformity, joint incongruity, or a combination of both. These problems usually result from trauma or disorders of growth and development.

6.1 Indications

Specific indications for osteotomy include:

1. Asynchronous growth of paired bones, such as radius and ulna, due to Salter type V injury
2. Asymmetric epiphysiodesis and angular deformity that result from a growth plate injury
3. Malunited diaphyseal and pelvic fractures
4. Torsional or angular deformities
5. Shortening deformities of a bone or an entire limb
6. Developmental joint diseases, such as hip dysplasia
7. Surgical approach to a bone or joint by osteotomy of a bone prominence, such as olecranon, in order to facilitate exposure

6.2 Planning

While the basic principles of internal fixation are the same as for fractures, considerable presurgical planning for an osteotomy is a prerequisite for success. It is essential to ensure that the bone is cut in the correct place(s), that soft tissues will tolerate repositioning of bone fragments, and that the fixation is biomechanically appropriate to allow union to occur. The aim of the operation should be total restoration of the bone's geometry by correction of angular, rotational, and length deformities. In examining the patient and radiographs, attention is paid to the entire limb, not just to the obviously deformed bone. Developmental deformities may affect several bones and may require multiple osteotomies. Furthermore, long-standing angular and rotational deformities alter joint loading and may produce ligament laxity, subluxation, cartilage erosion, and secondary osteoarthritis. These complications can adversely effect the prognosis after corrective osteotomy.

Currently, radiographs provide the most useful information for planning an osteotomy in animals. At least two views that include the proximal and distal joints are needed. Radiographs of the contralateral normal bone provide a valuable reference for determination of normal length and curvature, the latter being a feature of most canine long bones. Angular deformity may be apparent in more than one radiographic view. If there is a significant degree of angular deformity in both the craniocaudal and mediolateral radiographic views, then the deformity lies in an oblique plane. Additional oblique views are needed to determine the actual direction of the angular deformity. The degree of angular deformity can also be calculated mathematically, but the degree of rotational deformity is best determined by computed tomography. However, some estimations can be made by clinical examination and by evaluating the relative positions of proximal and distal joints on one or more radiographs. A trigonometric calculation is used for calculation of femoral anteversion.

Tracings of radiographs, made with felt-tip pens on clear acetate sheets, are used to determine the angle of deformity, the optimal position for the osteotomy, and the type and placement of internal fixation implants. Use of tracings obviate the need to cut up the radiograph or to make paper cutouts, and the tracing technique can be utilized in several ways. One method is to make a tracing of the deformed bone and then to draw in the normal axes of the proximal and distal parts of the bone. Ideally, the position of the osteotomy is marked at the point of maximum curvature of the deformity. The acetate sheet is then moved so that the distal fragment on the radiograph is anatomically aligned with the tracing of the proximal fragment. The distal fragment is again drawn on the acetate sheet to give a view of the corrected deformity. Adequacy of correction can be checked by superimposition of the tracing over the corresponding radiograph of the normal bone. In chronic deformities, local alterations in bone structure, such as cortical thickening due to remodeling according to Wolfe's law, will render the correction less than perfect.

Internal fixation implants are then drawn on the tracing. The number and position of screws are determined by measurements made from bony prominences or joint spaces that are palpable intraoperatively. Some slight correction in implant size is needed to account for radiographic magnification of the bone, which is normally about 10%–15%. If adequate stability cannot be achieved with the proposed fixation, the osteotomy may have to be relocated. This method of planning from radiographs is valuable as long as the limitations of the technique are recognized. Each radiographic view and tracing provides only two-dimensional information. In addition, calculations of the degree of angular deviation are rendered quite inaccurate if there is concurrent rotational deformity. However, alignment of the limb, following correction, can be evaluated during surgery if the field is draped so that the entire limb is visible.

In mature animals, autologous cancellous bone graft, packed into the defect or around the osteotomy, stimulates bone union. Preparation of graft donor sites should form part of the surgical plan.

6.3 Operative Considerations

Having completed the planning, the proposed osteotomy should be successful if the following basic questions can all be answered in the affirmative:

1. Can the osteotomy be accomplished by a standard surgical exposure?
2. Can Kirschner wires be used as guides intraoperatively?
3. Will the osteotomy be performed through viable bone that is free of disease, such as osteoporosis or infection?
4. Can the bone be adequately stabilized with implants?
5. Will the soft tissues withstand altered strain? Consider a one-stage correction versus progressive lengthening.

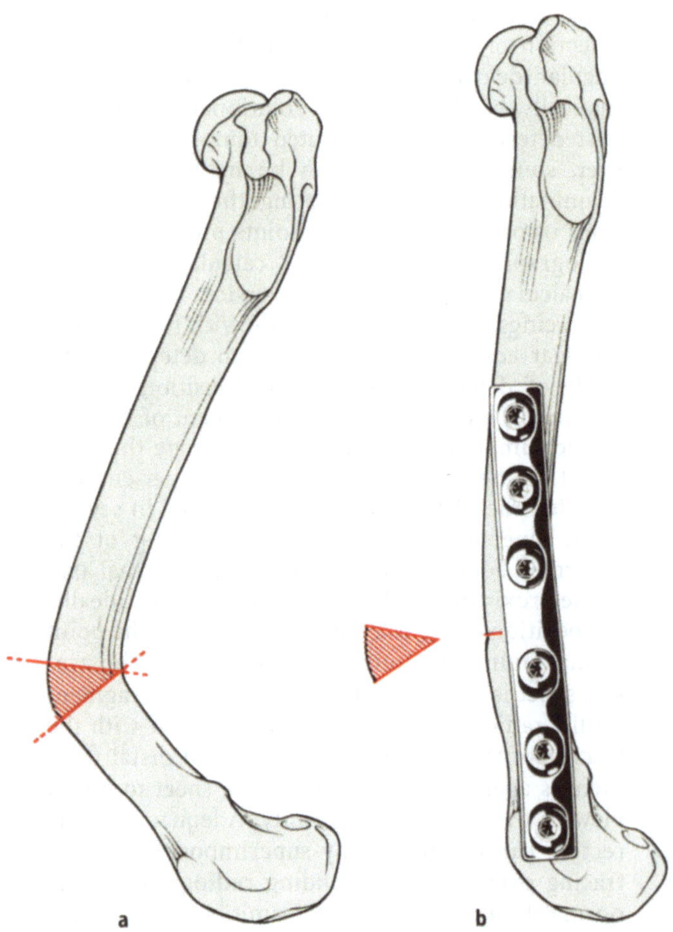

Fig. 6.1a,b. Cuneiform osteotomy, closing wedge type. **a** A wedge of bone of predetermined size is removed and the gap is closed. **b** Compression fixation is applied

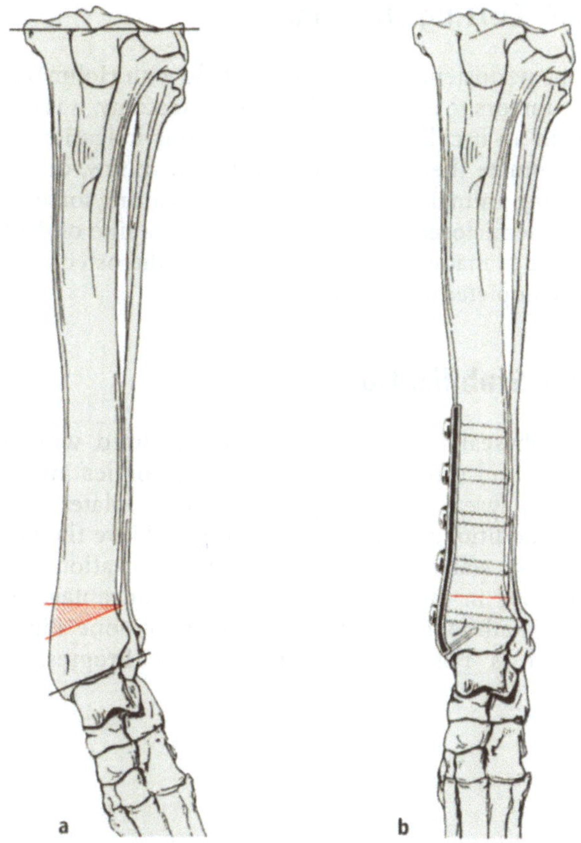

Fig. 6.2a–e. Cuneiform closing wedge osteotomy for correction of valgus angular deformity of the distal tibia. **a** Preoperative plan of the osteotomy wedge. **b** Stabilization of the osteotomy with a five-hole hook plate. **c** Valgus angular deformity of the distal tibia in an 11-month-old rottweiler dog. The deformity was due to asymmetric premature growth plate closure after trauma at 4 months of age. **d** Radiographs immediately following a 30° closing wedge osteotomy of the distal tibia, with stabilization with a five-hole hook plate. **e** Follow-up radiograph taken 3 months after the operation

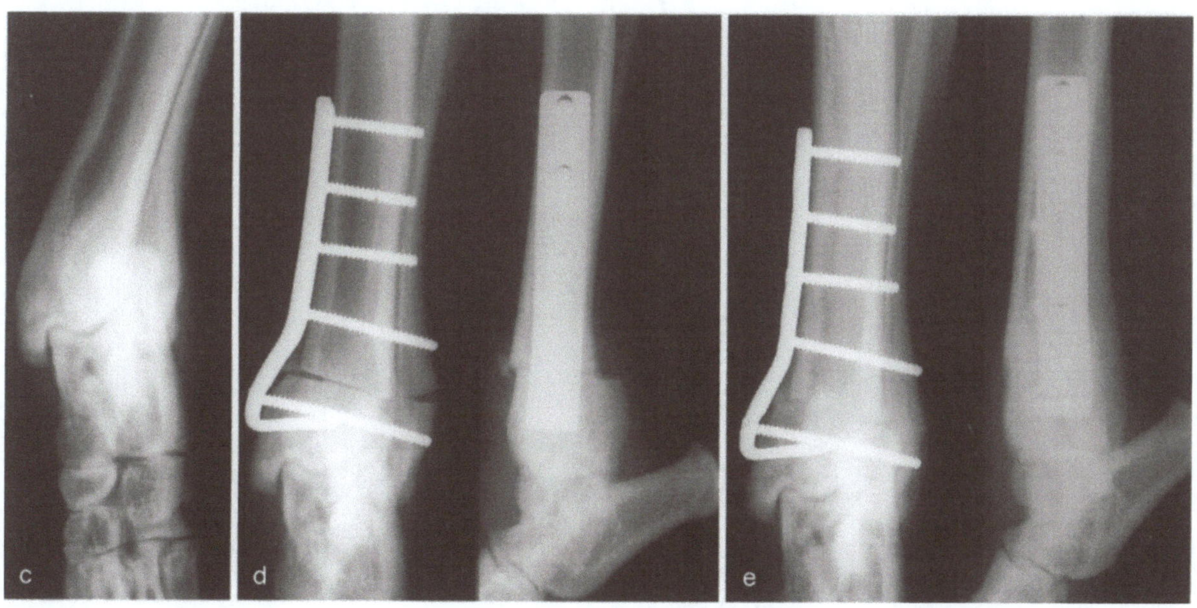

6.4 Cutting the Bone

The periosteum is elevated and held with Hohmann retractors to expose the bone for osteotomy. It is cut with an oscillating blade under saline irrigation to minimize thermal necrosis, a Gili wire saw, or (in young animals) double-action bone cutting forceps. For semiclosed or dome osteotomies, a line of drill holes is made in the bone, and then the osteotomy is completed with an osteotome.

6.5 Stabilization

Diaphyseal osteotomies can be stabilized with a plate and screws. However, for osteotomies in the metaphyseal region, T plates and hook plates permit additional points of fixation to achieve the necessary stability. External fixator stabilization can be used in the distal limb bones. An advantage of this method is that some adjustment of bone alignment is possible following surgery. Progressive lengthening and stabilization after osteotomy is accomplished with the small distractor or an external fixator. Application of each method of stabilization is illustrated in the following section on osteotomy types.

6.6 Types of Osteotomies

6.6.1 Closing Wedge (Cuneiform) Osteotomy

The closing wedge technique is used primarily to correct axial deformity, but may be used for coexistent rotational conditions. Closing wedge osteotomy is accomplished by removing a predetermined wedge of bone from the point of maximal deformity. The base of the wedge is at the convex surface of the deformity. After removal of the wedge, the resulting gap is closed and a compression plate is applied (Figs. 6.1, 6.2). This procedure shortens the bone, but maximizes bone to bone contact, which aids healing and stability.

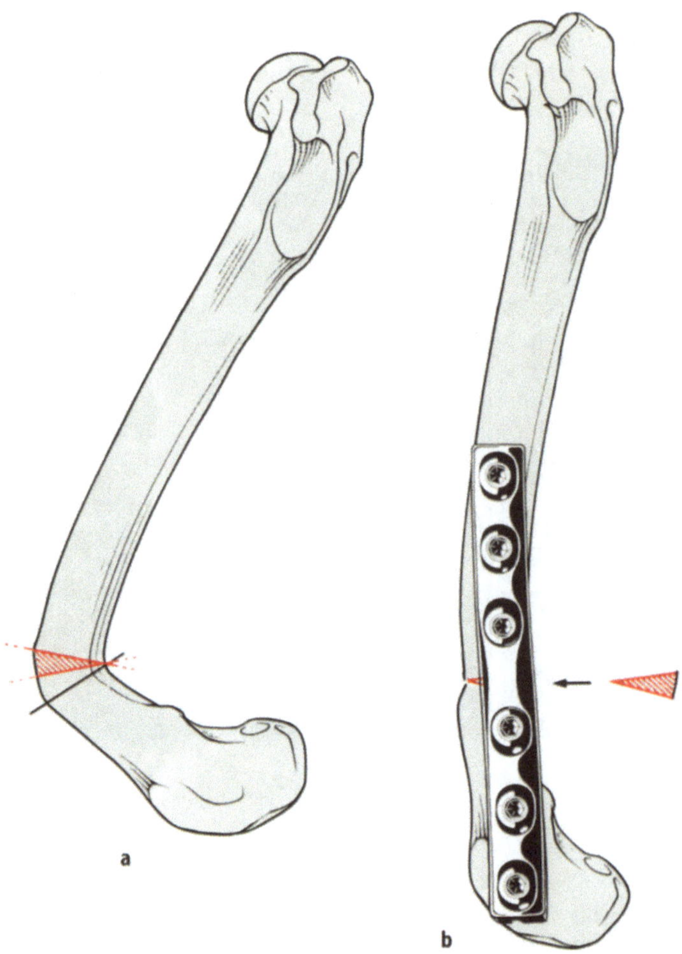

Fig. 6.3a,b. Cuneiform osteotomy, combined opening/closing wedge type. **a** The wedge size is predetermined and divided by two. The osteotomy is carried out. **b** The removed wedge is rotated 180° and reinserted, and a compression plate is applied

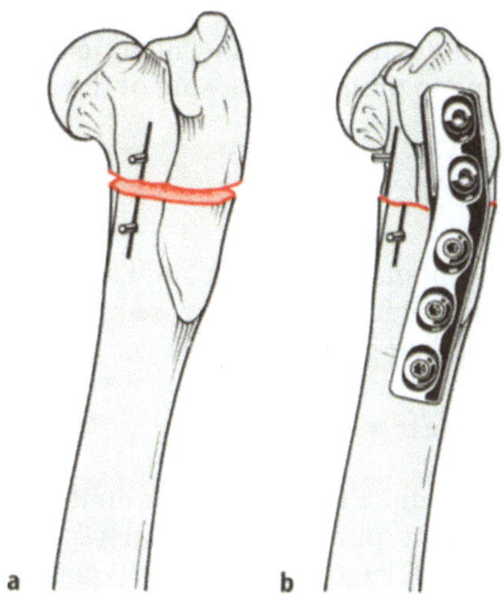

Fig. 6.4a,b. Transverse osteotomy of the proximal femur to accomplish rotational correction of the femoral head. **a** The angle of derotation is predetermined and marked, and a transverse osteotomy is performed. **b** The bone fragments are rotated to correct the alignment and fixed with a compression plate

6.6.2 Reverse Wedge Osteotomy

Where angulation needs correction but limb length should not be compromised, combination opening/closing wedge osteotomy is performed. Using this technique, the predetermined correction angle is bisected and the wedge of bone is removed from the convex side and inserted in the concave side (Fig. 6.3). The correction is thus completed, and bone shortening does not result. Rigid stabilization is necessary to maintain alignment and retain the wedge graft.

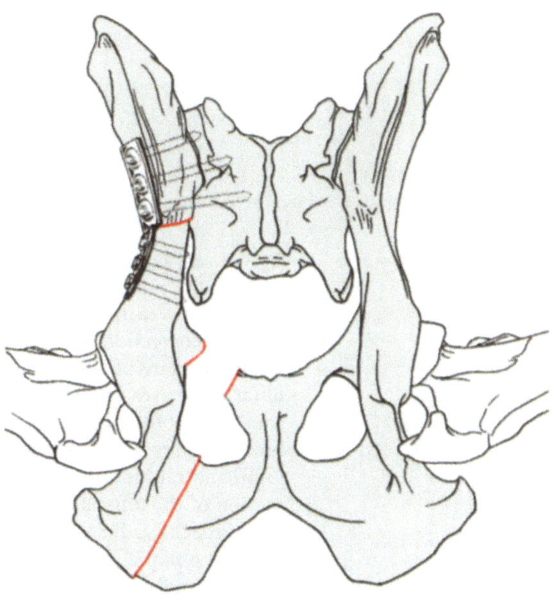

Fig. 6.5. Triple pelvic osteotomy for canine hip dysplasia. A segment of the pubic ramus is removed, and the ischium is osteotomized. A transverse osteotomy of the iliac shaft, just caudal to the sacral wing, allows the acetabular segment to be outwardly rotated to increase coverage of the femoral head dorsally. The iliac osteotomy is stabilized with a six-hole, 2.7-mm triple osteotomy plate

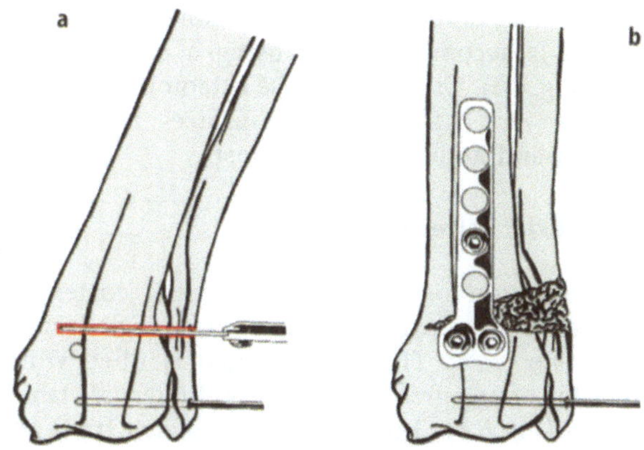

Fig. 6.6a,b. Transverse osteotomy and opening wedge with T plate fixation. **a** A corrective osteotomy of a distal radial malformation with the application of a T plate should be done only in cases with very distal valgus or varus deformation and minimal caudal angulation. Normally this malformation results from asymmetric premature closure of the distal radial physis. The opening wedge osteotomy is made from lateral in valgus deformation and medial in varus deformation. The level of the osteotomy line is about at the vertex of the proximal and bone axes and should be parallel to the joint axis of the antebrachiocarpal joint to ensure that the resulting distal segment is large enough to accept the bone screws through the plate head. Otherwise the osteotomy line has to be more proximal. A Kirschner wire is inserted parallel to the joint axis as a guide. The radius is cut with an oscillating saw in the planned osteotomy line, leaving a few millimeters of the medial cortex intact. The first screw hole for the head of the plate is drilled 5 mm distal to the osteotomy. An osteotome is inserted in the saw cut, and the distal segment is aligned by careful levering. **b** The plate is applied without any compression, and the gap filled with cancellous bone graft

6.6.3 Transverse-Opening Wedge Osteotomy

A single transverse osteotomy may be used for rotational, angular, and lengthening corrections (Fig. 6.4).

6.6.3.1 Rotational Correction

The osteotomy is performed in the region of major rotation by cutting in a transverse plane through the bone. Determination of the angle of derotation correction can be monitored by the use of Kirschner guide wires or by scoring the bone. Osteotomy fixation is accomplished by using a compression plate (Fig. 6.5). Using transverse osteotomy, the fixation is very stable, as flat surfaces are being opposed and no bone length is lost.

6.6.3.2 Axial Correction

For correction of axial deformity, the cortex is opened on the concave surface after a single transverse osteotomy. The resulting gap is filled with cancellous bone graft following rigid internal stabilization (Fig. 6.6). The bone length gained from an isosceles triangle is one half of the length to the base. The disadvantage of the method is that the plate has buttress function.

6.6.3.3 Lengthening

Lengthening of the bone may be accomplished by transverse osteotomy, distraction of the bone segments, and stabilization. In mature animals, the bone deficit should be filled with cancellous bone graft. This technique is especially applicable to paired bones, such as the radius and ulna, to correct shortening due to premature closure of the distal radial physis.

6.6.3.4 Shortening

Shortening of the bone may be accomplished by making two parallel cuts, removing a segment of bone, and then stabilizing with a compression plate.

6.6.4 Oblique Osteotomy

Oblique osteotomy can be used to correct multiplanar deformities. In its purest form, it allows two bones to be separated, lengthened, and still permit point contact (Fig. 6.7). In rotational and varus or valgus deformity, it can be used to provide total correction by placing the proximal obliquity into the medullary cavity of the distal fragment, thus providing a pivotal point for derotation and varus or valgus realignment.

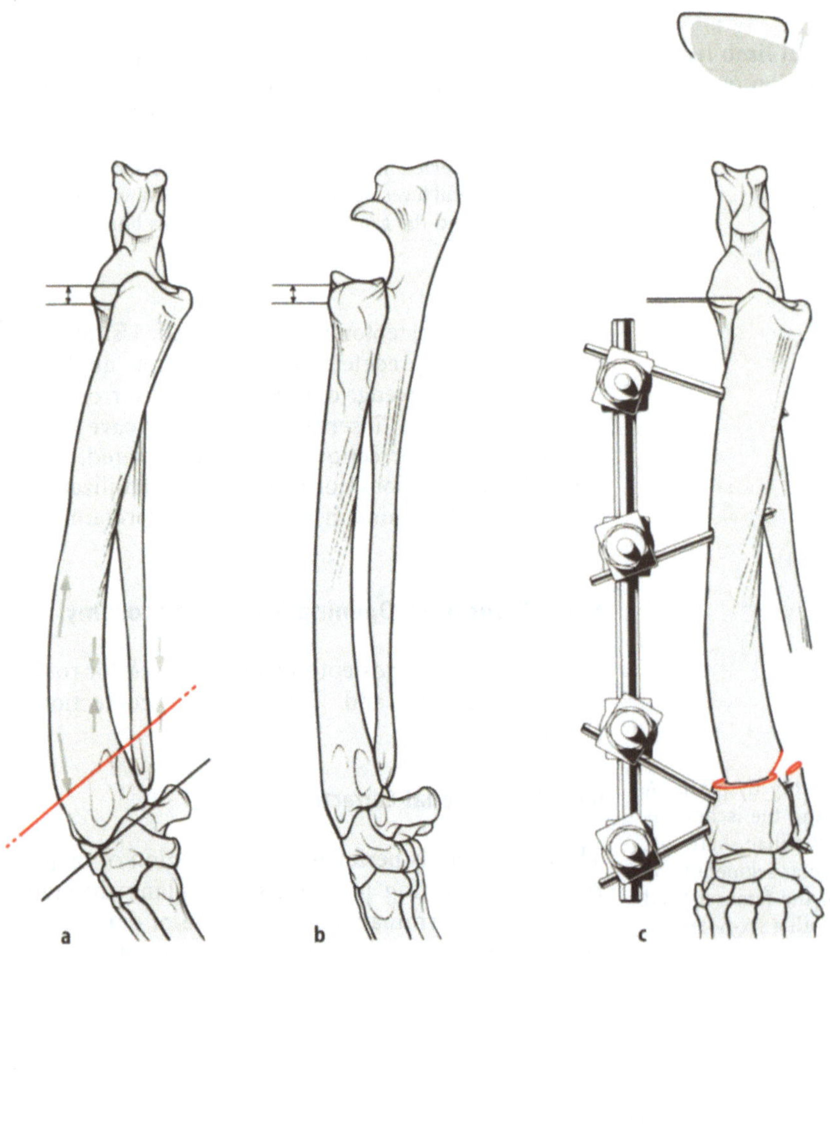

Fig. 6.7. a,b Oblique osteotomy of the radius and removal of a section of the ulna for correction of a premature closure of the distal ulnar physis resulting in shortening of the ulna, incongruency of the elbow joint, and radius curvus. **c** A section of the ulna is removed, the radius is osteotomized obliquely, and the fragments of the radius are realigned and placed in proper rotation. An external fixator is applied to the radius for stabilization. Invariably the proximal segment of the ulna moves proximally, and congruency is reestablished at the elbow joint

Arthrodesis is the surgical fusion of a joint for the treatment of painful instability of severe joint disease unresponsive to medical therapy. Indications for arthrodesis in small animals include severe degenerative joint disease secondary to ligamentous instability or trauma, intra-articular fractures, immune-mediated joint diseases, septic arthritis, joint luxations, and postural abnormalities caused by neurological dysfunction.

Strict adherence to the principles of arthrodesis is essential if joint fusion is to be successful. The articular cartilage is removed to expose subchondral bone. This is performed using currettes, rongeurs, or power-driven burrs. If the subchondral bone is sclerotic, it must be removed to expose bleeding cancellous bone. In many cases, the articular surfaces may be removed with a saw, providing exposure of subchondral bone and creating two flat, opposing surfaces. The flat surfaces maximize bony contact and eliminate shear stress when compression is applied to the bone ends. Autogenous cancellous bone graft is placed at the arthrodesis site to promote bony union across the joint. Rigid internal fixation is then applied to immobilize the joint and allow bone healing. Where possible, compression should be applied between the exposed subchondral bone surfaces to enhance healing.

7.1 Shoulder Arthrodesis

Shoulder arthrodesis is indicated for traumatic joint injuries, chronic subluxation unresponsive to surgical repair, severe degenerative joint disease, and congenital abnormalities. The angle of fusion should allow advancement of the limb and weight bearing without overextension of the elbow. A common angle for shoulder arthrodesis is 110°; however, the angle should be individualized for each patient. The correct angle is best determined by evaluating the animal preoperatively in a normal standing position. A spica bandage is applied to the limb for 4–6 weeks after surgery, and exercise should be restricted until union has occurred (Fig. 7.1).

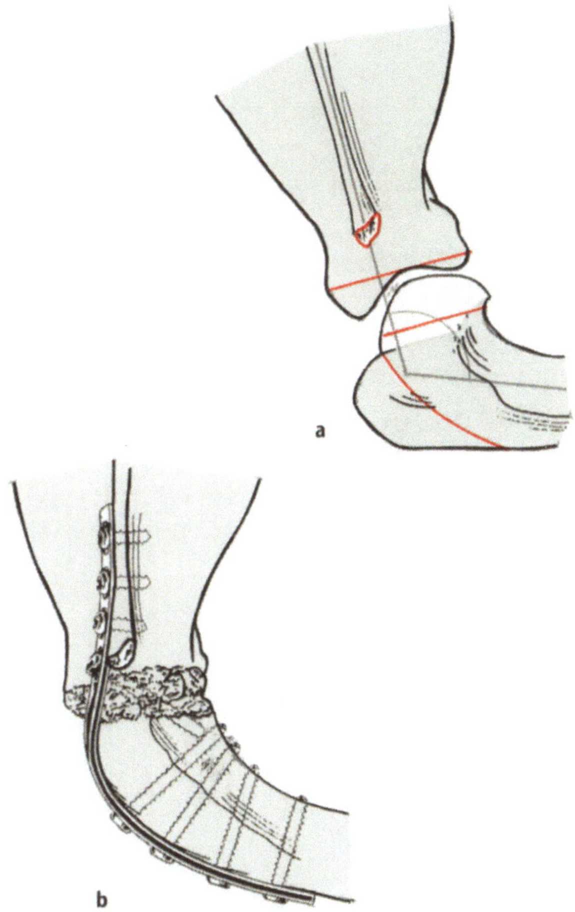

Fig. 7.1a,b. Surgical procedure for arthrodesis of the shoulder joint. **a** The joint is exposed through a combined cranial and craniolateral approach, including osteotomy of the acromion and greater tubercle and tenotomy of the biceps brachii, infraspinatus, and deltoideus. Injury to the suprascapular nerve should be avoided. The articular surfaces of the humeral head and glenoid are removed with an oscillating saw at the correct angle. Lateral or medial angulation of the ostectomies should be avoided. **b** The distal scapula and proximal humerus are opposed and temporarily fixed with Kirschner wires. A dynamic compression plate (eight to ten holes) is contoured and applied to the cranial aspect of the proximal humerus and the dorsocranial junction of the spine and body of the scapula. One screw is placed in lag fashion through the plate and across the joint. Cancellous bone collected from the ostectomized humeral head and glenoid is placed around the ostectomy site

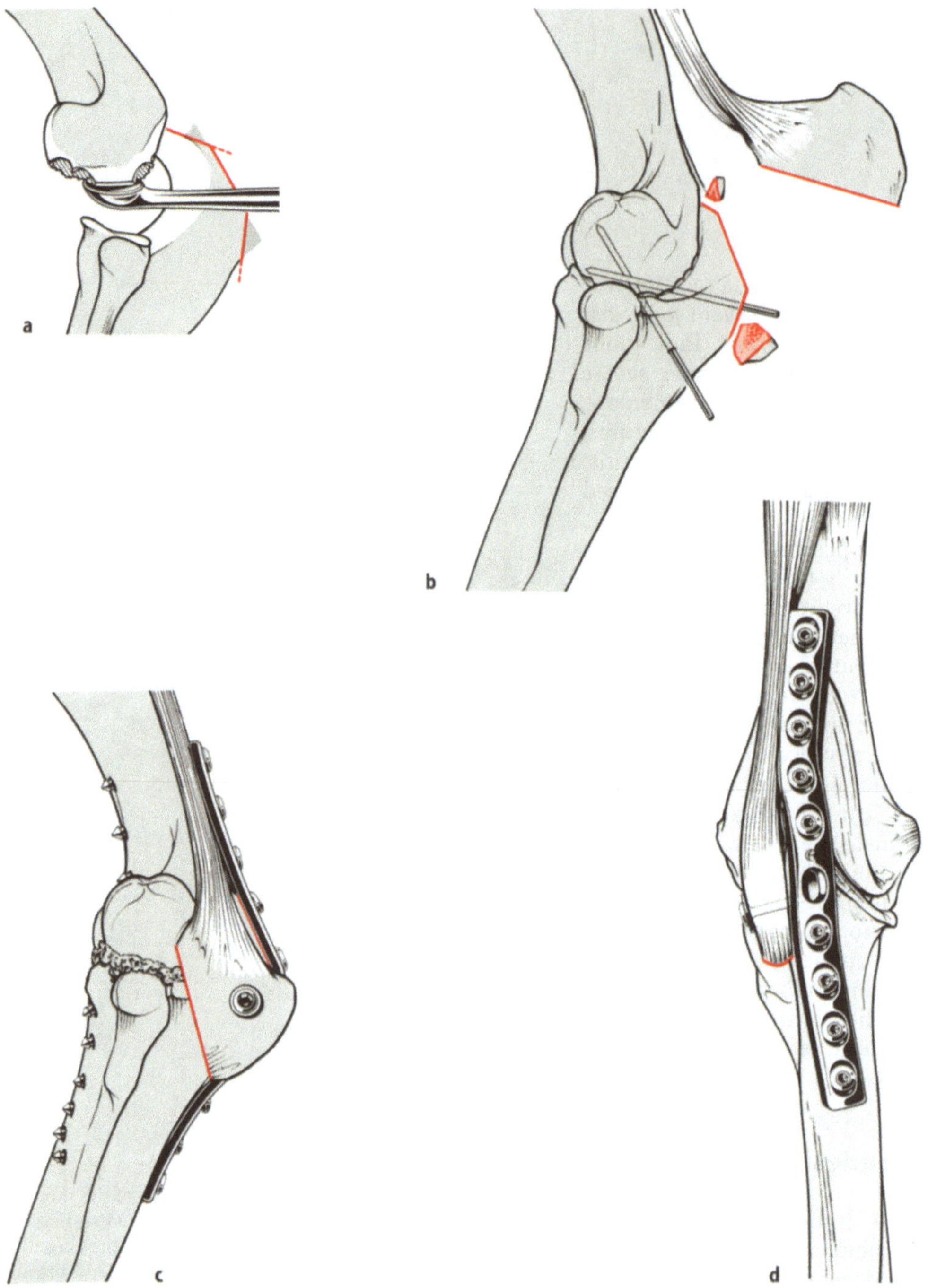

Fig. 7.2a–d. Surgical procedure for arthrodesis of the elbow joint. **a** The joint is exposed by a combined lateral approach and caudal approach with osteotomy of the olecrenon process. Transection of the ulnaris lateralis, lateral collateral ligaments, and the joint capsule allows removal of the articular cartilage from the radial head, humeral condyles, and the trochlear notch of the ulna using bone currettes. **b** A temporary pin is placed across the joint to maintain reduction at the desired angle. An eight- to ten-hole plate is contoured to the caudal surfaces of the humerus and ulna. The proximal ulna is shaped to allow the plate to seat smoothly. The plate should be positioned to allow a minimum of four screws to be placed in each bone. One screw is placed in lag fashion through the plate and lateral epicondyle into the radial head. A second screw is placed in lag fashion through the plate and ulna into the medial epicondyle of the humerus. Autogenous cancellous bone graft is packed around the joint. **c,d** The olecranon process is reattached medial to the plate using a screw in lag fashion

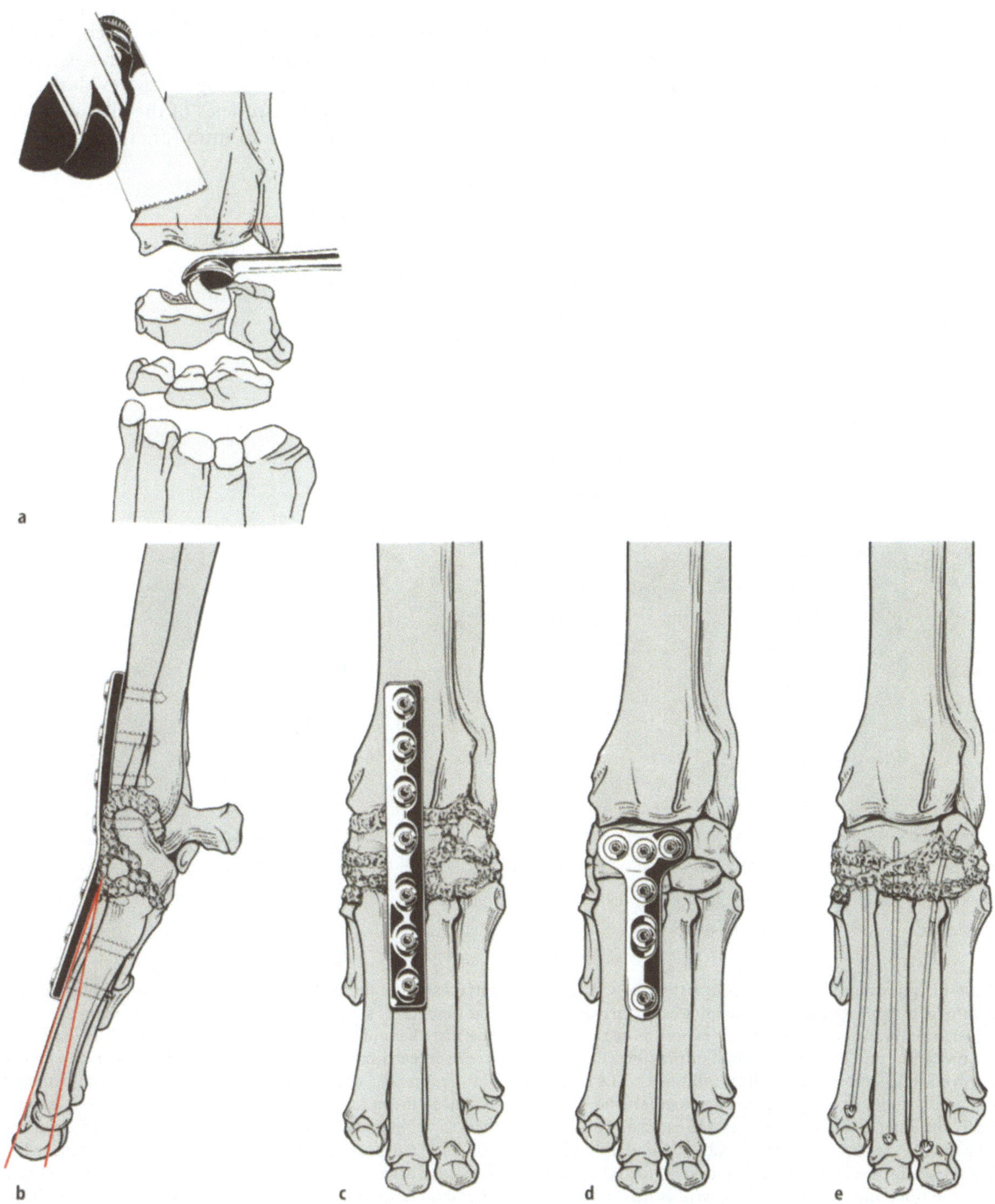

Fig. 7.3a–e. Surgical procedures for arthrodesis of carpal joints. **a** The distal radius, carpus, and proximal metacarpals are exposed through a dorsal midline approach. The articular cartilage is removed from the joints to be fused and the area packed with autogenous cancellous bone graft. **b,c** Pancarpal arthrodesis is achieved by placing a bone plate on the dorsal or palmar surface of the carpus. Three to five screws should be placed in the radius, one in the radial carpal bone and three to four in metacarpal III. Several screws are loaded to produce compression. **d** Partial arthrodesis may be performed by application of a T plate to the dorsal surface. The plate must be positioned distally on the radial carpal bone to prevent contact with the distal radius. The distal portion of the plate is affixed to metacarpal III. **e** Other plates, such as the veterinary cuttable plate and the veterinary T plate, can be used for this procedure. Partial carpal arthrodesis may also be achieved by placing intramedullary pins from metacarpals III and IV across the joint and into the radial carpal bone. The pins are inserted with the carpus in full flexion to minimize subluxation of the middle or carpometacarpal joints

7.2 Elbow Arthrodesis

Arthrodesis of the elbow is indicated for irreparable comminuted intra-articular fractures, chronic luxation unresponsive to surgical stabilization, and severe degenerative joint disease from a variety of causes. The elbow is usually fused at 110°, but the angle should be individualized for each patient (Fig. 7.2). Exercise must be restricted for 4–6 weeks after surgery or until radiographic evidence of fusion is observed. Arthrodesis of the elbow results in a significant decrease in limb function.

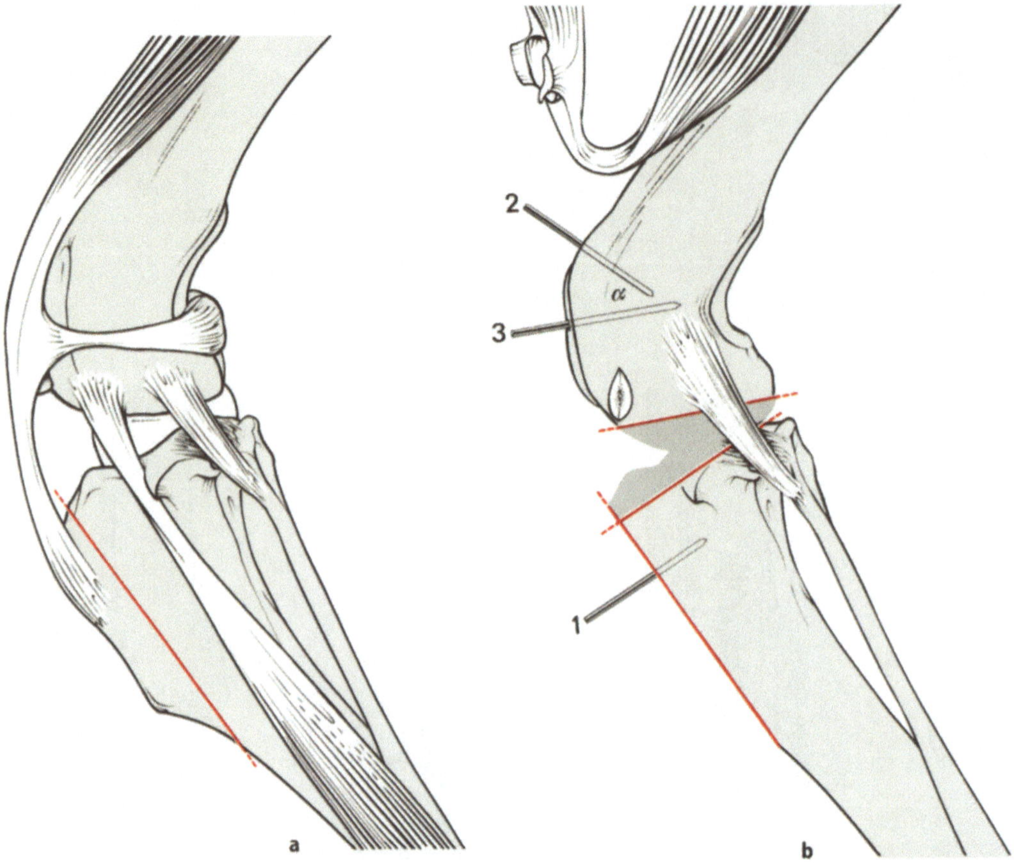

Fig. 7.4a–f. Surgical procedure for stifle arthrodesis. A bilateral parapatellar approach to the stifle joint is performed. The lateral incision is extended to provide exposure of the distal half of the femur and the proximal half of the tibia. Exposure is improved by osteotomy of the tibial tuberosity. The fat pad, cranial and caudal cruciate ligaments, medial and lateral menisci, and intermeniscal ligaments are excised. The collateral ligaments are preserved to facilitate manipulation of the limb. **a** Kirschner wires are used as markers for the ostectomies of the tibia and femur. The first wire is inserted in the sagittal midline plane of the proximal tibia, perpendicular to the long axis of the bone. A second wire is similarly placed in the distal femur. A third wire marker is inserted into the femur distal to the second. The angle between the second and third wires is equal to the complementary angle (α, i.e., 180° – arthrodesis angle). Ostectomy of the femur is then performed parallel to the third marker wire; ostectomy of the tibial is performed parallel to the first wire. **b** The femur and tibia are apposed and held in reduction with one or two Steinmann pins. Alignment of the wire markers is used to prevent rotation. **c, d** A bone plate is applied to the cranial surfaces of the femur and tibia. The femoral trochlear ridges and tibial crest should be removed to accommodate the plate. The plate should be of sufficient length to allow at least four screws in each fragment and should ideally cover one half of both femur and tibia. One or two of the plate screws should be placed in lag fashion across the joint to increase interfragmentary compression. Cancellous bone is removed from the ostectomized portions of the femur and tibia and placed at the site of arthrodesis prior to compression of the bone ends. The tibial tuberosity is then reattached medial to plate with a screw to restore normal quadriceps tension. **e, f** The contoured dynamic compression plate (DCP) is applied to the cranial surface of the femur and tibia. Cancellous bone-grafting is unnecessary if there is good apposition of the osteotomized cancellous surfaces. The ends of the crossed Kirschner wires are bent. The wires will increase the rotational stability and are left in place. The osteotomized tibial tuberosity is reattached to the tibia medial to the bone plate to restore normal quadriceps tension and a more anatomically pleasing end result

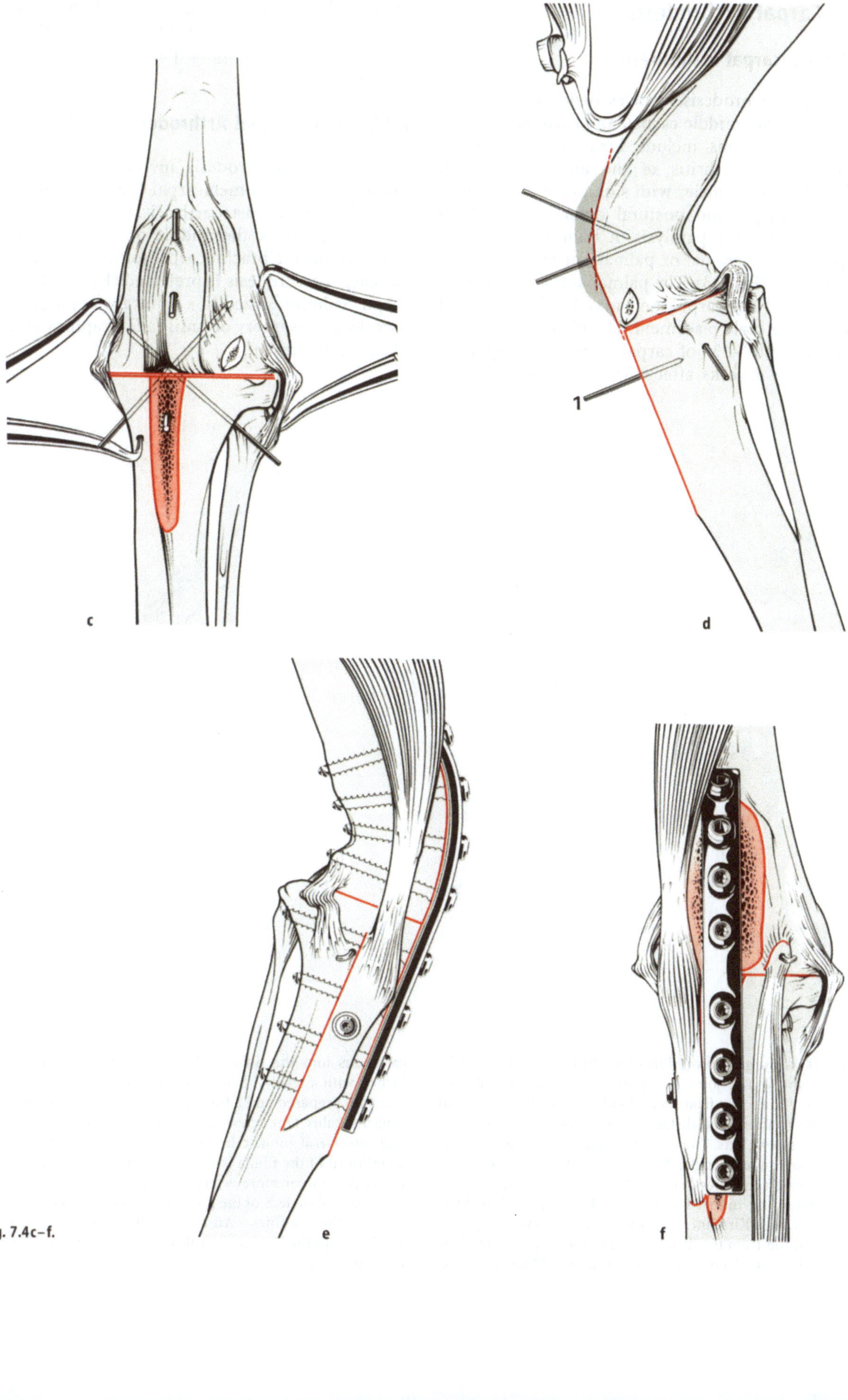

Fig. 7.4c–f.

7.3 Carpal Arthrodesis

7.3.1 Pancarpal Arthrodesis

Pancarpal arthrodesis involves fusion of the antebrachiocarpal, middle carpal, and carpometacarpal joints. Indications include luxation, hyperextension, or osteoarthritis of the antebrachiocarpal joint, shearing injuries with significant loss of articular cartilage, and postural deformity resulting from radial nerve paralysis. A bone plate may be applied to the cranial or palmar surface to achieve arthrodesis (Fig. 7.3). The palmar surface is the tension side of the carpus and may be the preferred location for plate placement. The plate is contoured to provide 10°–12° of carpal extension. A splint is applied for 6 weeks after surgery, particularly if a cranial plate is used. Arthrodesis of the antebrachiocarpal joint alone results in the eventual breakdown of the remaining carpal joint and is not recommended.

7.3.2 Partial Carpal Arthrodesis

Partial carpal arthrodesis involves fusion of the middle and carpometacarpal joints. Indications include trauma, osteoarthritis, and luxation or hyperextension of the middle or carpometacarpal joints. If the antebrachiocarpal joint is normal, partial carpal arthrodesis is preferred (Fig. 7.3d,e). The carpus is immobilized in a splint for approximately 6 weeks after surgery or until radiographic evidence of fusion is present.

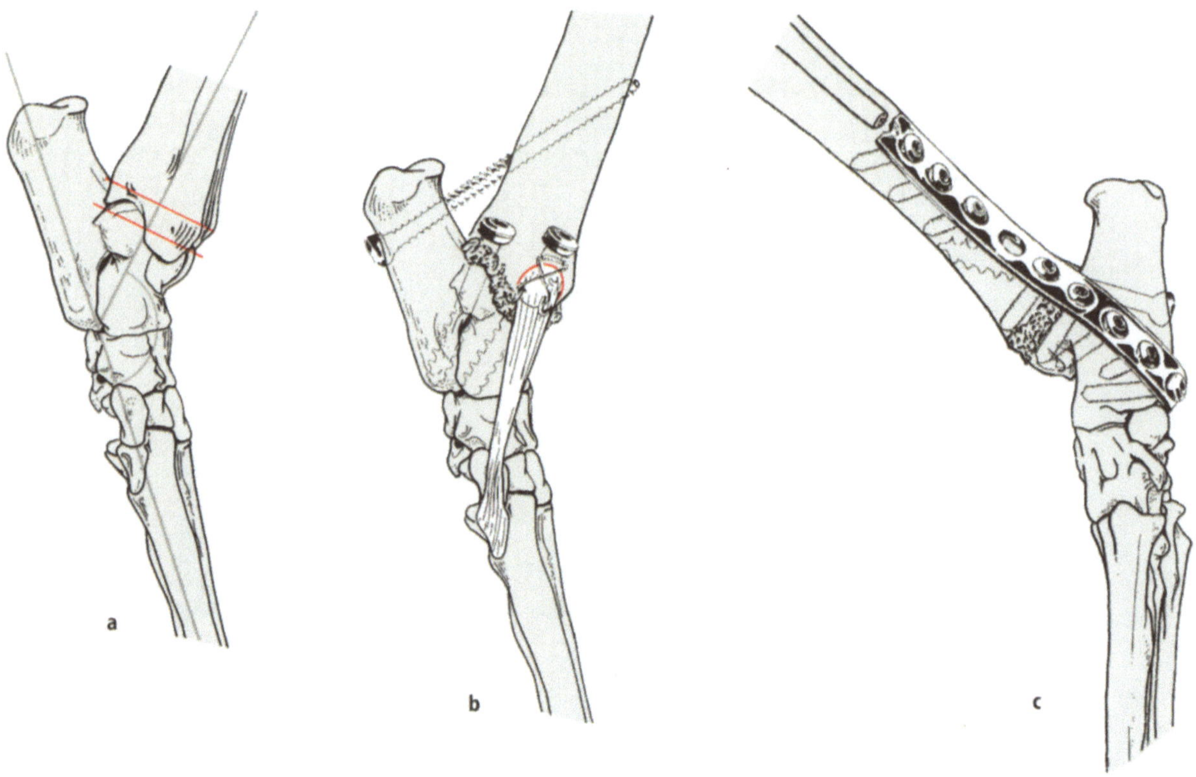

Fig. 7.5a–c. Surgical procedures for arthrodesis of the tibiotarsal joint. **a** The joint is exposed by a medial malleolar osteotomy for screw fixation and either cranially or laterally for plate fixation. The distal tibia is ostectomized at a 90° angle to its long axis. The proximal talus is cut to achieve the desired arthrodesis angle. Alternatively, the cartilage can be removed with currettes or burrs. Autogenous cancellous bone graft should be inserted at the site. **b** The joint is held in reduction with Kirschner wires while two screws are placed in lag fashion from the distal tibia into the talus and the base of the calcaneus. A positional screw is inserted from the tuber calcaneus into the tibia, and the medial malleolus is reattached with a tension band wire. Alternatively, the joint surfaces are prepared and a bone plate is placed cranially on the tibia and talus. One screw should not interfere with the proximal intertarsal joint. **c** In the lateral plating technique, the distal third of the fibula is resected and the joint surfaces are prepared. One or more veterinary cuttable plates are applied to the lateral surface of the joint. The plates may be stacked to increase their stiffness. An additional screw is placed in lag fashion from the base of the calcaneus, through the talus, and into the distal tibia

7.4 Stifle Arthrodesis

Indications for stifle arthrodesis include severe degenerative joint disease, comminuted intra-articular fractures, fracture disease, and irreparable joint luxation. The angle at which the stifle is fused is 135°–140° for dogs and 120°–125° for cats. The appropriate angle should be determined in the standing patient prior to induction of anesthesia. In order to compensate for bone shortening caused by osteotomy of the femur and tibia, it is advisable to add 10° to the stifle measurement in large dogs and 5° in small dogs and cats. Results of stifle arthrodesis are best if the stifle is fused at an angle that allows the foot to contact the ground without causing excessive flexion or extension of the opposite limb. The animal's activity must be restricted until radiographic union is achieved (typically 8–10 weeks). Supplementary external coaptation is usually unnecessary after plate fixation (Fig. 7.4).

7.5 Tarsal Arthrodesis

7.5.1 Tibiotarsal Arthrodesis

Indications for arthrodesis of the tibiotarsal joint include severe shearing injury, comminuted intra-articular fractures, joint laxity or hyperextension, irreparable damage to the calcanean tendon, and degenerative joint disease. The joint may also be fused along with transposition of the long digital extensor tendon for injury to the sciatic nerve. The angle of tibiotarsal arthrodesis is 135°–145° for dogs and 115°–125° for cats. Lag screws or bone plates can be used for arthrodesis of the tibiotarsal joint (Fig. 7.5). The joint should be immobilized in a splint or cast for 6 weeks after surgery or until radiographic evidence of fusion is noted. Degenerative disease may develop in the more distal tarsal joints after tibiotarsal arthrodesis.

7.5.2 Intertarsal and Tarsometatarsal Arthrodesis

Arthrodesis of the proximal intertarsal, distal intertarsal, or tarsometatarsal joints is indicated for hyperextension injuries, comminuted intra-articular fractures, shearing wounds, and osteoarthritis. Lateral plate fixation with autogenous cancellous bone grafting provides stability (Fig. 7.6). External coaptation is recommended for approximately 6 weeks after surgery.

7.5.3 Pantarsal Arthrodesis

Pantarsal arthrodesis involves fusion of the tibiotarsal, proximal and distal intertarsal, and tarsometatarsal joints. Indications include shearing injuries, osteoarthritis, and painful unstable conditions unresponsive to reconstruction. Because of the degenerative joint disease that often develops in the more distal tarsal joints, pantarsal arthrodesis may be preferred over tibiotarsal arthrodesis alone for diseases of the talocrural joint (Fig. 7.7).

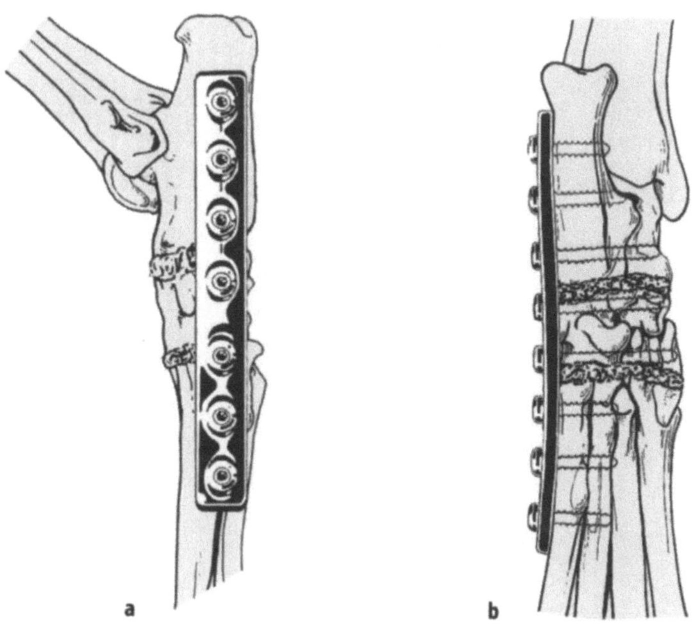

Fig. 7.6a,b. Surgical procedure for arthrodesis of the intertarsal and tarsometatarsal joints. The joints are exposed through a lateral approach. The articular cartilage is removed from the joints to be fused and cancellous bone graft is packed around the site. A bone plate is applied to the lateral surface of the joints. The base of metatarsal V and the calcaneus may be smoothed to improve seating of the plate. Three screws are placed into the calcaneus, the third engaging the talus. One or two screws span the tarsus, and three screws are placed into the metatarsal bones

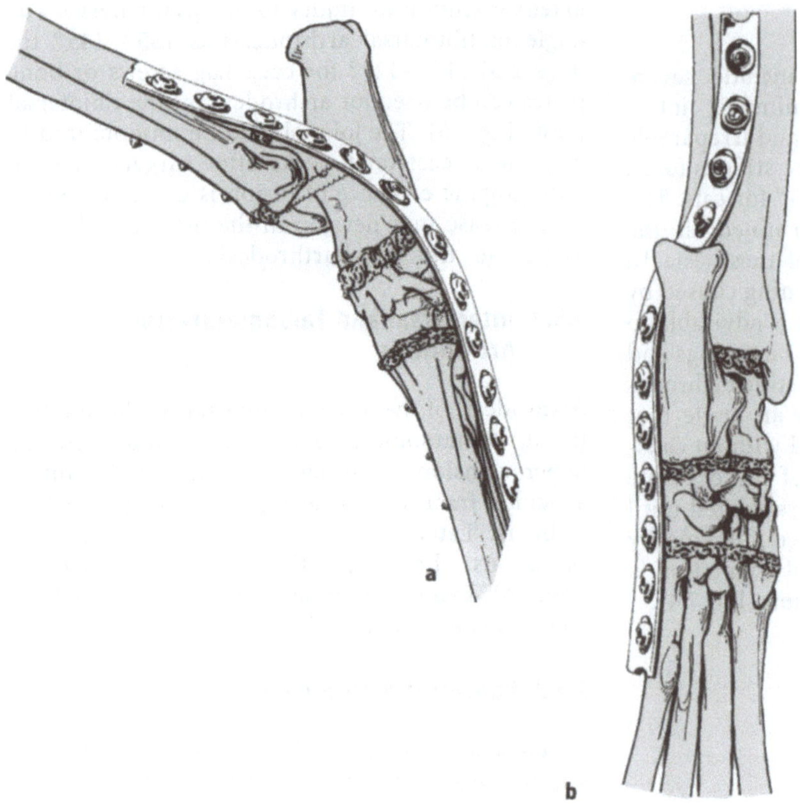

Fig. 7.7a,b. Surgical procedure for pantarsal arthrodesis. The joint is exposed through a lateral incision from the distal third of the tibia to the metatarsus. The joints are prepared as described for tibiotarsal, intertarsal, and tarsometatarsal arthrodesis, and cancellous bone graft is placed. A bone plate is applied to the caudolateral surface of the distal tibia, tarsus, and metatarsals. The plate is contoured to provide the desired angle of arthrodesis. The lateral surfaces of the bones may be smoothed to improved seating of the plate

8 Bone Transplantation

Bone transplantation (bone grafting) is frequently used in association with internal fixation of fractures and nonunions. Transplanted bone functions to enhance fracture healing in three ways. The transplanted bone is a source of osteoprogenitor cells. Surface cells on transplanted autogenous cancellous bone will survive under optimal conditions and participate in the total early osteogenic response around the graft. The transplanted bone stimulates the formation of new bones of host origin by recruitment and differentiation of the host mesenchymal cells. This process of osteoinduction is modulated by bone-inducing factors present in the matrix. The transplanted bone also serves as a trellis for the ingrowth of capillaries, perivascular tissue, and osteoprogenitor cells, a process called osteoconduction. In addition, transplanted cortical bone serves as a mechanical support for the fracture and internal fixation.

A bone graft is defined by the type of bone transplanted and the relationship of the donor to the host. Cancellous bone, cortical bone, and corticocancellous combinations such as ribs are used as bone graft material. Autografts are transplanted from donor site to recipient site within the same animal. Allografts are transplanted from a donor site in one animal to a recipient site in a different animal of the same species. An alloimplant is an allograft which has been treated or preserved in a manner which destroys the cells. The most commonly used transplanted bone is the autogenous cancellous graft. This graft material is easy to harvest and extremely effective in promoting healing of bone defects in fractures which are openly reduced and rigidly fixed with internal fixation. Cortical allografts or alloimplants are used to support the fixation in fractures with a large amount of cortical bone loss.

8.1 Cancellous Bone Autograft

8.1.1 Indications

Any fracture treated with open reduction and internal fixation is a candidate for cancellous bone autograft. In particular, the graft should be used to fill cortical defects remaining after fracture reconstruction or corrective osteotomy. The cancellous bone autograft promotes rapid healing of the defect, thus eliminating instability, which could otherwise cause failure of the metal implants. In addition, cancellous bone autograft laid along anatomically reconstructed fracture lines promotes rapid bone bridging of the fracture, increasing the strength of the healing bone.

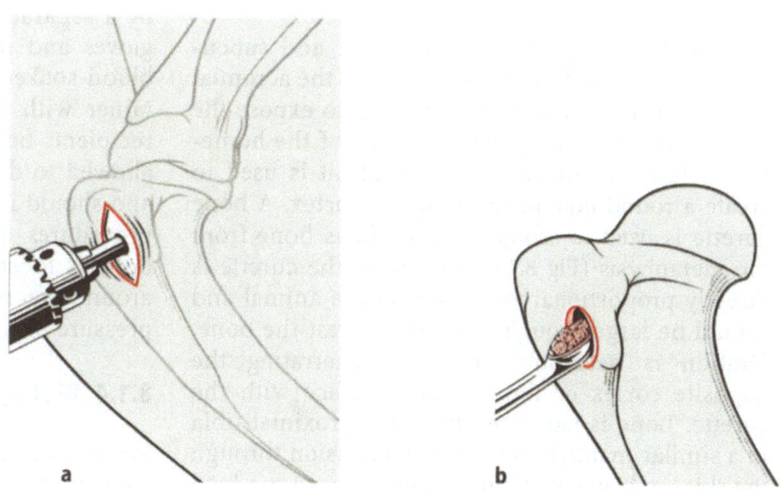

Fig. 8.1a,b. Greater tubercle of the humerus. **a** A 2- to 3-cm craniolateral skin incision will expose the periosteum, and a 1- to 2-cm incision exposes enough bone to allow perforation of the cortex with a Steinmann pin, drill, or trephine of sufficient size. **b** With a sharp curette of proper size, the cancellous bone can be removed and collected in a stainless steel cup or kept between sponges moistened with blood or Ringer's solution. Undermining of the joint cartilage should be avoided. In growing dogs, care must be taken to avoid the physis in the harvesting procedure

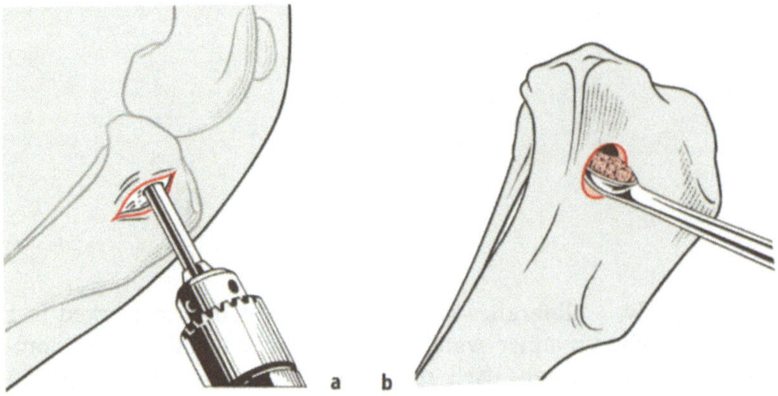

Fig. 8.2a,b. Proximal tibia. **a** A 2- to 3-cm longitudinal incision through skin and subcutaneous tissues on the medial surface of the proximal end of the tibia and 2–4 cm below the joint space, at a point between the middle and caudal third of the width of the tibia, will give easy access to the cancellous bone. **b** Here, too, harvesting is done by curetting. Closure in layers is routine. In small breeds, wide holes and accidental perforation of the opposite cortex should be avoided, since this may result in an iatrogenic fracture

Cancellous bone autograft is used to stimulate healing in nonunions which are reduced and stabilized with internal fixation. Grafting with cancellous bone is especially indicated for biologically inactive nonunion sites. A graft can also be effectively used in infected nonunions and chronic osteomyelitis. Cancellous bone autograft is packed into bone defects caused by curettage of bone cysts or benign tumors. Finally, cancellous bone autograft is essential for rapid bone union of arthrodeses.

8.1.2 Sources

Prerequisites for a donor site include easy accessibility and the presence of large amounts of cancellous bone. The most common donor sites for cancellous bone autograft are the proximal humeral metaphysis, the proximal tibial metaphysis, and the wing of the ilium (Figs. 8.1, 8.2). Donor sites are preselected and prepared for aseptic surgery when the fracture site is prepared. If large amounts of cancellous bone are required, multiple donor sites may be harvested.

8.1.3 Technique

A craniolateral incision through skin and subcutaneous tissue and caudal retraction of the acromial portion of the deltoid muscle is used to expose the lateral surface of the greater tubercle of the humerus. A large Steinmann pin or drill bit is used to create a round hole penetrating the cortex. A bone curette is used to scoop the cancellous bone from the metaphysis (Fig 8.1). The size of the curette is directly proportional to the size of the animal and should be large enough to easily harvest the bone. Caution is necessary to avoid penetrating the opposite cortex or the articular surface with the curette. Bone is harvested from the proximal tibia in a similar manner after a medial incision through the skin and subcutaneous tissue has been made to expose the medial surface of the proximal metaphysis (Fig. 8.2).

A dorsal incision through skin and subcutaneous tissue over the wing of the ilium is followed by elevation of the gluteal musculature to expose the cranial dorsal iliac spine. An osteotome is used to remove a wedge of the ilium. The wedge of corticocancellous bone is crushed into small particles with a rongeur. A bone curette is used to harvest additional cancellous bone from within the body of the ilium (Fig. 8.3). Closure of all donor sites is accomplished by apposition of the subcutaneous tissue and skin.

To ensure optimum survival of the donor cells, the bone should be transplanted directly from donor to hose site. In most cases, the cancellous bone is harvested after fracture reduction and fixation is complete and the recipient site has been lavaged. It is advantageous to mix the cancellous bone with autologous blood. The blood clots and forms a moldable composite, with the graft simplifying handling and placement in the recipient bed. When transplanting bone to tumor sites or infected fracture sites, all the bone graft should be harvested prior to approaching the primary site or by a separate surgical team using uncontaminated gloves and instruments. The bone is stored in a blood-soaked sponge or in a stainless steel container with autologous blood until placed in the recipient bed. Cancellous graft should not be allowed to dry, should not be immersed in saline, and should not be treated with antibiotics, as these procedures are toxic to the cells. The cancellous bone is loosely packed into the bone defects and around fracture lines and is held in place by the pressure of the surrounding soft tissues (Fig. 8.4).

8.1.4 Biology

Revascularization of the graft is complete within 2 weeks. New bone is deposited on the trabecular

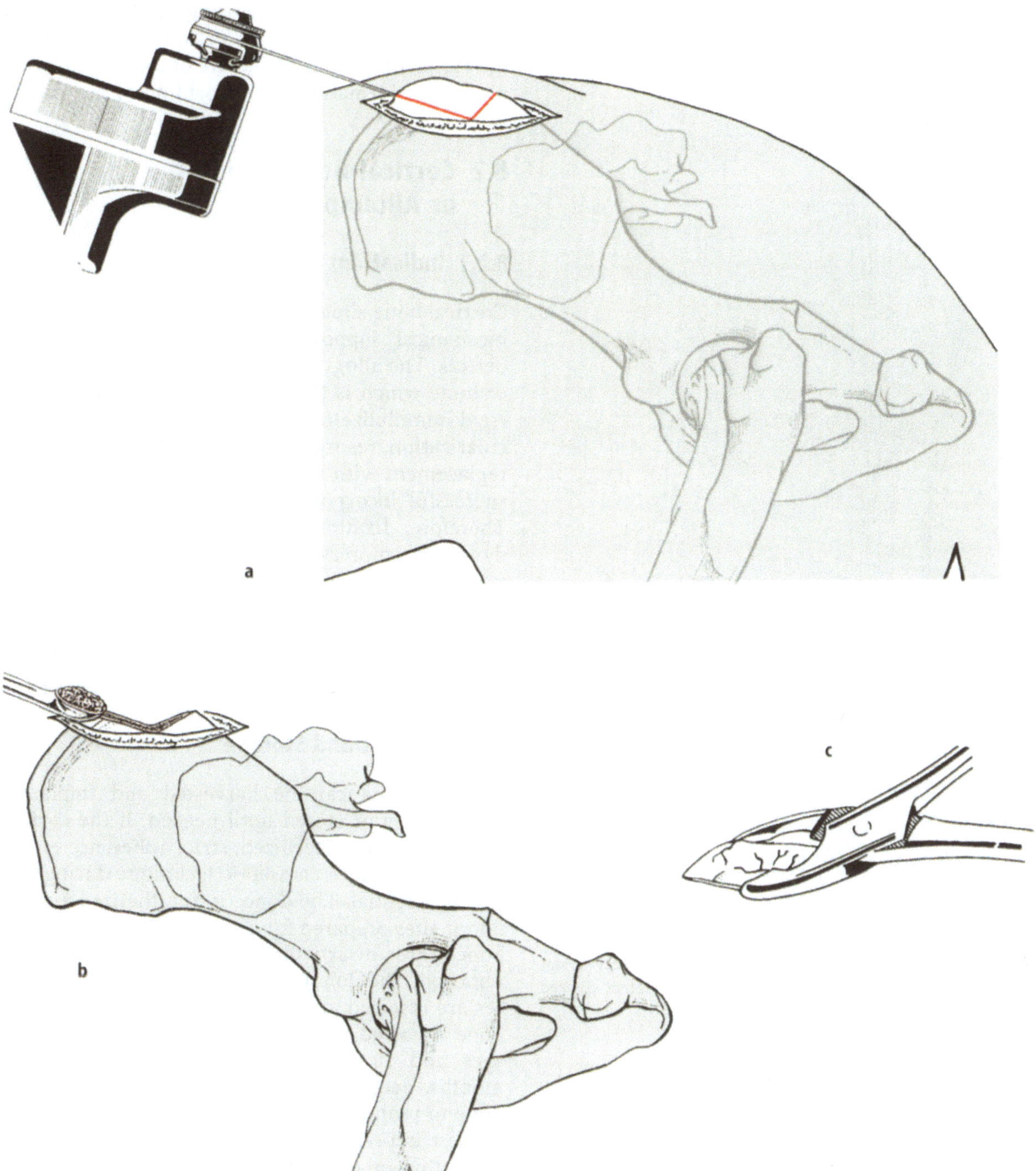

Fig. 8.3a–c. Ilial wing. A dorsal incision through skin and subcutaneous tissue over the wing of the ilium is followed by elevation of the gluteal musculature to expose the cranial dorsal iliac spine. **a** An oscillating saw or **b** an oscillating osteotome is used to remove a wedge of the ilium. **b** A bone curette is used to harvest cancellous bone from within the body of the ilium. **c** The wedge of cortico-cancellous bone is crushed into small particles with a rongeur. Closure of the site is accomplished in layers by apposition of musculature, subcutaneous tissue, and skin

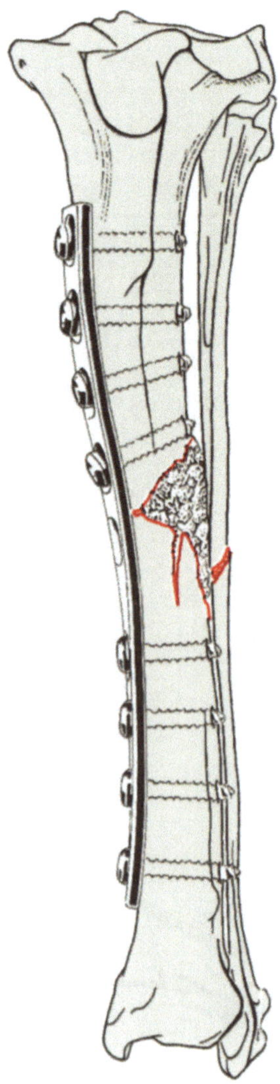

Fig. 8.4. Cortical defects. After reduction, the fracture is stabilized with a buttress plate and the cortical defect packed with cancellous bone

cores of the graft and at the fracture surfaces by surviving osteoblasts and differentiated host mesenchymal cells. Resorption of the necrotic transplanted bone occurs. Radiographically, the grafted site will initially become more radiopaque and then lose density as the necrotic bone is resorbed. The graft is completely resorbed and the newly formed bone remodelled into cortical bone in response to the mechanical environment within 3–6 months after implantation.

8.1.5 Complications

Complications associated with harvesting cancellous bone are rare. Donor site complications include seroma, wound disruption, fracture through the cortical entry site, and seeding of the donor site with bacteria or malignant cells. Complications at the recipient site include failure of the graft to stimulate bone formation and resorption of the graft.

8.2 Cortical Bone Allograft or Alloimplant

8.2.1 Indications

Cortical bone allografts or alloimplants are used for mechanical support in fixation of large cortical defects. The allograft or alloimplant is a large piece of bone which is foreign to the host and requires rigid immobilization for a long period to allow vascularization, resorption of the graft or implant, and replacement with host bone, which is essential for successful incorporation into the healed fracture. Therefore, fixation must be done using proper dynamic compression plate (DCP) application for a two-level fracture. In addition, the technique, graft or implant, and recipient bed must be aseptic. Specific indications include mid-diaphyseal segmental bone replacement after severely comminuted fracture, tumor resection, or lengthening osteotomy.

8.2.2 Harvest and Storage

Cortical bone can be harvested and implanted immediately or stored until needed. If the cortical bone is not to be sterilized, strict adherence to guidelines to achieve an aseptic technique during harvest is essential. The donor is anesthetized and the donor sites prepared for aseptic collection; the long bones are disarticulated and the soft tissues removed. The donor is euthanatized. The metaphyses are resected and the marrow removed, and the bone is sealed in presterilized impermeable packages and stored in a freezer (−20 °) for 6–12 months. Bacterial culture of representative bone is done to monitor the technique. Alternatively, clean harvest is performed and the bones are sterilized with ethylene oxide before storage (Johnson 1988). Cortical bone can be implanted directly into the recipient site; however, freezing or freeze-drying improves incorporation of the implant.

8.2.3 Technique

Radiographs of the corresponding contralateral bone are made to identify the size of the graft or implant required and to serve as a template for correct contouring of the plate.

An aseptic technique is essential for successful fracture treatment with a cortical allograft or

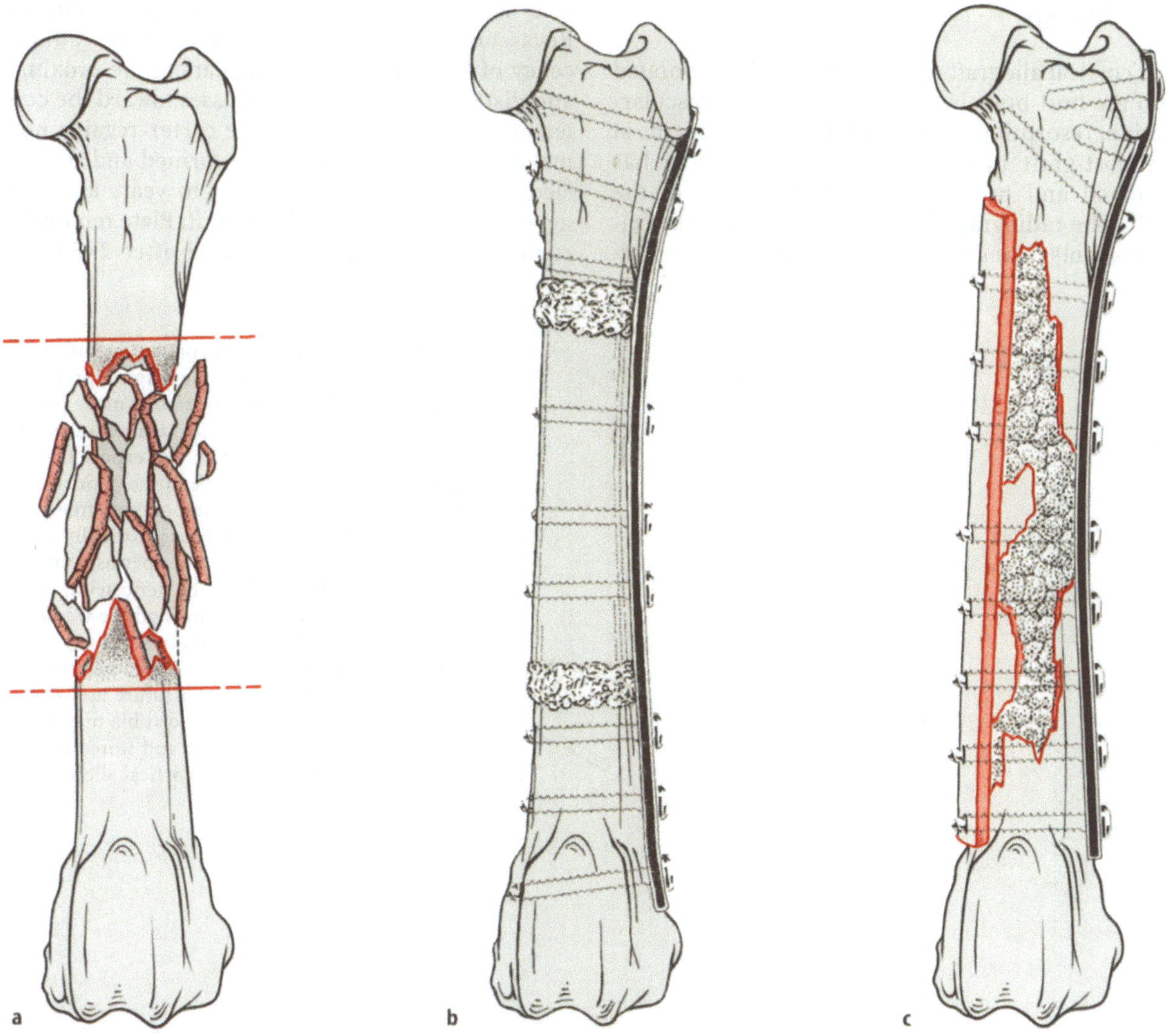

Fig. 8.5a–c. Cortical bone graft. **a,b**Tubular bone graft. In a badly comminuted midfemoral fracture, the fracture ends are trimmed with an oscillating saw. A frozen alloimplant is used to bridge the defect, applying compression according to the principles of a technique for fractures at two levels. The screws are placed in sequence and in a loaded or neutral position. An autogenous cancellous graft may be added at the host-graft interfaces. **c** Onlay graft as an alternative to the tubular graft. A longitudinally split rib is placed on the side opposite the plate, and the plate screws are anchored in the rib. Unvascularized small fragments may be removed and replaced with cancellous bone graft

implant. The appropriate graft is allowed to thaw in warm saline during the preparation of the recipient site. The fracture is approached and the comminuted fragments removed. The fractured ends of the proximal and distal bone segments are resected perpendicularly to the long axis of the bone and shaped to allow 360° contact with the graft. The graft is cut to the appropriate length and attached with screws to the precontoured plate using the neutral drill guide to position the screw holes. The plate graft composite is reduced to the proximal segment of the bone, and the load drill guide used through the first plate hole proximal to the host-graft interface. The hole is drilled, measured, and tapped and the screw is inserted, causing compression of the proximal host-graft interface. The distal bone fragment is reduced and the procedure repeated to create compression at the distal host-graft interface. The remaining plate holes are filled with screws placed in the neutral position. There must be adequate space for screws to be placed through three plate holes above and below the graft, and two plate holes in the graft (Fig. 8.5a,b). The recipient site is lavaged and cancellous bone autograft placed around the host-graft interfaces to encourage early bone bridging.

8.2.4 Biology

The cortical allograft or alloimplant is incorporated into the host bone by a slow process of revascularization, resorption, and remodeling which begins at the host-graft interfaces after bone bridging has occurred and proceeds toward the center of the graft. The radiographic appearance reflects the cellular events. Consolidation of the host-graft interface is observed by 3–4 months after surgery. Revascularization and resorption causes radiolucency of the cortex, which appears at the proximal and distal interfaces and progresses toward the center of the graft. Eventually, the cortex regains normal density as the host bone is formed and remodeled. This process takes months to years and may never completely remodel the graft. Plate removal is currently not recommended until after 2–3 years,

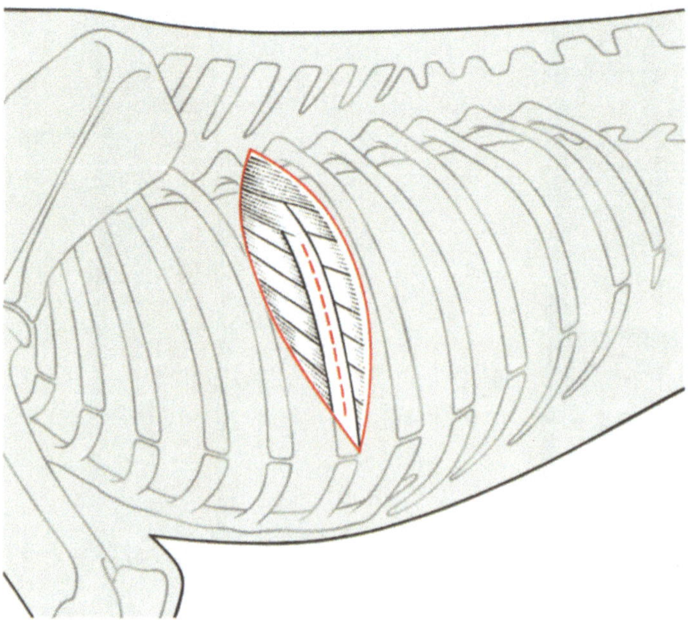

a

Fig. 8.6a–d. Rib. **a** With the patient in lateral recumbency and after routine surgical preparation and draping, a skin incision is made parallel to the sixth or seventh rib. Ligation of small vessels and simple dissection will expose the rib. **b** A midline incision is made in the periosteum. **c** The rib is then carefully and entirely freed from the periosteum and **d** cut proximally and distally. Perforation of the inner periosteum and pleura should be avoided. The periosteum is closed with absorbable suture, and the wound is closed routinely in layers. In nonsurviving donors, several of all of the ribs can be removed and stored in a bone bank for future use. The diaphyseal shaft of the femur or tibia may be collected in a similar manner and stored for future use as a full-cylinder cortical alloimplant

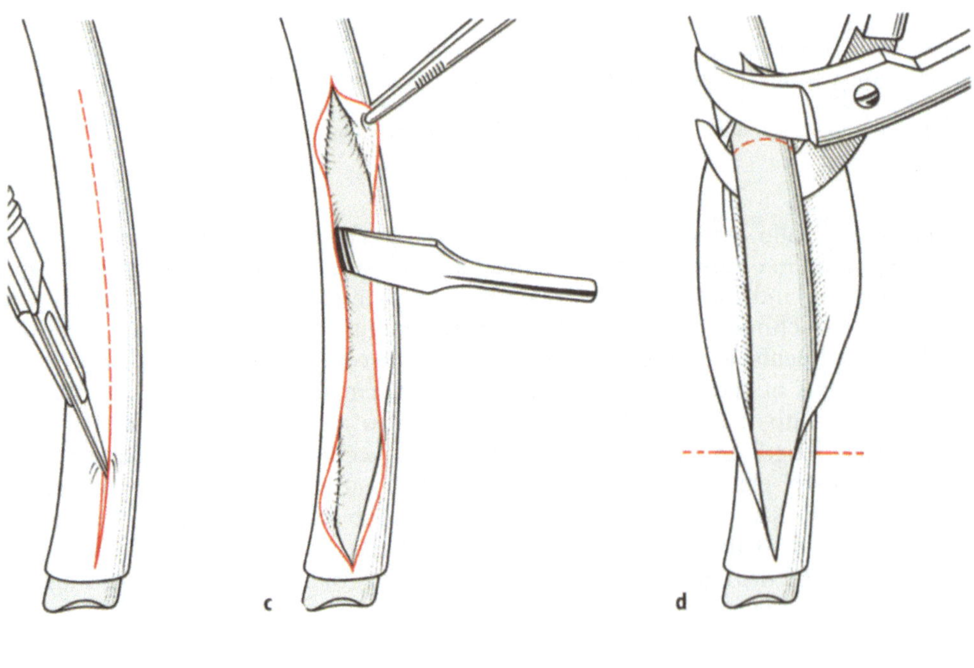

b c d

and in most cases it may be preferable to leave the plate in place indefinitely.

8.2.5 Complications

Infection and instability cause most of the complications associated with cortical allografts or alloimplants. The sequela is osteomyelitis with sequestration of the graft. Treatment involves removal of the graft, treatment with appropriate antibiotics, and buttress plate stabilization of the fracture with massive cancellous bone autografting of the cortical defect. Host rejection of the graft is evidenced by either sequestration of the donor tissue or resorption of the graft without replacement. Fracture of the unremodeled graft can occur with premature plate removal or plate failure.

8.3 Cortico-cancellous Bone Grafts

Either autogenous or allogenic cortico-cancellous bone grafts such as ribs (Fig. 8.6) or whole iliac crest can be used as chips for structural support.

9 Guidelines for Selecting Plate and Screw Size

The most important factors to be considered in choosing the size of implant include size of bone, weight of animal, type and location of fracture, activity, and condition of soft tissue. Some of the more common causes of failure include use of a plate which was too short or undersized, an insufficient number of screws, vascular impairment, induced infection, and failure to graft large architectural defects. If the basic principles of implantation are observed, the most consistent factor in choosing the size of the implant is the weight of the patient. However, the surgeon must evaluate each case on its individual merits.

Data has been compiled on more than several thousand clinical plate and screw fixation cases (AO/ASIF equipment) in which these techniques were used as the primary method of fixation. The summation of data collected is presented in the figures in the Appendix (Figs. A1–A5). As expected, there is some overlapping of appliance sizes for a given weight. This takes into account the other factors given above for choosing plate or screw size.

Application of the veterinary cuttable plate (VCP) is shown in Appendix A5.

10 Removal of Implants

Prior to removal of an implant used for fixation of a fracture, the following factors should be considered in arriving at the decision that clinical union is present:

1. Age of patient (see Table 10.1)
2. Location and type of fracture
3. History of fracture treatment: single or multiple operations, interrupted or inadequate fixation, impaired circulation, inadequate reduction and infection
4. Lapse of time since reduction and fixation: has there been sufficient time for healing to occur?
5. Type of fixation: optimal or less than optimal stabilization?
6. Radiographic examination (at least two views): clinical union

10.1 Indications for Removal of Bone Plates

The indications for removal of bone plates are as follows:

1. *Nonfunction.* Loose, bent, or broken plates, no longer serving a useful purpose and possibly causing discomfort or lameness or impeding healing.
2. *Thermal conduction.* Some owners have observed animals limping after being out in the cold. When they came back into a warm room, normal function returned. Removal of the plate after clinical union corrected the temporary intermittent lameness. This phenomenon is most frequently observed with fractures of radius and tibia.
3. *Irritation.* Infrequently, lesions characteristic of lick granulomas develop near the end of the plate closely adjacent to a joint, when the plates are covered only by subcutaneous tissue and skin. Plate removal is necessary in order to resolve the problem. This is usually carried out after clinical union.
4. *Infection.* The presence of low-grade infection is usually only resolved by removal of the implant, after the fracture has united. Fistulous tracks, if present, promptly resolve after plate removal. In some cases, sequestra which were not observed on the radiograph may be found under the plate. These are removed.
5. *Stress protection.* Plates are more rigid than bone. When applied for fixation of fractures, they may prevent the bone from responding to normal physiological stimuli, bringing about alterations in architecture and density which can be observed histologically and radiographically. The number which give rise to clinical problems is small and can usually be traced to the use of too large an implant or one left in place for a prolonged period. There is considerable evidence that this phenomenon is due to interference with the local vasculature.
6. *Accomplishment of objective.* After the fractured bone reaches the stage of clinical union, the implant does not serve any further purpose and may impede full functional performance, especially in field and racing animals. Many of the screws loosen after the fracture has healed. If a relatively long lever arm of bone extends beyond the last screw in the plate, a fracture may occur at this point, due to a difference in elasticity between the bone and plate, even though the original fracture has healed.

10.2 Suggested Time for Removal of Plates

Data on the age and plate removal time were collected from over 500 cases. From this, a schedule for approximate removal time was constructed (Table 10.1).

10.3 Surgical Removal of Implants

The skin incision and muscle separation used to remove the plate is usually the same as used for its insertion. In most cases, the cicatrix needs to be incised over the entire length of the plate. A portion

Table 10.1. Suggested time for removal of bone plates

Age (months)	Time (months)
≤3	1
3–6	2–3
6–10	3–5
>10	5–14

The removal period may need to be lengthened in more complicated and problematic cases.

of the plate may be covered with bone layer, which requires the use of an osteotome for removal. Build-up of bone along the edges of the plate is not removed. Following plate removal, hemorrhage is controlled and the wound closed by layers. It is always advisable to take a radiograph of the bone after implant removal; this allows a more accurate assessment of bone healing. The animal is usually released from hospital on the following day with instructions to the owner to restrict activity for at least 4 weeks. This may vary according to the radiographic appearance and activity of the patient.

In general, where bone screws are used as the primary method of fixation, they are left in place and not removed unless otherwise indicated.

10.4 Refracture

Refracture is defined as a fracture occurring in the region of a previous fracture which appears to have undergone sound union, both clinically and radiographically. In a documented series (Michigan State University Veterinary Hospital, unpublished), an incidence of approximately 1 % has been encountered following implant removal. Most refractures result from premature implant removal, poor anatomical reduction resulting in a fracture gap, osteoporotic bone, or failure to graft an architectural defect. This unfavorable sequela can be kept to a minimum if the basic principles of applying and removing implants are followed. In those cases in which the fracture appears to have healed radiographically, but the diameter of the fracture site area has decreased, improvement in bone structure and diameter usually follows removal of all but the end screws securing the plate to the bone. It may be months before the plate can be removed. In some instances, the addition of a cancellous bone graft is necessary.

10.5 Postoperative Care Following Removal

Much of the care needed after removal depends upon the appearance of the radiographs and activity of the patient. In general, postremoval care should consist of:

1. Supportive measures if the bone healing on the radiographs appears to be less than adequate
2. Restriction of activity for 1–6 weeks, which may mean confinement to a kennel or house, walking on a leash, or other limitations.

11 Appendix

1 Fractures of the Humerus

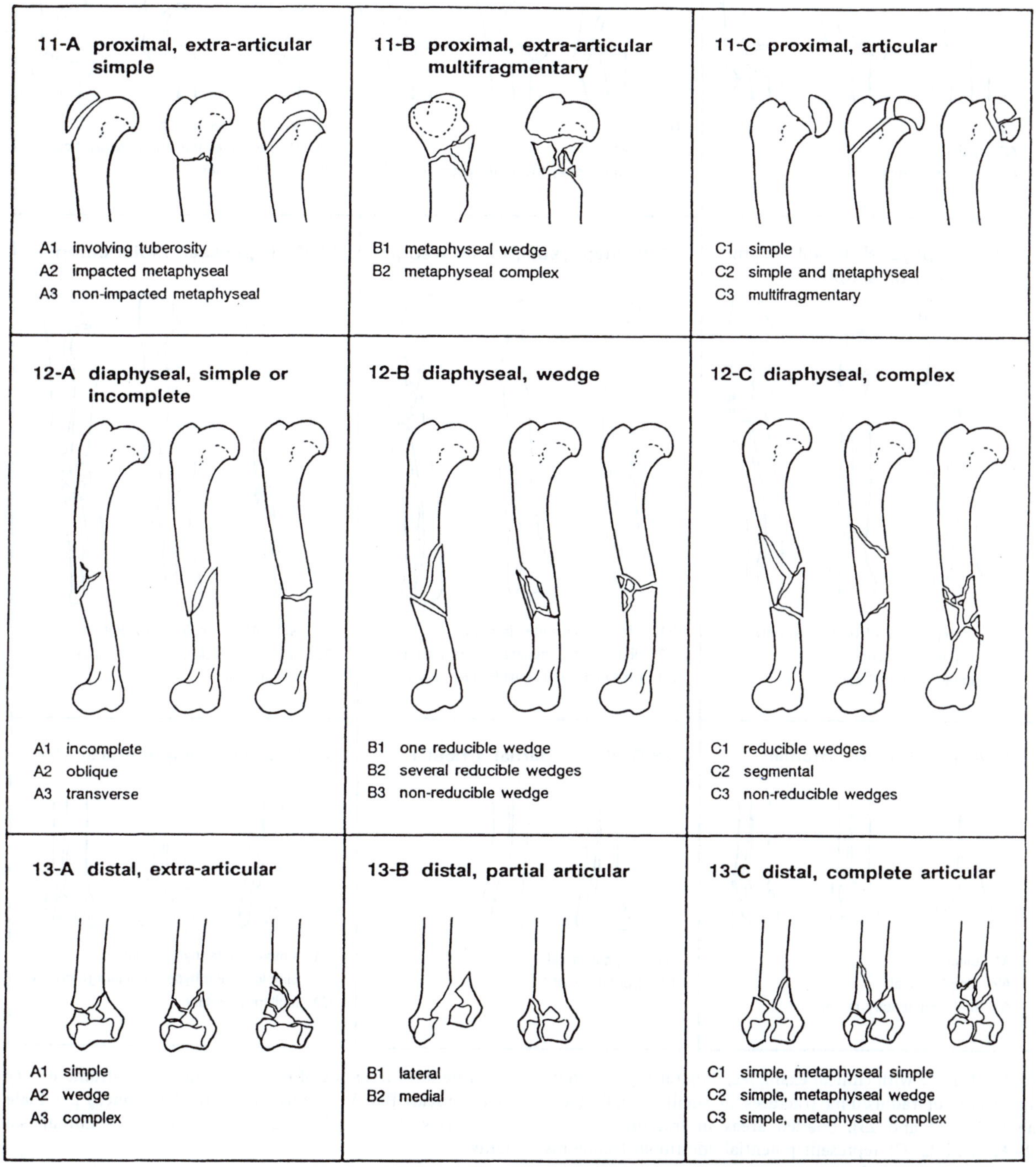

Fig. A1. **a** The broad dynamic compression plate (DCP) used with 4.5-mm cortex screws. **b** The narrow DCP. **c** The broad 3.5 DCP used with 3.5-mm cortex screws. **d** The 3.5 DCP to be used with 3.5-mm cortex screws. **e** The 2.7 DCP to be used with 2.7-mm cortex screws

Treatment – Circle one of the following: IM – Intramedullary (Diaphyseal) Pin, W – Wire, S – Screw(s) Alone, PL – Plate and Screw, P – Pin, EF – External Fixator, E – Euthanasia Only

2 Fractures of the Radius/Ulna

21-A proximal, extra-articular

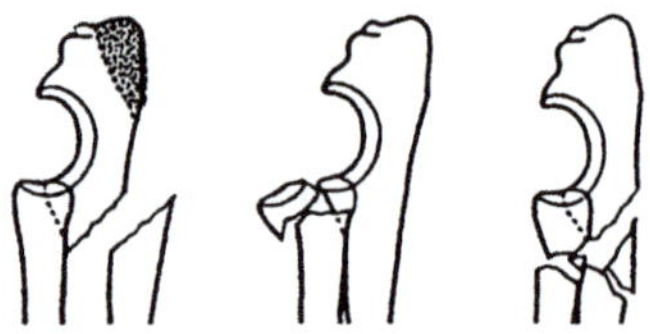

A1 ulnar
A2 radial
A3 of both bones

21-B proximal, simple articular

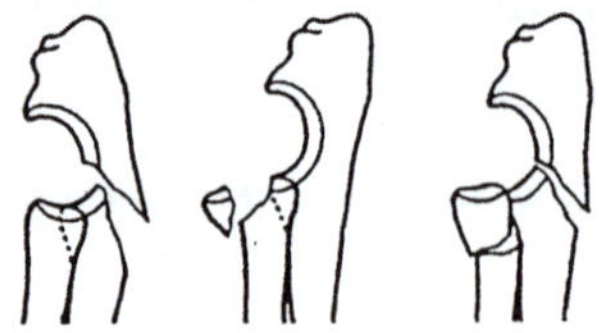

B1 ulnar
B2 radial
B3 of one bone, the other extra-articular

21-C proximal, multifragmentary articular

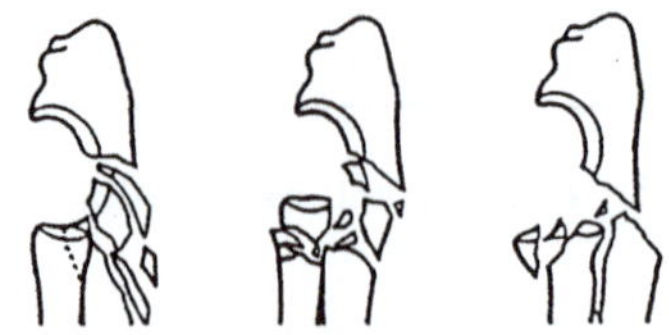

C1 one bone remains intact
C2 of one bone, the other extraarticular
C3 of both bones

22-A diaphyseal, radial incomplete or simple

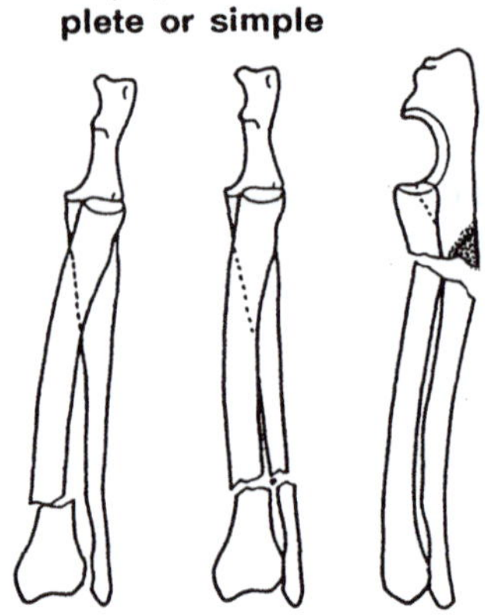

A1 incomplete or of one bone only
A2 simple, distal zone
A3 simple, proximal zone

22-B diaphyseal, radial wedge

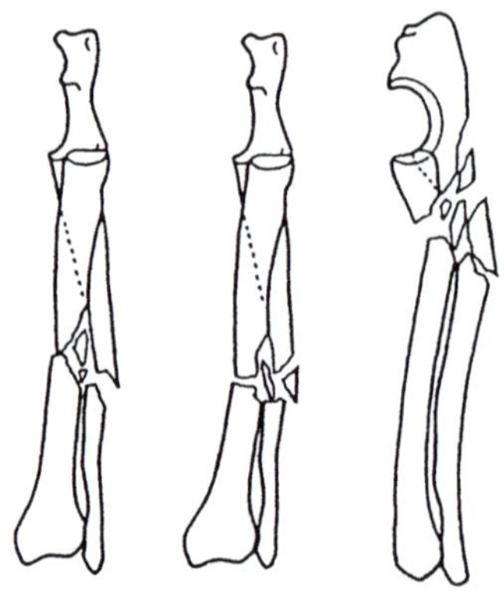

B1 with simple ulnar fracture
B2 distal zone, multifragmentary ulnar
B3 proximal zone, multifragmentary ulnar

22-C diaphyseal, radial complex

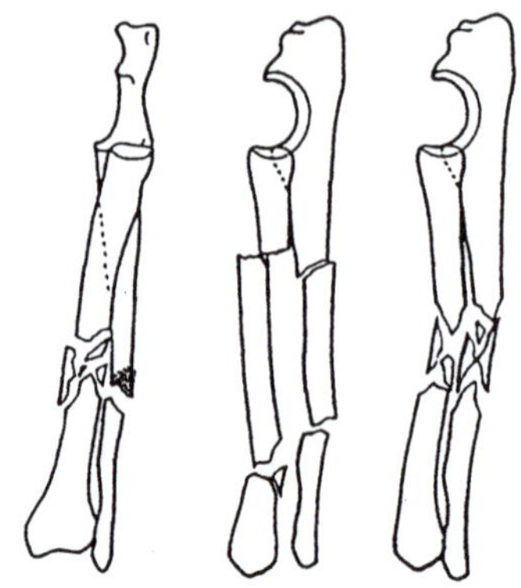

C1 with ulnar simple or wedge fracture
C2 segmental radial, complex ulnar
C3 complex ulnar

23-A distal, extra-articular

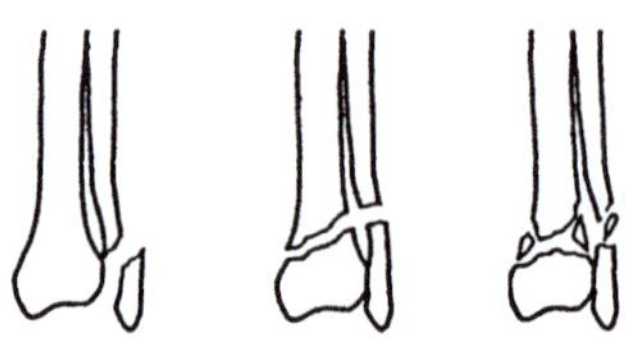

A1 ulnar
A2 simple radial
A3 multifragmentary radial

23-B distal, partial articular

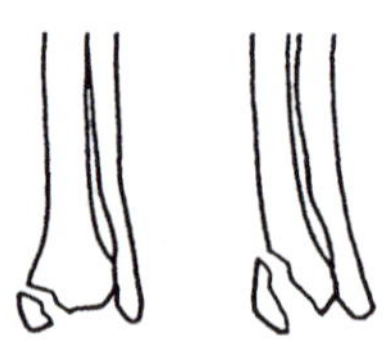

B1 sagittal radial
B2 frontal radial

23-C distal, complete articular

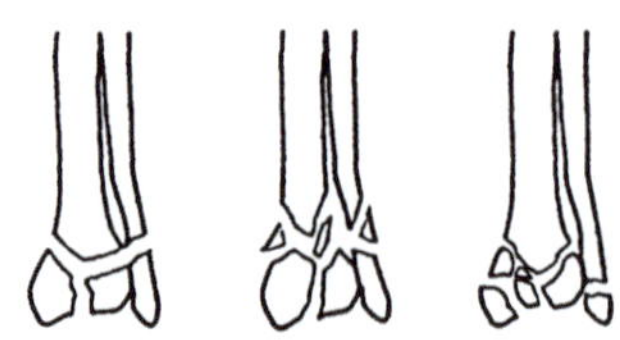

C1 simple, metaphyseal simple
C2 simple, metaphyseal multifragmentary
C3 multifragmentary

Fig. A1. b Table with clinical examples; illustrating the different groups of radius/ulna fractures in small animals (segments 21, 22 and 23). Shaded areas in fractures 21-A1, 22-A3, and 22-C1 represent potential additional fragments to be classified with the same code

Treatment – Circle one of the following: IM – Intramedullary (Diaphyseal) Pin, W – Wire, S – Screw(s) Alone, PL – Plate and Screw, P – Pin, EF – External Fixator, E – Euthanasia Only

3 Fractures of the Femur

31-A proximal, trochanteric region

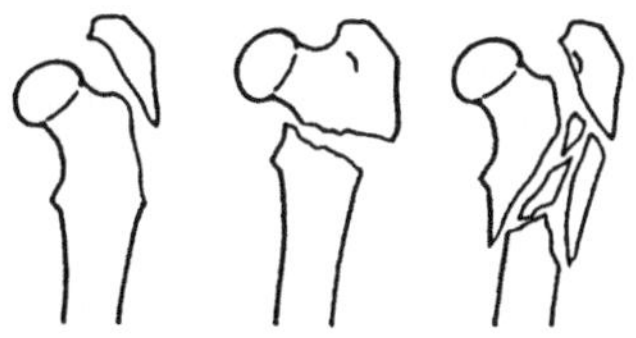

A1 avulsion
A2 intertrochanteric simple
A3 multifragmentary

31-B proximal, simple cervical

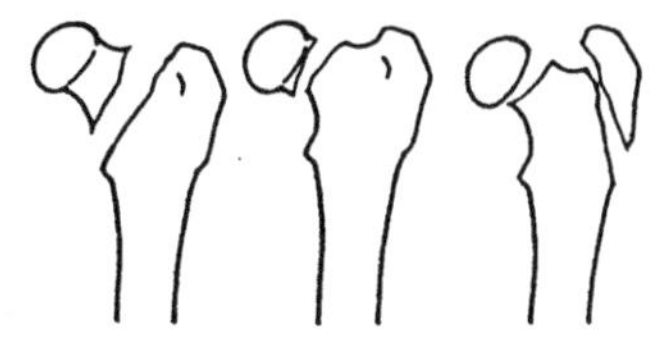

B1 basicervical
B2 transcervical
B3 with trochanteric avulsion

31-C proximal, capital or multi-fragmentary cervical

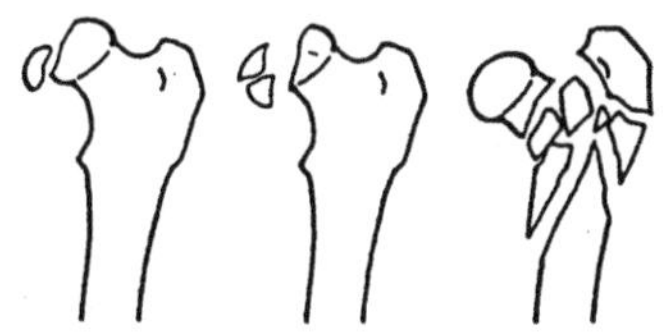

C1 articular simple
C2 articular multifragmentary
C3 multifragmentary cervical and trochanteric

32-A diaphyseal, simple or incomplete

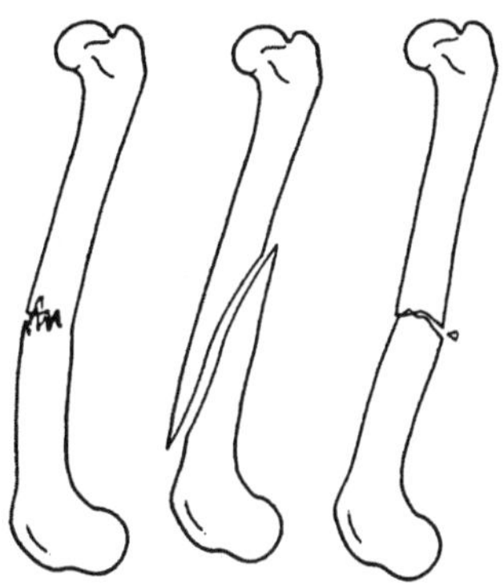

A1 incomplete
A2 oblique
A3 transverse

32-B diaphyseal wedge

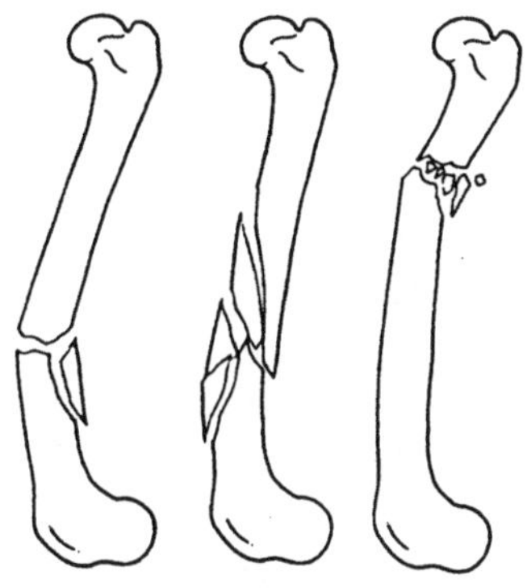

B1 one reducible wedge
B2 several reducible wedges
B3 non-reducible wedge

32-C diaphyseal, complex

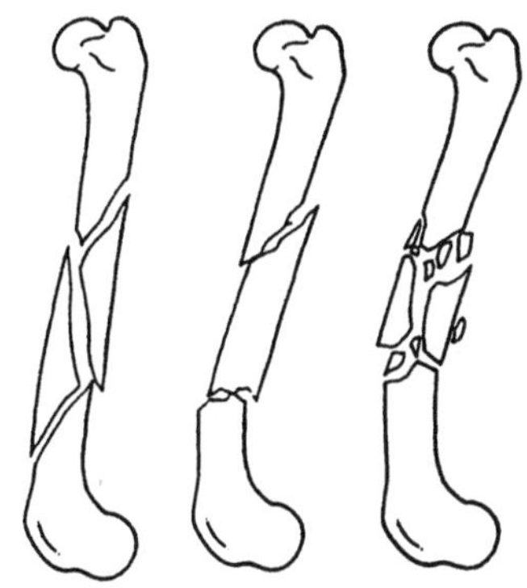

C1 reducible wedges
C2 segmental
C3 non-reducible wedges

33-A distal, extra-articular

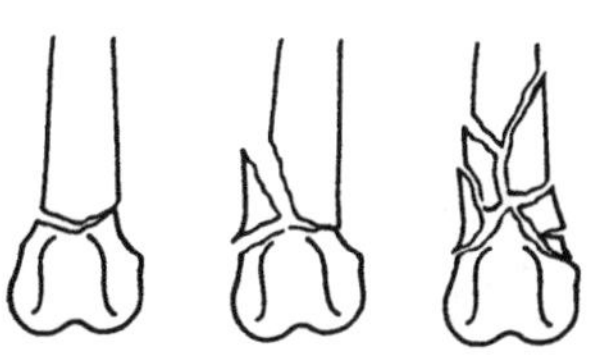

A1 simple
A2 wedge
A3 complex

33-B distal, partial articular

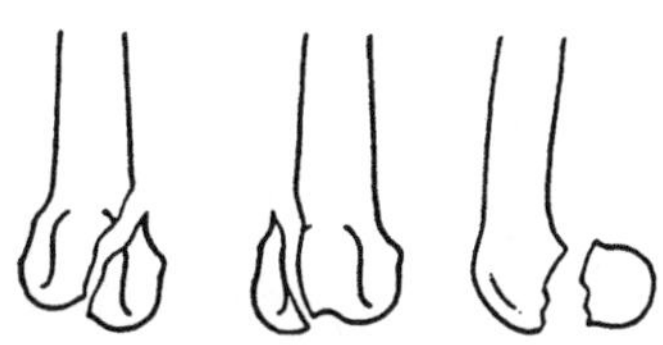

B1 lateral condyle, sagittal
B2 medial condyle, sagittal
B3 frontal, unicondylar

33-C distal, complete articular

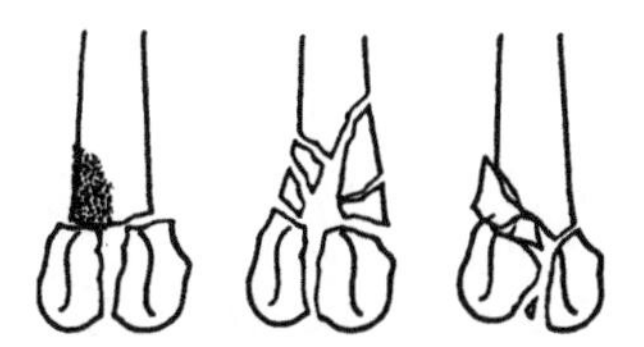

C1 simple, metaphyseal simple or wedge
C2 simple, metaphyseal complex
C3 multifragmentary

Fig. A1. c Table with clinical examples; illustrating the different groups of femur fractures in small animals (segments 31, 32 and 33). The shades area in fracture 33-C1 represent potential additional fragments to be classified with the same code

Treatment – Circle one of the following: IM – Intramedullary (Diaphyseal) Pin, W – Wire, S – Screw(s) Alone, PL – Plate and Screw, P – Pin, EF – External Fixator, E – Euthanasia Only

4 Fractures of the Tibia/Fibula

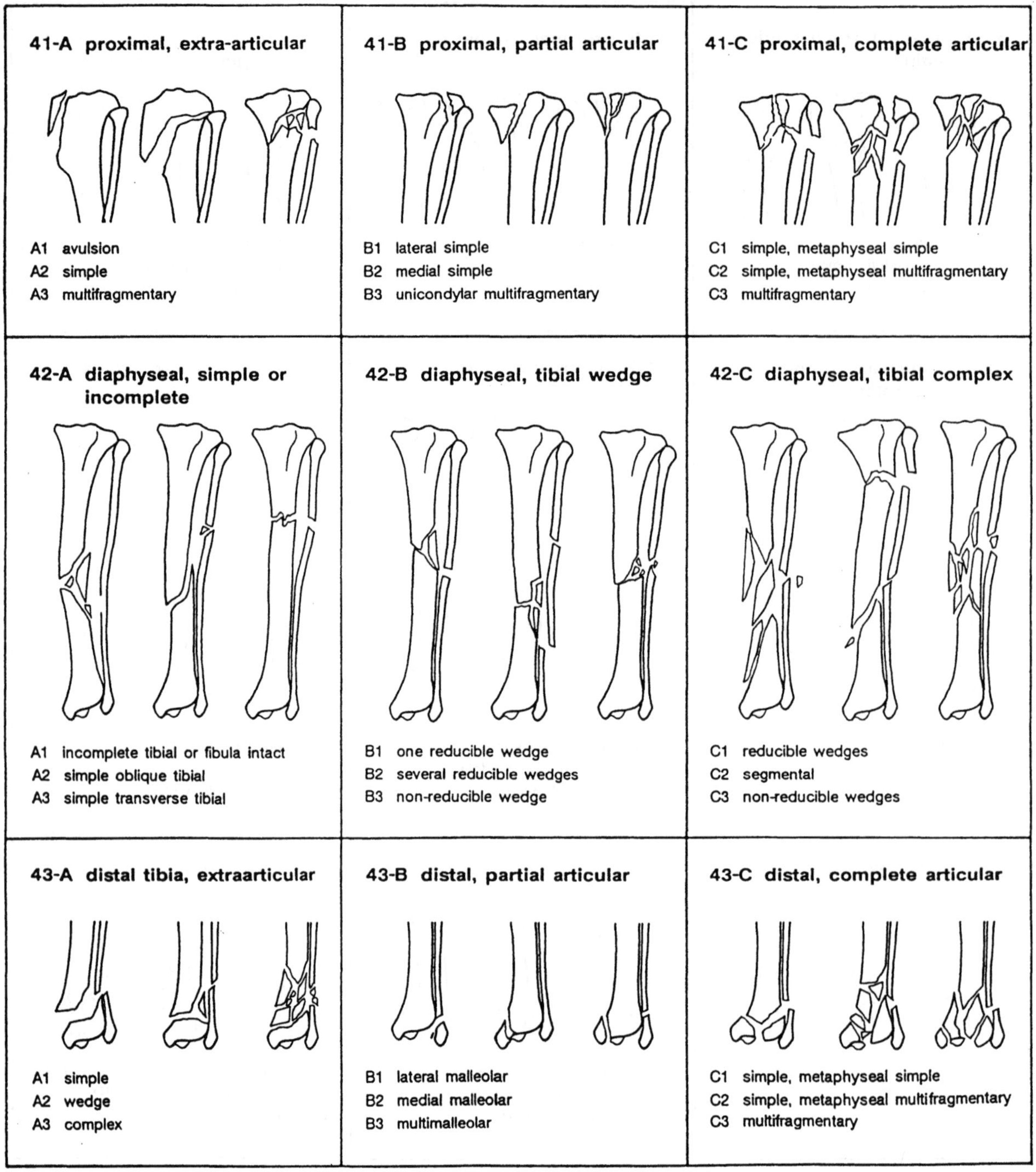

Fig. A1. d Table with clinical examples; illustrating the different groups of tibia/fibula fractures in small animals (segments 41, 42 and 43)

Treatment – Circle one of the following: IM – Intramedullary (Diaphyseal) Pin, W – Wire, S – Screw(s) Alone, PL – Plate and Screw, P – Pin, EF – External Fixator, E – Euthanasia Only

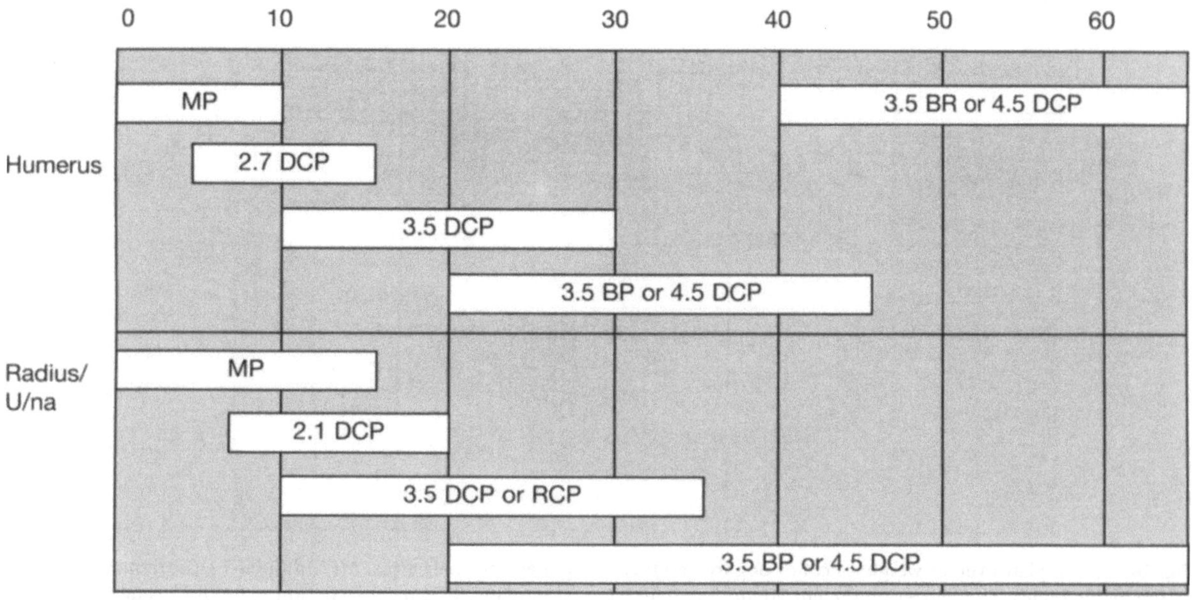

Fig. A2. Size of plate versus weight of cat or dog for fractures of the forelimb. The figures on the *horizontal line* for each anatomical structure refer to the approximate weight (in kg) of the animal for use of the various plates and their sizes. *MP*, miniplate; *DCP*, dynamic compression plate; *RCP*, reconstruction plate; *BR*, broad plate. Plates referred to are standard AO/ASIF implants

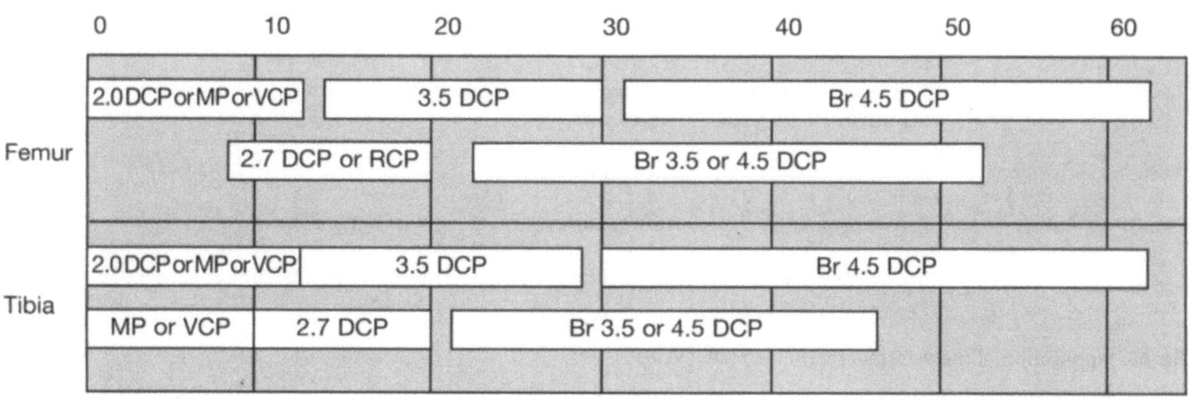

Fig. A3. Size of plate versus weight of cat or dog for fractures of the hindlimb. The figures on the *horizontal line* for each anatomical structure refer to the approximate weight (in kg) of the animal for use of the various plates and their sizes. *MP*, miniplate; *DCP*, dynamic compression plate; *RCP*, reconstruction plate. Plates referred to are standard AO/ASIF implants

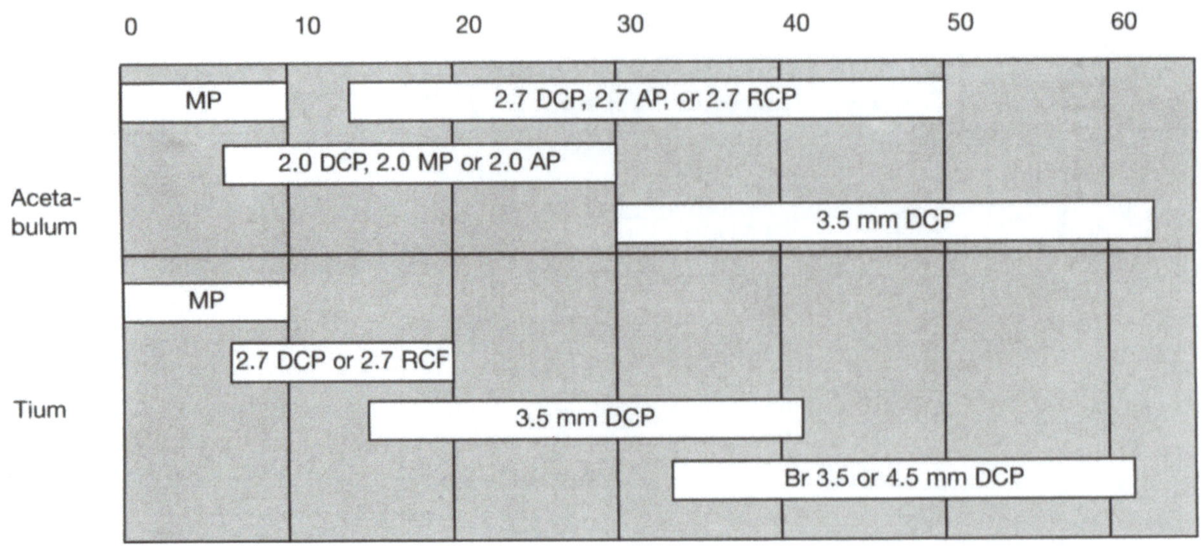

Fig. A4. Size of plates versus weight of cat or dog for fractures of the pelvic bones. The figures on the *horizontal line* refer to the approximate weight of the animal for use of the various plates and their sizes. *MP*, miniplate; *DCP*, dynamic compression plate; *RCP*, reconstruction plate; *AP*, acetabular plate

Patient	Weight (kg)	Bone	Fracture type	VCP	Screw
Cat	3–5	Humerus, femur, tibia	Transverse	Single 2.0/2.7	2.0
Cat	3–5	Humerus, femur, tibia	Multifragment, comminuted	3/4 sandwich 2.0/2.7–2.0./1.5	2.0
Dog	<5	Humerus, femur, tibia	Transverse or oblique	Single 2.0/2.7	2.0
Dog	<5	Humerus, femur, tibia	Multifragment, comminuted	3/4 sandwich 2.0/2.7–2.0/1.5	2.0
Dog	5–7	Humerus, femur, tibia, radius/ulna	All fracture types	1/1 sandwich 2.0/2.7–2.0/1.5	2.0
Dog	7–12	Humerus, femur, tibia, radius/ulna	All fracture types	1/1 sandwich 2.0/2.7–2.0/2.7	2.0 2.7
Dog	5–20	Pelvic, scapula	All fracture types	Single 2.0/2.7	2.0 2.7
Dog	>20	Metacarpus, tarsus, mandibula, skull, ulna	All fracture types	Single, 2.0/2.7 2.0	2.0 2.7

Fig. A5. Application of the veterinary cuttable plate (VCP)

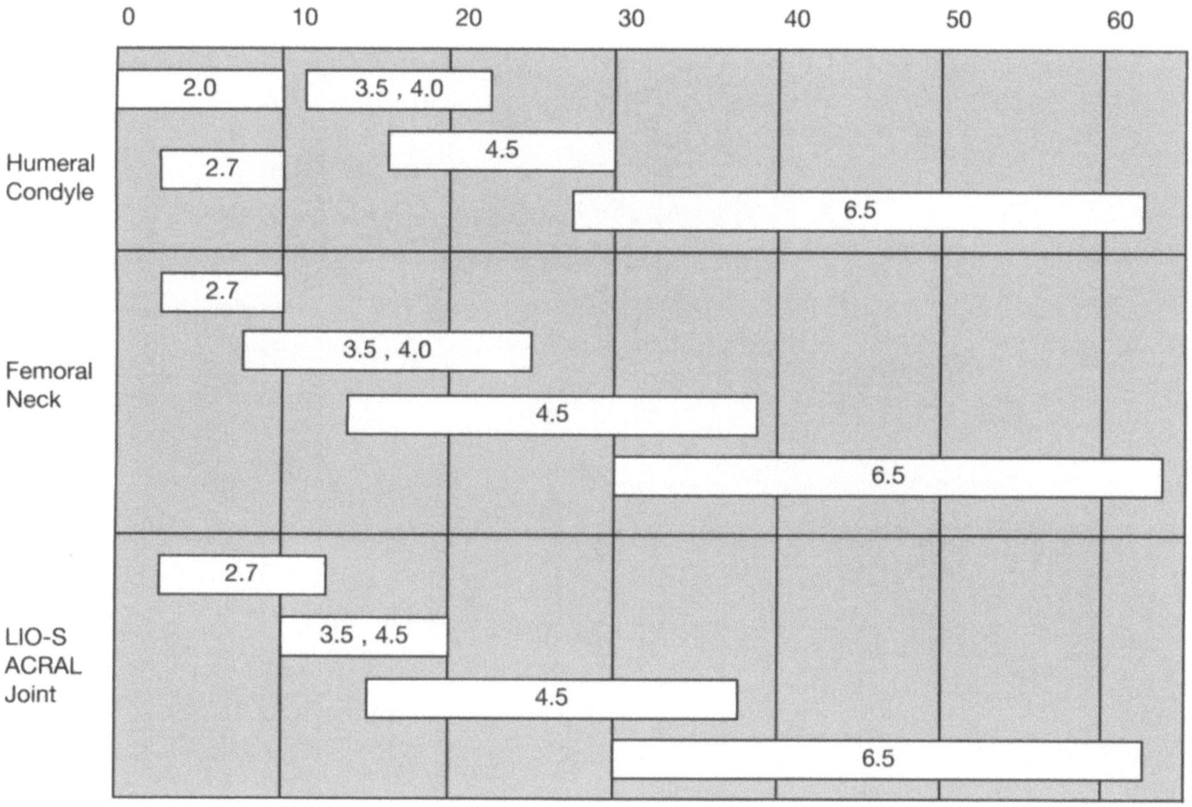

Fig. A6. Guide for selection of screw diameter (in mm) with respect to the weight of the animal. All screws referred to are standard AO/ASIF implants

12 References

Aeberhardt HJ (1973) Der Einfluß der Platten-Überbiegung auf die Torsionsstabilität der Osteosynthese. Inaugural dissertation, University of Bern

Allgöwer M (1978) Cinderella of surgery - fractures? Surg Clin North Am 58:1071-1093

Allgöwer M, Ehrsam R, Ganz R, Matter P, Perren SM (1969) Clinical experience with a new compression plate "DCP". Acta Orthop Scand [Suppl] 125:45-63

Allgöwer M, Matter P, Perren SM, Rüedi T (1973) The dynamic compression plate. Springer, Berlin Heidelberg New York

Allgöwer M, Durig M, Wolff G (1980) Infection and trauma. Surg Clin North Am 60:2

Anderson R (1936) Femoral bone lengthening. Am J Surg 31:479

Ansell RH, Scales JT (1968) A study of some factors which affect the strength of screws and their insertion and holding power in bone. J Biomech 1:279-302

Ashhurst DE (1986) The influence of mechanical conditions on the healing of experimental fractures in the rabbit. A microscopical study. Phil Trans R Soc Lond 313:271-302

Bagby GW, James JM (1957) An impacting bone plate. Staff meeting. Mayo Clin 32:55-57

Barraud GE (1982) De la stabilité des osteotomies spiroides in vitro fixées par différents vissages avec ou sans plaque de protection. Inaugural dissertation, University of Bern

Bassett CAL (1972) Clinical implications of cell function in bone grafting. Clin Orthop Rel Res 87: 4-59

Baumgart F (1991) The "mixing" of implant systems. Vet Comp Orthopaed Traumatol 4:38-45

Beaupre GS, Schneider E, Perren SM (1984) Stress analysis of a partially slotted intramedullary nail. J Orthop Res 2:369-376

Behrens F (1989) General theory and principle of external fixation. Clin Orthop 241:15-23

Behrens F, Searls K (1986) External fixation of the tibia. Basic concepts and prospective evaluation. J Bone Joint Surg [Br] 68:246-254

Berg P (1985) Wound ballistics. In: Newton CD, Nunamaker DM, (eds) Textbook of small animal orthopaedics. Lippincott, Philadelphia, pp 486-497

Bertoy RW, Johnson AL, Weigel RM (1989) Organ system injury and post-operative complications in dogs and cats with two long bone fractures: a matched case design. Vet Comp Orthopaed Traumatol 4:140-143

Bier A (1918) Beobachtungen über die Regeneration beim Menschen. Dtsch Med Wochenschr 44:281-284

Biliouris T, Schneider E, Rahn BA, Gasser B, Perren SM (1989) The effect of radial preload on the implant-bone interface: a cadaveric study. J Orthop Trauma 3:323-332

Blümlein H, Cordey J, Schneider UA, Rahn BA, Perren SM (1977) Langzeitmessung der Axialkraft von Knochenschrauben in vivo. Med Orthop Tech 97:17-19

Böhler L (1938) Technik der Knochenbruchbehandlung. Maudrich, Vienna

Bonin JG(1942) Time of union in the fractured tibia. Lancet 2:439

Bookbinder DF, Flanders JA (1992) Characteristics of pelvic fracture in the cat. A 10-year retrospective study. Vet Comp Orthopaed Traumatol 5:122-127

Border J, Allgöwer M, Hansen T, Rüedi T (1990) Blunt multiple trauma: comprehensive pathophysiology and care. Dekker, New York

Braden TD (1991) Post-traumatic osteomyelitis. Vet Clin North Am Small Anim Pract 21:781-811

Braden TD, Johnson CA, Gabel CL et al (1987) Posologic evaluation of clindamycin, using a canine model of post-traumatic osteomyelitis. Am J Vet Res 48:7

Braden TD, Johnson CA, Wakenell P et al (1988) Efficacy of clindamycin in the treatment of Staphylococcus aureus osteomyelitis in dogs. J Am Vet Med Assoc 192:12

Braden TD, Tvedten H, Mostosky UV et al (1989) The sensitivity and specificity of radiology and histopathology in the diagnosis of post-traumatic osteomyelitis. Vet Comp Ortho Trauma 3:98

Braden TD, Eicker SW, Abdinoor D, Prieur WD (1995) Characteristics of 1,000 femur fractures in the dog and cat. Vet Comp Orthopaed Traumatol 8:203-209

Brennwald J, Matter P, von Arx C, Cordey J, Perren SM (1975) Peroperative Messung des Drehmomentes an Knochenschrauben. Unfallmed Berufskr 3:123-126

Brinker WO (1990) Suggestions for the reduction of fractures. Vet Comp Orthopaed Traumatol 1:27-30

Brinker WO, Hohn RB, Prieur WD (1984) Manual of internal fixation in small animals, 1st edn. Springer, Berlin Heidelberg New York, p 216

Brinker WO, Piermattei DL, Flo GL (1990) Handbook of small animal orthopedics and fracture treatment. Saunders, Philadelphia, pp 68-69

Brunner CF, Weber BG (1981) Besondere Osteosynthesetechniken. Springer, Berlin Heidelberg New York

Brunner U, Schweiberer L, Cordey J, Rahn B, Perren SM (1990a) Treatment of large bone defects using segment bone transportation with nail fixation: experimental study. Transactions of the 36th Annual Meeting of Orthopaedic Research Society, New Orleans, 1990

Brunner U, Kessler S, Cordey J, Rahn B, Schweiberer L, Perren SM (1990b) Defektbehandlung langer Röhrenknochen durch Distraktionsosteogenese (Ilizarov) und Marknagelung. Theoretische Grundlagen, tierexperimentelle Ergebnisse, klinische Relevanz. Unfallchirurg 93:244-250

Brutscher R, Rueter A, Perren SM (1989) Der Stellenwert der Corticotomie und Osteotomie nach Segmentverschiebung bei der Behandlung von Knochendefekten. 53nd Annual

Meeting of the Deutsche Gesellschaft für Unfallheilkunde, Berlin

Bruse S, Dee J, Prieur WD (1989) Internal fixation with a veterinary cuttable plate 1989. Vet Comp Orthopaed Traumatol 1:40–46

Burchardt H, Enneking WF (1978) Transplantation of bone. Surg Clin North Am 58:403–427

Burwell RG (1969) The fate of bone grafts. In :Apley AG (ed) Recent Advances in orthopaedics. Williams and Wilkins, Baltimore, pp 115–207

Cameron BM (1966) Shaft fractures and pseudarthrosis. Thomas, Springfield

Caywood DD, Wallace LV, Braden TD (1978) Osteomyelitis in the dog: a review of 67 cases. J Am Vet Med Assoc 172:943–946

Claes L, Burri C, Kinzl L, Fitzer E, Hüttner W (1980) Less rigid fixation with carbon fibre reinforced materials: mechanical characteristics and behavior in vivo. In: Uhthoff HK, Stahl E (eds) Current concepts of internal fixation of fractures. Springer, Berlin Heidelberg New York, pp 156–159

Claes L, Palme U, Palme E, Kirschbaum U (1982) Biomechanical and mathematical investigations concerning stress protection of bone beneath internal fixation plates. In: Huiskes R, van Campen DH, de Vijn JR (eds) Biomechanics: principles and applications. Nijhoff, The Hague, pp 325–330

Claudi B, Schläpfer F, Cordey J, Perren SM, Allgöwer M (1979) Die schräge Plattenzugschraube - In-vitro-Messungen der Stabilität an queren Osteotomien des Tibiaschaftes. Helv Chir Acta 46:177–182

Cochran GVB (1969) Effects of internal fixation plates on mechanical deformation of bone. Surg Forum Orthop Surg 20:469–471

Cordey J (1987) Analyse mécanique de l'ostéosynthèse par plaque. PhD thesis, University of Lausanne

Cordey J, Schnetzer M, Brennwald J, Regazzoni P, Perren SM (1980) Direct in vivo measurements of torque and bending in sheep tibiae. In: Uhthoff HK, Stahl E (eds) Current concepts of internal fixation of fractures. Springer, Berlin Heidelberg New York, pp 78–87

Cordey J, Schwyzer HK, Brun S, Matter P (1985) Bone loss following plate fixation of fractures? Helv Chir Acta 52:181–184

Cordey J, Perren SM, Steinemann S (1987) Parametric analysis of the stress protection in bone after plating. In: Bergmann G, Kölbel R, Rohlmann A (eds) Biomechanics: basic and applied research. Nijhoff, Dordrecht, pp 387–392

Coutts RE, Akeson WH, Woo S, Matthews JV, Gonsalves M, Amiel D (1976) Comparison of stainless steel and composite plates in the healing of diaphyseal osteotomies of the dog radius: report on a short term study. Orthop Clin North Am 7:223–229

Danis R (1947) The operative treatment of bone fractures. J Intern Chir 7:318–320

Danis R (1979) Theorie et pratique de l'ostéosynthèse. Masson, Paris

Danckwardt-Lilliestrom G, Grevsten S, Olerud S (1972) Investigation of effect of various agents on periosteal bone formation. Ups J Med Sci 77:125–128

deHaan JT, Roe SC, Lewis DD, Renberg WC, Kerwin SC, Bebchuk TN (1996) Elbow arthrodesis in twelve dogs. Vet Comp Orthopaed Traumatol 9:115–118

DeMuth WF Jr (1966) Bullet velocity and design as determinants of wounding capability: an experimental study. J Trauma 6: 222–232

de Oliviera JC (19971) Bone grafts and chronic osteomyelitis. J Bone Joint Surg 53B: 672–683

Diehl K (1975) Stabilität und Beanspruchung von Osteosynthesen des Ober- und Unterschenkels bei der Frühmobilisation. Unfallheilkunde 79:81–89

Egger EL, Histand MB, Noridin RW, Kouds LJ, Schwarz PD (1993) Canine osteotomy healing when stabilised with decreasingly rigid fixation compared to constantly rigid fixation. Vet Comp Orthopaed Traumatol 6:182–187

Eisner HP, Barraud GE, Johner RT, Cordey J (1985) Optimal insertion of lag screws for internal fixation of spiral fracture of the tibia. Biomechanics 1:543

Elek SD, Conen PE (1957) The virulence of Staphylococcus pyogenes for man; a study of the problems of wound infection. Br J Exp Pathol 38:573

Feng TS, Ma Y, Fu RX, Li M (1988) The wounding characteristics of spherical steel fragments in live tissues. J Trauma 28(1):37–40

Fernández Dell'Oca AA (1989) Modular external fixation in emergency with the AO tubular system. Intergraf, Montevideo

Fox SM, Machon RG (1992) Use of double hook plates to correct bilateral tibial deformity in a Borzoi. J Am Anim Hosp Assoc 28:125–128

Francis DJ, Johnson KA (1990) Interfragmentary stability influence of intra-articular fractures. A radiographic study of canine femoral condyle fractures repaired with lag screws. Vet Comp Orthopaed Traumatol 3:71–77

Fries CL, Binnington AG, Cockshutt JR (1988) Quadriceps contract use in four cats: a complication of internal fixation of femoral/fractures. Vet Comp Orthopaed Traumatol 2:91–96

Fruchter AM, Holmberg DL (1991) Mechanical analysis of the veterinary cuttable plate. Vet Comp Orthopaed Traumatol 4:116–119

Frost HM (1989) The biology of fracture healing - an overview for clinicians, part II. Clin Orthop Rel Res 248:294–309

Ganz R, Brennwald J (1987) L'ostéosynthèse à compression du tibia du lapin. Etude de la revascularisation du canal medullaire et de la corticale sous fixation stable. In: Boitzy A (ed) Ostéogenèse et compression. Huber, Bern, pp 166–173

Ganz R, Perren SM, Rüter A (1975) Mechanical induction of bone resorption. Fortschr Kiefer Gesichtschir 19:45–48

Gautier E (1988) Belastungsveränderung des Knochens durch Plattenosteosynthese. Dissertation, University of Bern

Gautier E, Cordey J, Lüthi U, Mathys R, Rahn BA, Perren SM (1983) Knochenumbau nach Verplattung: biologische oder mechanische Ursache? Helv Chir Acta 50:53–58

Gautier E, Cordey J, Mathys R, Rahn BA, Perren SM (1984) Porosity and remodelling of plated bone after internal fixation: result of stress shielding or vascular damage? Elsevier Science, Amsterdam

Gautier E, Rahn BA, Perren SM (1986) Effect of steel versus composite plastic plates on internal and external remodeling of intact long bones. Orthop Trans 10:391

Genge M, Schneider E, Michel MC, Genge H, Perren SM (1988) Hochauflösende implantierbare Telemetrie-Anlage für statische Belastungsmessungen. European Telemetry Conference. Döring-Druck, Braunschweig, pp 288–296

Goldberg VM, Stevenson S (1987) Natural history of autografts and allografts. Clin Orthop Rel Res 225:7–16

Goldsmith S, Johnson KA (1991) Complications of canine tibial tuberosity avulstion fractures. Vet Comp Orthopaed Traumatol 4:54–58

Goodship AE, Kenwright J (1985) The influence of induced micromovement upon the healing of experimental fractures. J Bone Joint Surg [Br] 67:650–655

Gotzen L, Huetter J, Haas N (1980) The prebending of AO plates in compression osteosynthesis. In: Uhthoff HK, Stahl E (eds) Current concepts of internal fixation of fractures. Springer, Berlin Heidelberg New York, pp 201–210

Gotzen L, Haas N, Strohfeld G (1981) Zur Biomechanik der Plattenosteosynthese. Unfallheilkunde 84:439–443

Gozna, ER, Harrington,IJ (1982) Biomechanics of musculoskeletal injury. Williams and Wilkins, Baltimore

Gray JC, Elves MW (1981) Osteogenesis in bone grafts after short term storage and topical antibiotic treatment. J Bone Joint Surg 63B: 441–445

Gunst MA, Suter C, Rahn BA (1979) Die Knochendurchblutung nach Plattenosteosynthese. Helv Chir Acta 46:171–175

Haas N, Gotzen L, Riefenstahl L (1985) Biomechanische Untersuchungen zur Plattenfixation an die Hauptfragmente. Orthopedics 123:591

Hayes WC (1980) Basic biomechanics of compression plate fixation. In: Uhthoff HK, Stahl E (eds) Current concepts of internal fixation of fractures. Springer, Berlin Heidelberg New York, pp 49–62

Hay CW, Muir P, Johnson KA (1995) Control tarsal bone fracture in two dalmations. Vet Comp Orthopaed Traumatol 8:218–221

Hayes WC, Perren SM (1971) Flexural rigidity of compression plate fixation of fractures. Proceedings of the 2nd Nordic Conference on Medical and Biological Engineering, pp 242–244

Hearn TC, Surowiak JF, Schatzker J (1992) Effect of tapping on the holding strength of cancellous bone screws. Vet Comp Orthopaed Traumatol 5:10–12

Heini PF (1988) Untersuchungen der Tibia-Innenform im Zusammenhang mit der Marknagelung. Inaugural dissertation, University of Bern

Heiple KG, Goldberg VM, Powell AE, Bos GD, Zika JM (1987) Biology of cancellous bone graft. Orthop Clin North Am 18:179–185

Heitemeyer U, Hierholzer G (1985) Die überbrückende Osteosynthese bei geschlossenen Stückfrakturen des Femurschaftes. Akt Traumatol 15:205–209

Henry WB, Wadsworth PL (1981a) Diaphyseal allografts in the repairof long bone fractures. J Am Anim Hosp Assoc 17:525–534

Henry WB, Wadsworth PL (1981b) Ranalysis of failures in the repair of severely comminuted long bone fractures using large diaphyseal allografts. J Am Anim Hosp Assoc 17:525–534

Hertel R (1984) Beanspruchung von Osteosyntheseplatten mit schraubenfreiem Plattenloch. Inaugural dissertation, University of Bern

Hoffmann R, Krettek C, Haas N, Tscherne H (1989) Die distale Radiusfraktur. Frakturstabilisierung mit biodegradablen Osteosynthese-Stiften (Biofix). Experimentelle Untersuchungen und erste klinische Erfahrungen. Unfallchirurg 92:430–434

Harari J, Dunning D (1993) Fractures of the scapula in dogs: a retrospective review of 12 cases. Vet Comp Orthopaed Traumatol 6:105–108

Huiming T, Guanggui D, Mingjing H, Fengguo T, Guanyi S, Yingiu L (1988) Quantitative bacteriological study of the wound track. J Trauma 28(1):215–216

Huiskes R, Chao EYS, Crippen TE (1985) Parametric analyses of pin-bone stresses in external fracture fixation devices. J Orthop Res 3:341–349

Hulse D, van Gundy T, Johnson S, Waldron D (1989) Compression screw stabilisation of oblique ilial fractures in dogs. Vet Comp Orthopaed Traumatol 4:162–167

Hunt CA, Litsky AS (1988) Stabilisation canine pelvic osteotomies with AO/ASIF plates and screws. Vet Comp Orthopaed Traumatol 1:52–57

Hutzschenreuter P, Perren SM, Steinemann S, Geret V, Klebl M (1969) Some effects of rigidity of internal fixation on the healing pattern of osteotomies. Injury 1:77–81

Hyldahl C, Pearson S, Tepic S, Perren SM (1988) Induction and prevention of pin loosening in external fixators in the sheep tibia. Orthop Trans 12:378

Ilizarov GA (1989) The tension-stress effect on the genesis and growth of tissues. Clin Orthop 238: 249–281

Johner RT, Joerger K, Cordey J, Perren SM (1989) Rigidity of pure lag-screw fixation as a function of screw inclination in an in vitro spiral osteotomy. Clin Orthop 178:74–79

Johnson AL (1988) Principles and practical applications of cortical bone grafting techniques. Comp Contin Educ 10:906–913

Johnson AL (1991) Principles of bone grafting. Semin Vet Med Surg 6:90–99

Johnson AL, Stein LE (1988) Morphologic comparison of healing patterns in ethylene oxide sterilized cortical allografts and untreated control autografts in the dog. Am J Vet Res 49:101–105

Johnson AL, Stein LE, Roe SC (1987) Evaluation of collagen and autogenous cancellous bone used in repair of full thickness cortical bone defects. Vet Surg 16:146–150

Johnson KA (1986) Cancellous bone graft collection from the tibia in dogs. Vet Surg 15:334–338

Johnson KA, Bellenger CR (1980) The effects of autologous bone grafting on bone healing after carpal arthrodesis in the dog. Vet Rec 107:126–132

Johnson KA, Piermattei DL, Davis PE, Bellenger CR (1988) Characteristics of accessory carpal bone fractures in 50 racing greyhounds. Vet Comp Orthopaed Traumatol 2:104–107

Jörger KA (1987) Akute intrakortikale Durchblutungsstörung unter Osteosyntheseplatten mit unterschiedlichen Auflageflächen. Inaugural dissertation, University of Bern

Katzsokepreuter P, Babeck JO, Bruemmer H (1988) Transverse deformation of long bones in vivo during lag screw application. Vet Comp Orthopaed Traumatol 3:146–147

Kempf I, Grosse A, Lafforgue D (1978) L'apport du verouillage dans l'enclouage centro-medullaire des os longs. Rev Chir Orthop 64:635–651

Kessler SB, Perren SM, Hallfeldt KKJ, Madelkow H (1988) Refrakturen nach operativer Frakturenbehandlung. Biologische Aspekte. Hefte Unfallheilkd 194:13–27

Kamibayashi L, Pfieffer S, Hearn T, Taves C, Thompson JJ, Binnington AG (1989) Vet Comp Orthopaed Traumatol 3:104–107

Kirschner M (1916) Die künstliche Verlängerung von Beinen, die nach Frakturen, namentlich nach Schußfrakturen, mit starker Verkürzung geheilt sind. Beitr Klin Chir 100:329–370

Klaue K (1982) The dynamic compression unit (DCU) for stable internal fixation of bone fractures. Dissertation, University of Basel

Klaue K, Perren SM (1982) Fixation interne des fractures par l'ensemble plaque-vis à compression conjuguée (DCU). Helv Chir Acta 49:77–80

Klaue K, Frigg R, Perren SM (1985) Die Entlastung der Osteosyntheseplatte durch interfragmentäre Plattenzugschraube. Helv Chir Acta 52:19–23

Klause JE, Gustafson SB, Blackketter DM, Schurz PD (1992) Holding strength of 4.5 mm cortical screws in polymethylmethacrylate filled medullary cavities of canine bone. Vet Comp Orthopaed Traumatol 5:109–113

Klause SE, Piermattei DL, Schwarz PD (1989) Tarso-capural arthrodesis: complications and recommendations. Vet Comp Orthopaed Traumatol 3:119–124

Klause SE, Schwarz PD, Egger EL, Piermattei DL (1990) A modification of the unilateral type I external skeletal fixator configuration for primary or secondary support of supracondylar humeral and femoral fractures. Vet Comp Orthopaed Traumatol 3:130–134

Klein M (1990) Aufbohren oder nicht aufbohren? Zirkulationsstörung durch Marknagelung an der Hundetibia. Dissertation, University of Basel

Klein M, Rahn BA, Frigg R, Kessler S, Perren SM (1989) Die Blutzirkulation nach Marknagelung ohne Aufbohren. Proceedings, Berhard Küntscher Kreis, Vienna

Knets IV, Pfafrod GO, Saulgozis JZ (1980) Deformation of hard biological tissue (in Russian). Zinatne, Riga

Koch DA, Hazenwinkel HAW, Nap RC, Meij BP, Wolvekomp WTC (1993) Radiographic evaluation and comparison of plate fixation after triple pelvic osteotomy in 32 dogs with hip dysplasia. Vet Comp Orthopaed Traumatol 6:9–15

Krompecher S, Kerner E (1979) Callus formation. Symposium on the biology of fracture healing. Academiai Kiado, Budapest

Küntscher G (1970) Das Kallus-Problem. Enke, Stuttgart

Lambe DW, Mayberry-Carson KJ, Ferguson KP et al (1984) Morphological stabilization of the glycocalyes of 23 strains of five Bacteroides species using specific antisera. Can J Microbiol 30:809–819

Lambe DW, Costerton JW (1985) The role of glycocalyx in osteomyelitis: current hospital topics. Upjohn, Kalamazoo, Michigan

Lambrechts NE, Verstraete FJM, Sumner-Smith G, Raath AD, van der Linde MJ, Groeneveld HT (1993) Internal fixation of femoral neck fractures in the dog – an in vitro study. Vet Comp Orthopaed Traumatol 6:188–193

Lane WA (1913) The operative treatment of fractures. Medical Publishing, London

Lanyon LE, Rubin CT (1985) Functional adaptation in skeletal structures. Belknap, Harvard University Press, Cambridge, pp 1–25

Laraya JSR (1973) Alkaline phosphates activity in the initial stages of healing of stable and unstable canine bone fractures. Thesis, University of Guelph

LaRue SM, Withrow SJ, Powers BE, Wrigley RH, Gillette EL, Schwarz PD, Straw RC, Richter SL (1989) Limb sparing treatment for osteosarcoma in dogs. J Am Vet Med Assoc 195:1734–1744

Latta LL, Sarmiento A, Tarr RR (1980) The rationale of functional bracing of fractures. Clin Orthop 146:28–36

Leger L, Sumner-Smith G, Gofton N, Prieur WD (1982) AO hook plate fixation for metaphyseal fractures and corrective osteotomies. J Small Anim Pract 23:209–216

Leu D, Bilat C, Rüedi T (1989) Refrakturen nach Metallentfernung. Eine Nachkontrolle von operierten Tibiafrakturen. Unfallchirurg 92:399–400

Levine NS, Linderg RB, Pruilt B (1976) The quantitative swab culture and smear: a quick, simple method for determining the number of viable aerobic bacteria on open wounds. J Trauma 16:89–94

Lewis DD, Reade BS, Dean PW, Kearney MT (1990) Ischioilial pinning for stabilization of coxo-femoral luxations: an anatomical study. Vet Comp Orthopaed Traumatol 3:31–35

Liu YQ, Wu BJ, Xie GP, Chen ZC, Tang CG, Wang ZG (1982) Wounding effects of two types of bullets on soft tissue of dogs. Acta Chir Scand Suppl 508:211–221

Lucas-Championnière J (1907) Les dangers de l'immobilisation des membres – fragilité des os – altération de la nutrition du membre – conclusions pratiques. Rev Méd Chir Pratique 78:81–87

Lüthi UK, Rahn BA, Perren SM (1982) Implants and intracortical vascular disturbances. Transactions of the 28th Annual Meeting of the Orthopaedic Research Society, p 337

MacDonald JM, Matthiesen D (1991) Treatment of forelimb growth plate deformity in 11 dogs by radial dome osteotomy and external coaptation. J Vet Surg 20:402–408

McLaughlin RM (1991) The evolution of the understanding of bone healing. Vet Comp Orthopaed Traumatol 4:16–20

McLaughlin RM, Cockshutt JR, Kuzma AB (1992) Stacked veterinary cuttable plates for treatment of comminuted diaphyseal fractures in cats. Vet Comp Orthopaed Traumatol 5:22–25

Mast J, Jacob R, Ganz R (1989) Planning and reduction techniques in fracture surgery. Springer, Berlin Heidelberg New York

Montavon PM, Dee JF, Weiss R (1993) Distal tibial articular fractures in racing greyhounds. Vet Comp Orthopaed Traumatol 6:146–152

Matushek KJ, Sumner-Smith G, Schatzker J, Hearn TC, Taves C, Hoare J (1988) Dynamic strain in the canine tibia; an in vivo strain gauge analysis. Vet Comp Orthopaed Traumatol 2:58–63

Mathys R, Cotting A (1986) USA patent, 4, 628, 920

Matter P, Brennwald J, Perren SM (1974) Biologische Reaktion des Knochens auf Osteosyntheseplatten. Helv Chir Acta [Suppl] 12:1

Michel M (1990) Die klinische Anwendung der Marknagel-Telemetrie. Dissertation, University of Bern

Montavon PM, Hohn RB, Olmstead ML, Rudy RL (1985) Inclination and anterversion angles of the femoral head and neck in the dog. Evaluation of a standard method of measurement. J Vet Surg 14:277–282

Montavon PM, Pohler EEM, Olmstead ML, Wendelburg KL (1988) The mini instrument and implant set and its clinical application. Vet Comp Orthopaed Traumatol 1:44–51

Miller CW, Kuzma AB, Sumner-Smith G (1989) The narrow lengthening plate for treatment of comminuted diaphyseal fractures in dogs. Vet Comp Orthopaed Traumatol 2:108–112

Moor R, Tepic S, Perren SM (1989) Hochgeschwindigkeits-Film-Analyse des Knochenbruchs. Z Unfallchir 82:128–132

Morgan PW, Miller CW (1994) Osteotomy for correction of premature growth plate closure in 24 dogs. Vet Comp Orthopaed Traumatol 7:129–135
Moyen BJ, Lahey PJ, Weinberg EH, Harris WH (1978) Effects on intact femora of dog of the application and removal of metal plates. J Bone Joint Surg [Am] 60:940–947
Müller KH, Witzel U (1984) Die Brückenplatte zur Osteosynthese bei ossären Schaftdefekten des Femur nach Fehlschlägen von Plattenosteosynthesen. Unfallheilkunde 87:1–10
Müller ME, Allgöwer M, Willenegger H (1963) Technik der operativen Frakturenbehandlung. Springer, Berlin Heidelberg New York
Müller ME, Schneider R, Allgöwer M (1984) 25 Jahre Schweizerische Arbeitsgemeinschaft für Osteosynthesefragen (AO). Swiss Med 6:51–54
Müller ME, Allgöwer M, Schneider R et al (1991) Manual of internal fixation, 3rd edn. Springer, Berlin Heidelberg New York
National Academy of Sciences – National Research Council, Division of Medical Sciences, Ad Hoc Committee of the Committee on Trauma (1964) Postoperative wound infections: the influence of ultraviolet irradiation of the operating room and various other factors. Ann Surg 160:1
Nye R, Egger EL, Hahta J, Histand M, Mallinckrodt JT (1996) Acute failure characteristics of six methods for internal fixation of canine femoral oblique fractures. Vet Comp Orthopaed Traumatol 9:106–110
O'Connell KJ, Clark M, Lewis RH, Christenson PJ (1988) Comparison of low-and-high velocity ballistic trauma to genitourinary organs. J Trauma 28 [Suppl 1]:139–144
Olds RB, Sinibaldi KR, DeAngelis MP, Stoll SG, Rosen H (1973a) Autogenous cancellous bone grafting in small animals. J Am Anim Hosp Assoc 9:454–457
Olds RB, Sinibaldi KR, DeAngelis MP, Stoll SG, Rosen H (1973b) Autogenous cancellous bone grafting in problematic orthopedic cases. J Am Anim Hosp Assoc 9:430–435
Olmstead ML (1995) (ed) Small animal orthopaedics. Mosby, St. Louis
Pauwels F (1965) Gesammelte Abhandlungen zur funktionellen Anatomie des Bewegungsapparates. Springer, Berlin Heidelberg New York
Pauwels F (1980) Biomechanics of the locomotor apparatus. Springer, Berlin Heidelberg New York
Perren SM (1971) Biomécanique de la compression interfragmentaire. In: Boitzy A (ed) Ostéogenès et compression. Huber, Bern, pp 136–145
Perren SM, Boitzy A (1978) La différenciation cellulaire et la biomécanique de l'os. Anat Clin 1:13–28
Perren SM, Cordey J (1977) Die Gewebedifferenzierung in der Frakturheilung. Monatsschr Unfallheilkd 80:161–164
Perren SM, Cordey J (1980) The concept of interfragmentary strain. In:Uhthoff HK, Stahl E (eds) Current concepts of internal fixation of fractures. Springer, Berlin Heidelberg New York, pp 63–77
Perren SM, Huggler A, Russenberger M, Straumann F, Müller SM, Allgöwer M (1969a) Cortical bone healing. A method of measuring the change in compression applied to living cortical bone. Acta Orthop Scand [Suppl] 125:5–16
Perren SM, Huggler A, Russenberger M, Allgöwer M, Mathys R, Schenk R, Willenegger H, Müller ME (1969b) Cortical bone healing. The reaction of cortical bone to compression. Acta Orthop Scand [Suppl] 125:17–28
Perren SM, Russenberger M, Steinemann S, Müller ME, Allgöwer M (1969c) A dynamic compression plate. Acta Orthop Scand [Suppl] 125:31–41
Perren SM, Hayes WC, Eliasson E (1974) Biomechanik der Plattenosteosynthese. Med Orthop Tech 94:56–61
Perren SM, Ganz R, Rüter A (1975) Oberflächliche Knochenresorption um Implantate. Med Orthop Tech 95:6–10
Perren SM, Rahn BA, Lüthi U, Gunst MA, Pfister U (1981) Aseptische Knochennektrose:sequestrie render Umbau? Orthopäde 10:3–5
Perren SM, Klaue K, Frigg R, Predieri M, Tepic S (1991) The concept of biological plating using the limited-contact dynamic compression plate. Injury 22 [Suppl 1]:1–41
Pfister U (1983) Biomechanische und histologische Untersuchungen nach Marknagelung der Tibia. Fortschr Med 101(37):1652–1659
Phillips JH, Rahn BA (1989) Comparison of compression and torque measurements of self-tapping and pre-tapped screws. Plast Reconstruct Surg 83:447–4556
Phillips L, Blackmore J (1991) Kirschner-Ehmer device alone to stabilize caudal lumbar fractures in small dogs. Vet Comp Orthopaed Traumatol 4:112–115
Piermattei DL (1993) An atlas of surgical approaches to the bones and joints of the dog and cat, 3rd edn. Saunders, Philadelphia
Poland MA, Schwartz PD, Salman MD (1991) The adjunctive use of half-pin (type 1) external fixators in combination with intramedullary pins for femoral fracture fixation. Vet Comp Orthopaed Traumatol 4:77–85
Prieur WD (1987) Intertrochanteric osteotomy in the dog: theoretical consideration and operative technique. J Small Anim Pract 28:3–20
Putti V (1918) La trazione per doppia infissione d l'allungamento operative dell'arto inferiore. Chir Org Mov II: 421
Rahn BA (1987) Direct and indirect bone healing after operative fracture treatment. Otolaryngol Clin North Am 20:425–440
Rahn BA, Perren SM (1975) Die mehrfarbige Fluoreszenzmarkierung des Knochenanbaus. Chem Rundschau 29:12–15
Rahn BA, Gallinaro P, Schenk R, Baltensperger A, Perren SM (1971) Compression interfragmentaire et surcharge locale de l'os. In: Boitzy A (ed) Ostéogenèse et compression. Huber, Bern, pp 146–153
Rahn BA, Bacellar FC, Trapp L, Perren SM (1980) Methode zur Fluoreszenz – Morphometrie des Knochenanbaus. Aktuell Traumatol 10:109–115
Regazzoni P (1982) Osteosynthesen an Röhrenknochen:technische und biologische Untersuchungen zur Stabilität und Heilung. Inaugural thesis, University of Zurich
Regazzoni P (1989) Das Ilizarov-Konzept mit einem modularen Rohrfixateur. Operat Orthop Traumatol 1:90–93
Reuter A, Brutscher R (1988) Die Behandlung ausgedehnter Knockendefekte am unterschenkel durch die Verschiebeostetomie nach Ilizarov. Chirurg 59:357
Rhinelander FW (1978) Physiology of bone from the vascular viewpoint. Transactions of the Society for Biomaterials, San Antonio, Texas 2:24–26
Rhinelander FW, Wilson JW (1982) Blood supply in developing mature and healing bone. In: Summer-Smith G (ed) Bone in clinical orthopaedics. Saunders, Philadelphia
Robins GM, Eaton-Wells R, Johnson KA (1993) Customize hook plates for metaphyseal fractures, nonunions and osteotomies in the dog and cat. Vet Comp Orthop Traumatol 6:56–61

Rokkanen P, Böstman O, Vainionpää S, Vihtonen K, Törmälä P, Laiho J, Kilpikari J, Tamminmäki M (1985) Biodegradable implants in fracture fixation:early results of treatment of fractures of the ankle. Lancet 1:1422–1424

Roush JK, Wilson JW (1989) Healing of mandibular body osteotomies after plate and intramedullary pin fixation. Vet Surg 18(3):190–196

Rüter A, Brutscher R (1988) Die Behandlung ausgedehnter Knochendefekte am Unterschenkel durch die Verschiebeosteotomie nach Ilizarov. Chirurg 59:357–359

Salter RB, Simmonds DF, Malcolm BW, Rumble EJ, MacMichael D (1980) The biological effects of continuous passive motion on the healing of full thickness defects in articular cartilage:an experimental investigation in the rabbit. J Bone Joint Surg 62A:1232

Salter RB, Hailton HW, Wedge JM, Tile M, Torode IP, O'Driscoll SW, Murnaghan J, Saringer JH (1986) Clinical application of basic reserch on continuous passive motion for disorders and injuries of synovial joints: a preliminary report of a feasibility study. Techniques Orthopaed I(I):74

Sarmiento A (1980) Nichtoperative funktionelle Frakturbehandlung. Springer, Berlin Heidelberg New York

Schatzker J (1987) Two intra-articular fractures. In: Schatzker J, Tile M (eds) Rationale of operative fracture care. Springer, Berlin Heidelberg New York

Schatzker J, Tile M (1996) The rationale of operative fracture care, 2nd edn. Springer, Berlin Heidelberg New York

Schatzker J, Sanderson R, Murnaghan P (1975a) The holding power of orthopaedic screws in vivo. Clin Orthop 108:115–126

Schatzker J, Horn JG, Sumner-Smith G (1975b) The effects of movement on the holding power of screws in bone. Clin Orthop 108:115–126

Schatzker J, Horn JG, Sumner-Smith G (1975c) The reaction of cortical bone to compression by screw threads. Clin Orthop 111:263–265

Schatzker J, Manley PA, Sumner-Smith G (1980) In vivo strain gauge study of bone response to loading with and without internal fixation. In: Uhthoff H (ed) Current concepts of internal fixation of fractures. Springer, Berlin Heidelberg New York, pp 306–314

Schena DJ, McCurvin DM (1983) The use of fresh cortical and cancellous allografts in the repair of a fractured femur in a dog. A case report. J Am Anim Hosp Assoc. 19:352–358

Schena DJ, Mitten RW, Hoefle WD (1984) Segmental freeze-dried and fresh cortical allografts in the canine femur I. A sequential radiographic comparison over a one-year time interval. J Am Anim Hosp Assoc 20:911–925

Schenk R (1987) Cytodynamics and histodynamics of primary bone repair. In: Lane JM (ed) Fracture healing. Churchill Livingstone, New York

Schenk RK, Willenegger H (1963) Zum histologischen Bild der sogenannten Primärheilung der Knochenkompakta nach experimentellen Osteotomien am Hund. Experientia 19:593

Schenk R, Willenegger H (1964) Histologie der primären Knochenheilung. Langenbecks Arch Klin Chir 308:440–452

Schneider E, Genge M, Wyder D, Mathys R Jr, Perren SM (1988) Telemetrized interlocking nail for in vivo load determination in the human femur. European Telemetry Conference. Döring-Druck, Braunschweig, pp 272–279

Schrader SC (1992) Pelvic osteotomy as a treatment for obstipation in cats with acquired stenosis of the pelvic canal:six cases (1978–1989). J Am Vet Med Assoc 200:208–213

Simpka D, Goldsmith S (1994) Pancarpal arthrodesis in a cat. A report and anatomical study. Vet Comp Orthopaed Traumatol 7:45–50

Sinibaldi KR (1989) Evaluation of full cortical allografts in 25 dogs. J Am Vet Med Assoc 194:1570–1577

Smith BA, Kerwin SC, Hosgood G, Voyjudjis Echle R, Strain GM (1996) Mechanical comparison of two methods for interfragmentary fixation in a short oblique fracture model. Vet Comp Orthopaed Traumatol 9:145–151

Stadler J, Brennwald J, Frigg R, Perren SM (1982) Induction of bone surface resorption by motion. An in vivo study using passive and active implants. Transactions of Second International Symposium on Internal Fixation of Fractures, Lyon, pp 62–64

Steinemann SG (1977) Corrosion of implants – in vivo and in vitro tests. Transactions of Société Européenne pour les biomatériaux, Lyon

Steinemann SG, Mäusli PA (1988) Titanium alloys for surgical implants – biocompatibility from physicochemical principles. Transactions of 6th World Conference on Titanium, Cannes

Stevenson S (1985) Bone grafting. In: Slatter D (ed) Textbook of small animal surgery. Saunders, Philadelphia, pp 2035–2048

Sumner-Smith G (1988) Nonunion. Vet Comp Orthopaed Traumatol 1:3–6

Swach RP, Park DD, Piermattei DL, Wingfield WE, Bartels KE (1979) Gunshot fractures of the extremities: classification, management, and complications. Vet Surg 8:57

Tayton K, Johnson-Nurse C, McKibbin B, Bradley J, Hastings G (1982) The use of semi-rigid carbon fibre reinforced plastic plates for fixation of human fractures. J Bone Joint Surg [Br] 64:105

Timoshenko S (1941) Strength of materials. van Nostrand, Princeton

Timoshenko S (1968) Résistance des matériaux. Dunod, Paris

Thommasini MD, Betts CW (1991) Use of "Ilizarov" external fixator in a dog. Vet Comp Orthopaed Traumatol 4:70–76

Tonino AJ, Davidson CL, Klopper PJ, Linclau LA (1976) Protection from stress in bone and its effects. Experiments with stainless steel and plastic plates in dogs. J Bone Joint Surg [Br] 58:107–113

Toombs JP, Wallace LJ (1985) Evaluation of autogeneic and allogeneic cortical chip grafting in feline tibial nonunion model. Am J Vet Res 46:519–528

Tvedten HW, Till GO (1985) Effect of povidone, povidone-iodine, and iodide on locomotion (in vitro) of neutrophils from people, rats, dogs, and rabbits. Am J Vet Res 46:1797

Uhthoff HK, Dubuc FL (1971) Bone structure changes in the dog under rigid internal fixation. Clin Orthop 81:165–170

Unger M, Montoavon PM, Heim UFA (1990) Classification of fractures of the long bones in the dog and cat. Introduction and clinical application. Vet Comp Orthopaed Traumatol 3:41–50

Urist MR (1980) Bone transplants and implants. In: Urist MR (ed) Fundamental and clinical bone physiology. Lippencott, Philadelphia, pp 331–360

Vattolo M (1986) Der Einfluß von Rillen in Osteosyntheseplatten auf den Umbau der Kortikalis. Dissertation, University of Bern

Verstraete FJM, Ligthelm AJ (1992) Dental trauma caused by screws in internal fixation of mandibular osteotomies in the dog. Vet Comp Orthopaed Traumatol 5:104–8

von Arx C (1975) Schubübertragung durch Reibung bei Plattenosteosynthesen. AO Bulletin, pp 1–34

von Recum AF (ed) (1986) Handbook of biomaterials evaluation (section on intra vitam staining techniques). Macmillan, New York

Walker MA, Lewis RE, Kneller SK et al (1975) Radiographic signs of bone infection in small animals. J Am Vet Med Assoc 166:908

Weber BG, Brunner C (1981) The treatment of nonunions without electrical stimulation. Clin Orthop 161:24–32

Weber BG, Cech O (1973) Pseudarthrosen. Pathophysiologie – Biomechanik – Therapie – Ergebnisse. Huber, Bern

Weber BG, Ceck O (1976) Pseudoarthrosis. Huber, Bern

Weller S (1989) Instability of osteosynthesis and disturbed fracture healing. Vet Comp Orthopaed Traumatol 3:92–97

Willer RL, Schwarz PD, Powers BE, Histand ME (1990) Comparison of cerclage wire placement in relation to a neutralization plate: a mechanical and histological study. Vet Comp Orthopaed Traumatol 3:90–96

Wolff J (1893) Das Gesetz der Transformation der Knochen. Hirschwald, Berlin

Wolff J (1986) The law of bone remodelling. Springer, Berlin Heidelberg New York

Woo SLY, Akeson WH, Coutts RD, Rutherford L, Jemmott GF, Amiel D (1976) A comparison of cortical bone atrophy secondary to fixation with plates with large differences in bending stiffness. J Bone Joint Surg [Am] 58:190–195

Yamada H, Evans FG (1970) Strength of biological materials. Williams and Wilkins, Baltimore

Subject Index

MIX
Papier aus verantwortungsvollen Quellen
Paper from responsible sources
FSC® C105338
FSC
www.fsc.org

If you have any concerns about our products,
you can contact us on
ProductSafety@springernature.com

In case Publisher is established outside the EU,
the EU authorized representative is:
Springer Nature Customer Service Center GmbH
Europaplatz 3, 69115 Heidelberg, Germany

Printed by Libri Plureos GmbH
in Hamburg, Germany